salon FUNDAMENTALS™

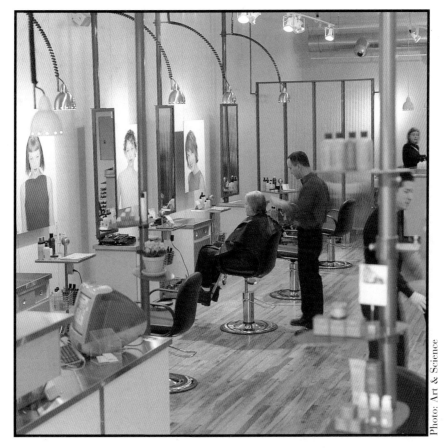

Photo: Art & Science

Learning is a treasure that will follow its owner everywhere.
– Chinese Proverb

A Resource for Your Cosmetology Career

ISBN 0-615-11288-9

Tenth printing September 2005
Updates included in this revision of
Salon Fundamentals™ can be
accessed by visiting
www.pivot-point.com/fundamentals.html

Pivot Point International, Inc.
1560 Sherman Avenue, Suite 700
Evanston, Illinois 60201
1.800.886.4247
www.pivot-point.com

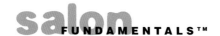

salon FUNDAMENTALS™

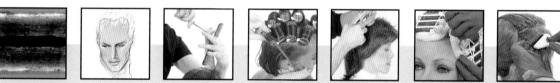

A Resource for Your Cosmetology Career

CONTENTS

PREFACE
Today's Stylist

The twenty-first century holds promise and unlimited opportunities for you, the professional cosmetologist, now a member of the ever-expanding, ever-changing, ever-fascinating Beauty Industry. New techniques, new products and new opportunities appear everyday. The numbers of people who require and visit beauty salons and the amount of money spent on beauty services are constantly increasing. If you are innovative and ambitious, there is no limit to your potential.

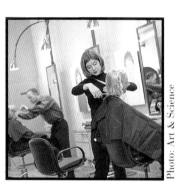

No other industry has such a constant demand for qualified, creative, well-trained graduates. None offers such bright opportunities for an individual to start a personal business and work toward financial independence. Another reward is the professional satisfaction that you gain with each client. Your artistic skills and training give you the potential of changing someone's life by making them look good and feel beautiful, possibly for the first time.

Set your goals high. The future is yours...just waiting for you to succeed!

Building Your Career

The professional beauty business has grown into a very sophisticated industry. Salon owners and stylists serve a new breed of consumer, one who makes knowledgeable demands and expects the salon to offer a full range of services and retail products. Cosmetologists must be highly educated, highly skilled professionals in order to meet these demands.

Personal commitment is a key ingredient in achieving professional success. Invest in yourself! Learn everything you can in school. Take an active part in school activities. Take advantage of extra classes and seminars. After graduation, continue to invest in your education by attending seminars, shows and workshops. Keep pace with what's happening in the industry. Become known for your willingness to share your knowledge and for your enthusiasm for the beauty business. There is no limit to the success you can achieve if you are willing to invest the time and energy success demands.

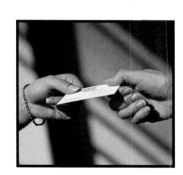

You made your first professional investment when you enrolled in this cosmetology school. Here you'll learn how to cut, perm and color, as well as how to communicate with clients, and much more. You can, and should, make another investment in your professional success even while you're in school...begin to "network."

In "networking," a professional creates communication opportunities with other professionals in the same or a related field. Through "networking," you can develop contacts that can be instrumental in your climb to success. You can discover opportunities for professional and personal growth and make new friends.

The ideal vehicles for "networking" in the professional beauty business are the outstanding professional associations that serve our industry. Some have student memberships available, and that means you can begin networking even now.

Professional Organizations
(CAF) Cosmetology Advancement Foundation

The Cosmetology Advancement Foundation mission is to develop a unified approach to issues and trends affecting the salon industry and to seek opportunities for contributing to the industry's image, growth and development. To achieve its mission CAF subscribes to the values of dedication to education, continuous communications, commitment to teamwork, trust and professionalism among all industry associations, organizations and their members.

CAF has led an all-industry task force in developing technical and non-technical skill standards for entry-level cosmetologists. These standards have been accepted by the industry and published at the end of each chapter in the Salon Fundamentals textbook ("It's Up to You") and Study Guide ("Show You Know").

(NCA) National Cosmetology Association

The National Cosmetology Association is the largest organized group of licensed beauty professionals in the United States. This non-profit group opens membership to all licensed cosmetologists, barbers, electrologists and estheticians and to non-licensed related professionals (educators, distributors and manufacturers). The group maintains a national executive office, state associations, and local or regional affiliates. Students may join the FCA or Future Cosmetologists Association by forming a local school club.

The educational branch of NCA is active in maintaining and upgrading the knowledge and skills of the styling professional. Hair America is a select group of educators within the NCA, who produce national, state and local educational events for the association. There are industry sections that include women's and men's hair design, esthetics and nails.

To become members, applicants must pass both written and practical exams that confirm their knowledge, skills and teaching ability. Hair America members donate time and effort to bettering the industry.

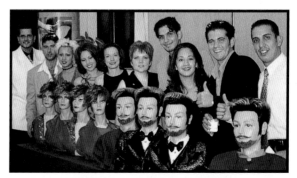

Another active role of the NCA is the sponsoring of international, national, regional and local competitions. The goal of these competitions is to prepare the participant to perform

1998 USA STUDENT TEAM

excellent salon work while building self-confidence and stage presence. The winner represents the United States in HairWorld championship competitions, held every four years.

Students may compete to become members of the Student Hairstyling Team. Information about how to get involved can be obtained from NCA Executive Office, 401 N. Michigan Ave., Chicago, IL 60611-4267. The U.S. student team has won numerous titles in international competitions in the last 10 years. For a student interested in developing skills needed to become a guest artist or an educator, this competition is an excellent training ground. After graduation, competitions are open to all licensed professionals and could be a personal opportunity for you.

(ABA) American Beauty Association

The American Beauty Association is the unified voice of the professional salon industry, representing manufacturers, manufacturer representatives and associated firms. Its mission is to expand, serve and protect the interests of the professional beauty industry. As the voice of the industry, the American Beauty Association represents its membership to the media, the consumer and the government, ensuring that those key groups are well informed on industry issues, news and trends. The American Beauty Association also offers its members opportunities for education, networking and fundraising at events including the all-industry DIALOG Conference, ABBIES Awards Program and Beauty Ball and Charity Auction.

(BBSI) Beauty & Barber Supply Institute Inc.

The Beauty & Barber Supply Institute Inc. is the international association of the professional salon industry comprised of distributors, and manufacturer representatives. BBSI strives to maximize the potential of the professional salon industry via alliances with all beauty-related industry associations; distribution of industry information to the salon community, media and public; education of beauty-related representation on key issues impacting the viability of the professional salon industry. The BBSI web address is www.bbsi.org.

(TSA) The Salon Association

A North American business association for owners of salons and spas, The Salon Association provides owner-to-owner networking, business education, industry statistics, economic benefits, and governmental representation for independent salon owners across the United States and Canada. Mission: "Owners soaring and sharing business solutions." The TSA web address is www.salons.org.

Intercoiffure

Intercoiffure is an organization that consists of 260 salons in the USA/Canada and 2000 internationally. It is a non-profit organization of elite salon, spa and school owners. The Intercoiffure members share educational and business ideas, customers and staff with each other around the world. The Intercoiffure web address is www.intercoiffure.net.

(NACCAS) National Accrediting Commission of Cosmetology Arts & Sciences

The National Accrediting Commission of Cosmetology Arts and Sciences (NACCAS) is an autonomous, independent accrediting commission constituted as a non-profit Delaware corporation, with its main offices located in Arlington, Virginia. The Commission's origins date back to 1969, when two accrediting agencies in the field merged to form the Cosmetology Accrediting Commission (CAC). CAC changed its name to "NACCAS" in 1981.

NACCAS is recognized by the U.S. Department of Education as a national agency for the institutional accreditation of postsecondary schools and departments of cosmetology arts and sciences, including specialized schools. It presently accredits approximately 1,000 institutions that serve over 100,000 students. These schools offer more than twenty courses and programs of study which fall under NACCAS' scope of accreditation. Please visit the NACCAS' Job Bank at www.naccas.org., the place where cosmetologists and salons come together.

(AACS) American Association of Cosmetology Schools

The purpose of the Association is to keep members abreast of changes in federal and state laws and regulations, to provide the membership with educational services, to promote the welfare of cosmetology education in the United States, to establish a unity of spirit and understanding among institutions and their instructional staff in pursuing the goals and resolving the problems related to postsecondary cosmetology education. The AACS web address is www.beautyschools.org.

(ACCSCT) Accrediting Commision of Career Schools and Colleges of Technology

ACCSCT is a private, non-profit, independent accrediting agency whose goal is maintaining educational quality in the career schools and colleges it accredits by striving to assure academic excellence and ethical practices. ACCSCT is dedicated to the more than 360,000 student who annually pursue career education at its accredited institutions. The ACCSCT web address is www.accsct.org.

(CCA) Career College Association

The Career College Association (CCA) is a voluntary membership organization made up of private, postsecondary schools and colleges which provide career-specific educational programs.

The association's primary objectives are to foster public policies that ensure equitable access for students to quality career and skill education; to assist member institutions in coping with a complex federal regulatory scheme; and to help member institutions achieve the highest possible standards of educational quality.

(NIC) National-Interstate Council of State Boards of Cosmetology

NIC is a not-for-profit organization whose membership consists of state board members of all 50 states, the District of Columbia, Guam and Puerto Rico. NIC provides for an interchange of ideas, promotes professionalism, encourages standardization of regulations and provides national examinations for licensure in cosmetology and related fields. The NIC web address is www.nictesting.org.

(ICSA) International Chain Salon Association

ICSA's membership is comprised of approximately 50 chain salon organizations throughout North America, Europe and Asia. Combined, ICSA members own and operate more than 15,000 salons, employing more than 150,000 people. ICSA was established to help chain salons grow in size and strength. ICSA is actively involved in a number of on-going projects, including: the first ever chain salon financial and employee performance operating survey, an employment opportunities study of the cosmetology industry; and cooperative work with other industry groups on such issues as state licensing reciprocity, all industry skills standardization, and in political initiatives that affect our entire industry. ICSA's members are actively working to enhance the image of the cosmetology industry through their commitment to following the highest professional ethics in their growing business practices. The ICSA web address is www.chainsalonassn.com.

Career Opportunities

A **licensed cosmetologist**, also referred to as a hair designer, hairstylist, beautician, stylist, or hairdresser, has completed a local, government-regulated number of hours of study (usually from 1,000 to 2,100) and has successfully passed a written and/or practical exam. There are approximately 200,000 salons in the U.S., at which the licensed cosmetologist can find employment.

The licensed cosmetologist is in daily contact with clients, performing all the services learned in cosmetology school. Your knowledge, image and all your professional skills, from cutting to communication, will be key components in determining your income.

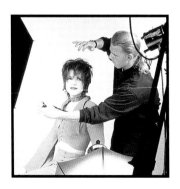

While most licensed cosmetologists are employed in salons, those stylists who want something different and, perhaps, a bit outside of the "routine" might explore more imaginative alternatives, including signing on as a ship's stylist for a passenger cruise line! A **cruise ship stylist** has no living expenses, can see at least a portion of the world and has a clientele in constant turnover as one cruise ends and the next begins! As a cruise ship stylist, you'd have no time to develop least-liked clients and you'd probably never be bored! The licensed cosmetologist can also work as a **photo stylist**, in hospital hair-care service areas, with modeling agencies, theater groups or, in Hollywood, even with major movie studios.

The cosmetology profession offers many opportunities beyond the entry-level position. Most of these jobs require experience, advanced training or a degree of some kind. Here is a sampling of those opportunities:

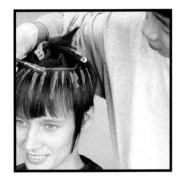

A **colorist** is someone who specializes in hair color services. This person is generally hired by a salon with a color department. Clients then go to another stylist in the salon for additional services. In 1985, 62% of all women with hair color applied their own at home. At the turn of the century, fewer than 50% of all women with hair color did their own color. That means exciting things for the cosmetologist whose specialty is color.

Most colorists take advanced training courses and/or attend color seminars. Color techniques change, as do fashion shades. "Hot" today may be slush-cold color by tomorrow. Color is, however, uniquely creative, providing the skillful stylist-colorist with the tools to "light up" and enhance a face. Color is also uniquely lucrative. Many color services command substantial fees.

A **Guest Artist** or **Platform Stylist** is self-employed by a professional beauty product manufacturer or by schools that offer continuing education courses in the beauty field. The position may be full or part time. Guest artists train licensed cosmetologists by teaching them about products, techniques, the newest trends and product sales. The experience, advanced-technique skills and stage presence necessary to be a platform stylist usually require a minimum of two to five years as a cosmetologist. Many stylists begin by helping other guest artists prep models, backstage, for shows. Success in this career is based on skill, creativity, personal charisma and luck. The position requires long-distance travel and is almost exclusively weekend work.

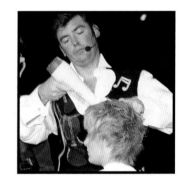

A **Salon Coordinator** is often an experienced cosmetologist acting as a director for the activities of a large salon. He or she is responsible for booking and scheduling appointments, greeting customers, public relations, retailing, inventory control, bookkeeping, recordkeeping and client retention.

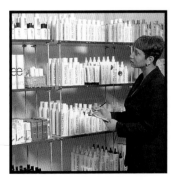

A **Salon Manager** is often a stylist who has shown superior styling skill and the ability to deal with clients. A manager may be employed by a non-cosmetologist or cosmetologist owner. Training in advertising, marketing, purchasing, client relations, budgeting, employee management techniques and finance or accounting is helpful.

A **Salon Owner** may, or may not, be a licensed cosmetologist. It's desirable for the salon owner to have had some business management experience before investing in a salon. For the individual to purchase a salon, a capital investment and a good credit rating are required. The owner is responsible for all salon operations, physical and financial.

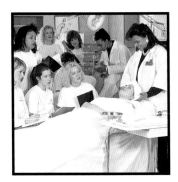

An **Instructor** is someone with proven styling skills, advanced training in products and techniques and specialized training in vocational education. Most area regulating agencies require instructors to be licensed. Some require a specific number of years of salon experience, others 400 to 2,500 hours of training and others a written and practical licensure examination. An instructor must have a superior personal image, enthusiasm, charisma and unflagging energy. He or she must be capable of dealing with people tactfully and with interest and concern. Instructing is an excellent training ground for future managers, owners, guest artists and manufacturer representatives.

A **Manufacturer Representative/or Field Technician** is usually a licensed cosmetologist with two to five years of successful salon experience. This position requires travel in a specific area of the country during which the representative holds in-salon or in-school workshops and classes on a variety of subjects. The representative also accompanies distributor sales consultants to salons to answer questions about products, techniques, etc., and helps in the backstage production of shows or seminars. Weekend and week-long travel is required.

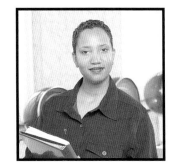

A **Distributor/Sales Consultant** may or may not be a licensed cosmetologist. The position of Sales Consultant involves travelling a "territory" and selling products to salon owners and managers and providing stylist training. The distributing house maintains contracts to sell professional products to licensed cosmetologists only. Salary is most often a guarantee-salary-plus-commission structure based on product sales.

A **School Owner or Director** is usually a licensed cosmetologist with experience as a stylist, salon manager, salon owner, instructor, manufacturer's representative or state board examiner. Many school owners start as stylists and work for years to gain the confidence, experience and capital needed to invest in a cosmetology school. School owners don't necessarily need to be licensed cosmetologists so long as they have a business degree or experience and have a passion for this industry.

A **Manufacturer's Spokesperson** is often a cosmetologist with a business or marketing degree. The opportunity to market new products for national distribution can be challenging and profitable.

A **Test Salon Cosmetologist or Product Analyst** is usually a licensed cosmetologist with specialized skills in a select type of product, such as perms, colors, relaxers or cosmetics. This person is responsible for the final product that cosmetologists use and sell in salons. All manufacturers test their products to varying degrees. Some maintain "company salons" or "laboratory salons" at the manufacturing plant. Others send products to salons for testing.

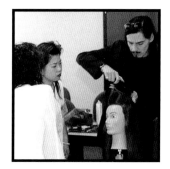

An **Education Manager or Trainer** may have a business or personnel management degree and/or may be a licensed cosmetologist with a good deal of experience similar to a long-term instructor's or school owner's. This person trains and manages manufacturer's representatives, chain salon staff, chain school staff or distributor staff for a company region or territory. Some are responsible for the company's entire sales or educational staff.

A **Sales, Marketing, or Management Consultant** is employed by a chain salon, distributor or manufacturer to "supplement" the company's existing educational staff. This consultant may not have any industry experience, but may have a personal reputation for helping companies overcome problems. Some cosmetologists have gained this kind of reputation based on combined business, styling and motivational skills. These skills are highly valued and usually well paid.

Chain Salon Employees are employed by chain salons. These chain salons make up a very large and growing segment of our industry and offer many opportunities for cosmetologists that include positions as salon coordinators, assistant and salon managers, district and area directors, local and company-wide technical educators, retail supervisors, product testing supervisors, warehouse managers and more.

A **Trade Publication Publisher, Writer or Editor** requires that individuals have a journalism background combined with knowledge of the cosmetology profession. These publications include magazines, newsletters and textbooks.

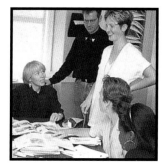

Commitment, ambition, technical skill and professional communication and networking pave the way to your success. Your opportunities are just waiting to happen.

Acknowledgements

Salon Fundamentals is designed to provide cosmetology education to meet the requirements of government agencies and the Skills Standards set for entry-level cosmetologists. An undertaking of such magnitude requires the expertise and cooperation of many people. Pivot Point International wishes to take this opportunity to acknowledge with gratitude and respect some of those many contributors.

Thank you to the reviewers across the country, models, outside consultants, individual and chain salons, industry manufacturers, Pivot Points' Educational Advisory Board and the dedicated Core Development Team that made this course possible.

In addition, we give special thanks to the North American Regulating agencies whose careful work protects our clients and thereby enhances the high quality of our work. These agencies include OHSA (Occupational Health and Safety Agency), EPA (Environmental Protection Agency) and ADA (Americans with Disabilities Act). The Salon Fundamentals program makes extensive use of their policies and procedures.

Following is a listing of the many individuals and organizations that made this program possible.

Vision, Approval and Support

Leo Passage
Chairman, Owner
Pivot Point International, Inc.

Robert Passage
Vice President School Division
Pivot Point International, Inc.

Core Development Team

Publishing/Editorial

Corrine Passage
Vice President, Publishing

Judy Rambert
Vice President,
Corporate Education

Janet Fisher
National Educational
Consultant

Subject Matter Experts

Vasiliki Stavrakis
Hair

Brian Fallon
Hair, Wigs

Benjamin Polk
Hair

Sabine Held-Perez
Hair

Lisa Fuentes
Hair

Production and Design

Jennifer Eckstein
Art Direction/Graphic Design

Denise Podlin
Graphic Illustrator

David Placek
Photographer

Editorial Consultants

Dr. Clif St. Germain	Mary Colgan McNamara	Joseph Miranda	Mark Reynolds
Educational Expert	*Copy and Development Editor*	*Development Editor*	*Test Consultant*

Additional Contributors

Subject Matter Experts – Pivot Point International, Inc.

Dora Brooks	Debbie Mack	Jean Harrity	Blanca Zapata
Skin, Nails	*Nails*	*Skin, Nails*	*Hair*
John Calabretto	Audry Pritchett	Francis Pugh	Markell Richards
Hair	*Hair*	*Hair*	*Hair*
Olivia Barr	Linda Randle	Theresa Pupillo	Steve Janssen
Hair	*Hair*	*Hair*	*Retail*

Subject Matter Consultants

Gerri Cevetillo	Kim Schottler	Dr. Keith Brown
Infection Control Specialist, Ultronics, Mahwah, NJ	*Great Clips, Inc Minneapolis, MN*	*Color Specialist/Chemist, Clairol New York, NY*
Theresa Lewis	Lori Neopolitan	Gloria DiSanza
Nail Specialist, OPI Chicago, IL	*Makeup Specialist Chicago, IL*	*Color Specialist, Clairol New York, NY*
RoseAnn Perea	National Interstate Council (NIC)	Mary Lee Krantz
Super Cuts Novato, CA	Michael Hill / Larry Walthers / Aurie Gosnell / Peggy Moon / Kitty Pierre	*Fantastic Sams Westchester, IL*
Dianna Kenneally		
Senior Scientist/P&G Beauty Cincinnati, OH		

Video Production

John Bernin	Paul Bernin	Frame One Communications
Video Development	*Video Script Writing/ Professor Pivot Illustration*	*Audiovisuals*

Illustration

Robert Richards
Makeup and Figure Illustration

Editorial Assistance

Yolanda Bryant	Connie Sloan
Assistant to Publishing	*Assistant to Publishing*

Narration

Xenon	Cara Torhan
Professor Pivot	*Narrator*

Reviewers

Judy Wait
Lytle's Redwood Empire Beauty College
Santa Rosa, CA

Fran Brown
Fran Brown College of Beauty Career Center
Layton, UT

Nicole M. Coppola
PB Cosmetology Education Center
Gloucester, NJ

Margy Wagner
Empire Beauty Schools
Pottsville, PA

Sue Sansom
Salon Ecology Expert
Phoenix, AZ

Debi Cline
McKenzie Career Center
Indianapolis, IN

Warren County Career Center
Jean Puckett (instructor) and students
Lebanon, OH

Grace Doran Francis
Pivot Point International, Inc.

Photo/Video Contributions

Ron Barris
Headstart Hair For Men
Winter Haven, FL

Great Lengths
Rome, Italy

Goldwell
Darmstadt, Germany

Olive Benson
Boston, MA

Celebrity Signatures International
Kansas City, MO

Art & Science
Chicago, IL

American Hairlines
Brooklyn, NY

Chicago Hair Goods
Chicago, IL

Cheryl Tricoci
Mario Tricoci Hair Salon and
Day Spa, Palatine, IL

Hairologi
Stockholm, Sweden

Garland Drake International
Costa Mesa, CA

Cornrows & Co.
Washington, DC

Surfacine Development, LLC

Marketing/Advertising

Gams
Marketing/Advertising

Kimberly Giles
Marketing Assistant

Thomas Greene
Promotional Design

Vi Nelson and Associates
Public Relations

Additional Members of Pivot Point Management Team

Jan Laan
Chief Executive Officer

Robert Sieh
Chief Financial Officer

Edward Nessel
Vice President, Marketing

Karol Thousand
Vice President, Corporate Schools

Overview

Cosmetology is the art and science of beauty care.

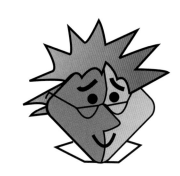

Hi! I'm Professor Pivot. You can call me Professor 'P' or "Pivot", for short. I'm your study companion for this course. I'm here to help you get all you can from every chapter in this book, go into your exams with confidence and become a top-notch, job-obtaining professional in cosmetology.

I've been a Professor too many years not to know how difficult studying can be on some days. You'll be trying to learn new things. You'll be doing new things. Sometimes you may get just plain discouraged. When you least expect it and most need it, there I'll be, popping up on the page near you, clarifying, explaining, giving hints, tips and shortcuts. You'll notice my hair, face and nails may change with each chapter, but my mission is always to help you.

Our special meeting place will always be the first two pages of each new chapter. There I give you a sneak preview of the whole chapter, the coming attractions, so to speak.

I list the major OBJECTIVES of the chapter, what you will know and be able to do after you complete the chapter.

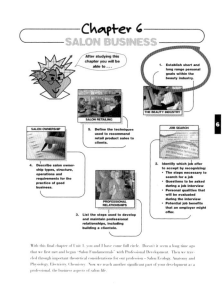

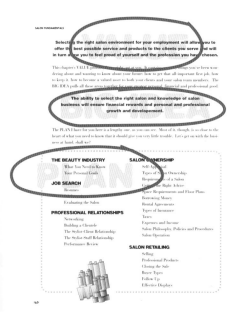

On the second page of each chapter, I give you a VALUE statement, an answer to the "What's in it for me?" question. Then I show you the BIG IDEA behind each chapter and a PLAN of action for making your way through it. For you personally, the PLAN can be of great assistance in guiding you through the major sections of the chapter.

When you know the chapter well enough, you can use the PLAN as a quick review of the main points.

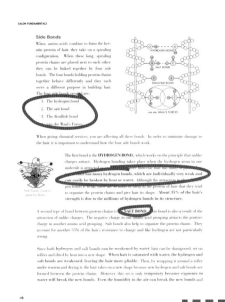

Side Bonds

When amino acids combine to form the keratin protein of hair, they take on a spiraling configuration. When these long, spiraling protein chains are placed next to each other, they can be linked together by four side bonds. The four bonds holding protein chains together behave differently and they each serve a different purpose in building hair. The four side bonds created are:

1. The hydrogen bond
2. The salt bond
3. The disulfide bond
4. van der Waal's Forces

When giving chemical services, you are affecting all these bonds. In order to minimize damage to the hair, it is important to understand how the four side bonds work.

The first bond is the **HYDROGEN BOND**, which works on the principle that unlike charges attract. Hydrogen bonding takes place when the hydrogen atom in one molecule is attracted to another that has many hydrogen bonds, which are individually very weak and can easily be broken by heat or water. Although the attraction in the hydrogen bond is weak, there are so many of them in the protein of hair that they tend to organize the protein chains and give hair its shape. About 35% of the hair's strength is due to the millions of hydrogen bonds in its structure.

A second type of bond between protein chains is the **SALT BOND**. This bond is also a result of the attraction of unlike charges. The negative charge in one amino acid grouping attracts the positive charge in another amino acid grouping. Salt bonds also help to organize the protein chains. They account for another 35% of the hair's resistance to change and like hydrogen are not particularly strong.

Since both hydrogen and salt bonds can be weakened by water, hair can be shampooed, set on rollers and dried by heat into a new shape. **When hair is saturated with water, the hydrogen and salt bonds are weakened, leaving the hair more pliable.** Then, by wrapping it around a roller under tension and drying it, the hair takes on a new shape because new hydrogen and salt bonds are formed between the protein chains. However, this set is only temporary because exposure to water will break the new bonds. Even the humidity in the air can break the new bonds and

06

I have worked ahead in each chapter and created some things to help call your attention to key points. Look for information that is:

- **Hightlighted in blue,** or in
- **Bold print,** or
- CAPITALIZED or
- Bulleted or
- **PLACED IN A CHART**

I designed these tools to help you recognize the important theory points to remember. (I also want to tell you that these are the items I think are most likely to be on a test!)

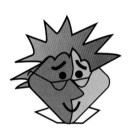

IMPLEMENT/SUPPLIES	FUNCTION
Master Sketcher Comb	Detangles and backcombs hair
Rake comb	Detangles; styles curly hair; defines texture
Lifter	Details; lifts; backcombs
Brushes	
Vent Brush	Achieves lift or volume when air forming smoother textures or creating directional emphasis
7 or 9-row Air Forming Brush	Smoothes wavy or curly textures; adds directional emphasis when air forming
Round Brushes (various diameters)	Impart varying degrees of curved or curled texture and volume
Cushion Brush	Relaxes sets; backbrushes; dry molds, styles or refines the form
Rollers, Pins And Clips	
Cylindrical Rollers	Create uniform curl formation/diameter across width of base; used in straight-shape roller setting
Conical or Cone-Shaped Rollers	Create progression of curl diameter from narrow end of base toward wide end. Used in curvature-shape roller setting
Picks	Secure rollers in place while hair dries; also secure perm rods
Single-Prong Clips	Secure pincurls
Double-Prong Clips	Secure molded shapes/sectioning; also secure rollers if picks are not used
Bobby Pins	Secure hair in place for finished style, especially in long hair designs
Hair Pins	Secure hair in place for finished style, especially in long hair designs
Long-Hair Pins	Define textural detail and movement
Wave or Styling Clamp	Keep fingerwaves in place
Thermal Styling	
Blow Dryer	Air forms in combination with various tools to create directional and textural changes
Thermal Irons	Add curled or waved texture to the hair
Hot Brush/Comb	Dries hair while creating waves or curls
Pressing Comb	Straightens overly curly hair

326

The first six chapters are strictly theory. After that some chapters will have procedures you need to learn in order to offer services to clients in the salon. These procedures all have a standard format, consisting of three components, which include the **PREPARATION** (announcing what needs to be done before you begin the service), **PROCEDURE** (the actual skills you will perform to create the service) and **COMPLETION** (the important final steps you do at the end of the service).

Scrunching Layered Form

Not all thermal styling and air forming techniques require the use of brushes, partings and base controls. Beautiful finishes can be achieved on naturally wavy, curly or permed hair using the scrunching technique. The scrunching technique uses a nozzle attachment on the blow dryer, called a diffuser, which creates a softer, spread-out (diffused) airflow. The diffuser allows you to dry the hair while maintaining the curl formation. Manipulating the hair as little as possible while air forming will result in a stronger curl formation and reduce the possibility of frizziness.

Your choice of styling products will be based on your client's hair type and the results that you wish to achieve. For this design, mousse was used for curl definition without excess weight. Speed and heat settings on the blow dryer can be adjusted according to the hair type. The finished design shows natural-looking, defined curl texture. More expansion in the form is achieved than natural air drying would have accomplished.

Scrunching Layered-Form Preparation

As with every professional service, it is important to prepare the area, products, implements and equipment in proper order. If the thermal styling service follows a haircutting service, note that most, if not all, of your preparation would have taken place prior to the haircut. This exercise assumes that the client is receiving only the thermal styling service. Before you begin the scrunching, layered-form procedure, be sure to satisfy the following points.

- Clean work station with disinfectant
- Arrange implements/supplies including blow dryer, diffuser, styling combs and appropriate styling products
- Ask the client to remove jewelry and store in a secure place
- Wash and sanitize hands; drape client for a wet service; perform scalp and hair analysis
- Shampoo and condition the hair using products appropriate for client's hair type
- Detangle and remove excess moisture from the hair

Scrunching Layered-Form Procedure

• Distribute mousse	• Dry ends, midstrand and then base
• Attach diffuser	• Work toward interior and complete back using same techniques
• Tilt head back	• Tilt head to either side and use same techniques
• Position diffuser beneath exterior strands	• Work toward interior and complete using same techniques
• Lift dryer up into lengths	
• Lift hair at scalp with your fingers	

346

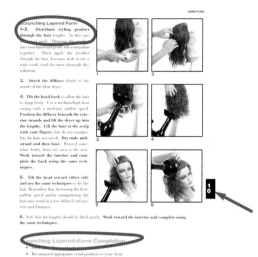

You'll notice that I have also created **step-by-step** photos to guide you through the 'hands-on' lesson. In addition, I placed in bold print the important steps, which were outlined in the **PROCEDURE**. These are the steps that are related to the Rubric found in your Salon Fundamentals Study Guide (your personal notebook for study). **Chapter numbers appear on the right hand side to help you quickly open the book to a selected chapter.**

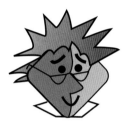

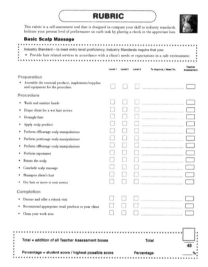

Here is a sample of a rubric from your Study Guide. A Rubric is a listing of the steps necessary to correctly complete the service and will help you and your teacher assess your progress.

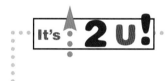

On the last page of each chapter you will find "It's up to you." This is your opportunity to show that you have mastered the information found in the chapter and can now meet the Industry Standards that have been established by the Cosmetology Advancement Foundation. It is here that you will find case scenarios that require you to use **"critical thinking skills"** to solve the case.

As I mentioned earlier, the Salon Fundamentals Study Guide is your personal notebook that goes right along with this textbook. The Study Guide will help you direct your thinking, manage the information presented in the chapter and assist you in tapping into your own natural intelligence! It will become the best friend to your long-term memory!

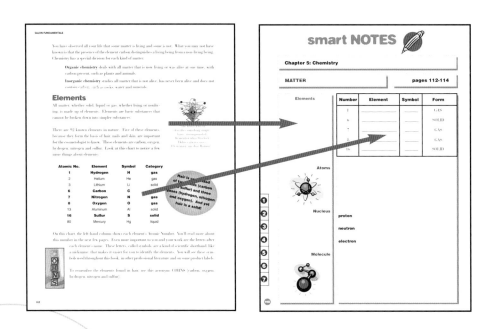

Now you know quite a bit about the Professor part of my name. What about the other part? Just what is a PIVOT? A PIVOT is a center point, a place of balance and rest, a place of quiet energy around which other things revolve and on which they depend. You can depend on me, your Pivot, as you move from lesson to lesson. I'll be there centering you until you yourself are ready to become your own center of energy and activity in the salon world and your first job.

The best place to start toward that world is with your development as a professional. That's where I want to guide you in Chapter 1, "Professional Development." See you on the next page!

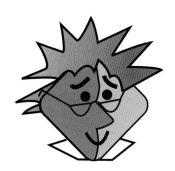

Chapter 1

PROFESSIONAL DEVELOPMENT

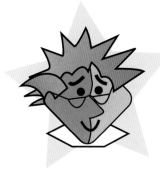

After studying this chapter you will be able to . . .

1. Establish routines to maintain a healthy body and mind.

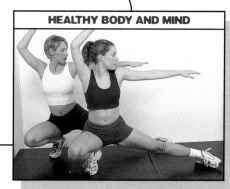

HEALTHY BODY AND MIND

2. Explain the elements of effective communication.

3. Develop and maintain positive human relations.

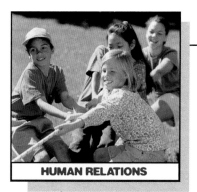

HUMAN RELATIONS

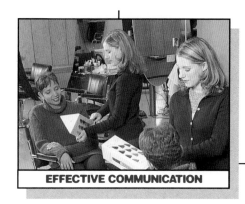

EFFECTIVE COMMUNICATION

Welcome to our briefing space! During our first time together as professor and student, let's consider two questions: The first, what is cosmetology? **Cosmetology is the art and science of beauty care.** The second question is, just what is a PROFESSIONAL? The word PROFESS comes from two words:

PRO = for + FESS = to speak, acknowledge, admit

Professionals are people who speak with their very lives about the value of what they have chosen to do. They are people who believe in something and work hard to achieve it. By entering this course, you are professing that you want to become one of these people, a professional.

Professional Development is a COMMITMENT to constantly improve yourself. Your dedication to professional development now as a student and soon as a cosmetologist will improve your health, elevate your professional status and foster positive relationships with clients and co-workers.

The core of any profession, the central VALUE it radiates to the world, involves *commitment*, the kind of inner promise you make to yourself. In every chapter, the BIG IDEA is a short statement that answers the question: "What will I learn in this chapter?" Understanding the BIG IDEA of this chapter and putting it into practice will bring your commitment alive in your life.

Success as a professional cosmetologist comes from your personal commitment to the development of a healthy body and mind, effective communication and positive human relations.

The PLAN gives you a visual summary of the important ideas in the chapter. In this chapter the plan, although both simple and practical, requires the kind of discipline that contributes to the growth of a true professional. It is my challenge to you not just to learn this material but to exemplify it in your life.

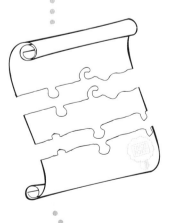

HEALTHY BODY AND MIND
Rest and Relaxation

Exercise

Nutrition

Hygiene

Image

EFFECTIVE COMMUNICATION
Nonverbal Communication

Verbal Communication

HUMAN RELATIONS
Personality

Teamwork

Ethics

HEALTHY BODY AND MIND

Establishing routines to maintain a healthy body and mind is the first step toward professional development. Dedication to each of these areas will help ensure that you are on the right track.

Rest and Relaxation

Sufficient rest and relaxation are as necessary as work for a healthy, happy life. Sleep helps relieve the frustrations and tensions that are a result of everyday activities. **Most people need six to eight hours of sleep or they become fatigued and cannot function properly. Rest and relaxation are necessary to prevent fatigue.** Being a "night person" will not help you with those early morning appointments. Your clients deserve a professional full of energy and vitality.

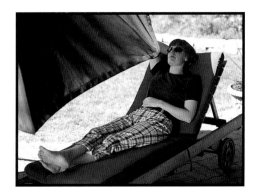

Being able to relax and "get away from it all" is also very important for a healthy body and mind. Reading a good book, listening to music, watching TV or going for a walk can all provide a relaxing change of pace, allowing you to return to work refreshed.

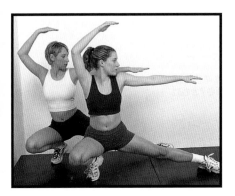

Exercise

A regular exercise program will help you feel better, look better and work better! Your muscles, heart muscles included, need to be in their best possible condition. Exercise is a proven method through which you can keep your muscles toned and equip your body to better cope with the stressful situations in your business and personal life. **Exercise also helps stimulate the blood circulation in your body and encourages proper functioning of organs.**

Take the time to set up an exercise program you will enjoy, such as a brisk daily walk, tennis a few times a week, bicycling or hiking on the weekend, aerobics or yoga to keep your body toned and in shape. Just getting out a few times a week to enjoy the fresh air will help! Remember that you have chosen a profession that is very physical and the better conditioning you give your body, the greater the chances of your success and health. Round out your exercise program by remem-bering to exercise your mind also. Reading is the best form of exercise for the mind.

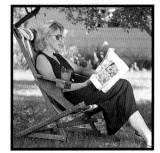

Exercise your mind . . . read.

Worry and fear are two emotions that can be injurious to mental health. Sometimes you may tend to get caught up in these two emotions and fail to exercise your choice to take charge of your life by controlling your thoughts and emotions.

Nutrition

A balanced diet is essential for your personal and professional well being as well as providing prevention for certain diseases. A typical day as a professional stylist can be demanding and your diet may be one of the most important factors for your success. You're going to need all the energy you can get!

Almost all foods contain mixtures of the three energy nutrients: carbohydrates, fats and proteins. The energy they contain is measured in calories. The body uses this energy in several ways: to heat itself, to build its structures and to move its parts during exercise and activities. The energy may also be stored in body fat for later use. In addition to the energy nutrients, other essential nutrients are vitamins, minerals and water.

RDA Guidelines for Daily Averages Based on % of calories:

Carbohydrates 60% (complex)

Fat 30% (10% or less saturated)

Protein 10%

You may have heard the term RDA - Recommended Dietary Allowances. The U.S. Government established the RDA as the appropriate nutrient intakes for people in this country in an attempt to help them select an adequate diet from the array of available foods. The human appetite cannot always be trusted to choose foods that are best for the individual or needed to complete the daily requirements. Many people tend to eat what they like rather than what is best for them.

Calories burned during exercise and activities

Activity (1 hour)	140 lb person	195 lb person
Aerobics, general	381	531
Basketball game	508	708
Bicycling, 10 mph, leisure	254	354
Bowling	191	266
Calisthenics (pushups, sit-ups), light/moderate effort	286	398
Cleaning house, general	222	310
Gardening, general	318	443
Golf, carrying clubs	350	487
Horseback riding, walking	159	221
Jogging	445	620
Judo, karate, kick boxing, tae kwon do	636	885
Mowing lawn	350	487
Rope jumping, moderate	636	885
Running, 6 mph (10 minute mile)	636	885
Ski machine	604	681
Skiing, snow, downhill, moderate	381	531
Tennis, singles	508	708

Data is based on research from Medicine and Science in Sports and Exercise, the "Official Journal of the American College of Sports Medicine."

Hygiene

Hygiene is the science that deals with healthful living. The practice of public hygiene is important because it helps to preserve the health of the community. The fact that you are in training to be a licensed professional says that you are ready to recognize that your clients can depend on you to protect them from health and safety hazards they might experience in the salon. Impure air from poor ventilation, inadequate lighting, improper disinfection practices and improper storage or use of food are the primary health hazards against which health officials expect you to protect clients. Your job as a professional is to protect and serve the public.

Your individual system for maintaining your cleanliness and health is your personal hygiene. In your work, you will constantly be very close to your clients. Scents that wouldn't ordinarily even be noticed or soil that wouldn't normally be detected can, therefore, offend. Obviously, establishing and maintaining a personal hygiene routine is essential if you expect your clients to enjoy your company and want to come back!

Oral Hygiene refers to maintaining healthy teeth and keeping the breath fresh.

Though you might like to believe otherwise, all bodies produce odors. Regular bathing using soap for cleanliness, followed by the application of a deodorant, plays a major role in preventing unpleasant body odors. Avoid excessive use of perfume or cologne. More and more clients have sensitivities to some fragrances. Soiled clothing accumulates odors. No article of clothing should be worn more than a few times before it's washed or your clothing will produce odors that offend no matter how often you bathe!

Few people consider the cleanliness of the inside of their shoes. Yet unclean shoes and the length of time you wear them in a day can create foot odor if not checked. A little talc or foot deodorant can often be of help!

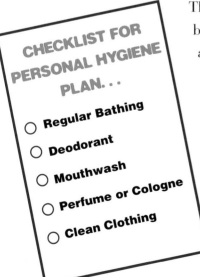

CHECKLIST FOR PERSONAL HYGIENE PLAN...

○ Regular Bathing
○ Deodorant
○ Mouthwash
○ Perfume or Cologne
○ Clean Clothing

The food you eat and the state of your health affect the condition of your breath. Most of you know that eating too much garlic results in unpleasant body smells from perspiration...and bad breath, referred to as halitosis (hal-eh-TOH-siss). Did you know, as well, that a sore throat often produces unpleasant odors from your mouth? Brush your teeth as often as you can each day - certainly after every meal - and use mouth wash. In other words, practice good oral hygiene. Your clients will be grateful.

Consider all potential hygiene problems and establish a personal hygiene plan that addresses them daily. Your personal hygiene contributes to (or detracts from!) your success.

Image

The salon business is a service business; therefore, close attention to personal grooming is a must. Care of your hair, skin, hands, feet and clothing needs to be of the utmost importance. Follow the basic guidelines listed in this section to help ensure your professional image.

Hair Care

The most beautiful hair is clean and healthy hair. As a cosmetologist, of course, the condition of your hair is of particular importance. A daily hair-care program is essential for the salon professional you are studying to become.

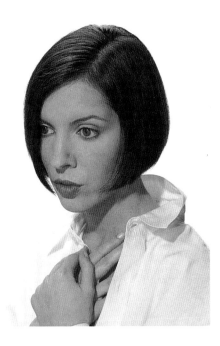

Your own hairstyle and color or perm design must communicate your professional expertise. Your hairstyle should be fashionable yet include any necessary modification that will allow it to better suit your face. If curly hair, for instance, doesn't flatter you or fit your style, don't curl it! Never wear a trendy style merely because it reflects the fashion of the day.

The way you wear color in your hair will help - or hinder - your efforts to introduce color to your clients. Fashion colors can be fun and, for some, flattering. However, if the fashion colors of the season are shades that are not flattering to you, don't wear them. Your ability to call attention to your personal use of hair color to flatter your complexion, "broaden" a narrow forehead or "narrow" a too-wide jaw will be a far greater help to you in encouraging your clients to try color than if you simply follow the current color fashion trends.

Skin Care and Makeup

The proper care of your skin isn't limited to the products you put on it. **Healthy, glowing skin is equally dependent on good nutrition, exercise and rest.** As a beauty business professional, you will need to keep your skin looking its best. Research the variety of skin care products now available and find the regimen best suited for your skin type. It will become increasingly apparent to you how personal skin care knowledge will be an advantage when recommending skin care products for your future clients.

Artfully applied, cosmetics enhance attractive facial features while balancing - to some extent - proportions that aren't quite right. Just as one can contour a face with creative hair color techniques, one can contour with the careful use of cosmetics.

When fashion trends change, the popular makeup look usually changes too. In your profession, it's as important to update your use of cosmetics as it is to wear a hairstyle that reflects the correct

CONTOUR TIPS

- **An overly wide jaw can be visually narrowed by applying darker contour creme on the outer areas of the jawline.**

- **Narrow foreheads can be visually broadened by applying lighter cosmetic shades along the hairline.**

- **Small lips can be made to appear larger by creating a lipstick line just outside the natural lip line.**

- **Large lips can be minimized by applying the lipstick line just inside the natural line of the lips.**

fashion look. It's important that you learn to modify current cosmetic trends into looks that are flattering for you. **The basics of makeup application never change:**

- **Foundation should match your skin tone.**
- **Contouring with light colors always broadens.**
- **Contouring with dark colors always narrows.**

Cosmetic shades change. So does the fashionable use of makeup...from obvious and dramatic to light and natural. Master the basic techniques and then you will be able to learn how to apply makeup to suit any fashion trend in the manner that will complement you best.

Hands

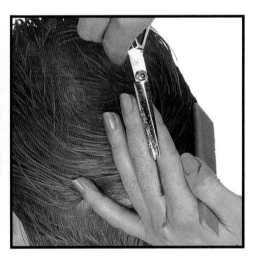

Your hands will touch many people during the course of your career, so they must be smooth, soft, immaculately clean and well manicured. Maintaining attractively manicured, well-cared- for hands is particularly challenging for a cosmetologist. The services you'll perform will often require the use of chemicals: perm solution and hair color, to name only two. **Wear protective gloves whenever performing chemical services.** Use moisturizing lotions frequently. Keep your nails attractively manicured. Avoid wearing rings that can chafe or irritate. Take the best care of your hands that you can.

Feet

A great deal of your time as a cosmetologist will be spent standing on your feet. In order to maintain a cheerful attitude, you will need to take proper care of your feet, practice good posture and wear good-fitting, low, broad-heeled shoes.

Make sure your feet are thoroughly dry after bathing to prevent fungus infections like athlete's foot.

To keep your feet at their best, schedule regular pedicures that will include cleansing, removal of calloused skin, massage and toenail trims. If you develop bunions, corns or ingrown toenails, etc., see a podiatrist (foot doctor).

Clothing

Your clothing must always be freshly washed, or cleaned, and pressed. No unsightly rings around the collar or the armpit can be accepted. Seams and hems must always be secure. Shoulder fit must be loose enough to allow easy movement. No article of clothing should be uncomfortably or unflatteringly tight. **Shoes must always be clean and polished.**

Dress for Success

Your clothing should be selected to incorporate current trends into a statement consistent with your personal sense of style. You're in an age of fashion that shows a variety of designer looks for any given season. Some will be more popular than others, but if the one that's popular doesn't look good on you, go on to something else! A very short woman, for instance, is often visually overwhelmed in a broad-shouldered, calf-length dress. A woman with heavy legs will not be flatteringly dressed in a mini-skirt. Exercise good sense by taking into consideration your height and silhouette when selecting fashions. For instance, wearing gaudy, overpowering jewelry could take away from the image of a well-groomed professional.

TIP:
Dress well 1st. Make money 2nd. Some people think they can't dress well until they make enough money. What they don't understand is that to make more money. . .you need to dress like those who do!

Many schools and salons have a dress code for their stylists or students. Follow it with careful consideration of your personal sense of style and fashion, and you'll look like the beauty business professional you aspire to be.

Posture

The need for good posture goes beyond just standing correctly. **Good posture enhances your physical well-being.** As a professional stylist, you'll be on your feet every day. As you shampoo and style your clients, you'll bend and stretch and stoop. As you restock inventory, *it may be necessary for you to lift boxes as heavy as 50 pounds.* Maintaining good posture and moving properly will:

- protect you from muscle strain and potential injury
- **reduce physical fatigue**
- present an attractive image

Dos and Don'ts for Good Posture

DO	DON'T
Do use the height adjustments styling chairs provide. Styling chairs are designed to raise and lower so you can work on your client's hair without stooping over or reaching up.	Don't slump over a shampoo bowl; bend forward at the waist holding your shoulders straight.
Do keep your head up, your chin level, your shoulders relaxed but straight and your abdomen held flat when standing.	Don't bend at the waist when lifting objects from the floor. Bend at the knees to lower your whole body.
Do keep your feet and knees together, feet on the floor, when sitting, and sit well back in the chair.	Don't, when standing, place more of your weight on one leg than the other. Choose positions that distribute your weight evenly.

EFFECTIVE COMMUNICATION

Throughout your career there will be one element that will propel you toward your goals of success faster than anything else. That element is your ability to communicate effectively.

communication
(kuh-myoo-nih-**KAY**-sh'n) *n.*
1. The act of communicating
2. Exchange of thoughts, information, etc., by conversation or writing
3. A message; news
4. A means of communication; connection
5. [*pl.*] System, as by telephone, for communicating

Every time you exchange ideas, thoughts or feelings with someone, you are communicating. Therefore, your communication skills are every bit as important to your success as your technical skills.

As a stylist, your primary responsibility is to use your knowledge and skills to make your clients look and feel their best. But remember, your advice and service are only as effective as your ability to convince clients of your sincerity and commitment to their well-being. Here your communication skills come into play.

Nonverbal Communication (Body Language)

In nonverbal communication (sometimes called "Body Language"), messages are exchanged without speaking. Appearance, posture, poise, touch, facial expression, eye contact, gestures and silence often "speak more loudly than words."

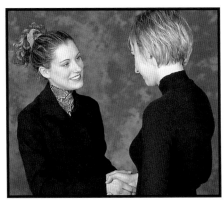
Positive Body Language

For example, a smile is a universal sign of approval. Another example, one who stands straight, shoulders squared, head held high and extends a hand to greet communicates self confidence. Bowed shoulders and sloping body posture convey uncertainty.

Eye contact tells your client - or anyone with whom you are talking - that he or she has your full attention. There will be times, even in the middle of styling a client's hair, that the importance of what that client is saying should cue you to pause and make eye contact. Simple eye contact can validate and reassure. It is a universal sign of acknowledgement.

In preliminary client consultations - or on any occasion when you're communicating face-to-face – leaning slightly forward conveys the unspoken message that the speaker has your complete attention and intense interest. A slightly forward lean communicates that you are interested in what is being said. A backward lean is an unspoken message that you are doubtful or uninterested.

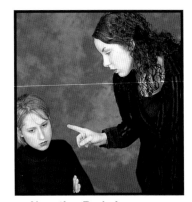
Negative Body Language

Become aware of the subtle ways posture can communicate your feelings about yourself and those around you. Be sure your posture conveys confidence and your movements indicate interest in what your client is saying.

List the messages that you feel the following body language sends:

Arms folded across the chest

Nodding head up and down

Shaking a pointed finger in someone's face

Shaking head back and forth

Can you think of other body language messages? Create a list here.

Language	Message

Verbal Communication (Voice and Tone)

How you speak is as important as what you're saying. A well-modulated voice gains greater positive attention than a voice that is unnecessarily - and often unattractively - high or shrill. A listener may well "tune out" an irritating voice and then miss the information being shared. Listen to your own voice in various situations. A voice that can carry very harmonious tones in normal conversation may become shrill during excitement. Be certain your voice always reflects the personal image you want to project.

Verbal communication (how you speak) can also influence the meaning of what you say. **The tone of your voice, inflection, level and rate of speech all play an important role in verbal communication.**

Grammar

Your language, used correctly, can clearly and beautifully communicate all your thoughts and needs. Used incorrectly, however, the beauty of the language may be marred. Worse still, your level of communication can be impaired.

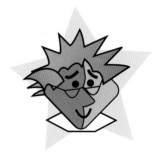

The use of poor grammar can begin accidentally, as you copy poor speech patterns used by those around you. It can also begin intentionally, when you choose to use it to imitate certain peers or to create particular effects. In either case, once the use of poor grammar has begun, it can become habitual and, therefore, difficult to recognize and correct.

"How you speak influences the meaning of what you say: tone, inflection, level and rate of speech play a key role in verbal communication."

The use of double negatives, certain slang words or words whose true meanings aren't quite appropriate to one's messages can all detract from the thought you are attempting to communicate. The listener can be confused by such communication and left with a completely incorrect understanding of the intended message. *No professional can afford to misuse language.*

Because the use of poor grammar may be habitual and not easily identified by the user, this, too, is an area in which you might ask for the help of teachers and friends. Ask people close to you to point out any words you may misuse and speech patterns that aren't appropriate. Many people have polished their use of language with the help of caring friends, relatives, teachers and/or spouses.

Two-Way Communication

Your success in providing your clients with exactly the service they desire depends on *how well you are able to understand and interpret their initial request.*

The best way to do this is, first, encourage them to give you enough information so that you perfectly understand their desires. Be a good listener and ask questions if necessary. *Second, practice reflective listening by repeating back to them in your own words what they just told you.*

For example: "Mrs. Jones, if I understand you correctly, today you would like me to give you more fullness on the top and shorten the back and sides. To do this I will layer the top and cut about one inch from the sides and back to achieve the look you want..."

When you have finished your explanation, always ask if the client understands what you will be doing and if he/she feels comfortable. Encourage questions. It is important that you are able to communicate comfortably and that you and your client understand each other. Here are several points that will help your communication skills become more effective:

Present a Pleasant Greeting
- Always greet a client by using the last name (Mrs. Brown, Mr. Smith, Ms. Johnson) unless the client offers permission for a first name basis and it is acceptable in the school and/or salon.
- Use a pleasing voice tone that projects your eagerness to offer your services.

Use Tact
- Tact is learning to say the proper thing to a person without giving offense. This skill requires sensitivity.
- Tact is a very important communication skill to use in building an honest professional relationship with your clients.
- It is your responsibility to communicate honestly with the client, without offending.
- Deciding whether your ideas or feelings should be expressed in public or private is considered being discreet.

- For example, a client may insist on a certain hair color, which you know will not be flattering. It is your responsibility to tactfully suggest otherwise:

> "Mrs. Jones, I have just returned from a training seminar where I took a special class on coloring and studied color as it relates to the natural tones of the complexion. If we make you a "cool brown," I believe it will tend to wash out your face and make your complexion a bit sallow. But if we weave some subtle warm blonde highlights…"

Express Your Ideas Clearly
- Think an idea through completely before you talk about it.
- Many good ideas fail because they are not thought through before they are expressed.

Define the purpose of your communication
Before you begin to express your idea, determine the purpose of your communication. Is it to:
- Gain information?
- Change an attitude?
- Seek support?
- Motivate?

Know the importance of your ideas
Be certain that the communication is valuable to others. When speaking:
- Consider the listener's needs and desires.
- Ask yourself…How will the listener benefit by what I'm saying?
- Be prepared to show visual representation of the ideas being suggested to the client by using style books, color charts, photographs, etc.

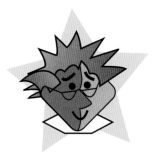

"Think before you speak!"

Be aware of your environment
- Be sure the timing is right for your communication.
- Decide whether your ideas or feelings should be expressed in public or private.
- Decide who should be the recipient of your communication.

Watch your overtones
- An overtone occurs when your tone of voice, inflection, expressions and reactions do not match your words. Example: You say, "I'm so happy to see you today," but you are not smiling or extending your hand in greeting.
- Be sure you are communicating the idea you want to convey.
- Be careful that your overtones aren't saying something entirely different from the words you speak.

Consult with others when necessary
- Be certain you have all the facts and information available.
- If you're in doubt, consult with others to gain new insights, ideas, opinions…and support.

Be a good listener
- Concentrate on understanding others first.
- **Listening is the important key to good communication.**
- The most successful business people and the best communicators are those who have learned to listen.

To be sure you succeeded in communicating, take the time to ask questions. Encourage others to express their opinions. Your success in communicating your thoughts is strongly related to how well you communicate your professionalism. Everything you speak and do should convey that you're a professional.

Avoid discussing the following topics with clients:
- Religion
- Politics
- Personal problems
- Other client's behavior
- Staff or competitor's workmanship
- Information given to you in confidence

For example, the **topics** you select to discuss with your clients **should be chosen with care. Avoid controversial topics.** Too many salon stylists rely on the weather, current movies and famous personalities to provide topics to discuss with clients. As a true salon professional, you'll want to focus your conversation on your client's lifestyle and beauty needs and then completely provide the beauty care direction that will help him or her meet those needs. A client's very active life, for example, would probably be well served with a short, easy-to-care-for style. You might, additionally, recommend a perm to further reduce time spent caring for his/her hair at home. You'll use particular products on each client for particular reasons. Explain what you're using and why. Your client will expect to receive your full attention while in your chair and to receive the full benefit of your professional expertise. Be sure that each client receives what he/she needs and your success will be guaranteed.

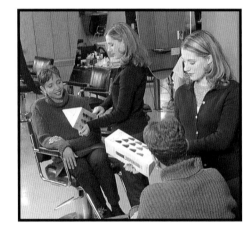

Be sure each client receives your full attention.

HUMAN RELATIONS

The psychology of **getting along with others** is referred to as **human relations.** Many factors influence good human relations in the workplace, including personality, teamwork and your professional code of ethics. Long hours of standing, high customer expectations and the need to increase the pace of work, may tend to cause added stress. Be cautious that this stress does not negatively reflect in how you deal with people.

Personality

Personality is defined as the outward reflection of your inner feelings, thoughts, attitudes and values. Your personality is the sum total of the emotional and behavioral characteristics that make you unique. Your individual personality consists of combinations of thousands of different human characteristics, such as emotions, attitudes, skills, beliefs, values and goals. All your many experiences influence the development of your personality, as well. These personality characteristics are not quickly changed - but can be modified over time.

A pleasing personality is a tremendous asset to a cosmetologist and includes personal attributes such as:

- **a good sense of humor**
- **a considerate nature**
- **a positive attitude**
- **emotional control**

- **vitality**
- **flexibility**
- **friendliness**
- **good manners**

Select three of the words or phrases from the graphic above and describe something that you have done or something that happened to you in the last three days that involved those personal attributes.

Chosen word or phrase

Good manners

Action

I opened the door for an elderly client yesterday.

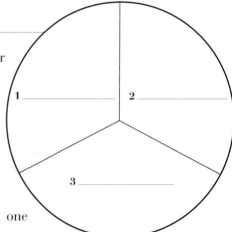

Using the pie chart to the right, fill in the blanks provided with your 3 best personality attributes. You can use those personality attributes listed in the graphic above as a reference or create your own descriptive words.

Attitudes

An "attitude" is the specific and identifiable emotion and/or reaction one experiences and projects in dealing with the demands of life. Because your attitude is projected, it can have an effect on those around you. **A negative attitude, obviously, can have a negative impact on others.** Conversely, projecting a positive attitude can have an uplifting effect on the people with whom you come in contact.

People are born with very few attitudes; attitudes, like habits, are "learned." Therefore, attitudes, like habits, can be "unlearned," changed and modified. Although attitudes are primarily learned, as parts of your personality they are very resistant to immediate change. "Positive" and "negative" are the two adjectives most often used to describe attitudes. Other descriptions include (but aren't limited to): enthusiastic, caring, confident, defensive, aggressive, fearful.

Attitudes like habits can be changed. It is not easy but is quite often the key to having your life run smoother!

All of us have attitudes. Some are so ingrained that we've come to accept them as unchangeable parts of our personalities. Too often, on questioning someone who constantly complains, for example, you'll hear, "Oh, don't mind me. That's just the way I am." Not true! It's the way that person has, consciously or unconsciously, CHOSEN to be. **Attitudes can be changed.** Because an attitude can be so deeply ingrained that it has become a way of life no longer even noticed - let alone examined - changing that attitude can be very hard to do. You must remember that an attitude is projected...it touches and affects others. Allowing yourself to project negativity in any form because "it's just the way I am" is grossly unfair to everyone around you. In the long run, you will suffer most.

Some self-assessment and management may be necessary merely to identify ingrained emotions as reactions that fall under any of the "negative" descriptions. Once identified, they can be changed. The process of such change can require frequent re-evaluation and continual focus. However, consider the rewards. Not only will you be happier within yourself, but other people will find greater pleasure in knowing you and spending time with you.

You may want to ask your friends if your attitude is generally positive or negative. If you find that you currently do not have a positive, healthy attitude toward life, yet success is important to you, you may want to start changing now.

Analyze your personality and attitude every few months to find out what progress you are making. Remember, **an attractive personality, including a positive attitude, is one of your greatest assets in life.** It is the charm revealed in your speech, appearance, behavior and manner - the total effect you have on other people.

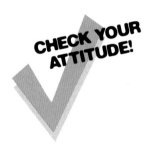

How would your best friend describe your attitude?

_____

How would your closest living relative describe your attitude?

_____

How would your instructor describe your attitude?

_____

How would you describe your attitude?

_____

As a salon professional, your potential success will be enormously enhanced if your peers and clients feel good in your presence. If you develop and nurture a positive attitude, not only will you have the ability to make your clients look good with your styling skills, you'll be able to make them feel good, too. That's a special gift, a goal worth working toward indeed!

Habits

Some people bite their nails, others bite their lips. Some people drum their fingers, others tap their feet. The only thing all these actions have in common is that the people performing them are probably not aware of doing so. These actions are very likely all habits.

Habits are "learned" and reinforced through events in your environment, which strengthen the habit. Like attitudes, habits become ingrained and are difficult to change. Most habits are harmless, inoffensive actions that others barely notice. *But some habits are annoying and unattractive.*

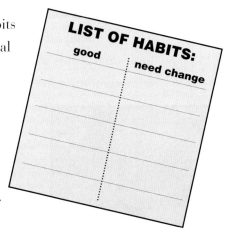

You're entering a service business and can't allow yourself to keep those habits that others may find annoying. Unattractive habits will limit your potential for success.

Sit down in a quiet room and make a well-considered list of all your habits. Because it's very possible to be completely unaware of personal habits, ask a few relatives or friends to review your list and add anything you've left out. Review each item on your list. Is each habit consistent with the personal image you want to present to others? If not, begin a program of change now!

Changing Habits

Have you changed a habit in the past? If so, list the efforts you put forth to make the change occur.

_____

_____

_____

_____

If you want to change a habit you currently have, can you apply these same efforts?

Having a positive attitude and practicing good habits will serve as fundamental principles in developing effective human relationships. Additional tips that will help along the way to your success include:

Maintain Attendance and Punctuality

- Manage your personal and professional schedule to avoid conflicts with time.
- Arrive at work on time. (Fifteen minutes prior to starting time is preferred by most employers.)

Connect with your Client

- Be sensitive to the mood of your client. Some clients need and want the appointment time to be quiet and relaxing, others will want to talk and visit. Be a respectful listener and keep your conversation within the realm of your client's needs. **Never gossip or tell off-color stories.**

Extend Courtesy

- **Courtesy is the key to success.** Your thoughtfulness of others will go a long way in allowing clients to feel comfortable and relaxed with you.

Teamwork

The emotional atmosphere of a salon has unique importance. The salon business is a service business...and a part of that service is the presence of a relaxed, peaceful environment. The existence of a harmonious salon environment depends heavily on teamwork.

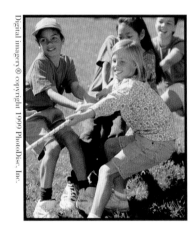

As an individual member of a team, you can bring certain valuable characteristics to it that will have a positive influence on the group. Your special behavior, skills and abilities are important to the success of the group. Strong, positive, professional relationships and team spirit will not be built overnight. You can begin by establishing a rapport with each person and continuing to work toward good communication, understanding and teamwork every day. The people you work with can become your friends as well as your professional associates.

Keeping your work station clean, with all your tools in place, is usually set forth by a regulating agency, but also adds visually to the overall atmosphere you'll be trying to create. Placing and storing salon tools after use avoids the potential frustration that can occur when another stylist needs the tool and it's not where it belongs. Respecting confidences shared by peers or clients is essential for an atmosphere of trust and sharing to exist. These are only a few of the many things a good team player will learn to do to help maintain the salon staff as a productive, happy team. **The key words for teamwork are consideration and cooperation.** If you're considerate and cooperative, you'll add to your team's success.

Ethics

Over the years your parents and teachers may have taught you to live by the "Golden Rule": "Do unto others as you would have them do unto you." The Golden Rule may have been your first introduction to a code of ethical conduct. As you grow older, you begin defining and learning what is good or bad, right or wrong, according to the rules of society. **As your personality develops, you establish your own personal system of moral principles and values, which become known as your personal ethics.**

Your personal ethics, how you live your life and demonstrate your positive values and beliefs, such as honesty and fairness, carry over into your profession as you apply them to your working environment and relationships. Professional ethics deal with proper conduct in relationships with your employer, co-workers and clients.

Most professions have associations that establish a "Code of Professional Ethics" for their individual members. It is important for you to familiarize yourself with the Cosmetology Code of Ethics in your area. Adherence to a professional code of ethics reflects your personal integrity. These codes are designed not only to protect the public and guarantee that they will be treated honestly and fairly, but also to help you build confidence and increase your clientele.

Some of the responsibilities and work ethics that will help you gain respect and build solid professional relationships with your clients and co-workers are listed on the sample "Professional Code of Ethics."

Professional Code of Ethics

- **Show respect for the feelings and rights of others. Remember the Golden Rule.**

- **Be fair and courteous to your co-workers. Don't attempt to win clients away from your fellow stylists.**

- **Be fair and courteous to your clients. Be consistent in pricing your services. Don't show favoritism to certain clients.**

- **Always be eager to learn new methods and techniques. Attend educational programs that provide updated information or help you to improve your skills.**

- **Represent yourself, your services and products honestly to the public. Do not advertise a service that you cannot perform.**

- **Set a good example of good conduct and good behavior. Always cherish a good reputation. It will carry you a long way.**

- **Be loyal to your employer and co-workers. A successful salon will aid in your success.**

- **Keep your word and fulfill your obligations. Never break the confidence entrusted to you by a client or co-worker.**

- **Practice only the highest standards of infection control as provided by your regulating agency laws. Keep your work area and tools spotlessly clean.**

- **Believe in and be proud of your profession, just as you believe in yourself!**

Commitment to Excellence

Invest in yourself! Learn everything you can in school. Take an active part in school activities. Take advantage of advanced education and seminars. After graduation, continue to invest in your education by attending seminars, shows and workshops. Keep pace with what's happening in the industry. Become known for your willingness to share your knowledge and your enthusiasm for the beauty industry. There is no limit to the success you can achieve if you are willing to invest the time and energy success demands of the true professional.

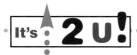

Build Your Critical Thinking Skills

In this chapter you have prepared yourself to meet the following Industry Standards for entry-level cosmetologists:

- Participate in lifelong learning to stay current with trends, technology and techniques pertaining to the cosmetology industry
- Use appropriate methods to ensure personal health and well-being

It's Up to You to know what to do. Using your training to this point, review the following case scenarios and think through how you would handle each challenge.

1. Last night your best friend visited you and it was 2:30 a.m. before you were able to go to sleep. That was the second night this week that you had fewer than 4 hours of sleep. Now, a new friend has just asked you to drive with her to see her brother's school play, which is being held in a city 3 hours from your home. If you go, it means that you will be home late again. You are scheduled with 5 appointments tomorrow and one is a spiral perm that you have not done before. Your new friend is counting on you. What would you do?

2. The students at your school have noticed an outbreak of theft recently. Things have been taken from their work stations and lockers and it seems that no one can be trusted. You think you saw someone look suspicious this morning as he picked up a pair of shears from a work station. You're not sure if the shears belonged to him or not. You just have an "inkling" that something is wrong. What would you do?

3. Your boss has just asked you to work a double-shift because a new employee is absent again. You saw this new employee at the same party you were at last night. You were able to get up and come in for your work shift, but the new employee did not make it. This is the third time this has happened in a 30-day period. What would you do?

Chapter 2
SALON ECOLOGY

After studying this chapter you will be able to . . .

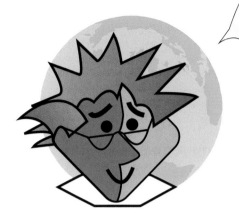

MICROBIOLOGY

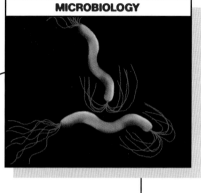

1. **Recognize the structure and function of bacteria and viruses by their**
   - **Types;**
   - **Classifications;**
   - **Growth and reproduction patterns;**
   - **Relationship to the spread of infection.**

FIRST AID

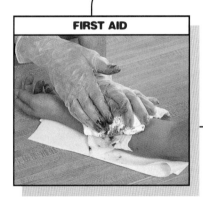

3. **List simple safety and first-aid applications for minor burns, cuts, choking, eye injury and fainting procedures.**

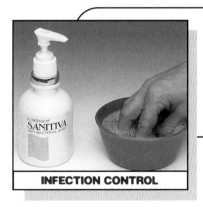

INFECTION CONTROL

2. **Identify the procedures and precautions for the infection control procedures used in schools and salons.**

I'm back! I hope you're joining me with good rest, good nutrition and good exercise. You'll need every bit of it to tackle this new material. You already know that you need a healthy mind and body to function as a respected professional. Now it's time to learn how to create and maintain a healthy, infection-free and safe environment for your work. That's the job of our second chapter, SALON ECOLOGY. Don't be scared off by the term ECOLOGY. It's simple enough when we look at its parts:

ECO = house, household + (O)LOGY = study of

In the world of cosmetology, your understanding of SALON ECOLOGY enables you to prevent the unnecessary spread of infectious diseases and to perform first-aid procedures as needed for the protection of the client.

Ecology is the study of households and the way they are kept in balance to ensure the well-being of those living there. SALON ECOLOGY studies ways to keep the larger, expanded environment of the salon in balance to guarantee the well-being and safety of all involved. That's the VALUE of this chapter to you and your clients alike and what the BIG IDEA has as its focus.

A healthy and safe environment requires an understanding of infection control and first-aid procedures.

The PLAN I have for you to put into action in this chapter starts under the heading "Microbiology." This chapter contains the theory you need to know to practice infection control and safety in the salon. After all, that's the goal of all my action plans – to help you transform the big idea into something of value to yourself.

MICROBIOLOGY

Bacteria
Growth of Bacteria
Viruses
External Parasites
Infection
Immunity

INFECTION CONTROL

Sanitation
Disinfection
Sterilization
Infection Control Guidelines

FIRST AID

Bleeding and Wounds
Burns
Choking
Fainting
Eye Injury

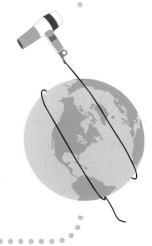

MICROBIOLOGY

Microbiology–what a big word to describe the study of small organisms! Yet that's exactly what microbiology is, the study (ology) of small (micro) living (bio) organisms called microbes, such as bacteria.

A basic knowledge of microbiology is important to you as a cosmetologist so that you can prevent the spread of disease through proper disinfection within the salon. As a stylist, it is your responsibility to protect your client's health and your own by taking the steps necessary to ensure that potentially infectious organisms aren't transmitted from one client to another - or to yourself and other stylists - via the use of contaminated (dirty) styling tools and implements.

Bacteria

Bacteria, sometimes called germs or microbes, are one-celled micro-organisms. The study of bacteria is referred to as bacteriology. While there are thousands of different kinds of bacteria, they can generally be classified into two types:

Here's a hint about how to remember these words. The Greek word pathos means suffering. Pathogenic bacteria cause disease and therefore suffering. Nonpathogenic =  suffering

1.   Nonpathogenic: nondisease producing bacteria
2.   Pathogenic: disease-producing bacteria

Nonpathogenic Bacteria

Nonpathogenic bacteria are harmless and can be very beneficial. Some bacteria have medical applications. Other bacteria, like some found in certain dairy products (such as yogurt), have health-enhancing properties. Still other bacteria cause the decay of refuse or vegetation and thereby improve the fertility of soil. **Saprophytes (SAP-ro-fights) are nonpathogenic bacteria that live on dead matter and do not produce disease. Approximately 70% of all bacteria are non-pathogenic and many live on the surface of the skin.**

Pathogenic Bacteria

Pathogenic bacteria live everywhere in your environment and even exist inside your body. There are several different types of pathogenic bacteria that are harmful because they cause infection and disease, and some produce toxins. These infectious bacteria can be easily spread in the salon by using unsanitary styling implements or via dirty hands and fingernails. Only in the last hundred years have scientists, such as Louis Pasteur, discovered these microscopic (seen only with the aid of a microscope) bacteria and invented solutions to destroy many of them and combat the spread of infection. Scientists found that these bacteria have distinct shapes that aid in their microscopic identification.

When a disease spreads from one person to another via contact, it is referred to as contagious or communicable. Examples are the common cold, hepatitis and measles.

Bacteria are single cells with one of three basic shapes as shown below. Remember that you won't be identifying them with a microscope in the salon. You need mainly to prevent their growth and spread. Listed below by shape and kind are the more common pathogenic bacteria that you might encounter as a stylist.

1) **Cocci** (**KOK**-si) are spherical (round)-shaped bacterial cells, which appear singularly or in groups. *To remember, think C = circle and Cocci.* There are three groups of Cocci:

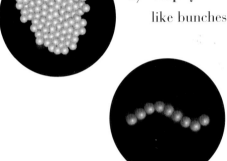

a) **Staphylococci** (staf-i-lo-**KOK**-si) are pus-forming bacterial cells that form grape-like bunches or clusters and are present in abscesses, pustules and boils.

b) **Streptococci** (strep-to-**KOK**-si) are also pus-forming bacterial cells that form in long chains and can cause septisemia (sometimes called blood poisoning), strep throat, rheumatic fever and other serious infections.

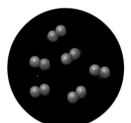

c) **Diplococci** (dip-lo-**KOK**-si) are bacterial cells that grow in pairs and are the cause of certain infections, including pneumonia. *Diplo means double.*

2) **Bacilli** (ba-**SIL**-i) are the most common form of bacterial cells. Bacilli are bar or rod-shaped cells that can produce a variety of diseases including tetanus, bacterial influenza, typhoid fever, tuberculosis and diphtheria. *To remember, think B = bar and Bacilli.*

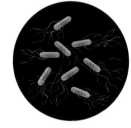

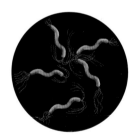

3) **Spirilla** (speye-**RIL**-a)are spiraled, coiled, corkscrew-shaped bacterial cells that cause highly contagious diseases such as syphilis, cholera and lyme disease. *To remember, think S = spiral and Spirilla.*

Keep in mind that this list is never complete. Through research, previously unknown pathogenic bacteria are discovered on an ongoing basis.

Bacteria can cause infections by invading the body through a break in the skin or through any of the body's natural openings (nose, mouth, etc.). An infection occurs when an insufficient number of antibodies are produced by the body's defense (immune) system to "fight" harmful bacteria.

2

Growth of Bacteria

Bacteria goes through a growth cycle that consists of two stages: an active stage and an inactive stage.

Active Stage

During the active stage, bacteria reproduce and grow rapidly. This reproduction usually takes place in dark, damp or dirty areas where a food source is available. As the bacteria absorb food, each cell grows in size and divides, creating two new cells. This activity is called mitosis. The process of cell division in bacteria is similar to the budding process in plants. Under favorable conditions, bacteria reproduce quickly, with as many as sixteen million offspring developing in twelve hours.

Inactive Stage

Bacteria are not always active; when conditions are unfavorable, the cells die or become inactive. Some bacteria, such as anthrax and tetanus, also have a normal inactive or dormant stage. When the environment makes the bacteria's survival difficult, some bacteria enter this inactive stage by creating spherical spores that are not harmed by disinfectants, cold or heat. Spore formation and other means by which bacteria can resist disinfection are factors to be considered when keeping the salon sanitary. Some bacteria can survive for a long time in extreme heat or cold. When conditions again become favorable for the bacteria's growth, the bacteria return to the active stage.

Over 1,500 of some types of bacteria will fit on the head of a pin.

Movement of Bacteria

Because of their tiny size, bacteria can travel easily from place to place through air or water, from you to your client and vice versa. Bacilli and spirilla have the ability to move by themselves by using hair-like projections called flagella (flah-**JEL**-ah) or cilia (**SIL**-ee-a), which extend from the sides of the cell. A wave-like motion of these projections can easily propel the cell through a liquid.

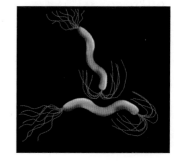

Viruses

Viruses are sub-microscopic particles (much smaller than bacteria) that cause familiar diseases like the common cold, which is caused by a filterable virus. Other familiar diseases caused by viruses include respiratory and gastrointestinal infections, chicken pox, mumps, measles, small pox, yellow fever, rabies, HIV (AIDS), hepatitis and polio.

"The National Centers for Disease Control (CDC) assigns the category titled Personal Service Workers to cosmetologists. Watch for the initials PSW as information is released."

Human Hepatitis B (HBV) is a highly infectious disease that infects the liver. Personal service workers (PSWs), such as nurses, doctors, teachers and cosmetologists, are asked to take precautions against HBV, which is a vaccine-preventable disease. Because these professionals work with the public, inoculation is often recommended. Check with your local health agency or doctor to determine if you are a candidate for this inoculation.

Acquired Immunodeficiency Syndrome (AIDS) is a disease caused by HIV (Human Immunodeficiency Virus). HIV interferes with the body's natural immune system and causes the immune system to break down. Scientists have gained a great deal of knowledge about HIV and how it is spread and how to prevent it. HIV is spread when body fluids from an infected individual are absorbed into the blood stream of an uninfected individual. The fluids from the infected person must contain sufficient amounts of the virus. Fluids known to contain sufficient amounts of HIV are blood, semen, vaginal fluids and breast milk. Body fluids must enter the uninfected person for that person to be infected. Infectious fluids can enter through sexual intercourse, sharing needles or syringes, childbirth, cuts or sores (that are exposed to the infectious materials) and other instances where the body fluid of one individual enters the body of another.

Adapted from "AIDS" - The War Within", Museum of Science and Industry, Chicago, IL

External Parasites

External parasites (**PAR**-ah-sights) are organisms that live on or obtain their nutrients from another organism. Parasitic fungi are molds and yeasts that produce such contagious diseases as ringworm (tinea capitis), honeycomb ringworm (favus) and nail fungus, and noncontagious conditions such as dandruff and seborrheic dermatitis. Parasitic mites are insects that cause contagious disease, such as itch mites (scabies) and head lice (pediculosis). Professionals prevent the spread of contagions (fungi, bacteria, and mites) through proper disinfection procedures.

Head Lice

Head lice are transmitted directly from one person to another, or by contact with articles that have come in contact with an infested person (such as combs and brushes, etc.). The presence of head lice is usually accompanied by head scratching, redness or small bite marks on the scalp. Close inspection of the hair and scalp with a fine-tooth comb, a strong light, and a magnifying glass will sometimes reveal the tiny grayish adult lice. But you are more likely to see their eggs, which are whitish, oval specks attached to the hair shafts about 1/4 inch (.75 cm) from the skin. The infestation is very easy to control, if detected, by using a pediculicide (lice-killing) shampoo.

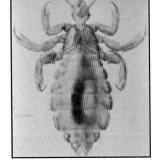
Magnified view of head lice

Infection

An infection occurs when disease-causing (pathogenic) bacteria or viruses enter the body and multiply to the point of interfering with the body's normal state. A contagious infection or communicable disease is one that can be transmitted from one person to another, usually through touch or through the air. Microorganisms that are spread to a new person frequently cause no infection unless they actually enter the body. **Bloodborne pathogens** are disease-causing bacteria or viruses that are carried through the blood or body fluids.

Common means of spreading infection in a salon include:

- **Open sores**
- **Unclean hands and implements**
- **Coughing or sneezing**
- **Common use of drinking cups and towels**
- **Use of same implements on infected areas and noninfected areas**
- **Unsanitary salon conditions**

Infections can be controlled by personal hygiene, public awareness and by practicing infection control procedures in the salon. If you have a contagious disease, it is important that you practice infection control procedures in order not to spread the infection. Check with your area's regulating agency for specific guidelines on dealing with contagious disease and refer a client with a contagious disease to a physician.

There are two basic classes of infection:

1. A local infection is located in a small, confined area. This is often indicated by a pus-filled boil, pimple or inflamed area. *To remember, think local = little.*

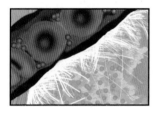

2. A general (or systemic) infection occurs when the circulatory system carries bacteria and their toxins to all parts of the body. *To remember, think general = giant.*

It is possible for a person to carry disease-producing bacteria or viruses with no recognizable symptoms of the disease. Such a person is called an "asymptomatic" carrier. For this reason the same infection control procedures should be used with all clients. This practice is called **"universal precautions."**

Immunity

Immunity is the ability of the body to destroy infectious agents that enter the body. *To remember, think immunity gives you ammunition to fight disease.* The body has remarkable defense mechanisms that fight infections in two basic ways:

1. Natural immunity is a partially inherited, natural resistance to disease. A healthy body produces white blood cells and antitoxins to fight disease. Also, the epidermis (outermost layer of skin) protects the body from microbes. If the skin is punctured, the cut must be treated to keep microbes from infecting the skin. It is often said that the unbroken skin is the body's first line of defense in regard to disease.

2. Passive (acquired) immunity is developed through the injection of antigens, which stimulate the body's immune response (e.g., inoculation for polio or flu).

INFECTION CONTROL

Now that you have read about the dangers of microbes, you are ready to learn how you can destroy them and prevent disease from spreading in the salon. As you know, microbes are everywhere, including in the air around you, so infection control is not an easy task.

Infection control is the term used to describe efforts to prevent the spread of disease and kill certain or all microbes. Infection control is divided into three main categories: sanitation, disinfection and sterilization. Sanitation standards apply to removing dirt to aid in preventing the growth of microbes. Disinfection standards require that all tools and implements, including those that have come in contact with blood or body fluids, must be free from a broad spectrum of microbes. Sterilization standards mean that all microbes must be killed or destroyed.

solution This upper reservoir to desired level. Use at a dilution of 1:64 (2 ozs. of this product per gallon of water or 16 ml per liter).

Beauty and Barber Shop, Instruments and Tools: Thoroughly pre-clean. Completely immerse brushes, combs, scissors, clipper blades, razors, tweezers, manicure and other shop tools for 10 minutes (or as required by local authorities). Wipe dry before use. Fresh solution should be prepared daily or more often when the solution becomes diluted or soiled.

*Virucidal: For Complete Instructions For Hepatitis B Virus (HBV) and Human Immunodeficiency Virus (HIV-1) DISINFECTION Refer To Enclosed Hang Tag.

Statement of Practical Treatment: In case of contact, immediately flush eyes or skin with plenty of water for at least 15 minutes. For eye contacts, call a physician. If swallowed, drink egg whites, gelatin solution or if these are not available, drink large quantities of water. Avoid alcohol. Call a physician immediately.

Note to Physician: Probable mucosal damage may contra-indicate the use of gastric lavage.

Note: Avoid shipping or storing below freezing. If product freezes, thaw at room temperature and shake gently to remix components.

Very important also to the area of infection control is the term efficacy, which means "ability to produce results" or "effectiveness." In relation to disinfectant products, standards have been established that require efficacy labels on all disinfectants to inform the user about what the product is "effective in fighting against." An example might be a disinfectant that states "effective against human Hepatitis B Virus and HIV-1." As you gain more information in this chapter, you will notice that you will be required to use products based on the efficacy label.

Reading the manufacturer's directions is another important step in ensuring infection control practices. You will notice that methods will vary from product to product. Times for immersion (soaking) in a disinfectant, storage practices and application methods will be different for each product. The only way you can be sure that a product will do what you want it to is to FOLLOW THE DIRECTIONS. It cannot be repeated often enough that two steps are necessary for effective infection control: READ THE LABEL and FOLLOW THE DIRECTIONS!

"Did I hear you say, 'Read the label and follow the directions'?"

Important Vocabulary

- **Infection control** involves the steps you take to prevent the spread of disease and kill certain microbes.
- **Sanitation, disinfection and sterilization** are the 3 main categories of Infection Control.
- **Sanitation means** to remove dirt and debris to aid in preventing the growth of microbes. **Sanitation practices** remove dirt, but do not kill microbes.
- **Antiseptics** arrest or prevent the growth of microorganisms on the skin.
- **Disinfection** means to destroy or kill a broad spectrum of microbes on nonporous surfaces, such as implements.
- **Sterilization** means to destroy or kill all microbes.
- **Bloodborne pathogen disinfection** is required for all tools and implements that have come in contact with blood or body fluids. This type of disinfection requires the use of an EPA-registered disinfectant labeled as effective against HIV and HBV or tuberculocidal.
- In relation to **disinfectant products**, standards have been established to require **efficacy labels** on all disinfectants to inform the user on what the product is "effective in fighting against." The only way you can be sure that a product will do what you want it to is to **READ THE LABEL AND FOLLOW THE DIRECTIONS.**

Sanitation

Sanitation is a term that means to remove dirt to aid in preventing the growth of microbes. Sanitation is the first level of infection control. It is important to note that **sanitation methods clean and reduce microbes on the surface, but do not kill germs.** Two ways to describe that to you would be first, to ask you to think of cleaning your house or apartment. If you are dusting an end table, you are removing dirt that has gathered on the surface, but you are not killing bacteria or germs that are possibly lurking there. Even if you used a furniture spray, you would not be killing the bacteria. Unless you use a product with an efficacy label stating it has the ability to kill specific microbes, the microbes would remain on the surface. Only the dirt or dust would be removed.

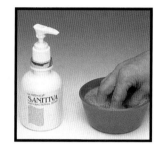

The second example involves giving a pedicure, manicure or other skin care procedure. Prior to any of these procedures, apply an antiseptic to clean the skin. **An antiseptic is a product that can be applied to the skin to reduce microbes.** In other words, you have a clean surface on which to perform procedures and you have helped to prevent the future growth of microbes. You may also use an antibacterial liquid soap as a manicure or pedicure soak to further reduce microbes on your client's skin before you begin your service. Remember, some of that bacteria might be good (nonpathogenic) and some may be harmful (pathogenic). Because you will not be breaking the skin, it is not necessary to use a product stronger than an antiseptic.

SANITATION GUIDELINES

1. Provide well-lit work areas.

2. Provide hot and cold running water.

3. Sanitize shampoo bowls before and after each use.

4. Clean and remove hair and debris from all implements before disinfecting.

5. Wash your hands with liquid soap and water immediately before serving each client. Antibacterial liquid soap is recommended since bar soaps can harbor and transmit microbes.

6. Remove all hair clippings after each service to prevent accumulation.

The Basics of Hand Washing

1. Moisten hands with warm water and antimicrobial, also called antibacterial, liquid soap.

2. Spend at least 15-20 seconds working up a good lather. Pay particular attention to the fingers and the spaces between them and the fingernails.

3. Rinse hands well in warm water. Position hands and fingertips downward so the rinse progresses from wrist to fingertips.

4. Dry hands well to remove any remaining microorganisms. A single-use paper towel or hands-free air blowers are the most effective and do not carry the risk of cross-contamination posed by communal cloth towels.

Infection control practices for sanitation of the school or salon require shared responsibilities from everyone on the team in order to provide a healthy environment. Review the Infection Control Sanitation Guidelines chart to gain knowledge in the steps taken to prevent the growth of microbes. Remember, preventing the growth of microbes and killing microbes are two different functions. Sanitation practices do not kill microbes, but do help in the prevention of the growth of microbes.

Rules of Infection Control are developed by area regulating agencies to protect the consumer. These rules require salons and cosmetology schools to keep the working areas, styling implements and all equipment in a sanitary condition. To do so, salons employ infection control methods to meet the required guidelines.

Ventilation

It is important that the salon be sufficiently ventilated so that the air does not have a stale, musty odor or contain the odor of sprays, bleaches and various chemical solutions. The average room temperature should be about 70° Fahrenheit (21° Celsius).

Care needs to be taken to maintain proper air conditioning and air safety in the salon. The following guidelines provide an overview of various ventilation and sanitation practices for a healthy environment:

- Air conditioners permit changes in the quality and quantity of air brought into the salon as they cool, dehumidify (remove moisture) and cleanse pollutants from the air. Remember to change air filters as needed.

- Forced-air furnaces heat the air and cleanse it, to a degree. Remember to change air filters as needed.

- Exhaust fans help circulate the air but do not clean it. Fans should always be positioned to draw air or blow air away from stylists' and clients' faces.

- Air should be mechanically supplied through vents and air returns and/or supplied by opening windows and doors and using blower fans to circulate the fresh air.

- Provide local exhaust ventilation for areas in which chemicals are mixed or artificial nails are applied. Always keep all bottles capped when not in use.

SANITATION GUIDELINES (CONT'D)

7. Provide clean restrooms, with well stocked toilet tissue and paper towels. Never use restroom areas for storage of chemicals.

8. Provide disposable drinking cups. Clean sinks and water fountains regularly.

9. Keep salon free from insects and rodents.

10. Never use the salon for cooking or living quarters.

11. Empty waste receptacles daily.

12. Wear clean, freshly laundered clothing.

13. Use freshly laundered or disposable towels on each client. Never allow the protective cape to touch the client's neck.

14. Never place tools, combs, rollers or bobby pins, etc., in your mouth or pockets.

15. Properly launder all client gowns and headbands before reusing.

16. Store soiled towels in a covered receptacle until laundered.

17. Launder towels/linens after each use with an approved disinfectant so they don't accumulate and present a safety hazard (due to chemicals that may be present).

18. Avoid touching your face, mouth or eyes during services.

19. Never allow pets or animals in service area, except for Service Animals as identified in the Americans with Disabilities Act.

20. Allow smoking only in designated areas.

21. Dispense all semi-fluids and powders with a shaker, dispenser pump, spray-type container, spatula or disposable applicator.

2

- For localized exhaust systems in chemical mixing areas, manicure areas or perm areas, etc., make sure the fan in the unit is powerful enough to draw or blow the chemical vapor or dust away in an attempt to improve the safety of the stylist and client.

Disinfection

Disinfection is the second level of infection control. Disinfection standards require products to destroy or kill bacteria and a broad spectrum of viruses. These standards apply to all tools and implements used by the cosmetologist. Note that disinfection products are toxic.

Disinfectants are chemical products used to destroy or kill bacteria and some viruses (except bacterial spores). Bactericidals (kill harmful bacteria), tuberculocidals (kill tuberculosis), fungicidals (destroy fungus), viricidals (kill viruses) and pseudomonacidals (kill pseudomonas) are all categories of disinfectant products designed to kill specific organisms. The disinfecting chemicals used to kill these microbes are very strong and work well to disinfect styling implements but could be harmful to your skin. Follow manufacturer's directions regarding their use.

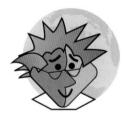

"Little things can hurt us even though we can't see them."

OSHA (The Occupational Safety and Health Administration) is the regulating agency under the Department of Labor that enforces safety and health standards in the workplace. OSHA Standards require that employees be informed of the dangers of the materials used in the workplace and the exposure they might have to toxic substances. **Material Safety Data Sheets (MSDS) and labeling of products are two important regulations that this group has put in place to assist in safe operations.** A Material Safety Data Sheet is designed to provide the key information on a specific product regarding ingredients, associated hazards, combustion levels, storage requirements, etc. Remember that for your protection and safety, it is your right as an employee to know what is contained in the product being used. OSHA standards are important to the industry and help ensure general safety, especially in regard to mixing, storing, labeling and disposing of chemicals.

The EPA (Environmental Protection Agency) approves the efficacy of products used for infection control. This means that a manufacturer submits a product to this agency for verification of effectiveness against the organisms listed on the label. Once that determination has been made, an EPA registration number is given to the product along with approval of the efficacy claims on the label, stating what the product will destroy or be effective against. This registered number ensures the product is both safe and effective.

Always follow the manufacturer's directions, and always wear protective gloves and safety glasses when mixing disinfectants.

Broad spectrum disinfectants, formerly known as hospital-grade or hospital-level disinfectants are a group of disinfectants that kill bacteria, viruses, fungi, and pseudomonas. These products are effective and quick-acting. The label on a broad spectrum disinfectant will have an EPA-registered number along with an efficacy label stating that the product is an effective bactericidal, virucidal, fungicidal and pseudomonacidal. The disinfectant may also be effective against HIV and HBV or tuberculocidal. Many regulating agencies have adopted this efficacy label for disinfection of all tools and implements. Check your area's rules and regulations for required usage.

ALERT!

The 1997 OSHA (Occupational Safety and Health Administration) Bloodborne Pathogens Standard requires the use of an EPA-registered disinfectant with an efficacy against HIV and HBV or tuberculocidal. This requirement applies to implements that accidentally come into contact with blood or body fluids.

The most important thing for you to know is that the efficacy label will tell you what the disinfectant is effective against. You will be guided by your area's rules as to what efficacy standard you need to use. One standard may guide you for disinfection of all tools and implements that **have not** come in contact with blood or body fluids, and another standard may guide you for disinfection of all tools and implements that **have** come in contact with blood or body fluids. Will one product work for both? Yes, a broad spectrum disinfectant with an efficacy label that reads "effective against HIV and Human Hepatitis B Virus or tuberculocidal" will meet both requirements.

Chemical disinfecting agents are available in varied forms, including liquid, capsule and powder. When choosing one from your beauty supplier, consider the following:

- Is it nonirritating to the skin?
- Is it in compliance with your area's regulating agency or Health Department?
- Is it economical and easy to purchase?
- Is it easy to use?
- Does it work quickly?
- Is it noncorrosive (harmless to metal or plastic implements)?
- What type of container is recommended for storage and usage?

PLEASE NOTE:
Many regulating agencies are very specific in their rules pertaining to precleaning metal instruments thoroughly with soap and water before immersing in any disinfectant solution. Precleaning instruments eliminates any minute particles that could cling and cause infection.

Read the directions carefully and follow recommended safety precautions! Always note and follow specific immersion times. Cleanse implements before disinfecting.

It is important to remember that disinfecting methods do not work instantly, but require some time to destroy microbes. Procedures and timing will vary, based on the product you are using. To familiarize you with a procedure used during general disinfection, an outline for disinfecting a brush or comb is listed on the next page.

2

Brush or Comb Disinfection Procedure

1. Remove all hair from the brush or comb.

2. Wash the brush or comb thoroughly with soap and water to remove any dirt, grease or oil.

3. Rinse the brush or comb thoroughly and pat dry to avoid dilution when immersed in disinfectant.

4. Immerse the brush or comb completely in disinfecting solution. Follow timing instructions from manufacturer.

5. Remove the brush or comb with forceps, tongs or gloved hands. Follow manufacturer's directions for rinsing and drying.

6. Store in a disinfected, dry, covered container or cabinet (referred to as a dry sanitizer) until needed.

Prior to using a disinfectant, ultrasonic cleaners can be used. Ultrasonic cleaners use high-frequency sound waves to create a cleansing action that cleans areas on implements or tools that are difficult to reach with a brush. Hand cleaning is eliminated through the use of ultrasonic cleaners.

Disinfection Guidelines and Procedures

An easy way to remember if you need to use sanitation or disinfection procedures is to tell yourself, "Implements that come in contact with the client must be discarded or disinfected." The following is an overview of the primary infection control procedures used for disinfection in the cosmetology environment:

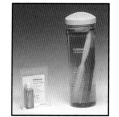

Wet disinfectant container

- Disinfect combs and brushes after each use.

- Change chemical solutions in disinfectant containers regularly as recommended by manufacturer.

- Disinfect unplugged electrical appliances by spraying or wiping with a with a regulatory agency-approved solution. This includes parts of tools such as the guards on hair clippers.

- Wash, rinse and disinfect by complete immersion, all cosmetology, nail care, esthetic and electrolysis tools and metal implements after each use in an approved, disinfectant solution mixed and used in accordance with the manufacturer's directions. In most cases, an EPA-registered, broad spectrum bactericidal, virucidal, fungicidal and pseudomonacidal disinfectant (which are effective against HIV, HBV or tuberculocidal) is used to ensure safety even in the case of exposure to blood or body fluids.

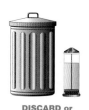

DISCARD or DISINFECT

- Discard emery boards, cosmetic sponges and orangewood sticks after each use or give to the client, unless the manufacturer has specified that the product used can be disinfected (based on your area's requirements). **Implements must be non-porous to be disinfected. Guiding principle here is discard or disinfect.**

- Store all disinfected tools in a disinfected, dry, covered container or cabinet.

- Dispose of sharp objects (razor blades, insulin needles, etc.) in a sealable, rigid container (puncture-proof) strong enough to protect you, the client and others from accidental puncture wounds that could happen during the disposal process.

- Ensure that all disinfecting products are labeled properly.

- Label and properly store prepared commercial disinfecting products, such as household bleach, to clean shampoo bowls, sinks, floors, working surfaces and bathroom fixtures. Even though your floor may be cleaned daily, never pick up and use an implement, cape, towel or anything that you have dropped. **Always continue your services with clean, disinfected materials and implements.**

Disinfection Precautions

Since the use of chemical disinfecting agents can be dangerous, they must be used cautiously to prevent mistakes and accidents. When using these chemical agents, always remember to take the following precautions:

- Tightly cover and label all containers.

- Store in a cool, dry area. (air, light and heat can weaken their effectiveness.)

- Purchase chemicals in small quantities.

- Do not inhale (or smell) the chemical solutions. Avoid contact with skin or eyes. Wear gloves. Refer to Material Safety Data Sheet for procedures if contact with the eyes or skin occurs.

- Wash hands with soap and water after handling all chemicals. Avoid using bar soap that can harbor and transmit microbes. Use a liquid-type pump for soap disbursement. Usually an antibacterial soap is recommended.

- Try to avoid spilling. Wipe up all spills at once. Refer to Material Safety Data Sheet for proper handling if spills occur.

- Use forceps, tongs or gloved hands to insert or remove objects if a holding basket is not provided.

- Always follow manufacturer's instructions.

- Keep a first aid kit on hand.

- Refer to sterilization guidelines for blood spill procedures for cuts or broken skin exposures.

- Dispose of any material coming in contact with blood or body fluids, such as discharge from open sores, pimples and sebaceous glands, in a sealable plastic bag and place inside a covered waste can liner for disposal. This process is referred to as "double bagging," meaning that the contaminated material is sealed in a bag, then placed in another bag (the waste can liner) for disposal. You may be required to label this bag with a red or orange marker to indicate that it is hazardous waste. Check with your area's regulating agency for disposal guidelines.

Decontaminated is free from dirt, oil and/or microbes.

Sterilization

Sterilization is the most effective level of infection control. Sterilization procedures kill or destroy all microbes. **You will be guided by your area's regulating agency for standards regarding cosmetology services and sterilization procedures.** Usually sterilization does not apply to cosmetology services because you are not puncturing or invading the skin when performing these services.

The amount of blood or body fluid that might be present during an offered service is a prime factor when regulators decide if sterilization procedures are required. Sterilization procedures are normally required for electrolysis and some esthetics services. For example, needles used by electrologists and lancets used by estheticians to invade (puncture) the skin must be sterilized, or they must be designed to be disposable. Sterilization standards require the use of a liquid sterilant and/or moist or dry heat, calibrated to various temperatures, to produce a surface free from all living organisms, even bacterial spores. Specific calibrations and time frames are normally required for sterilization procedures. In addition, periodic checks by manufacturer representatives or approved technicians are assigned to ensure that procedures and equipment are being used in the proper way. Sterilization methods are costly, time-consuming and require a high degree of quality control to ensure results.

Infection Control Guidelines

ITEM	LEVEL OF INFECTION CONTROL	PROCEDURE
	Sterilization	**kills all**
Tools and implements that are used to puncture or invade the skin		Use a liquid sterilant and/or moist or dry heat, calibrated to various temperatures to produce a microbe-free result.
	Disinfection	**kills certain bacteria**
Tools and implements that **have** come in contact with blood or body fluids	more	Use antibacterial, EPA-registered disinfectant effective against HIV and human Hepatitis B Virus or tuberculocidal mixed and immersed according to manufacturer's directions or as required by your area's regulating agency.
Tools and implements that **have not** come in contact with blood or body fluids	POWER	Use broad-spectrum, EPA-registered bactericidal, virucidal, fungicidal, pseudomonacidal disinfectant, mixed and immersed according to manufacturer's directions or as required by your area's regulating agency.
	Sanitation	**removes dirt**
Countertops Sinks Floors Toilets Towels Linens	KILLING	Use EPA-registered cleaning product. Efficacy label will state "appropriate for floors, countertops, sinks, toilets, towels and/or linens."
Your hands before each service		Use liquid soap. Avoid bar soaps. Antimicrobial (antibacterial) is recommended.
Your hands and client's hands and/or feet prior to manicuring or pedicuring service	less	Use antiseptic designed for hands and/or feet.

FIRST AID

Up to this point you have studied the health considerations involved in operating a salon. Safety precautions are equally important. Most states have enacted Good Samaritan Laws to encourage people to help others in emergency situations. These laws give legal protection to people who provide emergency care to ill or injured persons. They require that the "good samaritan" use common sense and a reasonable level of skill not to exceed the scope of the individual's training in emergency situations. As a licensed professional, you are in contact with many people during the course of your career. Being prepared will help make the most of a serious situation. Following are some basic first aid techniques that can be used in the workplace or at home:

Bleeding and Wounds

1. Place a clean cloth or gauze and gloved hand over the wound. Apply firm steady pressure for at least 5 minutes.
2. Call 9-1-1 or other emergency personnel if bleeding is severe.
3. Elevate an injured arm or leg above the level of the victim's heart if practical.
4. When bleeding stops, secure the cloth with a bandage. DO NOT lift the cloth from the wound to check if bleeding has stopped. Be sure the bandage is not too tight. It may cut off circulation.
5. Never use a tourniquet unless you cannot control the bleeding. Tourniquets may result in subsequent medical amputation.
6. Have emergency personnel check the victim for shock if necessary.

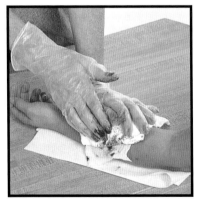

Cover wound, **apply** pressure

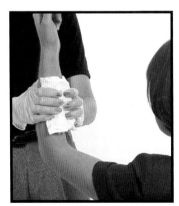

Elevate injured limb above heart

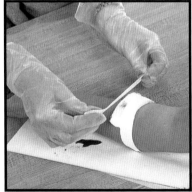

When bleeding stops - **apply** bandage

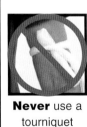

Never use a tourniquet

Burns
Chemical Burns

1. Rinse away all traces of chemicals while moving away any contaminated clothing from burn area.
2. Cover the burn loosely with a clean, dry cloth.
3. Refer person to medical attention if necessary.

Heat or Electrical Burns

1. If the skin is not broken, immerse the burned area in cool (not ice) water or gently apply a cool compress until pain is relieved. Bandage with a clean, dry cloth.

2. Do not break a blister if one forms. Do not apply ointments or creams.

3. If skin is broken or if burns are severe:
    *   Call 9-1-1 or other emergency personnel.
    *   Do not clean the wound or remove embedded clothing.
    *   Cover the burn loosely with a clean, dry cloth.

Choking

1. Determine if the victim can speak or cough forcibly and is getting sufficient air. Do not interfere with the victim's attempts to cough the obstruction from his/her throat. If victim cannot speak or is not getting sufficient air, have someone call 9-1-1 while you perform abdominal thrusts.

2. Stand behind the victim and wrap your arms around his/her stomach.

3. Make a thumbless fist with one hand and place that fist just above the navel and well below the ribs, with the thumb and forefinger side toward the victim.

4. Perform an upward thrust by grasping this fist with the other hand and pulling it quickly toward you with an inward and slightly upward movement. Repeat if necessary.

Note: These instructions are for choking victims over one year of age. There are specific guidelines for treatment of infant choking that are not outlined in this text.

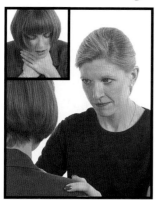

Determine if victim can talk or cough

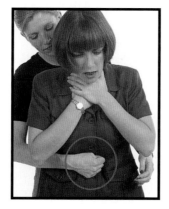

Wrap your arms around victim from behind and **make** a thumbless fist

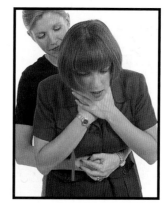

Perform an upward thrust

Fainting

1. Lay the victim down on his/her back and make sure he/she has plenty of fresh air.

2. Reassure the victim and apply a cold compress to his/her face.

3. If the victim vomits, roll him/her on his/her side and keep the windpipe clear.

Note: Fainting victims regain consciousness almost immediately. If this does not happen, the victim could be in serious danger and you should call 9-1-1 as soon as possible.

Eye Injury
Chemical

1. Hold the eyelids apart and flush the eyeball with lukewarm water for at least 15-30 minutes. Be careful not to let runoff water flow into the other eye.
2. Place a gauze pad or cloth over both eyes and secure with a bandage.
3. Get to an eye specialist or emergency room immediately.

Cut, Scratch or Embedded Object

1. Place a gauze pad or cloth over both eyes and secure with a bandage.
2. Do not try to remove an embedded object.
3. Get to an eye specialist or emergency room immediately.

Material Safety Data Sheets

A separate Material Safety Data Sheet (MSDS) for potentially hazardous products used in the salon should be kept readily available in a file in case of an emergency. The MSDS provides information on the contents, including potential hazards, which may be helpful if an allergic reaction or injury occurs related to the product's usage.

The safety, protection and welfare of the clients you serve is the reason you are licensed as a professional. This chapter holds valuable information for you to utilize and practice. Remember that your health and safety are important issues as well. Make sure you know the procedures necessary for a clean, healthy, safe environment. Your clients will respect your efforts and trust in your services.

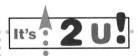

Build Your Critical Thinking Skills

In this chapter you have prepared yourself to meet the following Industry Standard for entry-level cosmetologists:

- Conduct services in a safe environment and take measures to prevent the spread of infections and contagious diseases

It's Up to You to know what to do. Using your training to this point, review the following case scenario and think through how you would handle the challenge.

Everything is going wrong for you today. You are running late and now just realized that your spray water bottle is missing. You go to the dispensary and find another spray bottle and return to your work station, ready to begin wrapping a perm. As you apply the first spray of what you thought was water in the bottle, you realize it was a cleaning product, due to the strong odor you are recognizing. What would you do?

Chapter 3
ANATOMY AND PHYSIOLOGY

After studying this chapter you will be able to . . .

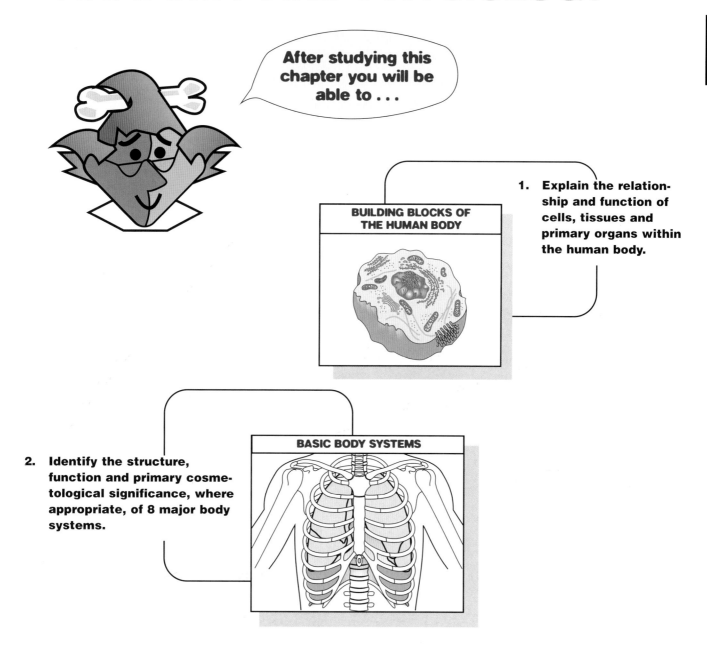

BUILDING BLOCKS OF THE HUMAN BODY

1. Explain the relationship and function of cells, tissues and primary organs within the human body.

2. Identify the structure, function and primary cosmetological significance, where appropriate, of 8 major body systems.

BASIC BODY SYSTEMS

Professor P here. By now you are beginning to understsand why Unit 1 is called "Theory Essentials." Professors have a reputation for loving theory, right? I hope I'm not the only one, though, and that you are also coming to appreciate the fact that theory plays an essential role in the practical, day-to-day life of a professional stylist. Without some knowledge of Anatomy and Physiology, you would not be thoroughly prepared to offer styling and massage services to your clients.

Because cosmetology is among one of the last few professions licensed to touch the public, you have a responsibility to know and understand the human body and its functions in order to make good judgement when providing services that touch your clients.

It's easy to see that the central VALUE of this chapter revolves around the power of human touch, the means by which you will enrich all communication and contact you have with your client. The BIG IDEA as always gives you the information you need to make this value a part of your life.

Knowledge of the human body and its systems provides the foundation for enhancing the quality of hair, nail and skin care services.

The PLAN for this chapter involves the careful study of the human body so that you will be prepared to perform styling and massage services on your clients. The chapter progresses from the simplicity of the single cell to the wondrous organization of each body system. Of particular importance to salon work will be the skeletal, muscular, circulatory and nervous systems. You're launched into the chapter. I'll meet you there.

BUILDING BLOCKS OF THE HUMAN BODY

Cells

Tissues

Organs

Body Systems

BASIC BODY SYSTEMS

The Skeletal System

The Muscular System

The Circulatory System

The Nervous System

The Digestive System

The Excretory System

The Respiratory System

The Endocrine System

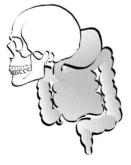

BUILDING BLOCKS OF THE HUMAN BODY

3

Few professions know and value the human body more than the profession you are entering. Cosmetologists, like doctors and nurses, are licensed to touch a client. Whether you are shampooing, massaging, styling, working on nails or skin, you have the privilege of bringing relaxation, well-being and personal enhancement to others.

Of particular interest to the cosmetologist are the muscles, nerves, circulatory system and bones of the head, face, neck, arms and hands. An understanding of muscles, circulatory system and nerves will help you develop beneficial facial and massage techniques. Knowledge of the bones of the skull is essential for the design of flattering hairstyles and for the proper application of cosmetics. The major groups of muscles, nerves and bones will receive the greatest focus in this chapter. However, you will also review other fundamental structures and functions of the human body to have a broader context for understanding the importance of touch within your profession.

The study of the human body can be conveniently divided into two general categories: **Anatomy, the study of the *organs* and *systems* of the body, and Physiology, the study of the *functions* these organs and systems perform. The study of structures that can be seen with the *naked eye* is called gross anatomy. The study of structures too small to be seen except through a microscope is called histology or microscopic anatomy.**

To understand anatomy and physiology you must first be aware of the building blocks of the human body, which are:

- Cells
- Tissues
- Organs
- Systems

Just for fun. . .

In reality you are building on information that you already know. In the various diagrams below, label any image that you can identify.

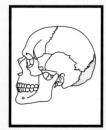 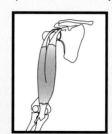 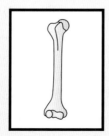 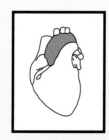 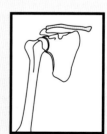

Cells

Your knowledge of muscles, nerves, bones and all bodily systems needs to start at the level of the single cell. **Cells are the basic units of living matter (life).** Cells are composed of **protoplasm (PRO**-to-plazm), a gel-like substance containing water, salt and nutrients obtained from food. Cells vary in size, shape, structure and function, but they have certain characteristics in common. A cell contains three basic parts:

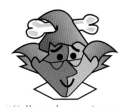

"Cells make up tissues and tissues make up organs and organs make up systems."

1. **The nucleus (NU-kle-us), or control center, of cell activities**

2. **The cytoplasm (SI-to-plazm), or production department of the cell, where most of the cell's activities take place**

3. **The cell membrane, or outer surface of the cell, which encloses the protoplasm**

The nucleus is located in the cytoplasm, and both are surrounded by the cell membrane. Cells with common properties or functions combine to form the various tissues of the body.

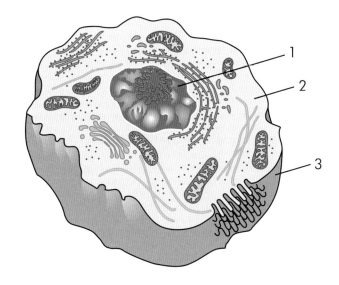

In order to grow and remain healthy, cells need adequate supplies of food, oxygen, water, proper temperature and the ability to eliminate waste products. If these criteria are not present, cell growth will be impaired. The chemical process in which cells receive nutrients (food) for cell growth and reproduction is known as **metabolism** (me-**TAB**-e-lism). There are two phases of metabolism:

1. **Anabolism (ah-NAB-oh-lizm), the process of building up larger molecules from smaller ones.** During this phase, the body stores water, food and oxygen for the times when they are needed by the body.

2. **Catabolism (kah-TAB-oh-lizm), the process of breaking down larger molecules or substances into smaller ones.** This phase causes a release of energy within the cell, necessary for the performance of specific body functions, including muscular movements and digestion.

Tissues

Groups of cells of the same kind make up *tissues*. There are four primary types of tissue in the human body:

1. **Epithelial** (ep-i-THE-le-el) **tissue** that covers and protects body surfaces and internal organs

2. **Connective tissue** that supports, protects and holds the body together

3. **Nerve tissue** that coordinates body functions in addition to carrying messages to and from the brain and spinal cord

4. **Muscular tissue** that contracts, when stimulated, to produce motion

3

Organs

Organs are separate body structures that perform specific functions. They are composed of two or more different tissues. Organs of primary importance include:

1. The **brain**, which controls all body functions

2. The **eyes**, which control vision

3. The **heart**, which circulates the blood

4. The **lungs**, which supply the blood with oxygen

5. The **stomach** and **intestines**, which digest food

6. The **liver**, which removes the toxic byproducts of digestion

7. The **kidneys**, which eliminate water and waste products

8. The **skin**, the body's largest organ, which forms the external protective layer of the body

Body Systems

A system is a group of body structures and/or organs that, together, perform one or more vital functions for the body. The eight body systems you will study in this chapter are listed below. You will study another system, the integumentary system, in Chapter 15, The Study of Skin.

Skeletal	Provides framework of the body
Muscular	Moves the body
Circulatory	Circulates blood through the body
Nervous	Sends and receives body messages
Digestive	Supplies food to the body
Excretory	Eliminates waste from the body
Respiratory	Controls breathing of the body
Endocrine	Controls growth and general health and reproduction of the body

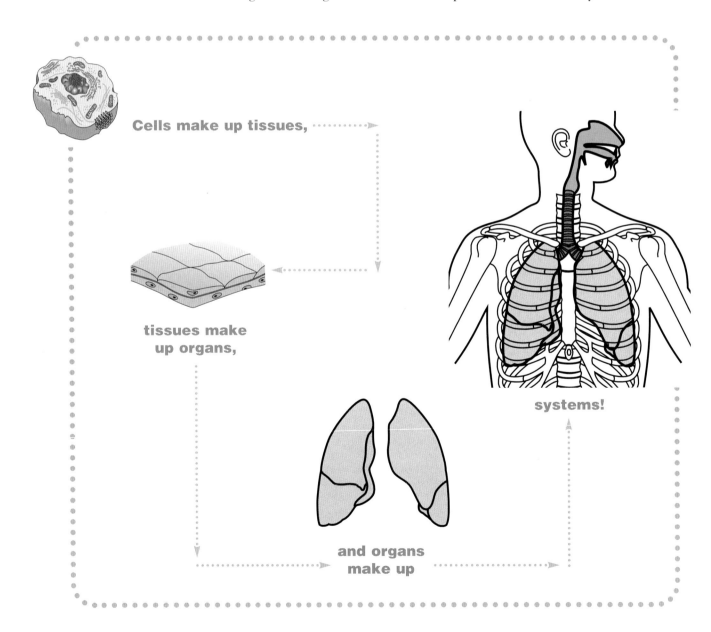

Cells make up tissues,

tissues make up organs,

and organs make up

systems!

BASIC BODY SYSTEMS

The Skeletal System

The physical foundation of the body, the skeletal system, is composed of **206 bones** of different shapes and sizes, each attached to others at movable or immovable joints. A joint is the point at which two or more bones are joined together.

Osteology (as-te-AL-e-je) **is the study of bone.** The term "Os" is the technical term for bone. Bones are described as either long, flat, or irregular in shape. **Long bones** are found in the arms and legs. **Flat bones** are plate-shaped and located in the skull. **Irregular bones** are found in the wrist, ankle, or spinal column (the back). **Bone, the hardest structure of the body,** is composed of 2/3 mineral matter and 1/3 organic matter and produces red and white blood cells and stores calcium.

The functions of the skeletal system include:

1. **Supporting the body by giving it shape and strength**
2. **Surrounding and protecting internal organs**
3. **Providing a frame to which muscles can attach**
4. **Allowing body movement**

The Skull

The skull is the skeleton of the head that encloses and protects the brain and primary sensory organs. Bones of the skull are divided into two groups: the *eight* bones of the cranium and the *fourteen* bones of the facial skeleton.

The Cranium

Of the *eight bones* that compose the *cranium*, only six are affected by scalp massage.

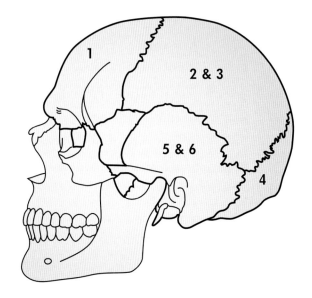

1. The **frontal** is the bone that extends from the top of the eyes to the top of the head and forms the forehead.

2-3. The **parietal** (pah-RI-e-tal) are the two bones that form the crown and upper sides of the head.

4. The **occipital** (ak-SIP-et-al) is the bone that forms the back of the skull, indenting above the nape area.

5-6. The **temporal** (TEM-poh -ral) are the two bones located on either side of the head, directly above the ears and below the parietal bones.

These bones, too, will frequently be referred to when directions are given for hair styling and cutting techniques.

The remaining two bones of the cranium have no part in either massage or styling techniques and are not labeled on the illustration on page 69.

- The **sphenoid** (**SFE**-noid) is located behind the eyes and nose and connects all the bones of the cranium.
- The **ethmoid** (**ETH**-moid) is the spongy bone between the eyes that forms part of the nasal cavity.

Facial Skeleton

Of the fourteen bones that compose the facial skeleton, only nine are involved in facial massage.

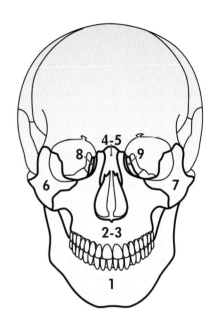

1. The **mandible** (**MAN**-di-bl) is the lower jaw and the largest bone of the facial skeleton.

2-3. The **maxillae** (mak-**SIL**-e) are the two bones of the upper jaw.

4-5. The **nasal** (**NA**-zel) are the two bones which join to form the bridge of the nose.

6-7. The **zygomatic** (zi-go-**MAT**-ik) or **malar** (**MA**-ler) are the two bones that form the upper cheek and the bottom of the eyesocket.

8-9. The **lacrimal** (**LAK**-ri-mal) are the smallest two bones of the facial skeleton and form the front part of the inner, bottom wall of the eyesocket.

The remaining five bones of the facial skeleton are unaffected by facial massage and are not shown on the illustration.

- The **turbinal** (**TUR**-bi-nal) are the two spongy bones that form the sides of the nasal cavity.
- The **vomer** (**VO**-mer) or Nasal System is the bone in the center of the nose that divides the nasal cavity.
- The **palatine** (**PAL**-ah-tin) are the two bones that form the roof of the mouth and the floor of the eyesockets.

The shape and size of all bones of the skull and their relationship to one another will help you determine the most flattering use of makeup and hair designs for individual clients.

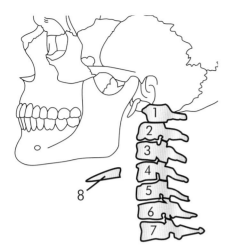

Neck Bones

1-7. The **cervical vertebrae** (**SUR**-vi-kel **VURT**-e-bray), the seven bones that form the top part of the spinal column, are often manipulated in extended scalp massage.

8. The **hyoid** (**HI**-oid) bone is the u-shaped bone referred to as the "Adam's apple" located in the throat.

Back, Chest and Shoulder Bones

The chest, or **thorax** (**THO**-raks), is the bony cage composed of the spine, or **thoracic** (tho-**RAS**-ik) vertebrae (1), and the **sternum** (2) and 12 **ribs** (3-14). It encloses and protects the heart, lungs and other internal organs. The bone that forms the area from the throat to the shoulder is known as the **clavicle** (**KLAV**-i-kel) (15) or collarbone. The large, flat bone extending from the middle of the back upward to the joint where it attaches to the clavicle is called the **scapula** (**SKAP**-yu-lah) (16).

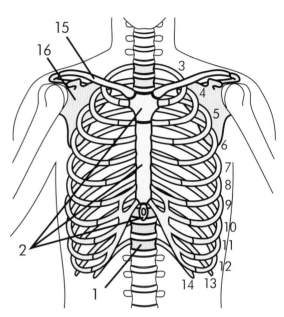

Arm, Wrist and Hand Bones

1. The **humerus** (**HU**-mur-us), the largest bone of the upper arm, extends from the elbow to the shoulder.

2. The **radius** (**RAD**-e-us) is the small bone on the thumb side of the lower arm or forearm.

3. The **ulna** (**UL**-nah) is the bone located on the little finger side of the lower arm.

4. The **carpals** (**KAR**-pels) are the eight small bones held together by ligaments to form the wrist or carpus.

5. The **metacarpals** (met-ah-**KAR**-pels) are the five long, thin bones that form the palm of the hand.

6. The **phalanges** (fah-**LAN**-jes) are the fourteen bones that form the digits or fingers. Each finger has three phalanges, while the thumb has only two.

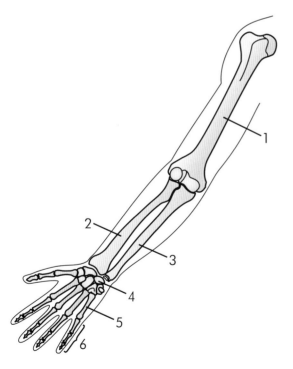

The Muscular System

Myology is the study of the structure, function and diseases of the muscles

Myology (mi-OL-o-je) is the study of muscles. There are more than 500 large and small muscles in the body, composing approximately 40% of the body's weight. Muscles are fibrous tissues that contract, when stimulated by messages carried by the nervous system, to produce movement. The functions of the muscular system include:

1. Support of the skeleton
2. Production of body movements
3. Contouring of the body
4. Involvement in the functions of other body systems (e.g., digestive, circulatory, and nervous systems)

There are two types of muscle tissues:

1. The voluntary or **striated** (**STRI**-at-ed) muscles respond to commands regulated by will.

2. The involuntary or **non-striated** muscles respond automatically to control various body functions including the functions of internal organs.

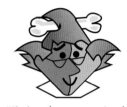

"Striated means striped, grooved or ridged."

The same muscles may function both voluntarily and involuntarily. For example, eye muscles respond to a conscious command to blink, but they also blink automatically to maintain eye moisture. The cosmetologist is primarily concerned with the voluntary muscles of the head, face, neck, arms and hands.

The cardiac (heart) muscle is the muscle of the heart itself and is the only muscle of its type in the human body. This rugged muscle functions involuntarily.

Special Terminology

The following common terms will be used to describe what a muscle does or where it is located.

anterior (an-**TER**-e-er) - in front of
posterior (pos-**TER**-e-er) - behind or in back of

superioris (su-per-e-**OR**-es) - located above or is larger
inferioris (in-**FIR**-e-or-es) - located below or is smaller

levator (le-**VA**-ter) - lifts up
depressor (de-**PRES**-er) - draws down or depresses

dilator (**DI**-la-ter) - opens, enlarges or expands

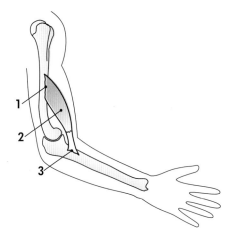

The three parts of the muscle are:

1. The **origin** is the nonmoving (fixed) portion of the muscle attached to bones or other fixed muscle. The term skeletal muscles refers to muscles attached to bone.

2. The **belly** is the term applied to the midsection of the muscle, between the two attached sections.

3. The **insertion** is the portion of the muscle joined to movable attachments: bones, movable muscles or skin.

3

Muscles produce movement through contraction (tightening) and expansion (relaxing). When a contraction occurs, one of the muscle attachments moves (insertion) while the other remains fixed (origin). All muscles (except those of the face) are attached at both ends either by bone or another muscle. Facial muscles are only attached at one end.

Stimulation of muscular tissue can be achieved by using the following methods:

1. Massage
2. Electric Current (high-frequency and faradic current)
3. Light Rays (infrared rays and ultraviolet rays)
4. Heat Rays (heating lamps and heating caps)
5. Moist Heat (steamers, warm steam towels)
6. Nerve Impulses (through nervous system)
7. Chemicals (certain acids and salts)

Scalp and Face Muscles

The scalp and face muscles are of primary interest to the cosmetologist as you perform scalp and neck massages and/or facials. The professional stylist will also often employ general massage techniques to the scalp and neck just before or during a shampoo. **Muscles affected by massage are generally manipulated from the insertion attachment to the origin attachment.** The cosmetologist who performs facials must know the position of the muscles in the face. Light facial massage, used when applying certain facial treatment products, should follow the muscle line. **NOTE:** Other services that may be performed by a trained salon professional and involve the stimulation of various muscles include electrotherapy and light therapy.

Scalp Muscles

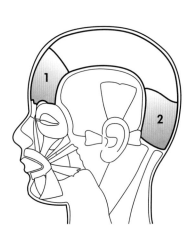

The scalp or **epicranium** (ep-i-**KRA**-ne-um) is covered by a broad muscle called the **epicranius** (ep-i-**KRA**-ne-us) or **occipito-frontalis** (ok-**SIP**-ih-to-fron-**TA**-les). The epicranius is formed by two muscles joined by the **aponeurosis** (ap-o-noo-**ROH**-sis) tendon:

1. The **frontalis** (frun-**TA**-les) muscle extends from the forehead to the top of the skull. It raises eyebrows or draws the scalp forward.

2. The **occipitalis** (ok-sip-i-**TAL**-is) muscle is located at the nape of the neck and draws the scalp back.

Ear Muscles

The three muscles of the ear are stationary and have no recognized function.

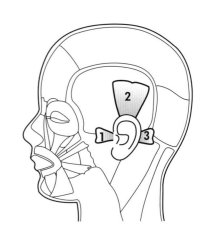

1. The **auricularis** (aw-rik-ya-**LA**-ris) **anterior** muscle is located in front of the ear.

2. The **auricularis superior** muscle is located above the ear.

3. The **auricularis posterior** muscle is located behind the ear.

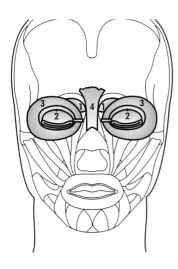

Eye and Nose Muscles

1. The **corrugator** (**KOR**-e-gat-er), located between the eyebrows, controls the eyebrows, drawing them in and downward.

2. The **levator palpebrae** (**POL**-pe-bra) **superioris**, located above the eyelids, functions to raise the eyelid.

3. The **orbicularis oculi** (or-bik-ye-**LAR**-es **AK**-yu-le) circles the eyesocket and functions to close the eyelid.

4. The **procerus** (pro-**SER**-us), located between the eyebrows across the bridge of the nose, draws brows down and wrinkles the area across the bridge of the nose.

Four muscles located inside the nose, called the **nasalis**, **posterior dilatator naris**, **anterior dilatator naris**, and **depressor septi**, control contraction and expansion of the nostrils.

Mouth Muscles

1. The **oris orbicularis** (**O**-ris or-bik-ye-**LAR**-es) circles the mouth and is responsible for contracting, puckering and wrinkling the lips, as in kissing or whistling.

2. The **quadratus labii superioris** (kwod-**RA**-tus **LA**-be) (also known as the Levator Labii Superioris) consists of three parts. It is located above the upper lip, raises both the nostrils and the upper lip, as in expressing distaste.

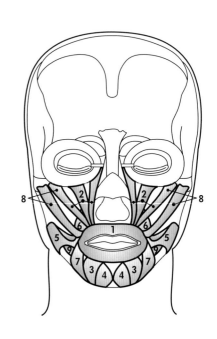

3. The **quadratus labii inferioris** (also known as the Depressor Labii Inferioris), located below the lower lip, pulls the lower lip down or to the side, as in expressing sarcasm.

4. The **mentalis** (men-**TAL**-us), located at the tip of the chin, pushes the lower lip up and/or wrinkles the chin, as in expressing doubt.

5. The **risorius** (re-**SOR**-e-us), located at the corner of the mouth, draws the mouth up and out, as in grinning.

6. The **caninus** (kay-**NEYE**-nus) (also known as the Levator Anguli Oris), located above the corners of the mouth, raises the angle of the mouth, as in snarling.

7. The **triangularis** (tri-an-gu-**LAR**-us) (also known as the Depressor Anguli), located below the corners of the mouth, draws the corners of the mouth down, as in expressing depression.

8. The **zygomaticus** (zi-go-**MAT**-ik-us), located outside the corners of the mouth, draws the mouth up and back, as in laughing and consists of zygomaticus major and minor.

9. The **buccinator** (**BUK**-si-na-ter), located between the jaws and cheek, is responsible for compressing the cheek to release air outwardly, as in blowing.

Mastication Muscles

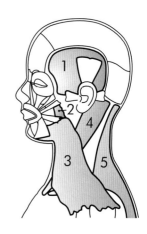

1. The **temporalis** (tem-po-**RA**-lis) is located above and in front of the ear and performs both opening and closing the jaw, as in chewing (mastication).

2. The **masseter** (**MAS**-se-ter) covers the hinge of the jaw and aids in closing the jaw, as in chewing (mastication).

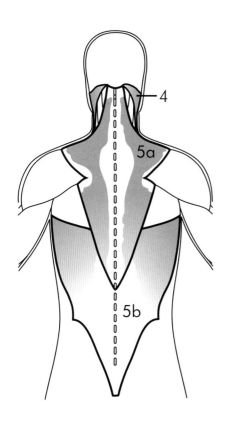

Neck and Upper Back Muscles

Refer to both diagrams for clarification.

3. The **platysma** (plah-**TIZ**-mah) extends from the tip of the chin to the shoulders and chest and depresses the lower jaw and lip, as in expressing sadness.

4. The **sternocleido mastoideus** (stur-no-**KLI**-do mas-**TOID**-e-us) extends along the side of the neck from the ear to the collarbone and causes the head to move from side to side and up and down, as in nodding "yes" or "no".

5. The **trapezius** (5a) (trah-**PE**-ze-us) and **latissimus dorsi** (5b) (lah **TIS**-i-mus **DOR**-se) cover the back of the neck and upper back. These muscles draw the head back, rotate the shoulder blades and control swinging of the arm.

Shoulder, Chest and Arm Muscles

1. The **pectoralis** (pek-to-**RAL**-us) major (1a) and pectoralis minor (1b) extend across the front of the chest. These muscles assist in swinging the arms.

2. The **serratus anterior** (ser-**RA**-tus an-**TER**-e-er) is located under the arm. This muscle helps in lifting the arm and in breathing.

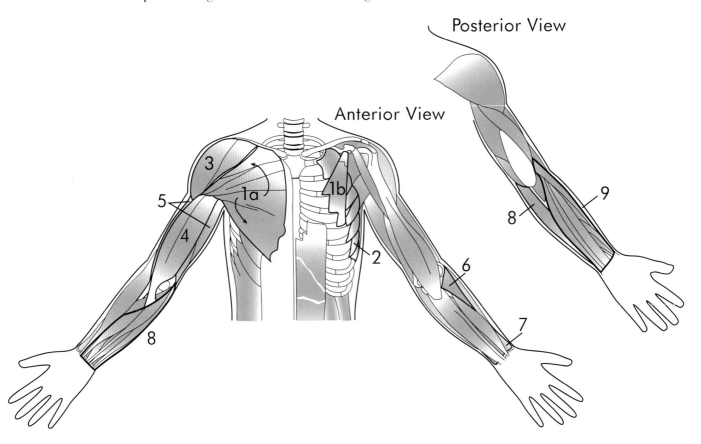

3. The **deltoid** (**DEL**-toid) covers the shoulder. This triangular-shaped muscle lifts the arm or turns it.

4. The **bicep** (**BI**-cep) is the primary muscle in the front of the upper arm. This muscle raises the forearm, bends the elbow and turns the palm of the hand down.

5. The **tricep** (**TRI**-cep) extends the length of the upper arm to the forearm. This muscle controls forward movement of the forearm.

6. The **supinator** (**SU**-pi-nat-or) runs parallel to the ulna. This muscle turns the palm of the hand up.

7. The **pronator** (**PRO**-nat-or) runs across the front of the lower part of the radius and the ulna. This muscle turns the palm of the hand downward and inward.

8. The **flexor** (**FLEX**-er) is located mid-forearm, on the inside of the arm. This muscle bends the wrist and closes the fingers.

9. The **extensor** (eks-**TEN**-sor) is located mid-forearm, on the outside of the arm. This muscle straightens the fingers and wrist.

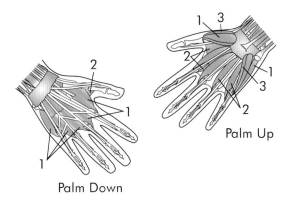

Palm Up

Palm Down

Hand Muscles

A number of small muscles stretch over the fingers, connect the joints and provide dexterity. **Abductor** (ab-**DUK**-tor) muscles (1) separate the fingers while **adductor** (ah-**DUK**-tor) muscles (2) draw them together. The **opponens** muscles (3) are located in the palm (palmor view) of the hand and cause the thumb to move toward the fingers, giving the ability to grasp or make a fist.

3

The Circulatory System

The circulatory or vascular system controls the circulation of blood and lymph through the body. As a professional cosmetologist, you will use massage treatments that will directly influence or stimulate this very important body system. The circulatory system is divided into two, interrelated subsystems called:

1. The **cardiovascular** or **blood-vascular** system, which is responsible for the circulation of blood, includes the heart, arteries, veins and capillaries.

2. The **lymph-vascular** system, which is responsible for the circulation of lymph through lymph glands, nodes and vessels.

The cardiovascular system, using **arteries**, **veins** and **capillaries** as blood-carrying vessels, combines with the lymph system to maintain steady circulation of the blood. Lymph is a product of the blood system and, after traveling through the lymph glands and vessels, moves back into the normal bloodstream. Lymph filters the blood by removing toxins (poisons). **The main function of lymph is to reach the parts of the body not reached by blood.**

The Cardiovascular System
The Heart

The heart, a cone-shaped, muscular organ located in the chest cavity, is normally about the size of a closed fist. The rugged muscle of this organ, entirely encased in a membrane called the **pericardium** (per-i-**KAR**-de-um) (1), contracts and relaxes to force blood to move through the circulatory system. **The interior of the heart contains four chambers: The upper chambers consist of the right atrium (AY-tree-um) (2) and the left atrium (3). The lower chambers consist of the right ventricle (VEN-tri-kel) (4) and the left ventricle (5). A normal heart**

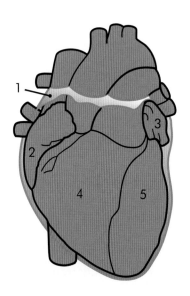

beats **60-80 times per minute**, according to impulses received from the sympathetic nervous system and the **vagus** (tenth cranial nerve), which regulate the heartbeat.

The Blood

Blood is the sticky, salty fluid that circulates through the body bringing nourishment and oxygen to all body parts and carrying toxins and waste products to the liver and kidneys to be eliminated. On the average, an adult has 8 to 10 pints of blood flowing through the circulatory system. The blood is made up of red and white corpuscles, platelets and plasma. These three components are referred to as the blood cells and compose the semisolid part of the blood. Additional details regarding these blood cells are listed below:

1. **Red blood cells (RBC) are also called erythrocytes (e-RITH-ro-sitz) or red corpuscles.** These cells carry oxygen and contain a protein called hemoglobin. **Hemoglobin (HE-mo-glo-bin)** attracts oxygen molecules through a process known as **oxygenation** (ok-si-je-NA-shun). The blood appears bright red in color when oxygen is being carried. As the red blood cell moves through the body, it releases oxygen molecules and collects molecules of carbon dioxide. When oxygen is low, the blood appears deep scarlet red.

2. **White blood cells (WBC) are also called leucocytes (LOO-ko-sitz) or white corpuscles.** These cells fight bacteria and other foreign substances and increase in number when infection invades the body.

3. **Blood platelets (PLAT-letz) or thrombocytes (THROM-bo-sitz) are responsible for the clotting of blood,** starting the process of coagulation (clotting) when they are exposed to air or rough surfaces (bruised skin).

4. **Plasma is the fluid part of the blood in which red and white blood cells and blood platelets are suspended, to be carried throughout the body by this liquid's flow. Plasma is about 90% water.**

Blood Vessels

Blood vessels are any vessels through which blood circulates through the body. There are three types of blood vessels:

Arteries are tubular, elastic, thick-walled branching vessels that carry pure blood from the heart through the body. Because arteries carry pure blood (blood containing oxygen), the color of the blood is bright red.

Veins are tubular, elastic, thin-walled branching vessels that carry the blood from the capillaries to the heart.

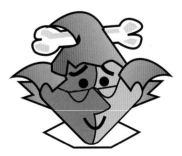

"Arteries take blood away from the heart and veins take blood to the heart."

Varicose veins may be one of the problems experienced by cosmetologists, due to long periods of standing.

Varicose veins are bulges that might form if veins stretch and lose their elasticity.

Preventive measures such as support hose and wearing the appropriate size shoes are recommended practices.

Veins contain cup-like valves to prevent back flow. Impure blood (blood containing carbon dioxide) is carried by the veins (dark red in color) back from capillaries to the heart. Veins are positioned closer to the outer surface of the body than arteries.

Capillaries are small vessels that take nutrients and oxygen from the arteries to the cells and take waste products from the cells to the veins.

Blood Flow Through the Heart

The entire process of blood traveling from the heart throughout the body and back to the heart is referred to as **systemic** or **general circulation**. The right and the left atrium are also known as the right and the left auricle.

- Oxygen-poor blood enters the right auricle through the **superior vena cava**.

- From the right auricle, blood is pumped through the **tricuspid** (tri-**KUS**-pid) valve into the right ventricle.

- From the right ventricle, blood is pumped into the **pulmonary** (**PUL**-mo-ner-e) **artery**.

- Blood travels through the pulmonary artery to the lungs where it is *oxygenated* (combined with oxygen). This phase of the circulation of blood is referred to as **pulmonary circulation**.

- From the lungs the newly oxygenated blood returns to the heart via the pulmonary vein and enters the heart's left auricle.

- Blood is pumped from the left auricle to the left ventricle by the bicuspid valve or mitral valve.

- From the left ventricle, blood pumps through the valve into the aorta.

- Blood then flows from the aorta to arterioles, capillaries, venules and veins as it circulates through the body, only to return to the superior vena cava and begin the circulatory process once again.

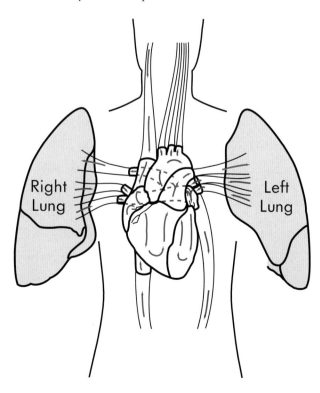

Right Lung

Left Lung

Arteries and Veins of the Face, Head and Neck

Blood is supplied to the head, face and neck by the **common carotid** (kah-**ROT**-id) **arteries** (**CCA**) (1) located on either side of the neck. These arteries split into the **internal carotid artery** (**ICA**) (2) and the **external carotid artery** (**ECA**) (3). The **internal carotid artery** supplies blood to the brain, eyes, and forehead. The **external carotid** branches into smaller arteries, supplying blood to the skin and muscles of the head. All blood from the head, face and neck returns through two veins, the **internal** (**IJV**) (4) and **external jugular** (**EJV**) (5) (**JUG**-u-lur) **veins**.

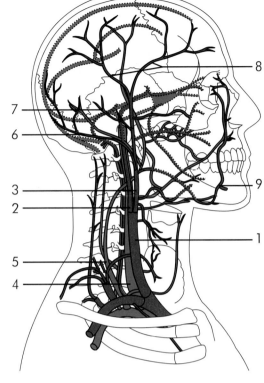

The **External Carotid Artery** branches into smaller arteries.

6. The **Occipital** (ak-**SIP**-et-el) supplies blood to the back of the head, up to the crown.

7. The **Posterior Auricular** (pos-**TER**-e-or aw-**RIK**-u-lur) supplies blood to the scalp above and behind the ears.

8. The **Superficial Temporal** (su-pur-**FI**-shul **TEM**-po-ral) supplies the sides and top of the head with blood and branches farther into five smaller arteries that supply more precise locations.

9. The **External Maxillary** (**EKS**-tur-nal **MAK**-si-ler-e) (facial artery) supplies the lower portion of the face, including the mouth and nose. Like the superficial temporal artery, the external maxillary breaks down into smaller branches with more specific destinations, including:

   - The **submental artery**, which supplies the chin and lower lip
   - The **inferior labial**, which supplies the lower lip
   - The **angular artery**, which supplies the sides of the nose
   - The **superior labial**, which supplies the upper lip and septum
   - The **frontal artery**, which supplies the forehead
   - The **parietal artery**, which supplies the crown and sides of the head
   - The **middle temporal**, which supplies the temples
   - The **transverse artery**, which supplies the masseter
   - The **anterior auricular**, which supplies the anterior part of the ear

The **Internal Carotid Artery** also separates into smaller branches, including the important **Supra-Orbital Artery** which supplies blood to parts of the forehead and eyes.

The Lymph-Vascular System

The **lymph-vascular system** (also referred to as the **lymphatic system**) is the second subsystem of circulation. Lymph is a colorless liquid produced as a byproduct in the process through which plasma passes nourishment to capillaries and cells. Lymph also nourishes the parts of the body not reached by blood, such as the far extremities.

Lymph travels through lymph nodes or glands that filter out toxic substances, like bacteria, and adds antibodies to the fluid. Swollen or tender lymph nodes indicate infection in the body.

The lymphatic system picks up leaked fluid and plasma proteins and returns them to the cardiovascular system.

3

There are over 100 lymph nodes in the body that act as barriers to infection from one part of the body to another. As the lymph nodes take on this protective task, they may swell and cause pain. The lymph nodes most often affected in this way are in the neck and under the arms. Many other circumstances may be causing the swelling, but a doctor should be consulted at the first sign of any swelling in these areas.

The Nervous System

The study of the nervous system is called Neurology. The nervous system coordinates and controls the overall operation of the human body.

The nervous system is divided into three subsystems:
1. The central or cerebrospinal nervous system
2. The peripheral nervous system
3. The autonomic or sympathetic nervous system

Primary components of the nervous system include the brain, spinal cord and nerves. The components of the nervous system, operating in harmony, receive and interpret stimuli and send messages away from the nerve cell to the appropriate tissues, muscles and organs.

The Central Nervous System

The central or cerebrospinal nervous system is composed of the brain, spinal cord and spinal and cranial nerves. The central nervous system is responsible for all voluntary body action.

The Brain

The brain controls all three subsystems of the nervous system. For that reason, it is referred to as the command center. The brain is the largest of the nerve tissues and is located in the cranium. **The average human brain weighs between 44 and 48 ounces** Anatomically, the brain can be conveniently divided into four parts.

1. The **Cerebrum** (se-**RE**-brum), responsible for mental activity, is located in the upper, front portion of the cranium.

2. The **Cerebellum** (ser-e-**BEL**-um), responsible for the control and coordination of muscle movement, is located in the occipital area directly below the cerebrum.

3. The **Pons** connects other parts of the brain to the spinal column and is located below the cerebrum and directly in front of the cerebellum.

4. The **Medulla Oblongata** (me-**DOOL**-ah ob-long-**GA**-ta) also connects parts of the brain to the spinal column and is located just below the pons.

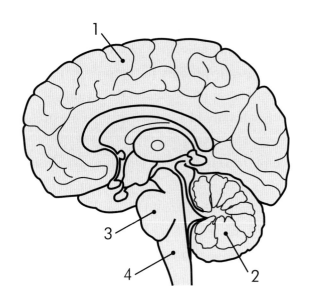

The Spinal Cord

The spinal cord, composed of long nerve fibers, originates in the base of the brain and extends to the base of the spine. The spinal cord holds 31 pairs of spinal nerves that branch out to muscles, internal organs and skin.

The Peripheral Nervous System

The peripheral (pe-**RIF**-ur-al) nervous system is composed of sensory and motor nerves that extend from the brain and spinal cord to other parts of the body. This network of nerve cells carries messages to and from the central nervous system.

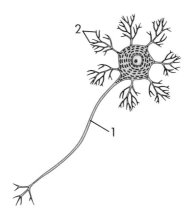

Nerve Cells

Like other cells, the **nerve cell** or **neuron** (**NU**-ron) has a nucleus, **cytoplasm** (**SI**-to-plazm) and membrane. Nerve cells, however, differ in appearance from other cells due to the long and short threadlike fibers, called **axons** (**AK**-sonz) (1), that extend from them. At the end of each axon is a **nerve terminal** (synapse). These terminals may connect the neuron to muscles, organs or other nerve cells. They are responsible for sending messages away from the nerve cell in the form of nerve impulses. The short fibers are called **dendrites** (**DEN**-dritz) (2). These structures receive the messages sent to the nerve cell.

The dendrite system is similar to over a million interstate highways traveling back and forth from nerve cell to nerve cell. Certain activities, such as harmful narcotic drugs or a prolonged lack of oxygen, can close the highways down, never to open again.

Types of Nerves

Nerves or nerve tissues perform two basic functions. **SENSORY** or **afferent nerves** carry messages to the brain and spinal cord. These are the nerves that determine our sense of smell, sight, touch, hearing and taste. Nerve cells called **receptors** are located in the papillary layer of the dermis. These cells react to outside stimulation by sending a sensory message to the brain.

3

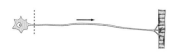

MOTOR or **efferent nerves** carry messages from the brain to the muscles. When the brain sends a message, motor nerves receive the message and cause a muscle to contract or expand.

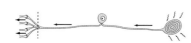

Sensory and motor nerves can work together or independently. For example, if you want to close this book, the brain simply sends a message to the **MOTOR** nerves of your hand. This is a conscious decision. You are in control of your hand movement. However, remember the last time you accidentally touched a hot curling iron? Your **SENSORY** nerves sent a rapid message to your brain transmitting the sensation you experienced. Your brain immediately responded by sensing "pain" and by sending impulses back to MOTOR nerves to move your hand away. This interaction of sensory and motor nerves is called a **reflex action**.

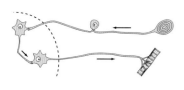

Many large nerves perform both sensory and motor functions. These are called **MIXED nerves**. Large nerves have many branches. One branch of the **trifacial nerve**, for instance, may be helping you chew, while another branch is sensing an "itch" in your eyebrow.

Face, Head and Neck Nerves

Two of the twelve pairs of cranial nerves exert primary control in the areas of the face, head and neck: the **trifacial (trigeminal or fifth cranial)** nerve and the **facial (seventh cranial)** nerve.

The Trifacial Nerve

The largest of the cranial nerves, the trifacial (fifth cranial) nerve is the mixed nerve primarily responsible for transmitting facial sensations to the brain and for controlling the muscle movements of chewing (mastication). The trifacial nerve divides into three main branches.

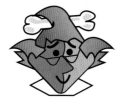

"That's why it's called TRI, for three, like TRIcycle and TRIplets."

The **ophthalmic** (of-**THAL**-mik) branch (green) is the main nerve branch to the top 1/3 of the face, which further divides into:

1. The supraorbital extending to the skin of the upper eyelid, eyebrow, forehead and scalp

2. The supratrochlear extending to the skin of the upper side of the nose and between the eyes

3. The nasal extending to the tip and lower side of the nose

The **maxillary** (**MAK**-si-ler-e) branch (pink) is the main nerve branch to the middle 1/3 of the face, which further divides into:

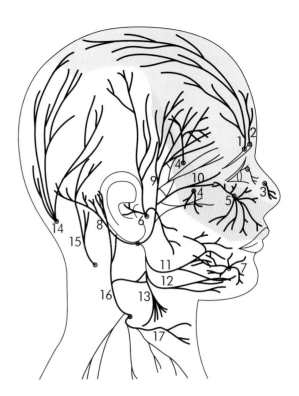

4. The **zygomatic** (zi-go-**MAT**-ik) extending to the side of the forehead, temple and upper part of the cheek

5. The **infraorbital** extending to the lower eyelid, side of the nose, upper lip and mouth

The **mandibular** (man-**DIB**-u-lur) branch (yellow) is the main nerve branch to the lower 1/3 of the face and further divides into:

6. The **auriculo temporal** (aw-**RIK**-u-lo **TEM**-po-ral) extending to the ear and to the area from the top of the head to the temple

7. The **mental** extending to the lower lip and chin

The Facial Nerve

The facial (seventh cranial) nerve emerges from the brain at the lower part of the ear and is the primary motor nerve of the face. Of its many branches, six are of particular importance.

8. The **posterior auricular** (pos-**TER**-e-er aw-**RIK**-u-lur) branch extends to the muscles behind and below the ear.

9. The **temporal** (**TEM**-po-ral) branch extends to the muscles of the temple, the side of the forehead, the eyebrow, eyelid and upper cheek.

10. The **zygomatic** (zi-go-**MAT**-ik) branch extends to the upper muscles of the cheek.

11. The **buccal** (**BUK**-al) branch extends to the muscles of the mouth.

12. The **mandibular** (man-**DIB**-u-lur) branch extends to the muscles of the chin and lower lip.

13. The **cervical** (**SUR**-vi-kal) branch extends to the muscles on the side of the neck.

Other cervical nerves originate in the spinal cord with branches into the scalp and neck.

14. The **greater occipital** (ak-**SIP**-et-el) nerve extends up the back of the scalp to the top of the head.

15. The **lesser occipital** nerve extends into the muscles at the back of the skull.

16. The **greater auricular** (aw-**RIK**-u-lur) nerve extends into the side of the neck and external ear.

17. The **cervical** (**SUR**-vi-kal) **cutaneous** (ku-**TA**-ne-us) nerve extends into the side and front of the neck to the breastbone.

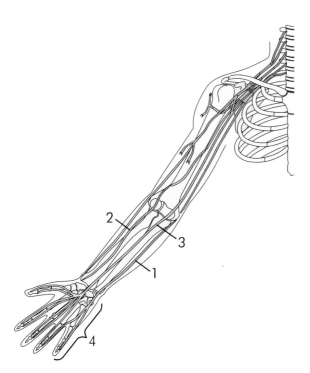

Arm and Hand Nerves

All four of the primary nerves found in the arm and/or hand are mixed nerves; they transmit sensations to the brain and carry impulses from the brain to the muscles.

1. The **ulnar** nerve extends down the little finger side of the arm into the palm of the hand.

2. The **radial** nerve extends down the thumb side of the arm into the back of the hand.

3. The **median** nerve extends down the mid-forearm into the hand.

4. The **digital** nerve extends into the fingers of the hand.

Nerves and Massage

The nerves of the face, head and neck, listed above and on the preceding pages, may be stimulated during facials and/or scalp massage. During full body massages and massage of the face, head and neck, manipulations can stimulate sensitive nerve tissues resulting in nerve impulses that expand and contract corresponding muscles. Through this process, tight muscles can be relaxed; fatigued muscles can be soothed.

The Autonomic Nervous System

The **autonomic** (aw-to-**NOM**-ik) or **sympathetic** nervous system is physically part of the central nervous system. The same nerve tissues are involved but perform different functions. **The autonomic system is responsible for all involuntary body functions.** It operates the respiratory, digestive, circulatory, excretory, endocrine and reproductive systems.

The Digestive System

The digestive system breaks food down into simpler chemical compounds that can be easily absorbed by cells or, if not absorbed, eliminated from the body in waste products. The digestive process begins as soon as food is ingested, when **enzymes** (**EN**-zimz) secreted by the **salivary** (**SAL**-i-ver-e) glands (1) start breaking down the food. Food travels down the **pharynx** (**FAR**-ingks) (2) and through the **esophagus** (e-**SOF**-ah-gus) (3) into the **stomach** (4), propelled by a twisting and turning motion of the esophagus called **peristalsis** (per-i-**STAL**-sis). In the stomach, **hydrochloric** (hi-dro-**KLO**-rik) acids and several other enzymes further break down food. One of these other enzymes called pepsin is responsible for the breakdown of protein into **polypeptide** (pol-e-**PEP**-tide) molecules and free amino acids, which are of particular importance to the production of hair, skin and nails.

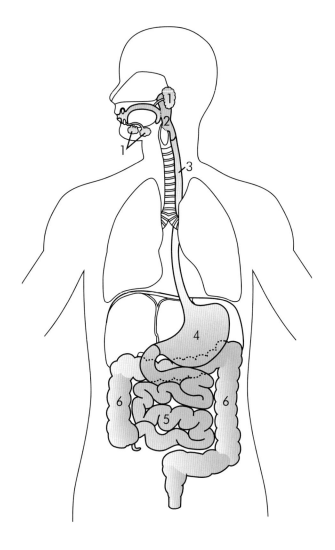

As partially digested food passes from the stomach into the **small intestine** (5), the assimilation of nutrients begins. Nutrients are absorbed by the **villi** (**VIL**-i), which are finger-like projections of the intestine walls, and transported through the circulatory system to the tissues and cells of the body.

Undigested food passes into the **large intestine** (6), or colon, which stores the waste for eventual elimination through the anal canal. This entire process of digestion takes about 9 hours to complete.

As a reminder, the digestive system, also known as the gastrointestinal system includes,

1. Salivary Glands
2. Phayrnx
3. Esophagus
4. Stomach
5. Small Intestine
6. Large Intestine

Perhaps you have heard it said, "The way to a man's heart is through his stomach!" Well, the truth is that **happiness and relaxation promote good digestion.** Good digestion helps keep all other bodily functions on track.

The Excretory System

The excretory system eliminates solid, liquid and gaseous waste products from the body.

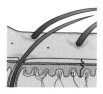
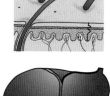
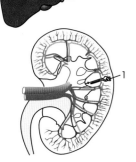

Organs of the excretory system include:

- The **skin** covers nearly 20 square feet of body surface and is the body's largest organ. The skin releases water, carbon dioxide and other waste through the sweat glands.

- The **liver** converts and neutralizes ammonia from the circulatory system to **urea** (u-**RE**-ah). Urea is then carried, through the bloodstream, to the kidneys for excretion.

- The **kidneys** receive urea from the liver and then pass the urea through small tubelike structures known as **nephrons** (NEF-ronz) (1). Nephrons filter out waste products and water, allowing usable nutrients to be reabsorbed into the blood. Excreted waste products travel through the **ureters** (U-re-turz) and bladder and are eliminated from the body in urine.

The Respiratory System

The primary functions of the respiratory system are:

- **The intake of oxygen to be absorbed into the blood**

- **The exhalation of oxygen's toxic byproduct, carbon dioxide**

Both of these functions take place every time you take a breath.

While it is possible to breathe through both the mouth and the nose, *breathing through the nose is the healthier option.* The nose contains mucus membranes, to filter out dust and dirt, and warms the inhaled air as it travels through the nasal passages.

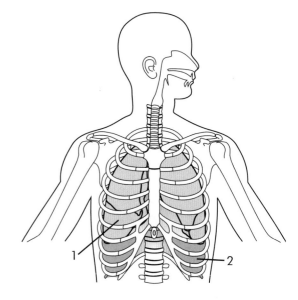

Primary respiratory system organs include:

1. The **LUNGS** are spongy muscles composed of cells into which air enters when you inhale. These cells process oxygen for absorption into the blood and release carbon dioxide as you exhale.

2. The **DIAPHRAGM** is a muscular organ that separates the chest cavity from the abdomen. The diaphragm expands and contracts automatically, forcing air into and out of the lungs.

The Endocrine System

The endocrine system is composed of a group of specialized ductless glands that regulate and control the growth, reproduction and health of the body. These glands manufacture chemical substances called hormones and secrete them directly into the blood stream.

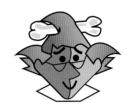

"You will learn more about the sebaceous and suderiferous glands in chapter 15, The Study of Skin."

The endocrine system is a carefully balanced mechanism that directly affects hair growth, skin conditions and energy levels. Nutrition plays a key role in the proper regulation of this system. **Signs of fatigue or changes in hair growth may signal the need for medical attention.**

Reproductive System

The reproductive system is responsible for the process by which a living organism procreates others of its kind.

Integumentary System

The skin and its layers make up the integumentary system of the body. The two primary glands of the integumentary system are the sebaceous (si-BAY shus) (oil) and the sudoriferous (soo-dohr-IF-er-us) (sweat) glands. These glands are referred to as duct glands because both secrete into canal-like structures (ducts) that deposit their contents on the surface of the skin.

Your understanding of the human body provides essential knowledge to aid you in making design decisions that will enhance your client's appearance. In addition, your review of the fundamental structures and systems of the body prepares you for learning massage techniques used in nail and skin care services.

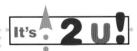

Build Your Critical Thinking Skills

In this chapter you have prepared yourself to meet the following Industry Standard for entry-level cosmetologists:

- Enhance the client's appearance using hair, nail and skin care services.

It's Up to You to know what to do. Using your training to this point, review the following case scenario and think through how you would handle the challenge.

When evaluating the bone structure of your client Bob, who has requested a close clipper cut, you determine that the occipital region is more predominant than normal. Should you cut the hair closer in this area, which would emphasize the occipital region, or would you leave the hair longer in the occipital area? What would you do?

Chapter 4
ELECTRICITY

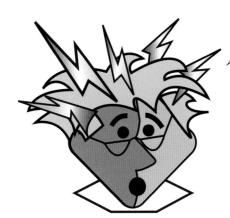

After studying this chapter you will be able to . . .

1. **Define the 10 major terms used in electricity; describe the safety measures to be followed when using electrical appliances.**

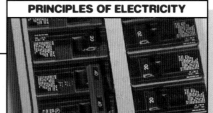

PRINCIPLES OF ELECTRICITY

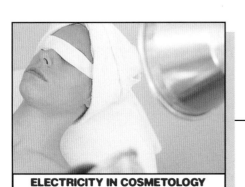

ELECTRICITY IN COSMETOLOGY

2. **Explain the three kinds of effects that can be created by electric current during cosmetology services; list three kinds of effects that can be created by electric current as it is used during electrotherapy and light therapy treatments.**

Don't mind my appearance! I've just received 'shockingly' good news – you're ready for more theory, this time about electricity. Look around the room in which you're reading this chapter. Can you imagine it without electricity? Even more impossible to imagine without electricity is the contemporary salon. In order to work smoothly and efficiently (without ending up looking like me!) in such an 'electric' environment, you will definitely need this chapter.

Understanding the "basics" of electricity will enable you to serve your clients more efficiently and safely, especially when working with electrotherapy and specialized electrical appliances.

Have you noticed a recurring theme developing in your theory chapters? The VALUE of safety to yourself and your client isn't hard to miss, is it? The BIG IDEA underlying this chapter also highlights safety. What you learn in this chapter guarantees that you know enough about electricity to use the appliances and forms of therapy offered in the salon.

Using electricity safely ensures the well-being of the stylist and client.

Electricity in a salon involves more than just on/off switches. That's why the PLAN my colleagues and I have designed for you includes some important electrical terms and a discussion of electric current as well as the exciting ways electricity is used in cosmetology.

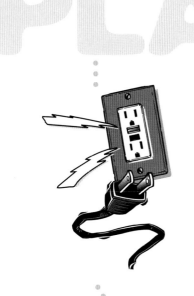

PRINCIPLES OF ELECTRICITY
Vocabulary of Electricity
Electric Current
Safety Measures

ELECTRICITY IN COSMETOLOGY
Effects of Electric Current
Electrotherapy
Light Therapy

PRINCIPLES OF ELECTRICITY

Electricity is a powerful and important form of energy. Anyone who has ever watched lightning crackle in a stormy sky has seen its power. Anyone who has felt an electric shock knows what that power feels like. All who remember "where they were when the lights went out" have a story to tell about how essential to modern life electrical energy is. No salon could function without it. Of course, as a salon professional you aren't expected to develop the knowledge and skills of an electrician, just an understanding of electricity's basic principles and its important uses in your future work.

4

Vocabulary of Electricity

Familiarity with some of the key terms used in this chapter will help you jump start your understanding of electricity. Keep this list handy as you move through this chapter.

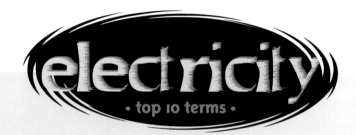

1. **Electricity** is a form of energy that produces light, heat, magnetic and chemical changes.
2. **Electric current** is the movement of electricity along a path called a conductor.
3. **Load** is the technical name for any electrically powered appliance.
4. **Conductor** is a material that allows electricity to flow through it easily.
5. **Insulator** is material that does not allow the flow of electric current.
6. **Amp** is a unit of electric strength.
7. **Volt** is a unit of electric pressure.
8. **Ohm** is a unit of electric resistance.
9. **Watt** is a measure of how much electrical energy is being used.
10. **Electrotherapy** is the application of electrical currents during treatments to the skin.

Electricity and Electric Current

Electricity is a form of energy that produces light, heat, magnetic and chemical changes. Most of the electricity you use daily consists of a flow of tiny, negatively charged particles called electrons. That flow of electrons is called an electric current, which moves along a path called a conductor.

Loads, Conductors and Insulators

A salon is full of loads (electrically powered appliances) just waiting to be activated by the flow of electric current. Just imagine all the blow dryers, curling irons and clippers that need electrical energy to work.

The materials that best transport electricity are called CONDUCTORS. The best conductors are silver and copper. However, other metals, carbon, graphite and water containing ions allow current to flow as well. Since our body is composed of 85% water, it too can be a conductor.

The purpose of a conductor is to transport current in a circuit to a load. This conductor is safely contained in an **INSULATOR, which is a material that DOES NOT allow a current to pass through it.** Insulators protect you from electric current and allow you to handle electricity safely. Examples of insulating materials include silk, plastic, rubber, wood, glass, paper, air, brick, cloth and certain liquids such as alcohol, oil and pure distilled water. Most currents in the salon are carried by copper wire (conductors) insulated with varying amounts of rubber. You know this combination of conductor and insulator as a cord. *Cords on appliances should be kept straight and free of knots, kinks, and tangles to prevent breaks.* **A break in any electrical cord can put you or your client in contact with an active current, causing electric shock.**

Amp

An AMP or AMPERE is a unit of electric *strength.* The amp rating indicates the number of electrons flowing on a line. Your house has a power box with a certain number of amps coming to it that enables you to use all the appliances in the house. The conductors (wires) in your home have the ability to carry a limited number of amps at a time. Circuits will have 10, 20, 30 or larger "AMP RATINGS." When buying or remodeling an older building, you may have to have new powerlines laid to run the appliances in the building. It has only been in the last 60 years that electricity has become a central element in our lives. Through the years, additional uses for electricity, such as the microwave, clothes dryer, computer, etc., have increased the amp requirements for the modern home. One ampere equals 1000 milliamperes.

AMP =	strength
VOLT =	pressure
OHM =	resistance
WATT =	electricity used

Volt

A VOLT, also called VOLTAGE, is a unit of electric *pressure.* In simple terms, a volt measures how hard the electrons are being forced or pushed by the source. AC generators force or push 110 or 220 volts in a circuit. Large motors, such as those found in clothes dryers and air conditioners, may require the higher electrical pressure of 220 volts to operate properly. 220-volt sockets look different from standard wall sockets, in that the prongs that plug into the wall are generally round and pointed into the shape of a "v" at the end. This precaution reduces the danger of someone attempting to plug a 220-volt appliance into a 110-volt wall socket. The cord carrying 220-volt current is also much thicker and there is a higher cost to install lines that carry higher voltage currents.

Ohm

An OHM is a unit of electric *resistance*. A German physicist named George Ohm discovered that every conductor has a specific rate at which it will allow electrons to move through it. The measure of how difficult it is to push electrons through a conductor is called impedance or RESISTANCE. The resistance to the motion of the electrons through a conductor is the OHM'S RATING. The manufacturer of an appliance determines the current needed to power the machine, then installs a conducting wire with an ohm's rating allowing the desired flow.

Watt

A WATT is a measure of how much electrical energy is being *used*. One watt is a small amount of energy. A blow dryer can use 1,000 watts per second. A light bulb can use 25, 60, or 100 watts per second. You can use thousands of watts in a short period of time. To deal with these large numbers, the power company describes watt use in larger terms. 1,000 watts equal one KILOWATT. With many appliances on at one time, thousands of kilowatts can be used in a short time. The power company defines how fast energy is used in hourly terms.

> A hertz rating provides the number of cycles, per second, a generator alternates the current from the source. One hertz unit indicates a frequency equal to one cycle per second.

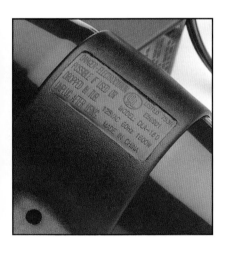

If you turned on a 500-watt dryer and let it run for 8 hours, you would have used 4,000 (500 x 8 = 4,000) watt hours (or 4 kilowatt hours) of power. You pay the electric company so many cents per kilowatt hour used. Energy conservation is important to the salon. When not in use, appliances should be turned off and stored safely.

> The nameplate of an appliance tells the frequency-Hertz (Hz needed), volts needed (110 or 220 V), and the watts this appliance consumes per second (100W, 200W, etc.). It may also have a UL or Underwriter's Laboratory designation. A UL rating means the appliance has been certified to operate safely under the conditions the instructions specify. Look for these ratings on your tools.

Electric Current

Electrical current exists in two forms:

1. **DC or Direct Current in which electrons move at an even rate and flow in only one direction.**
2. **AC or Alternating Current in which electrons flow first in one direction and then in the other.**

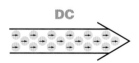
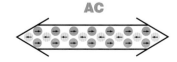

Special instruments can be used to change alternating current (AC) to direct current (DC) or direct current (DC) to alternating current (AC). A converter changes direct current to alternating current. A rectifier changes alternating current to direct current. In Cosmetology, certain currents (as explained later in this chapter) are used to produce certain effects on the skin.

LIGHT UP YOUR CREATIVITY

Here is an activity to help you remember the meaning of the terms you have read about so far. Draw a picture of the following "electric" words. Refer to pages 91-93. A sample is provided to jump start your creativity.

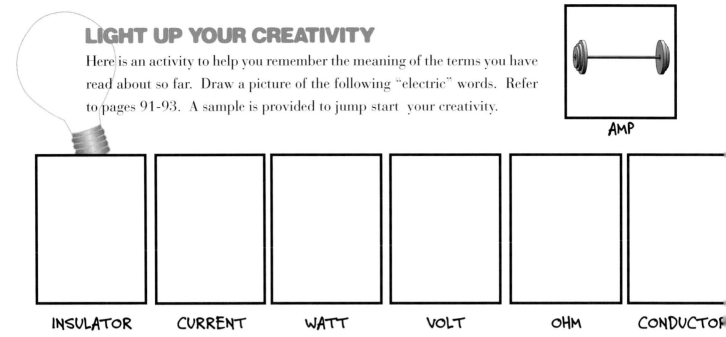

AMP

INSULATOR   CURRENT   WATT   VOLT   OHM   CONDUCTOR

Sources of Electric Current

Electrons cannot move through a conductor without help. A SOURCE provides the force to move the electrons in the conducting material. Two common sources of electric current are batteries and generators. A BATTERY has a positive terminal (+) and a negative terminal (-) and produces DIRECT CURRENT ONLY. The negatively charged electrons are both attracted to the positive terminal and repelled by the negative terminal of the source. This means the electrons flow toward the positive terminal in a circuit.

A GENERATOR is the power source most often used in a salon. Generators produce ALTERNATING CURRENT. When you want to turn on a dryer, you plug it into a wall socket. The wall socket itself is not the source of current. The source is the generator, a machine that uses mechanical energy to produce a flow of electrons. A separate form of energy–nuclear, hydroelectric, solar, thermal or wind–propels the generator, usually from a source located many miles away. Engineers have devised ways for these sources of energy to force generators to mechanically pump huge numbers of electrons into power lines that bring electricity to our homes and businesses.

The generator has two terminals (one positive and one negative). During the operation of the generator, these terminals mechanically alternate their charges, producing an ALTERNATING CURRENT. They switch (or cycle) from positive to negative and back. The number of times this cycling occurs per second is called the FREQUENCY. A generator is built to "cycle" at a specific rate. The rate of cycling or frequency is measured in cycles per second.

In the United States, generators are built at a frequency of 60 cycles per second or 60 hertz (60 Hz). The nameplate of an appliance will indicate the frequency of the source into which the appliance must be plugged to operate safely. Appliances from other countries have different hertz (Hz) or cycle ratings and cannot be operated in the U.S. without an adapter. The same is true of appliances made for U.S. use but are taken out of the country.

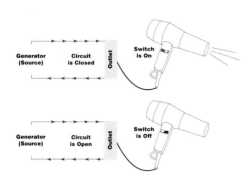

Closed vs. Open Circuit

How Electric Current is Produced

Two conditions must exist for electric current to be produced. First, as you just read, there must be a source. Second, there must be a CLOSED PATH, called a CIRCUIT, through which the electrons travel. A closed path is a path on which the electrons leave the source and operate an appliance. When this path is broken, it is called an OPEN CIRCUIT. If you plug in a blow dryer, turn it on and air begins to flow, you have an example of a closed or completed circuit. When you turn the switch off, the circuit breaks and is now an open circuit.

There are two ways circuits can be connected to power loads. PARALLEL WIRING allows the user to power several loads at different times or at once. With parallel wiring, a blow dryer, curling iron and blow comb can be plugged into the same circuit. Each can be run alone or all three can be run at once. SERIES WIRING forces the user to have all loads running at the same time, since the circuit travels from one load to the next. An example of this would be many connected strings of Christmas tree lights. If one string of lights is malfunctioning, the electric current cannot flow to the next string. The malfunction causes an open circuit, and none of the strings work. In the salon, only parallel wiring should be installed.

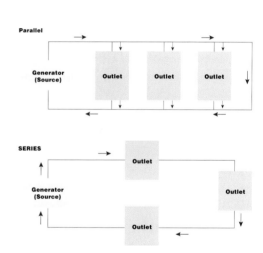

Parallel vs. Series Wiring

Overload and Short Circuit

When a building is constructed, an electrician normally wires it with a certain number of circuits (each capable of carrying 20 or 30 amps). When you turn on an appliance, such as a hair dryer, the appliance causes current to flow on the line to meet its power needs. A problem can occur when too many appliances are put on one circuit and are operated all at the same time. More current flows than the line is designed to carry. This situation is called an OVERLOAD. Although there are safety devices to detect overloading, they can fail. If they do, the lines of the circuit will heat up and may burn.

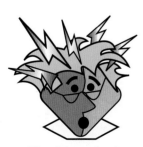

"Careful, overloading a circuit can cause fires."

In general, it takes 1 amp on the circuit to operate every 100 watts of an appliance. So, to operate a 1,000-watt blow dryer, a 10-amp circuit is required. If you operated a 1,000-watt dryer on a 5-amp circuit, it would overload. **Fires can occur when an extension cord with multiple plugs is used to attach 4 or 5 appliances to one wall socket.** If all the appliances are turned on, that extension cord (if not rated for the amps flowing) can melt and burn in seconds. It is essential to hire a qualified electrician to install adequate wiring. The number of amps demanded by each appliance (dryers, air conditioner, washer) during a normal working day must be determined to safely predict the number of amps needed by the salon. Part of salon design is planning salon energy use and safety. Knowledge of electricity is essential.

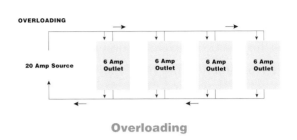

Overloading

A second problem that frequently occurs in the salon is called a SHORT CIRCUIT. A short circuit can occur any time a "foreign conductor" comes in contact with a wire carrying current to a load (appliance). A classic short circuit occurs when a child tries to plug in an appliance and gets a finger between the wall socket and the plug. The child's finger becomes the foreign conductor and receives the electrical current instead of the appliance for which the current was intended.

Dropping an appliance into water will cause the current to flow through the water, in this case a foreign conductor. If you tried to retrieve the appliance, you would be electrocuted. With dry hands, remove the plug from the wall socket first.

ELECTRIC SHOCK CAN BE FATAL.

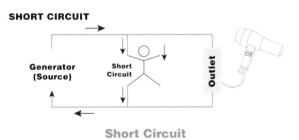

Short Circuit

Short circuits commonly occur in thermal styling tool cords. Twisting and bending of cords can eventually break the copper wires. If you touch the break, you'll get an electrical shock.

Safety Measures

Because of the possibility of overloads and short circuits, safety devices are installed in many appliances and buildings. Two of these devices, fuses and circuit breakers, connect directly to the circuits in the power box, the carefully insulated location where the electric current enters a building from a generator or power plant. From the power box, many circuits continue throughout the building.

Fuse

A FUSE is a device that contains a fine metal wire that allows current to flow through it. If an overload occurs (too much current flowing), the fuse will heat up and the wire will melt, breaking the circuit and cutting the flow of electricity. Fuses cannot be reused. A new fuse of the same amp rating (10, 20, or 30) must be installed.

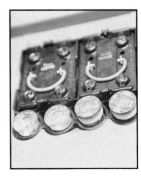

Before installing a new fuse:

1. Turn off all appliances operating on that circuit.

2. Go to the power box and turn off the main power handle on the side of the box.

3. Remove the burned-out fuse and replace it with a new one.

4. Close the box and switch on the main power handle.

Have an ample supply of fuses on hand. Remember, too many appliances on one circuit caused the problem. Change your appliance use or switch to a different circuit.

Circuit Breaker

A CIRCUIT BREAKER is simply a reusable device that breaks the flow of current when an overload occurs. It contains two pieces of metal that make contact with each other. Like a fuse, these pieces of metal conduct electric current unless too much current flows on the line. If the flow is too high, there is

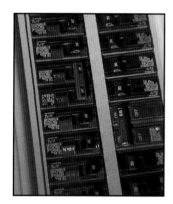

a heat-sensing device that causes the two pieces to separate, and the circuit is broken. In order to restore power when circuit breakers are being used:

1. Turn off appliances.

2. Go to the power box and open it.

3. Find a row of switches that look just like wall light switches.

4. Look for a switch that has a color marker (red or yellow) showing. Turn this switch completely to the "off" position, then immediately to the "on" position. This resets the breaker. The circuit is now operating.

It will be wise to become familiar with the power box in your salon. Know where it is and how to safely operate it. Each circuit should be clearly labeled, and you should have a flashlight available in case it is dark when a circuit breaks.

Grounding Wire

Another safety device is called a three-wire system. Wall sockets contain three holes for plugging in an appliance. Two of the holes are long and rectangular. Some appliances use only these two. The third hole is circular. This circular opening is connected to a wire that runs directly into the ground below the building. This GROUNDING WIRE is designed to protect you when operating certain kinds of appliances. Some appliances have conducting mechanisms inside that could accidentally come in contact with the outside case, for example, a hooded dryer, vacuum cleaner or hair clipper. The manufacturer installs a special wire for conducting high and sudden flows of electric current out of the appliance, into the cord and to the plug. Any appliance requiring this protection has a three-prong plug. If this grounding wire did not exist, your body would receive the excess flow of electric current.

Shock

Human contact with an electric current causes a shock. If someone comes in contact with an electric current, it is most important to break the circuit carrying the power. You can:

1. Knock the person out of the circuit by using an INSULATOR like a broom, a plastic brush or a plastic garbage pail.

2. Unplug the appliance. Be careful to use an insulator to keep yourself out of the circuit.

3. Rush to the power box and turn off all the circuit breakers.

A *local shock* passes through a small part of the body, causing burns and muscle contractions. Immerse the burn in cold water immediately and, if severe, take the person to a hospital or physician. If minor, keep the affected area immersed. Wait until the burn is completely "cold" and has stopped swelling. Blot dry and apply an antiseptic cream. Blistering can sometimes be prevented if the skin is cooled fast enough. If blistering occurs, scarring may occur also.

A *general shock* passes through the nervous system. Again, break the circuit before touching the person. This type of shock causes the heart to stop, the breathing to cease and the muscles to convulse. Emergency help should be called. Dial 911. Start CPR (cardiopulmonary resuscitation). CPR is the only procedure that can save the victim's life. Don't stop CPR until an emergency team arrives.

If a fire results from an overload of an electric circuit and an appliance melts and burns, DO NOT PUT WATER ON IT!!! Turn off the circuit. Smother the fire with a rug, a heavy towel, or a powder, such as cornstarch or laundry detergent, or a fire extinguisher.

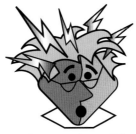

"Be sure to have all fire extinguishers checked periodically."

KNOW YOUR EQUIPMENT

There are three types of electrically-powered equipment typically used in the salon: thermal, mechanical or a combination of the two.

THERMAL EQUIPMENT is used to generate heat. Curling irons, heat lamps, color machines, manicure heaters, facial steamers and scalp steamers are thermal appliances. Facial steamers and scalp steamers produce moist heat at a constant temperature.

MECHANICAL EQUIPMENT has a motor. Clippers and massagers are mechanical appliances.

COMBINATION EQUIPMENT generates heat and produces a flow of air. Hooded dryers, blow dryers and blow combs fall into this category.

ELECTRICITY IN COSMETOLOGY

From operating the lights in your salon to running your blow dryer, electricity is critical to you as a professional cosmetologist. Now that you understand the principles of electricity, you can take a look at how it is used in the salon.

4

Effects of Electric Current

Three kinds of effects can be created by electric current during cosmetology services. They are HEATING effects, MECHANICAL or MAGNETIC effects and ELECTROCHEMICAL effects.

Heating effects

Every conductor has some resistance to the flow of current through it. The more resistance, the more "drag or friction" in the line. The result is increased heat. A curling iron, a light bulb and a blow dryer all create heating effects because they contain special conductors (heating elements) that heat up when current flows through them. A low setting simply cuts the amount of current allowed to pass through the special conductor. This fact explains why a blow dryer can have a "cold" setting. This setting stops all flow of current to the heating element but still allows current to flow to the blower.

Mechanical or Magnetic Effects

As you've learned, electrical generators push alternating current through the conductor. Alternating current flows first one direction and then the other. Manufacturers of mechanical equipment – clippers, massagers, electrodes, etc., – design motors with magnetic fields with positive and negative polarity. When the current travels through the conductor and into the magnetic field of the motor, a push-pull effect is created as the negative and positive charges interact. This push-pull effect causes the motor to turn, creating a mechanical motion like the rotating blades of a fan.

Electrochemical Effects

Electrochemical effects are created when electric current travels through a water-based solution (a liquid conductor) in order to produce relaxing or stimulating results.

ALERT!

A person with any potentially restrictive medical condition should always consult a physician before receiving electrotherapy treatment.

Electrotherapy

So far you've learned about electricity in general and about some of the electrical equipment you'll be using as a stylist. Electric currents can also be used during skin care services. ELECTROTHERAPY is the application of special currents (or modalities) that have certain effects on the skin. The benefits of these currents are not always agreed upon by all cosmetologists. It is important, however, to know what they are promoted to do so you are familiar with their potential in the salon. There are four types of current you should know: Galvanic, Faradic, Sinusoidal and Tesla.

In order to be safely used in GALVANIC, FARADIC, SINUSOIDAL and TESLA current electrotherapy, electric current must be reduced from the 120 volts of electric power carried through a wire-conductor to a level safely handled by the human body. This reduction of power is accomplished by a portable appliance known as a wall plate. The wall plate is available in various sizes and styles and plugs into the stationary wall outlet. The current conductors to be used in electrotherapy applications are plugged into and operated through the wall plate, allowing voltage regulations as necessary for a particular treatment or current. A current conductor called an ELECTRODE is used to bring the current from the appliance to the client's skin. The most common electrodes are:

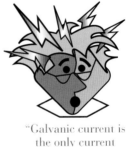

RAKE ELECTRODE

1. A comb electrode (for use on the scalp)
2. A rake electrode (for use on the scalp)
3. A wrist electrode (for the cosmetologist)
4. A carbon electrode (for the patron to hold)
5. A massage roller electrode (for application to the client by the stylist)

An electrode, like those listed above, is the only safe contact point through which the current can pass to the client.

Galvanic Current

Galvanic current has an electrochemical effect and is the oldest form of electrotherapy in the salon. **Galvanic current is a direct current (DC) of low voltage and high amperage.** Because galvanic current is a direct current and generally only alternating current is available in the salon, a special appliance is necessary to convert the salon's alternating current to the direct current.

"Galvanic current is the only current that is direct and has an electrochemical effect."

Galvanic current has chemical effects that are caused by passing the current through particular acid or alkaline solutions and/or by passing the current through body tissues and fluids.

All electrotherapy applicators have both a negatively charged electrode (called a *Cathode*) and a positively charged electrode (called an *Anode*). The cathode is usually black in color or displays a large "N" or negative sign (-). The anode, usually colored red, displays a large "P" or a positive sign (+).

If the electrodes are not visibly marked as negative or positive, test for polarity. You can determine polarity by separating the tips and submerging the tips only into a glass of water. Salt water is best but tap water will do. Keep tips from touching each other. Slowly turn up the Galvanic current using the wall plate's regulator. The negative electrode will create more and smaller bubbles than will the positive electrode.

The process of forcing an acid (+) or alkali (-) into the skin by applying current to the chemical is called PHORESIS and is probably the most typical application of galvanic current. ANAPHORESIS uses a negative pole (cathode) or electrode to force negatively-charged (alkaline) solutions into the skin without breaking the skin. CATAPHORESIS uses a positive pole (anode) or electrode to force positively-charged (acidic) solutions into the skin without breaking the skin.

4

Anaphoresis

The **negative pole of galvanic current** is believed to have the following temporary effects on the area of the body to which it is applied:

1. Produces an alkaline reaction, which can force alkaline solutions to penetrate the skin
2. Increases the blood flow by expanding the vessels to aid circulation
3. Softens tissues
4. Stimulates nerves

Cataphoresis

The **positive pole of galvanic current** is believed to have temporary effects opposite to those produced by the negative pole, including:

1. Produces an acidic reaction, which can force acidic solutions to penetrate the skin.
2. Slows the blood flow by contracting the vessels to decrease redness or inflammation when applied to simple blemishes on the skin.
3. Hardens tissues, closing pores after facial treatment.
4. Soothes nerves.

Galvanic Current Electrotherapy

- The salon professional applies the ACTIVE electrode to the client. The active electrode is connected to either the positive or negative pole, depending on the therapeutic reaction desired.

- The client holds the inactive electrode, which is connected to the opposite pole.

- Both the active and inactive electrodes should be wrapped lightly in moist cotton. While the comfort level for the current will vary from one client to the next, never use more than one milliampere of current.

A galvanic current machine is also used for a process called iontophoresis (eye-on-to-fo-**REE**-sis). Iontophoresis introduces water-soluble treatment products into the skin. Desincrustation is a treatment in which sebum is broken down or blackheads are liquefied, as in deep-pore cleansing.

ALERT!

Do not use the galvanic current over an area having many broken capillaries.

Faradic Current

FARADIC CURRENT is an alternating current (AC), interrupted to produce a mechanical, non-chemical reaction. Faradic current stimulates nerve and muscle tissue. Benefits believed to be derived from the application of faradic current include:

1. Improved blood circulation
2. Improved muscle tone
3. Stimulation of hair growth
4. Increased glandular activity

Used chiefly to cause muscle contractions during scalp and facial massage, faradic current can be soothing and relaxing and is believed to help preserve muscle tone.

The most frequently used application of the faradic current is the INDIRECT METHOD of faradic current electrotherapy. In the Indirect Method, the salon professional usually wears a wrist band with a moistened electrode. The second electrode is wrapped in moist cotton and either held by the client or, better, attached to the client's lower neck between the shoulders. The salon professional's fingers are then placed on the client's face before the current is turned on to prevent shock. When the current reaches the desired level, a facial massage is given, with particular focus on motor points. The current is gradually decreased and finally turned off completely BEFORE the cosmetologist's fingers are removed.

The DIRECT METHOD of application, used less often for faradic current electrotherapy, places both electrodes on the client's skin, BEING CERTAIN THAT THEY NEVER TOUCH. The current is turned on and slowly increased only after the electrodes are in place. In this application, the current travels through the motor nerves between the two electrodes, causing muscle stimulation.

Sinusoidal Current

SINUSOIDAL CURRENT is an alternating current (AC) with a mechanical effect, much like the faradic current that produces muscle contractions. (Machines that cause muscle contraction are illegal in some areas. Be sure to read your area's rules and regulations.) Sinusoidal current electrotherapy is performed by using the Indirect Method application.

ALERT!

Sinusoidal current electrotherapy should not be used on unhealthy and/or broken skin.

Some users believe sinusoidal current to be superior to faradic current because sinusoidal current penetrates more deeply and can provide greater stimulation to the treated area. For this reason, it is most often preferred to faradic current for middle-aged and older clients. Treatments using sinusoidal current generally last no longer than 30 minutes.

Tesla Current

TESLA, HIGH FREQUENCY CURRENT, known as the "violet-ray," is an alternating current which can be adjusted to different voltages to produce heat. Because the Tesla is a high oscillation current, its use does not produce muscle contractions. Use of the Tesla current can result in relaxation or stimulation, depending on method of application.

There are three methods for using the Tesla current:

1. When using DIRECT APPLICATION of the Tesla High Frequency current, the salon professional applies the electrode directly to the client's scalp or face.

2. When using INDIRECT APPLICATION, the cosmetologist hands the glass electrode to the client before activating the current to avoid the electrical shock that could result in passing an active current from one person to another. The client then holds the activated electrode while the cosmetologist manually stimulates the area being treated. The current is turned off before the client returns the electrode to the stylist after the treatment.

3. In GENERAL ELECTRIFICATION, the cosmetologist hands the electrode to the client before activating the current. The power is switched on and a generalized tingling or vibration effect is experienced by the client.

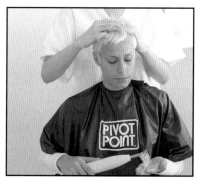

Direct

Indirect

4

To create soothing or relaxing effects, the electrode must be kept in direct contact with the areas being treated. To stimulate an area through rapid vibration, during a direct application, a towel is placed over the skin and the electrode is applied over the towel. The slight separation of the electrode from the skin creates a mild, stimulating sensation.

Benefits believed to be derived through application of the High Frequency or Tesla current include:

1. Improved blood circulation

2. Increased rate of metabolism

3. Increased sebaceous (oil glands) glandular activity

Cosmetology Uses for Tesla Current

Dry Skin Facial Treatment - Indirect Application

1. Cleanse client's face.
2. Have the client hold the glass rod electrode.
3. Place the tips of your fingers against skin on client's face before turning on the High Frequency current.
4. Turn on the current, slowly increasing strength. Perform usual facial massage manipulations, being careful not to lift fingers from client's skin.
5. Massage according to manufacturer's directions, in most cases for no more than 7 minutes per treatment. Your fingertips may tingle slightly during contact. This is normal.
6. Turn off current before removing your fingers from client's face to avoid shock.
7. Complete facial treatment.

Mild Acne and/or Blackhead Facial Treatment - Direct Application

1. Cleanse client's face.
2. Apply the facial electrode directly to the skin and turn on current.
3. Move the electrode gently across skin, in small circular rotations, while slowly increasing strength of the current.
4. Repeat until entire face has been covered at least once, but do not exceed a total of 5 minutes for the entire treatment.
5. Turn the current down slowly until it's turned off completely.
6. Remove the electrode from your client's skin and proceed with the rest of the facial.

Dry Scalp - Indirect Application

1. Apply moisturizing scalp treatment cream.
2. Have client hold glass rod electrode.
3. After putting your hand on the client's scalp, turn on the current.
4. Perform normal scalp massage, being careful not to break contact with the client, while gradually increasing current.
5. Time treatment according to manufacturer's directions, massaging entire scalp.
6. Turn off the current, maintaining contact with client.
7. Complete scalp treatment.

Scalp Treatment - Direct Application

1. Apply moisturizing scalp treatment cream.
2. Apply scalp electrode (rake) to scalp and turn on current.
3. Using push-pull movements, manipulate rake electrode over entire scalp while slowly increasing strength of current.
4. Continue treatment for approximately 5 minutes.
5. Turn off current.
6. Remove electrode rake from scalp and complete scalp treatment.

Electrotherapy Precautions

General

- Always read the manufacturer's directions and follow them carefully.
- Electrodes should never touch each other.

Galvanic/Faradic/Sinusoidal

- Never take the current over one milliampere.
- Make sure the current is off before beginning indirect application and before breaking contact with client at the end of the treatment.
- Sinusoidal electrotherapy treatment should never exceed 30 minutes.

Tesla High Frequency

- Begin each treatment with a mild current, increasing strength slowly.
- Keep client out of contact with metal during treatment.
- Limit treatment duration to approximately 5 minutes.
- If you use cream during scalp or other high frequency treatments, be sure the cream contains NO ALCOHOL. Alcohol-based creams may be flammable and could be ignited by a spark.
- Turn the current on only after the client is holding the electrode. Turn the current off before removing the electrode from client's contact.

Heat Energy

Heat always moves from a hotter body to a cooler body and can be transferred from one object to another in one of three ways:

1. Conduction - the transfer of heat via direct contact
2. Convection - the transfer of heat via liquid or gas
3. Radiation - the transfer of heat through a vacuum (empty space)

Effects of Heat

Heat can be mild and pleasant or intense and damaging. Mild heat relaxes the muscles, causes blood circulation to increase and helps stylists perform many hair and skin care services. Intense heat destroys cells and tissues. You can observe this chemical breakdown of the skin (called pyrolysis) when you are burned and a blister forms.

Short Wavelength

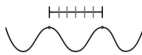

Long Wavelength

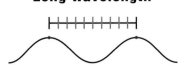

Light Therapy

Light therapy is the production of beneficial effects on the body through treatments using light rays or waves. Radiation is the transfer of heat energy through an empty air space (a vacuum). Heat energy is simply movement of electrons. When heat energy is transferred by radiation, these electrons move in wave-like patterns. These waves of electrons are called electromagnetic radiation. The waves can be long or short. They are measured from the crest of one

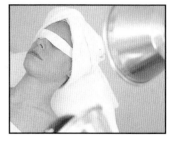

wave to the crest of the next. This measurement is a wavelength. The range of all the wavelengths that can be produced by radiant energy is called the electromagnetic spectrum. The shorter the wavelength, the more energy the wave is carrying. X-rays have a short wavelength.

Longer wavelengths are very helpful. TV and radio broadcasts are examples of long wavelengths of radiant energy. Heat lamps used in chemical services have long wavelengths as well.

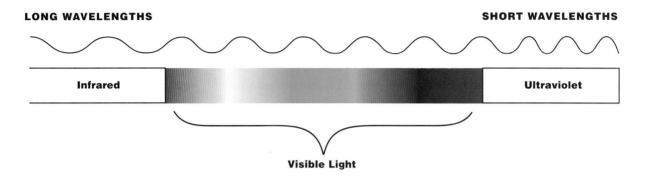

LONG WAVELENGTHS   **SHORT WAVELENGTHS**

Infrared   Ultraviolet

Visible Light

Visible Light

The portion of the electromagnetic spectrum humans can see is called visible light. This range of wavelengths produces visible color. When these waves hit an object, they are either absorbed or reflected. Our eyes pick up the reflected waves and interpret them as color.

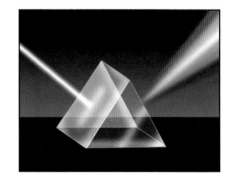

White light is referred to as combination light. This visible light can be broken into its individual wavelengths by a prism. A prism is a three-sided glass object. If white light (sunlight or light from a light bulb) passes through a prism, the wavelengths are separated and become visible to the eye as seven colors: Red, orange, yellow, green, blue, indigo and violet. Raindrops act as prisms, breaking up white light into the colors of the rainbow. **The wavelengths that produce red are the longest waves of the visible spectrum.** The wavelengths that produce violet are the shortest.

Two kinds of light in the salon produce "white light":
1. Fluorescent light
2. Incandescent light

Fluorescent Light

Fluorescent light is an economical and long-lasting light source. However, depending on its design, fluorescent light can create "blue" tones or "cool" casts in the objects it lights. In the salon, fluorescent light can create hair coloring problems unless natural sunlight is available, or the fluorescent bulbs are balanced for daylight.

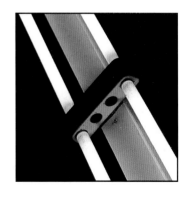

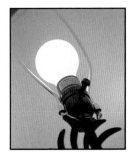

Incandescent Light

To balance the tones of light in the salon, a second source of light can be used. This source is called incandescent light. This kind of light is provided by an ordinary light bulb. Normally this light produces redder tones or warmer casts in the objects it lights. Although more expensive to operate and replace than fluorescent light, incandescent light creates the closest substitute for natural sunlight.

Salon owners need to plan a balance of incandescent and fluorescent lighting in the salon design. Proper lighting systems can have a pleasant psychological effect on staff and clients. Fluorescent light can be irritating to some people, while incandescent light can create excessive heat. Lighting should be comfortable to work under and easy to adjust.

Invisible Light

Cosmetologists use invisible light to produce physical effects in the skin. Since this range of light is not visible to the human eye, you can be overexposed to invisible light in natural sunlight without knowing it.

Eighty percent of sunlight is composed of invisible rays beyond red, which are called infrared. Eight percent of natural sunlight is composed of invisible rays beyond violet, which are called ultraviolet.

Small doses of infrared or ultraviolet light can produce beneficial effects. Using either ultraviolet or infrared light to treat the skin is called light therapy.

Infrared Light

Just as infrared rays produce pure heat rays, any infrared light produces heat. Heat lamps or infrared bulbs can be purchased for use in processing chemical services. Take care to position the lamps according to the manufacturer's instructions.

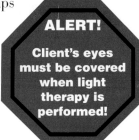

ALERT!

Client's eyes must be covered when light therapy is performed!

Benefits of using infrared light during a facial include:

1. Increased circulation
2. Increased skin gland secretions
3. Relaxation of muscles
4. Stimulation of cell and tissue activity

Exposure times range from 5 to 15 minutes. The light must be placed at least 30 inches from the client's face. Eye pads or protective eye forms must be used to cover the client's eyes.

Ultraviolet Light

Ultraviolet rays, also known as actinic rays, have a shorter wavelength and can be more damaging than infrared rays. Ultraviolet light, or UV, produces both positive and negative effects on the skin, depending on the exposure time. Small doses of UV light can tan the skin and may help the body produce Vitamin D. UV light is germicidal and can kill bacteria that

cause skin infections. It can also produce harmful chemical effects on the skin. Skin can be sunburned, eyes can be damaged, and hair can be photochemically damaged by UV rays. Studies prove overexposure to UV light can result in skin cancer. Conversely, it is believed that ultraviolet rays may promote healing and are used in the treatment of acne.

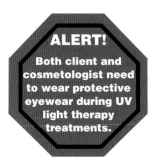

ALERT!
Both client and cosmetologist need to wear protective eyewear during UV light therapy treatments.

During facials or scalp massage, UV light can be used effectively. The skin or scalp should be cleansed before using ultraviolet light on the client. The client's eyes should be covered with protective eyewear, such as cotton eye pads, goggles, etc. The cosmetologist should wear protective eyewear also. For germicidal treatments, place the lamp at least 12 inches from the area to be treated. This distance allows the strong "short waves" to penetrate intensely. Expose the skin initially for 1 minute. Check for reactions. 1 to 5 minutes of total exposure time is often recommended.

For larger areas, like the scalp, place the lamp 20 to 30 inches from the area. Exposure can be up to 10 or 15 minutes. This exposure time would include the normal scalp massage.

The current trend of tanning beds or booths in styling salons poses serious questions for the professional cosmetologist. Reasonable tanning can be healthy looking and cause minimum damage, but any tanning does cause damage. Dry, leathery skin, peeling, itching, wrinkling, sagging and permanent discoloration are all common reactions to long exposure. **When using ultraviolet rays you and your client should wear protective eyewear.**

Electricity plays a key role in the successful operation of every salon. Your understanding of the safe use of electricity will provide an environment that is safe and efficient, whether you are using it to perform basic client services, such as blow drying or thermal styling, or to provide a relaxing or stimulating effect during skin care services.

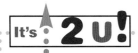
It's **2 U!**

Build Your Critical Thinking Skills

In this chapter you have prepared yourself to meet the following Industry Standards for entry-level cosmetologists:

- Use appropriate methods to ensure personal health and well-being
- Provide basic hair, nail and skin care services

It's Up to You to know what to do. Using your training to this point, review the following case scenario and think through how you would handle the challenge.

You are the last stylist in the salon, finishing your last client. You have just started to blow dry your client following a perm service, when all the lights go off and your blow dryer stops. What would you do?

Chapter 5
CHEMISTRY

After studying this chapter you will be able to . . .

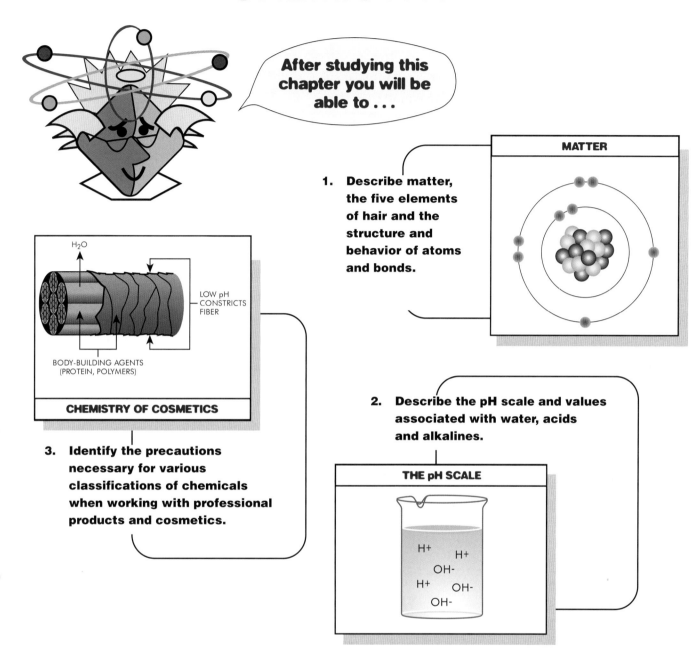

1. Describe matter, the five elements of hair and the structure and behavior of atoms and bonds.

MATTER

CHEMISTRY OF COSMETICS

H₂O

LOW pH CONSTRICTS FIBER

BODY-BUILDING AGENTS (PROTEIN, POLYMERS)

3. Identify the precautions necessary for various classifications of chemicals when working with professional products and cosmetics.

2. Describe the pH scale and values associated with water, acids and alkalines.

THE pH SCALE

H+ H+
OH-
H+ OH-
OH-

"Eureka!" Isn't that what absent-minded cartoon professors (not like me, of course) say as they stand in the midst of smoking test tubes and broken glass? In many minds, science labs, chemistry and disaster just seem to go hand in hand. You've recently studied chapters on Salon Ecology, Anatomy and Electricity. You probably learned more about disinfection, skull bones and short circuits than you ever dreamed there is to know. Then, you run into this chapter on Chemistry. Have no fear. Professor P is here!

In the world of cosmetology, CHEMISTRY helps you use a variety of products to improve the personal well-being of your client.

You may think chemistry is complicated, but it's not as difficult as it seems. Together we'll tackle what you must know to truly understand hair, its properties and characteristics, how to protect hair and scalp during chemical services and how to understand product ingredients. Then, through the BIG IDEA you will experience the VALUE of this material for your career.

Understanding the principles of chemistry helps in marketing products, making sound decisions about appropriate services and guarding the safety of your client.

Would you believe that many people out there think that shampoo is shampoo is shampoo...? Wrong! – and it's chemistry that makes the difference. Putting this PLAN into action, you'll gain, among other things, a deeper understanding of products – shampoos, rinses, conditioners and cosmetics. I can see you now on the floor of the salon, a walking storehouse of information for your clients. Way to go! Maybe someday a chemist will invent something to tame even my wild hair.

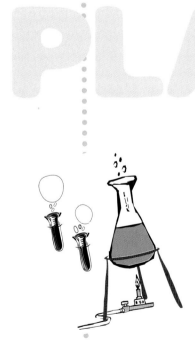

MATTER

Elements

Chemical Bonds

THE pH SCALE

CHEMISTRY OF COSMETICS

Cosmetic Classifications

Shampoos

Rinses and Conditioners

Perms

Relaxers

Curl Reformation

Hair Color

Product Information

MATTER

Matter is anything that occupies space. Look around. Matter is everywhere. Nails, hair and skin are matter. Water is matter. Yes, even oxygen is matter. All of these things occupy physical space.

Chemists (scientists who study matter, its properties and changes) teach that matter exists in three basic forms:

Solids – matter with definite weight, volume and shape

Liquids – matter with definite weight and volume but no definite shape

Gasses – matter with definite weight but indefinite volume and shape

For example, hair is a solid because it has definite weight, volume and shape. Conditioners, perm solutions and most shampoos are liquids. They have weight and volume but no definite shape. In fact, as you have observed many times, liquids take the shape of the solid container into which they are poured. Oxygen is a gas. It has weight, even though it may not seem to, but no definite volume or shape.

Matter can be changed from one of these forms (solid, liquid or gas) to another in two ways:

1. **Physical change** – a change in the physical characteristics of a substance without creating a new substance.

2. **Chemical change** – a change in a substance that creates a new substance with chemical characteristics different from those of the original substance.

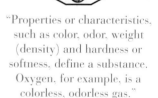

"Properties or characteristics, such as color, odor, weight (density) and hardness or softness, define a substance. Oxygen, for example, is a colorless, odorless gas."

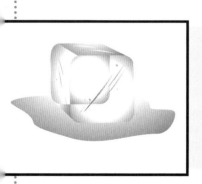

An example of a physical change in matter would be when water freezes and becomes ice. It is still water, but now it's a solid instead of a liquid.

An example of a chemical change occurs when hydrogen combines with oxygen to form a new substance, water.

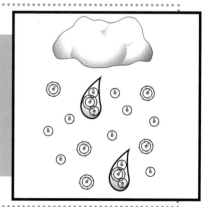

Now you know enough to understand the definition of chemistry, the overall subject of this chapter. **Chemistry is the scientific study of matter and the physical and chemical changes of matter.**

You have observed all your life that some matter is living and some is not. What you may not have known is that the presence of the element carbon distinguishes a living being from a non-living being. Chemistry has a special division for each kind of matter:

Organic chemistry deals with all matter that is now living or was alive at one time, with carbon present, such as plants and animals.

Inorganic chemistry studies all matter that is not alive, has never been alive and does not contain carbon, such as rocks, water and minerals.

Elements

All matter, whether solid, liquid or gas, whether living or nonliving, is made up of elements. Elements are basic substances that cannot be broken down into simpler substances.

As of this printing, there are 118 known elements. Those above the 92nd element are synthetic and do not occur naturally. Five of these elements, because they form the basis of hair, nails and skin, are important for the cosmetologist to know. These elements are carbon, oxygen, hydrogen, nitrogen and sulfur. Look at this chart to notice a few more things about elements:

All matter is composed of atoms, which make up elements.

Atomic No.	Element	Symbol	Category
1	**Hydrogen**	**H**	**gas**
2	Helium	He	gas
3	Lithium	Li	solid
6	**Carbon**	**C**	**solid**
7	**Nitrogen**	**N**	**gas**
8	**Oxygen**	**O**	**gas**
13	Aluminum	Al	solid
16	**Sulfur**	**S**	**solid**
80	Mercury	Hg	liquid

Hair is comprised of two solids (carbon and sulfur) and three gases (hydrogen, nitrogen and oxygen). And yet hair is a solid!

On this chart, the left-hand column shows each element's Atomic Number. You'll read more about this number in the next few pages. Even more important to you and your work are the letters after each element's name. These letters, called symbols, are a kind of scientific shorthand, like a nickname, that makes it easier for you to identify the elements. You will see these symbols used throughout this book, in other professional literature and on some product labels. **Oxygen is the most abundant element in the earth's crust and the second most abundant element in the earth's atmosphere.**

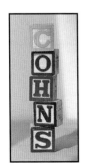

To remember the elements found in hair, use this acronym: COHNS (carbon, oxygen, hydrogen, nitrogen and sulfur).

Atoms

Atoms are the smallest complete unit of an element. Each element consists of a certain kind of atom different from the atoms of any other element.

Atoms have three main parts: protons, neutrons and electrons. Protons and neutrons are packed together tightly to form a dense core, or nucleus, at the center of the atom. Electrons move about this nucleus on orbiting paths or shells at nearly the speed of light.

> **Protons** have a positive electrical charge (+) and identify the atom as, for example, a hydrogen atom or an oxygen atom, etc.
>
> **Neutrons** have no electrical charge. They are neutral, hence their name, neutron. The neutron determines the weight of the atom.
>
> **Electrons** have a negative electrical charge (-). Under certain circumstances, they make it possible for atoms to unite with other atoms to form bonds.

5

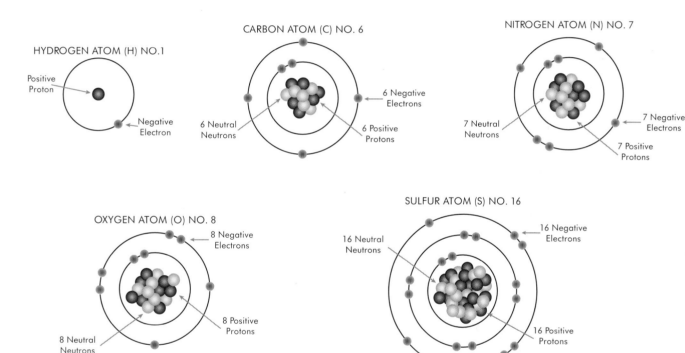

On this page you see a diagram of the atomic structure of the five elements important to you as a cosmetologist. Notice how different one atom is from another in terms of number of protons, neutrons and electrons.

This diagram can help you begin to understand what an element's atomic number means. (Refer to the chart on page 112.) The atomic number indicates how many protons are in a single atom of a particular element. For example, the atomic number of hydrogen is 1, which means it has only 1 proton and 1 electron. **Hydrogen is the simplest atomic structure.** Carbon, as you can see, has an atomic number of 6, which means it has 6 protons, 6 neutrons and 6 electrons. Nitrogen has 7, oxygen 8 and sulfur 16.

The chemical behavior of an atom depends mostly on the number of electrons in its outermost orbiting path or shell. Some atoms by their very structure are not missing any electrons in their outer shell. These atoms are considered stable and are electrically neutral.

If the outer shell of the atom is missing electrons, however, the atom is considered unstable or reactive. Unstable atoms seek other atoms with which they can share electrons to complete their outer shell. When they combine, they make more complex units, known as molecules.

Molecules

When unstable atoms combine chemically by sharing electrons, they form molecules. **A molecule is two or more atoms joined together by a chemical bond.** If the atoms that combine are different, for example, an atom of hydrogen and an atom of oxygen, the resulting molecule is a **compound**. Different atoms joined together as molecules become the smallest parts of a compound.

With an element, the atoms are the same. With a compound, the atoms are different.

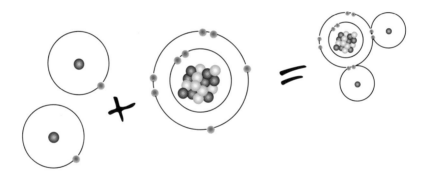

When two hydrogen atoms, each with one electron, combine with one oxygen atom and its eight electrons, the result is a water molecule of the compound H_2O. This is an example of two gasses – hydrogen and oxygen – uniting and becoming a liquid.

Chemical Bonds

You are now somewhat familiar with the diagrams of the atoms of the five elements of hair – carbon, oxygen, hydrogen, nitrogen and sulfur. These atoms combine chemically to create compounds that eventually create the protein of hair. To see how they join to form hair, you'll need to learn a little about chemical bonds, starting with amino acids.

Amino Acids

Amino acids are compounds consisting of carbon, oxygen, hydrogen and nitrogen. There are 22 common amino acids. These amino acids join together in chains to become proteins, which provide the chemicals the body needs for growth and repairing tissues.

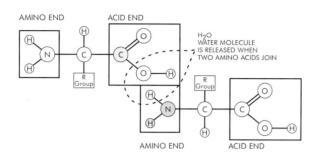

Although amino acids create all proteins, each protein is different because of the way it is put together. **Hair is a form of protein called keratin.** Keratin in hair contains 19 of 22 common amino acids. In fact, **hair is made of 97% keratin protein and 3% trace minerals.**

The chain, or the order in which the amino acids link together, makes each type of protein one of a kind. Also, the number of amino acids in the chain is important. For example, the 19 amino acids found in hair must all be present or the structure won't be hair.

Peptide Bonds (End Bonds)

The amino acids that create protein are linked together end to end by a peptide bond, also known as an end bond. The peptide bond is the backbone of all protein molecules. When two amino acids are positioned end to end, the acid end of one amino acid attaches to the amino end

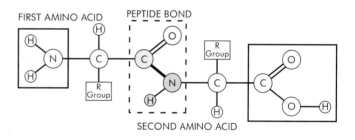

of another amino acid. **The peptide bond forms when these two ends join.** The polypeptide bond ("poly" means many) connects thousands of amino acids lengthwise to form a chain.

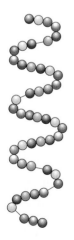

In other words, **hair is the linking together of protein groups.** You, as a stylist, will be altering these links. You need to know how your techniques and tools will affect your client's hair. **It's very important not to disturb peptide bonds.** For instance, if you put a sodium hydroxide relaxer under a hair dryer, **the combination of the alkaline chemicals and heat could break these critical peptide bonds and destroy the protein structure.** If they are broken, the protein chains separate into small fragments, or revert to groups of amino acids that no longer have the characteristics of hair.

Side Bonds

When amino acids combine to form the keratin protein of hair, they take on a spiraling configuration. When these long, spiraling protein chains are placed next to each other, they can be linked together by four side bonds. The four bonds holding protein chains together behave differently and they each serve a different purpose in building hair. The four side bonds created are:

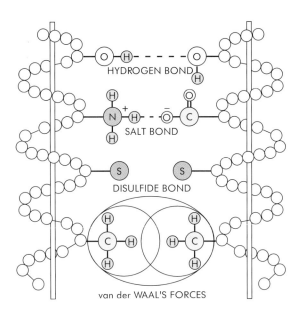

1. The hydrogen bond
2. The salt bond
3. The disulfide bond
4. van der Waal's Forces

When giving chemical services, you are affecting all these bonds. In order to minimize damage to the hair, it is important to understand how the four side bonds work.

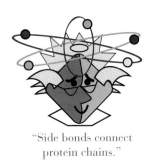

"Side bonds connect protein chains."

The first bond is the **HYDROGEN BOND,** which works on the principle that unlike charges attract. Hydrogen bonding takes place when the hydrogen atom in one molecule is attracted to an atom of another molecule that has many negative electrons. **Hair has many hydrogen bonds, which are individually very weak and can easily be broken by heat or water.** Although the attraction in these hydrogen bonds is weak, there are so many of them in the protein of hair that they tend to organize the protein chains and give hair its shape. **About 35% of the hair's strength is due to the millions of hydrogen bonds in its structure.**

A second type of bond between protein chains is the **SALT BOND**. This bond is also a result of the attraction of unlike charges. The negative charge in one amino acid grouping attracts the positive charge in another amino acid grouping. Salt bonds also help to organize the protein chains. They account for another 35% of the hair's resistance to change and like hydrogen are not particularly strong.

Since both **hydrogen and salt bonds can be weakened by water**, hair can be shampooed, set on rollers and dried by heat into a new shape. **When hair is saturated with water, the hydrogen and salt bonds are weakened, leaving the hair more pliable.** Then, by wrapping it around a roller under tension and drying it, the hair takes on a new shape because new hydrogen and salt bonds are formed between the protein chains. However, this set is only **temporary because exposure to water will break the new bonds. Even the humidity in the air can break the new bonds** and restore the original ones. Styling the hair on rollers or performing a thermal style with blow dryer and curling iron is referred to as a physical change since it is only the physical characteristics of the hair that changes.

The sulfur-containing side bond, the DISULFIDE BOND is the most important to your work. When these sulfur-type side chains join with other sulfur-type side chains, they form the disulfide bond. This bond is a chemical bond that forms between protein structures. A lot of your chemical services, particularly perming and relaxing, directly affect the disulfide bond by either breaking the disulfide bond or reforming it in a new shape. This process is a chemical change and creates lasting results.

The side bond known as **van der Waal's Forces** is based on the theory that atomic groups prefer an environment with other groups that have structures similar to theirs. This type of bonding is not important for your work as a stylist other than to know that it exists and plays a role in bonding protein chains.

5

In Other Words. . .

1. Hair begins with individual atoms, the smallest unit of matter.

2. These atoms unite by sharing electrons to become molecules of amino acids.

3. One end of one amino acid bonds to the opposite end of another amino acid to form the peptide or end bond.

4. The amino acids create polypeptide protein chains.

5. The individual protein chains bond, side-to-side, to other chains by hydrogen bonds, salt bonds, disulfide bonds and van der Waal's Forces.

6. The bonding of protein chains to other protein chains makes human hair.

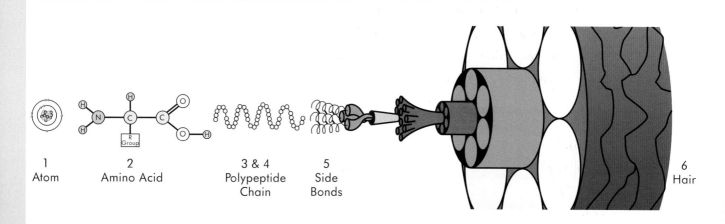

1	2	3 & 4	5	6
Atom	Amino Acid	Polypeptide Chain	Side Bonds	Hair

STAGES OF HAIR FORMATION

THE pH SCALE

pH (potential hydrogen) is a unit of measurement that indicates whether a substance is acidic, neutral or alkaline. Alkaline is sometimes called "base." Just as degrees measure temperature and inches measure distance, **pH numbers measure the amount of acid or alkali in a water-based solution.** As a professional cosmetologist, you need to understand pH and its effects on hair, skin and scalp. This means knowing which products have high or low pH and why. **Only solutions containing water and/or which dissolve in water can have an acidic or alkaline nature.** A solution is acidic or alkaline depending on the number of negative hydroxide ions or positive hydrogen ions it contains (an ion is an atom that has gained or lost electrons). If a solution has more *positive* hydrogen ions than negative hydroxide ions, it is *acidic*. If it has more *negative* hydroxide ions, it is *alkaline*. **When a solution has an equal number of hydrogen and hydroxide ions, it is neutral.**

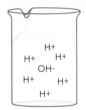

A solution is acidic if it has more positive hydrogen ions than negative hydroxide ions.

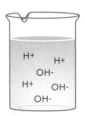

When a solution has an equal number of positive and negative ions, it is neutral.

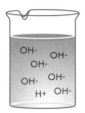

A solution is alkaline if it has more negative hydroxide ions.

The pH measurement scale ranges from 0 to 14 with number 7 as neutral. Numbers less than seven indicate acid while numbers greater than seven indicate alkaline. The scale is **logarithmic**, which means *each step or number increases by multiples of 10.* pH 6 is 10 times more acidic than neutral 7; however, 6 is 10 times less acidic than 5, which falls in the range of the average pH of hair, skin and scalp. So, when you are using products that are pH 6 or "only one number" away from the average pH of hair, it is actually 10 times less acidic. That is a big difference. For example, have you ever peeled an orange and, as the juice from the orange came in contact with your skin, you felt a slight tingle? The pH of an orange is approximately 2, which is 3 steps away from the pH of your skin (4.5 – 5.5).

0 - 6.99 = Acid
7 = Neutral
7.01-14 = Alkaline

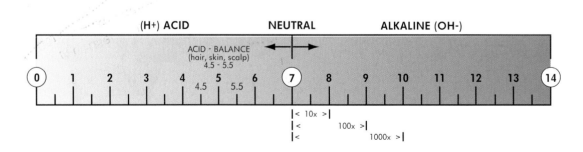

Another type of logarithmic scale is the Richter Scale. This scale measures the power of earthquakes. Using this system of measurement we can see that a 6.2 earthquake is 100 times more powerful than one that measures 4.2. Logarithmic scales enable us to work with very large numbers in a more simplified manner.

At the top of the scale is 14, which is 10 million times more alkaline than 7. As you can see, a very slight variation in pH will greatly affect the acidity of any salon product.

pH balanced and acid balanced are two terms that are sometimes confused in the cosmetology industry. pH balanced means the pH is balanced at a certain number, but not necessarily at 4.5 to 5.5 (average pH range of hair, skin and scalp). **Acid balanced means just that, balanced within the acid range of 4.5 to 5.5.** Acid balanced is the term applied to most professional shampoos and conditioners. Your task as a professional cosmetologist is to use products that will help maintain the acid balance of the hair and skin at the 4.5 to 5.5 acid range level.

Understanding pH measurements and values will greatly assist your ability to keep the hair, skin and scalp in the best condition possible. Reading labels correctly, selecting the right products for clients and recommending products for home hair care will also be based on a good understanding of pH values.

Three methods of testing any product to determine the pH level include pH (Nitrazine) paper, pH pencil or a pH meter. The acid mantle that coats the skin and hair can also be measured with these.

5

ITEM	pH VALUE (approx.)	ACID, ALKALINE OR NEUTRAL
Lemon Juice	2.5	Strong Acid
Diet Cherry Coke	3.0	Weak Acid
Distilled Water	7.0	Neutral
Toothpaste	8.5	Weak Alkaline
Ammonia	12.5	Strong Alkaline

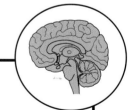

BRAIN BALANCING

Unscramble these words from the pH section for a "brain-balanced" feeling!

oaiiclgthmr   **eiaanlkl**   **cdneaalb**   **dcai**   **eualrtn**   **oedngyrh**

_____   _____   _____   _____   _____   _____

CHEMISTRY OF COSMETICS

The Food and Drug Act of 1938 defines cosmetics as "articles intended to be rubbed, poured, sprinkled, or otherwise applied to the human body or any part thereof for cleansing, beautifying, promoting attractiveness or altering the appearance." As a professional cosmetologist it is important to understand the physical and chemical characteristics of cosmetics in order to better serve your clients.

Cosmetic Classifications

Six general classifications are assigned to categorize cosmetics used in the cosmetology industry. Knowledge of these cosmetic classifications will help you understand product labels and directed use. These classifications are based on how well the substance combines with another as well as the physical characteristics of each. The six classifications are:

1) Solutions   4) Ointments
2) Suspensions   5) Soaps
3) Emulsions   6) Powders

A mixture is two or more substances that are physically combined.

Solutions

Solutions are mixtures of two or more kinds of molecules, evenly dispersed. For example, a solution is made by mixing a package of instant soup and a cup of hot water. The dry soup would be called the solute, which is any substance that dissolves into a liquid and forms a solution.

Water is considered a universal solvent because it is capable of dissolving more substances than any other solvent. Only oil and wax can not be dissolved in water.

The water would be called a solvent, which is any substance that is able to dissolve another substance. The soup would be called the solution. Solutions do not separate when left standing and are generally clear mixtures. Stirring is usually required when dissolving a solute. Solutes can be either solid, liquid or gas. Hydrogen peroxide would be an example of a gas mixed with a liquid to form a solution. There are three classes of solutions:

Dilute solution contains a small quantity of the solute in comparison to the quantity of solvent.

Concentrated solution contains a large quantity of the solute in comparison to the quantity of solvent.

Saturated solution cannot take or dissolve more of the solute than it already holds at a given temperature.

Suspensions

Suspensions are also mixtures of two or more kinds of molecules. Unlike solutions, however, suspensions have a tendency to separate when left standing and therefore need to be shaken before using. An example of a suspension would be vinegar and oil as a salad dressing preparation. If left standing, the mixture of vinegar and oil separates and needs shaking before being used. Many lotions used in the cosmetology industry are suspensions. Calamine lotion is another example.

Emulsions

Emulsions are formed when two or more nonmixable substances (like oil and water) are united with the help of a binder or gum-like substance. The gum-like substance might be a soap. General classifications of emulsions are oil-in-water (perm solutions) and water-in-oil (cold creams). Most emulsions used in the cosmetology industry are classified as oil-in-water.

Immiscible = liquids not able to be mixed

Miscible = liquids able to be mixed together without separating

Ointments

Ointments are mixtures of organic substances and a medicinal agent, usually found in a semi-solid form. Water is generally not present in this mixture. Ointment-type preparations come in the form of sticks (like lipstick), pastes (like some eye shadows or blush) and mucilages (thick liquids, such as styling lotions).

Soaps

Soaps are mixtures of fats and oils converted to fatty acids by heat and then purified. Soaps used in the cosmetology industry generally fall into the categories of deodorant soaps, beauty soaps, medicated soaps and antibacterial soaps.

Powders

Powders are equal mixtures of inorganic and organic substances that do not dissolve in water and that have been sifted and mixed until free of coarse gritty particles. Perfume and shades of color are usually added for purposes of enhancement.

Shampoos

You are now ready to take a look at the chemistry of products and procedures for services in the salon. The natural place to start is with the service most often performed...shampooing. **You shampoo primarily to clean the hair and scalp and to remove all foreign matter, including dirt, sebum (natural scalp oil), cosmetics, hair spray and skin debris without adversely affecting either the scalp or hair.** Shampooing the hair is an important function for the stylist as it is often the first impression the client has of the salon and of the stylist. Shampooing, as part of a salon service, can be a highly therapeutic experience when done in a caring, organized and confident manner. Remember, **the shampoo should be a soothing, relaxing experience, as it sets the climate for all future services.**

Hair should be shampooed as often as necessary depending on how quickly the scalp and hair become soiled. Frequency varies from individual to individual. **Improper or irregular cleansing allows a breeding place for disease-causing bacteria** and can lead to scalp disorders and even hair loss. Generally, oily hair needs to be shampooed more often than normal or dry hair. Strong alkaline shampoos are not recommended as they may make the hair dry and brittle.

How Shampoo Works

Even though the hair fiber beyond the scalp is dead (i.e., biologically inactive), a mixture of secretions from the sebaceous glands and perspiration from the sweat glands helps maintain the hair and scalp at its natural pH of 4.5 to 5.5, allowing a shiny, alive appearance. These scalp secretions can be spread by simply running the fingers through the hair or by brushing or combing. Failure to remove these scalp secretions on a regular basis will allow a build-up of oily film. The oily film is an emulsion, a combination of oil, sweat, dead epidermal cells and dirt particles.

emulsion (ee-**MUL**-shun), n. a substance formed when two or more non-mixable substances, such as oil and water, are united with the aid of a binder or an emulsifier.

Most shampoo is water-based and contains an ingredient known as a **surfactant** or *cleansing agent*. **Surfactants, also called surface active agents, are used to remove oil from the hair.**

A surfactant is necessary because water alone cannot attack and dissolve oil. For example, if you just wet the remains of a greasy dinner plate of spaghetti, the water simply beads up. Once you add soap, the grease breaks up and is easily washed away. It is necessary to add detergents, soaps or other surface active agents (surfactants) to do the job.

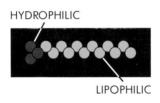

HYDROPHILIC

LIPOPHILIC

The molecule of a surface active agent is a two-part molecule. **It has a water-loving part (hydrophilic) and an oil-loving part (lipophilic).** During a shampoo, the water-loving part is attracted to water, while the oil-loving part is attracted to oil on the hair. The resulting "push-pull" action causes the oil to "roll up" into droplets, which are then lifted into the water and washed away. By removing the oil from the hair shaft and scalp, the water can wet the hair and scalp and the debris can be washed away.

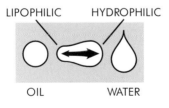

LIPOPHILIC   HYDROPHILIC

OIL   WATER

Some shampoos contain both a surfactant and conditioner. Together they not only cleanse the hair but help condition it as well. These conditioners can contain many ingredients, including hydrolyzed protein derivatives. These derivatives strengthen damaged areas of the hair by depositing protein fragments along the hair shaft.

The Role of Water

Water plays an important part in the success of your shampoo. Water can be classified as either hard or soft, depending on the amount and kinds of minerals present. Hard water contains certain salts of calcium, magnesium

Water is usually the first ingredient listed on most shampoos, which indicates it is the primary ingredient. This is usually pure or deionized water. Remember water is electrically charged, neutral on the pH scale and earns the title of "universal solvent."

Water (H₂O) makes up 85% of the human body and covers 75% of the earth's surface.

and other metals that prevent the shampoo from lathering. It can be softened by a chemical process. Soft water contains very small amounts of minerals and is preferred for shampooing as it lathers more freely.

Water Purification

Sedimentation and filtration are two methods used in the purification of water. During sedimentation undesirable substances, such as clay, sand, etc., sink to the bottom and then during filtration, pass through a porous substance. Chlorine is added to kill bacteria and complete the purification process. Water boiled at a temperature of 212° (100° Celsius) will also destroy most microbic life.

Key points to remember about shampooing:

- The natural pH of hair, 4.5 to 5.5, is maintained by the mixture of secretions from the sebaceous glands and perspiration.
- Shampoos contain surfactants, which remove oil from the hair.
- Hard water contains certain minerals which prevent shampoo from lathering; soft water is preferred due to its low amount of minerals.
- Shampoos should be formulated to conform to the natural pH of the acid mantle of the hair and scalp.

Types of Shampoos

Many varieties of shampoos are available today to the professional stylist. It is important that you familiarize yourself with all of them to learn which will bring the best results to your individual clients. Remember to always read and follow the recommended directions for successful results.

1. **All-purpose shampoos** contain a low alkaline content and a low concentration of surface active agents. They are designed to cleanse the hair without correcting any special condition. They do not strip color and are very mild. Some even include anti-fungus and anti-dandruff agents.

2. **Acid-balanced (non-stripping) shampoos** are formulated to have the same pH as the hair and skin (4.5-5.5) and can be used on almost all types of hair. They are made especially to cleanse chemically treated hair without removing permanent hair coloring or toners. Always use a mild non-stripping shampoo on bleached hair and dry, damaged hair.

3. **"Plain" shampoos** are usually strong and contain a high alkaline or soap base. They can be used successfully on virgin hair in good condition, but are not recommended for chemically treated or damaged hair. When using this type of shampoo, always follow with an acid rinse to restore the acid balance of your client's hair and scalp.

4. **Soapless shampoos** are able to lather without harsh alkaline ingredients. They are made by a process in which the oils from synthetic detergents have been treated with sulfuric acid, resulting in substances known as wetting agents. These soapless shampoos or surfactants are effective in both soft and hard water and rinse out easily.

5. **Medicated shampoos** may be available from your local beauty supply house, but often can be obtained only by prescription from your client's doctor. They contain ingredients designed to treat scalp and hair problems or disorders.

6. **Clarifying shampoos** often have a higher alkalinity in order to be able to remove residue, such as product build-up, dirt, etc.

7. **Anti-dandruff shampoos** are formulated for either a dry or oily scalp and contain an anti-fungus or germicide ingredient and conditioners to control dandruff conditions or other scalp conditions that could breed infections. When using an anti-dandruff shampoo, always follow the manufacturer's directions, massage the scalp vigorously and rinse thoroughly.

8. **Liquid dry shampoos** are used to cleanse the scalp and hair when the client is unable to receive a normal shampoo. The shampoo loosens the dirt and oil from the hair and scalp when applied with saturated cotton. Liquid dry shampoos are effective in cleaning wigs and hairpieces because ordinary shampoos deteriorate the wefting (base material to which the hair is sewn). The basic procedure is to apply the solution to the scalp and small strands of hair, rubbing briskly along each section. Follow the application by blotting with a towel. Any remaining solution will evaporate. Liquid dry shampoos are very drying to the hair and should be used only when necessary. They are highly flammable and should be used with CAUTION. Always use in a well-ventilated room away from open flames or appliances. Never smoke cigarettes or allow clients to smoke when using liquid dry shampoos.

9. **Powder dry shampoos** are formulated for clients who are bedridden and cannot wet their hair. These shampoos contain orris root powder that absorbs soil and oil as the product is brushed through the scalp and hair. After applying the powder, brush it out of the hair with a long-bristled brush until all traces of powder are removed. Between strokes wipe the brush with a clean towel. Do not give a powder dry shampoo before a chemical service.

10. **Conditioning shampoos** contain small amounts of animal, vegetable or mineral additives that penetrate into the cortex or coat the cuticle layer of the hair. These additives can improve the tensile strength and porosity of hair and will usually be removed with the next shampoo. Protein substances found in penetrating shampoos/conditioners can last through several shampoos.

11. **Color shampoos** contain temporary color molecules that adhere to the outer cuticle of the hair and deposit color. The effects of these shampoos, available in enhancing and vivid colors, last from shampoo to shampoo.

12. **Shampoos for thinning hair** are formulated as gentle shampoos, with a lighter molecular weight that does not cause damage or weigh hair down. These shampoos may also contain ingredients to provide a healthy environment for the maximum amount of hair growth.

This wide variety of shampoos has one desired result – a satisfied customer with healthy hair. It is essential for you, as a cosmetologist, to realize that not all shampoos that claim pH balance are necessarily acid balanced. An acid-balanced shampoo has the natural 4.5-5.5 pH of the hair and scalp. If the natural acidic conditions are maintained during a shampoo, the cuticle scales are kept in a more compact state and therefore a minimal amount of swelling of the cuticle fibers occurs. Hair is strongest at a pH of 4.5-5.5 because it is compact and least swollen. If the pH of a shampoo is too alkaline (or too acidic), the hair fiber can swell. This swelling weakens the hair, making it more susceptible to other forms of distress, such as dryness and cuticle damage. Strong, compact hair is more pleasing in appearance and easier to manage.

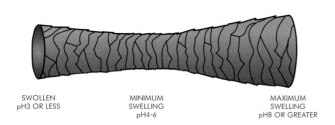

SWOLLEN
pH3 OR LESS

MINIMUM
SWELLING
pH4-6

MAXIMUM
SWELLING
pH8 OR GREATER

5

Rinses and Conditioners

Shiny hair...healthy hair...hair in optimum condition is rarely seen in today's salons. Hair's chemical composition is changed with perm and color services. Bonds are broken that can never be rejoined. Hair becomes chemically and mechanically damaged through daily care. The tools of your profession - thermal styling irons, blow dryers, teasing combs, brushes and even rollers - can cause a degree of damage. Other factors that can affect hair condition are the environment and products such as alkaline shampoos. Once the natural bonds in the hair are broken, nothing can be done to actually reconnect them and repair the hair.

As a stylist, it is your responsibility to be aware of products that can strengthen hair, add body and protect it from further damage. Scientists have formulated products that can smooth rough hair cuticles, add protein molecules to the hair shaft and add humectants (moisturizers) to replace moisture to dry hair. It is important for you to investigate these products, to help your clients' hair to be as cosmetically pleasing as possible and to prepare their hair properly for chemical services. To achieve this, it is important for you to know why and when each product type is used and the results you can expect to achieve.

COSMETIC APPEARANCE is the luster or shine of the hair. If the layers of the outer cuticle stand away from the hair shaft, the hair will appear rough and dull.

POROSITY refers to the amount of moisture the individual hair strand can absorb.

MANAGEABILITY is determined by how easily a comb can pass through wet or dry hair.

ELASTICITY is the ability of the hair to stretch and return to its natural shape without breaking. Healthy hair can be stretched about 50% when wet and up to 40% when dry. Tensile strength measures the amount of tension that can be applied before the hair breaks.

Rinses

Rinses affect mostly the surface of the hair. Rinses are usually applied to the hair and rinsed off immediately. They sometimes leave a coating that surrounds each hair strand. Some rinses can actually be detrimental to the hair because they contain ingredients that "build up" on the hair's surface. This "build up" can make the hair feel limp, attract dirt and make it difficult to control. Rinses are applied to the hair to help close the cuticle and make hair feel soft and manageable.

There are several superior rinses available in the marketplace today. Many rinses (and conditioners) are formulated for specific types of hair by chemists who have made a science of the study of hair. At one time, however, all rinses had to be painstakingly prepared by the salon or the consumer "at home." Rinses you should be familiar with include:

1. **Vinegar and lemon (acid) rinses** help keep the cuticle compact. The vinegar rinse is mixed by using two tablespoons of white vinegar with a pint of tepid water. Lemon rinse uses the strained juice of two lemons or 15 drops of concentrated lemon extract. Adjust with water to a pH 4.5-5.5. Acid rinses usually have a very low pH (2-3) and are designed to dissolve soap scum and curds, untangle and separate the hair and add sheen. Soap scum, caused by the combination of the minerals in the water and the fatty acids of soap, is the residue remaining on the surface of the hair after shampooing. An acid rinse can also be used to counteract the alkalinity present after a chemical service.

2. **Creme rinses** soften and add luster, making tangled hair easier to comb. A creme rinse is creamy in appearance and adheres to the hair shaft, even after ordinary rinsing, thus leaving the hair with a soft feel and much easier to comb and handle. Creme rinses are only slightly acidic and do not have the same function as acid rinses. In selecting a creme rinse, be sure to select one with a proper pH level for your needs.

3. **Medicated rinses** are designed with ingredients that control minor dandruff and scalp conditions. They can usually be applied with cotton or poured over the scalp followed by a one-minute scalp massage, but be sure to follow manufacturer's instructions. Their active ingredients, such as benazlkonium chloride, lauryl isoquinolinium bromide and polysorbate leave the hair lustrous and manageable.

Conditioners

Conditioning is an important step in your client's hair needs. Sometimes a client's hair may be in great condition and only require a rinse to smooth the cuticle. But in many cases the hair has been dried out and damaged by strong alkaline shampoos, chemical damage or heat styling. Any amount of heat can damage the cuticle layer over time, leaving a rough, dry feeling. In these cases, a conditioning treatment may be needed.

Conditioners usually penetrate deep into the hair so they are formulated differently from rinses. In order to achieve maximum penetration, they are usually kept on the hair for a specific length of time.

The length of time a conditioner should be left on the hair depends on its formulation and purpose. Sometimes the addition of heat is recommended to open the cuticle, which allows for better penetration. Read the manufacturer's instructions before applying.

Remember, hair "damage" generally refers to bonds (disulfide, etc.) that have been broken through the application of chemical services or thermal styling. Conditioners don't actually repair broken bonds, but rather fortify the damaged areas of the hair and protect it against further damage from chemical services or heat. They may also alter the way hair behaves, giving it less stretch or reducing the relaxation of a set. Conditioners provide a temporary remedy for existing hair problems.

1. **Instant conditioners** coat the hair shaft and restore moisture and oils, but do not penetrate into the cortex or replace keratin in the shaft. Instant conditioners usually have a vegetable oil base, an acidic pH and are not recommended for fine and limp hair. They are generally left on the hair for 1-2 minutes, then rinsed off.

2. **Normalizing conditioners** also usually contain a vegetable protein and have an acidic pH which causes the cuticle to close after alkaline chemical services. They are generally applied for approximately 2 minutes and rinsed off.

3. **Body-building conditioners** are required when hair is fine and limp and contains too much moisture to maintain a good style. The formula, with protein, will penetrate into the damaged hair shaft and deposit proteins into the cortex. The proteins displace the excess moisture, providing more body to the hair. This modifies the delicate moisture/protein balance and makes the hair more manageable and able to hold a style for a longer period of time. Protein conditioners may be used before chemical services to help ensure their success. They are usually left on about 10 minutes. However, always follow manufacturer's instructions.

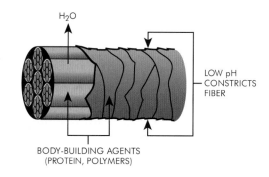

H₂O

LOW pH
CONSTRICTS
FIBER

BODY-BUILDING AGENTS
(PROTEIN, POLYMERS)

4. **Moisturizing conditioners** contain hydrolyzed animal proteins and are recommended for dry, brittle hair that has been mechanically or chemically damaged. The humectants (moisturizing ingredients) in a moisturizing conditioner will penetrate into each hair shaft to bind and hold moisture in the hair. These conditioners form a thin film on the cuticle, acting as a barrier to keep moisture from escaping. Moisturizing conditioners should not be used for several days after a perm or it will go limp. Follow manufacturer's directions for the length of time to leave on the hair after shampooing.

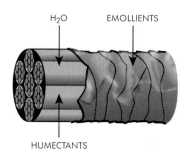

H₂O   EMOLLIENTS

HUMECTANTS

5. **Customized conditioners** are formulated to meet special needs. When a client's hair requires a combination of moisturizing and body-building properties, you may customize the

treatment, mixing a moisturizing conditioner with a body-building protein product to improve the condition of your client's hair.

Ingredients for Conditioners

Most protein conditioners are derived from animal or vegetable materials, and a few come from minerals. A common animal protein found in conditioners is bovine serum, a refined and sterilized cattle tissue such as blood and bone marrow. The refined placenta of female cattle and sheep and collagen are also popular animal proteins found in hair conditioners.

The vegetable proteins found in conditioners are usually made from soybeans, balsam trees, olives, wheat germ and tong beans. These vegetable and animal proteins are refined through a very complex method (with various combinations of chemicals into the formulation of a conditioner). A conditioner need not contain protein. However, since hair is largely made up of protein, it becomes the logical choice and a major component in most conditioning products.

Additional ingredients found in conditioners include:

- **Amines/Quats** make hair easier to comb and control static.
- **Dimethicones** give softness to the feel of hair without weighing it down. They are a form of silicone.
- **Fatty alcohols** and acids give hair a smooth feel when dry and make it easier to comb. Fatty alcohols are creamy in texture and help retain moisture.

Conditioners should be used sparingly and only when necessary for clients with fine, thin hair. However, a heavier conditioner may be needed for thick or curly hair. In some cases, a leave-in product may be used to help control curl and waves. Some clients may be concerned that using a conditioner will make their hair "too soft" or "weigh it down." Just remember, the right conditioner for each client should provide the needed result, great looking, healthy and well-conditioned hair.

Perms

The three major chemical services, perm (also known as permanent waving), chemical relaxing and hair color, are covered in depth in each respective chapter of Unit 2. In this section of Chemistry, you are given an overview of the information that pertains to the chemical ingredients with which you will be working when performing these services. Preparation guidelines and complete procedures for perm services begin on page 446.

Perms allow stylists to chemically reform hair into a wavy or curly formation.

- First the client's hair is wrapped around perm tools chosen to reflect the desired curl pattern.
- Then, a processing lotion (also called waving lotion) is applied to break disulfide bonds. This softens the protein structure and allows the protein chains to assume the shape of the perm tool.

Original Straight Hair

- Rinsing removes the processing lotion.

- A second chemical, the neutralizer (also called rebonding lotion), reforms the disulfide bonds into the new configuration. The resulting chemical change in the hair holds the hair in its new position.

Perms fall into two primary categories:

1. Alkaline waves (cold waves), which are processed *without* heat and have a pH of approximately 8.0-9.5.

2. Acid waves (heat waves), which are processed *with* heat and must be wrapped with tension. Acid waves have an approximate pH of 6.9 to 7.2.

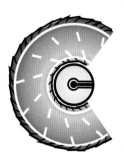

Shifting and breaking of disulfide bonds

The main chemical ingredient found in alkaline waves is *thioglycolic acid* **or its derivatives and ammonium hydroxide.** *Ammonium hydroxide* **is added to the formula to shorten the processing time.** It is also responsible for the swelling that occurs during this process, which makes it easier for the thioglycolic acid to penetrate the hair structure and break the disulfide bonds. Processing begins as soon as the chemical has been applied to the hair.

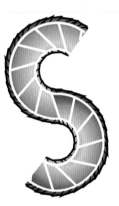

Disulfide bonds reformed

The main chemical ingredient found in **acid waves** is *glyceryl monothioglyco-late*. In acid waving, speed is sacrificed for a more controlled curl and less damage to the hair when procedures are carefully followed. Heat is sometimes used to assist in the penetration of the hair structure.

The main ingredient found in most neutralizers (or bonding lotions) is either hydrogen peroxide, sodium perborate, or sodium bromate. All three of these ingredients can cause additional damage to the hair if left on longer than specified by the manufacturer.

Relaxers

Just as a perm adds curl and body to hair by changing its molecular structure, a chemical relaxer reduces curl in excessively curly or wavy hair by changing its molecular structure.

- The reforming (relaxing) product, which is usually formulated in a heavy cream base, is applied to the hair and holds the hair in a straight position while it is being processed. In addition a smoothing or pressing action is applied to the softened hair, causing the entire protein structure to relax to the straighter position.

- The neutralizing (bonding) step utilizes a neutralizing shampoo or lotion to reduce the swelling caused by alkaline formulas. This chemical change causes the hair to be held in the new straight configuration.

There are two popular types of products used to chemically relax hair:

1. Sodium hydroxide type - formulated with 2% to 3% sodium hydroxide in a heavy cream base with an alkaline pH of anywhere from 10.5 to 14.

2. Ammonium thioglycolate type - formulated with 4% to 6% thioglycolic acid or its derivatives with 1% ammonium hydroxide and an 8.8 to 9.5 pH. A cream base is also usually added.

It is important to remember that the chemical action of sodium hydroxide is irreversible. Once the bond has been broken in this manner, it cannot be reformed. The straightened hair must grow out before additional chemical services can be performed.

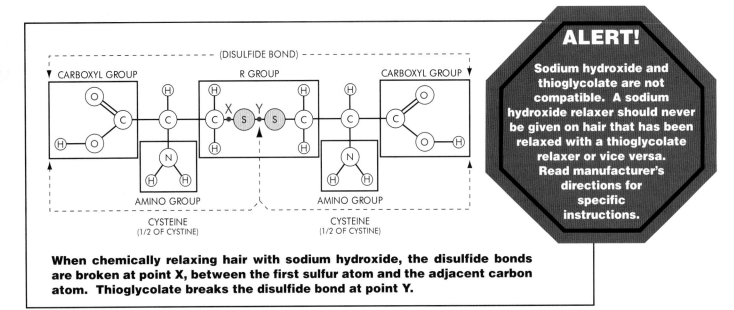

ALERT!

Sodium hydroxide and thioglycolate are not compatible. A sodium hydroxide relaxer should never be given on hair that has been relaxed with a thioglycolate relaxer or vice versa. Read manufacturer's directions for specific instructions.

When chemically relaxing hair with sodium hydroxide, the disulfide bonds are broken at point X, between the first sulfur atom and the adjacent carbon atom. Thioglycolate breaks the disulfide bond at point Y.

Curl Reformation

A soft curl perm (which will be referred to as curl reformation or curls) is a service used to loosen the texture of overly curly hair. The hair is first smoothed into a relaxed shape by using the back of a comb and fingers combined with the application of a thioglycolate-based product in a gel or cream form. Once the hair has achieved a straightened shape, the thioglycolate product is rinsed from the hair. A curl booster is applied and perm rods are used to achieve the curl formation. **Once the test curl displays the desired curl formation, the hair is rinsed and a neutralizing (bonding) lotion is applied to reform (fix) the curl into a lasting shape.**

The chemical change that occurs with this service is the same as in a perm service. **The application of the processing solution prior to wrapping the hair on perm rods serves to soften and rearrange the disulfide bonds. The chemical rearranger is rinsed before a complete relaxation (straightening) of the hair takes place, allowing the disulfide bonds to take on the shape of the selected perm rod.**

Extreme care must be taken during this service to ensure satisfactory results. **Extended processing time, combined with dual application of processing solution can damage the hair.** Follow manufacturer's directions closely.

Hair Color

Manufacturers create an array of colors and lighteners that give the stylist the ability to create subtle to dramatic hair color changes. Haircolor products fall into the following general categories:

- Nonoxidative Color
- Oxidative Color
- Lighteners
- Developers
- Vegetable, Metallic and Compound Dyes

> **Oxidants (often called developers) are products that have the ability to release oxygen, which is needed for a chemical change. Oxidative colors are mixed with an oxidant (developer) such as hydrogen peroxide. Nonoxidative colors are not mixed with oxidants and are used straight from the bottle. In the oxidation process a substance loses an electron and oxygen is acquired. When a substance gains an electron and oxygen is released the process is called reduction. This process not only occurs in hair color services, but in perming/relaxing services as well.**

Nonoxidative Colors

1. **Temporary Colors** are non-reactive, direct dyes that only coat the surface of the hair shaft. There's nothing to lighten the hair and no chemical changes occur in the solution. These colors are called certified colors and are accepted by the government for use in foods, drugs and cosmetics. Temporary colors last only until they are shampooed out.

2. **Semi-permanent colors** last through several shampoos, then the color molecules generally shampoo out. Semi-permanent colors are dye molecules in a solution that are able to penetrate the cuticle layer of the hair versus coating the hair shaft as with temporary colors. Semi-permanent color molecules are smaller in size and weight than the molecules found in temporary color products, and they are slightly alkaline in pH. Semi-permanent colors use a direct dye process, which means the color is present without the need to chemically develop it. Direct dye colors need no mixing and the color you see in the bottle is the color that is deposited on the hair.

Oxidative Colors

1. **Long lasting semi-permanent colors** (sometimes referred to as demi-permanent or oxidative without ammonia) use a low volume peroxide to develop the color molecules and aid in the color depositing. Ammonia is a colorless gas with a strong odor, composed of hydrogen and nitrogen. Peroxide alone does not lift color from the hair. It needs an alkaline substance such as ammonia to lift color. Therefore, long lasting semi-permanent or demi-permanent colors are only able to add color to the hair. They cannot subtract, lift or lighten. Long lasting semi-permanent colors are available in liquid, cream and gel forms.

2. **Permanent hair colors** (sometimes referred to as oxidative with ammonia) use an oxidation system that starts out with colorless molecules. When these molecules are combined with peroxide, a chemical reaction (change) occurs, building colored molecules. The small molecules enter the hair with the aid of an alkaline substance such as ammonia and then, as they oxidize in the cuticle and the cortex, they link together to form a permanent colored molecule. When this happens, they are permanently anchored in the hair. It is the combination of the ammonia and hydrogen peroxide that is also responsible for the permanent color's ability to both lighten the hair's natural color and deposit artificial color.

Permanent hair colors are also referred to as analine derivative tints. These colors penetrate the cuticle and the cortex, remaining in the hair until they are removed by chemical means or the hair grows out and is cut off. Their primary ingredient is usually paraphenylene diamine or a related chemical. It's usually possible to reproduce human hair shades without losing shine or condition when using an analine derivative color. Analine derivative colors can safely be applied over hair that has been previously permed or colored.

ALERT!
Because allergies to analine tints are unpredictable, manufacturer labels prescribe a patch test to be given 24 hours before any application.

Lighteners

Lightening the hair is also referred to as bleaching or decolorizing. It is one of the oldest methods used in a hair color service. Before permanent tints were formulated to lift and deposit color in one application, bleaching was the first step to any permanent hair coloring service in which lighter hair was desired.

Lightening hair always involves oxidation of the natural melanin in the hair. Oxidation in the lightening process means that peroxide is mixed with an alkaline product such as ammonia. The release of oxygen from the peroxide chemically alters other molecules, changes the melanosome (pigment) structure of the hair and lightens the color of the hair. It does this by breaking down pigment granules into tiny fragments that are no longer able to absorb light to the same degree as they did before. The longer this lightening solution remains in contact with the hair, the more the melanin is changed. This process is called oxidation. The melanin doesn't immediately lose its color when oxidized. The hair goes through several color changes as the pigment disperses and each change lightens the hair to a new level.

Lighteners or bleaches are made up of a combination of ingredients including an alkaline substance such as ammonia. Some also contain conditioning and thickening agents for control in application. They need to be mixed with peroxide immediately before application because only then is the oxidation process at full strength. The solution quickly begins to weaken.

1. **On-the-scalp lighteners** are gentle enough to be applied directly on the scalp and are available in two forms.

   Oil lighteners use a certain amount of ammonia to give high lift. Because of the added oil, this is a mild form of lightener. For this reason it can be used directly on the scalp with no ill effects. When mixed with peroxide, its pH is around 9.

   Cream lighteners are the most popular form of lightener because added conditioners make them gentler and the creamy consistency keeps them in place on the hair and

prevents running or dripping. They are also used directly on the scalp. Their pH is about the same as that of the oil lighteners.

Activators can be added to oil or cream lighteners to boost their strength. These activators increase the pH of a lightener toward the alkaline side, thus increasing the speed of the oxidation process. The pH is increased by chemicals called alkali salts and persulfates. Since activators can double the strength of hydrogen peroxide, no higher than 20 volume is recommended when mixing for an on-the-scalp application.

2. **Off-the-scalp lighteners** (powder bleaches) contain alkaline salts and a strong oxidizing agent that, when mixed with peroxide, become a strong lightening product. These lighteners are much stronger than the oil or cream lighteners and lighten the hair faster.** Because they have no added oils or cream, they can irritate the scalp causing burns and blisters. For this reason they are usually used for off-the-scalp lightening procedures such as highlighting.

Conditioning agents provide some protection to the scalp and the hair, however. Some off-the-scalp bleach powders have protein conditioning agents that help prevent chemical damage to the hair during the lightening process. This type of powder bleach has a distinct advantage over ones that do not contain conditioning agents. During the bleaching process, the conditioner can protect the hair's internal protein structure and the surface of each hair shaft. The pH of powder lighteners when applied to the hair is about 10.3.

Developers

Hydrogen peroxide (H_2O_2) is the most common developer or oxidizing agent used in hair coloring and in hair lightening. It is mixed in various proportions and various strengths. The strength most often used is a 20 volume solution. Volumes refer to the amount of oxygen gas that would be removed from a peroxide solution if **the molecule was broken into its components, water and oxygen. Hydrogen peroxide is also called a developer or oxidizing agent** because permanent colors require peroxide to develop their color molecules. Peroxide comes in different forms such as clear, cloudy, creamy and gels. Its pH is between 2.5 and 4.5.

In hair lightening, ammonia or other alkalis are used to activate or raise the peroxide's pH, therefore making it more alkaline. Once activated by the higher pH substance, the peroxide can then act as an oxidizer and lift or subtract hair color.

A hydrometer is used to measure the strength (volume) of hydrogen peroxide. A hydrometer indicates the potency (strength) of hydrogen peroxide and allows you to dilute higher strength liquid peroxide to lower volumes. A hydrometer is also beneficial if there is a question about whether hydrogen peroxide that has been stored over a long period of time is still potent. Manufacturer recommendations will indicate **shelf life (usually 3 years) of hydrogen peroxide and instruct that it be stored in a cool, dry place.**

Vegetable, Metallic and Compound Dyes

A less professional category of hair color includes natural vegetable dyes, metallic salts and the combination of the two called a compound dye. Henna is an example of a vegetable dye and, in its purest form, produces reddish highlights in the hair. It is one of the oldest forms of hair coloring and is derived from the Egyptian privett plant. Natural colors other than the characteristic henna reds are produced by combining henna with metallic salts, such as lead, silver and copper. There are problems when using henna and henna compounds because repeated use coats and builds up, causing damage to the hair.

The more these colors are used the more color change takes place. For this reason these dyes are called progressive colors. Hennaed hair sometimes cannot be permed because the reforming solution can't penetrate evenly through the buildup. In addition, the metals in a henna compound may react violently with other chemicals used in salon chemical services causing hair breakage or discoloration. There are certain formulas designed to remove henna build-up, but they are not very effective. The best solution is to let it grow completely out before any chemical service.

Pure metallic dyes seem relatively harmless but can also cause complications. They too are incompatible with other chemical services such as perms and oxidative hair coloring. These colors, depending on the metals used, may fade into peculiar or unnatural shades. With exposure to the sun and chlorine, silver dyes may appear to have a green cast, lead dyes a purple cast, and copper may turn green. Metallic coatings have a tendency to look and feel dry.

Metallic colors can be purchased over the counter at local drug stores or supermarkets. Some clients might not know they are using metallic dyes. That makes the consultation before chemical services very important. If you suspect that your client has used metallic colors and doesn't know it, perform the test for metallic salts featured in Haircoloring, Chapter 13. Metallic dyes are toxic and both you and your client should wash your hands thoroughly after exposure.

Product Information

The understanding of specific ingredients in the products you use and what effects they have will mark you as an above ordinary stylist. Material Safety Data Sheets from the manufacturer are the best source of specific information about a product. Additional resources can include the Federal Drug Administration (FDA), which regulates cosmetics in the United States, and the United States Pharmacopeia (U.S.P.), which is a book that lists and standardizes drugs. Information can also be found in the International Cosmetic Ingredient Dictionary, which is published by the Cosmetic, Toiletries and Fragrance Association and is available at many public libraries.

Cosmetic Ingredients

When you read a product label, the ingredients are listed in order of their concentration. The first ingredient on the list appears in the largest amount and so on. At present, the cosmetic industry selects from more than 5000 different ingredients. Here are some common ingredients and their usual function:

MOISTURIZERS function as a moisture barrier or to attract moisture from the environment:

- Cetyl alcohol (fatty alcohol) - keeps oil and water from separating; also a foam booster
- Dimethicone silicone - skin condition and anti-foam ingredient
- Isopropyl lanolate, myristate, and palmitate
- Lanolin and lanolin alcohols and oil - used in skin and hair conditioners
- Octyl dodecanol - skin conditioner
- Oleic acid (olive oil)
- Panthenol (vitamin B-complex derivative) - hair conditioner
- Stearic acid and stearyl alcohol

PRESERVATIVES and antioxidants (including vitamins) prevent product deterioration:

- Trisodium and tetrasodium edetate (EDTA)
- Tocopherol (vitamin E)

ANTIMICROBIALS fight bacteria:

- Butyl, propyl, ethyl, and methyl parabens
- DMDM hydantoin
- Methylisothiazolinone
- Phenoxyethanol (also rose ether fragrance component)
- Quaternium-15

THICKENERS and waxes used in stick products such as lipsticks:

- Candelilla, carnauba, and microcrystalline waxes
- Carbomer and polyethylene thickeners

SOLVENTS used to dilute:

- Butylene glycol and propylene glycol
- Cyclomethicone (volatile silicone)
- Ethanol (alcohol)
- Glycerin

EMULSIFIERS break up and refine:

- Glyceryl monostearate (also pearlescent agent)
- Lauramide DEA (also foam booster)
- Polysorbates

COLOR additives:

- Synthetic ORGANIC colors derived from coal and petroleum sources (not permitted for use around the eye):

  D&C Red No. 7 Calcium Lake (lakes are dyes that do not dissolve in water)

- INORGANIC pigments - approved for general use in cosmetics, including for the area of the eye:

  iron oxides
  mica (iridescent)

HAIRCOLOR - phenol derivatives used in combination with other chemicals in permanent hair colors:

- Aminophenols

pH ADJUSTERS stabilize or adjust acids and bases:

- Ammonium hydroxide in skin peels and hair waving and straightening
- Citric acid - adjusts pH
- Triethanolamine pH adjuster used mostly in transparent soap

OTHERS:

- Magnesium aluminum silicate - absorbent, anti-caking agent
- Polymers and plasticizers - hair stiffening agents used in hair sprays
- Silica (silicon dioxide) - absorbent, anti-caking, abrasive
- Sodium lauryl sulfate - detergent
- Stearic acid - cleansing, emulsifier
- Talc (powdered magnesium silicate) - absorbent anti-caking
- Zinc stearate - used in powder to improve texture, lubricates.

U. S. Food and Drug Administration
Center for Food Safety and Applied Nutrition
Office of Cosmetics Fact Sheet
February 3, 1995

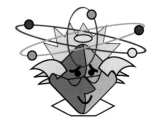

"Did you know that hair sprays contain polymers. One type is also used to glue the layers of wood in plywood together!"

Salon Products and Their pH Ranges

Today's professional cosmetologist needs to understand the pH of the chemicals they use and its effects on hair, skin and nails. Remember that there are three ways of testing pH in professional products: nitrazine paper, pH pencil and the pH meter.

Nitrazine paper, or pH paper, is one of the most familiar methods. To use this testing method, just dip the paper into the solution. A product with a 4.5 pH or below will not change the paper from its original yellow shade, while a higher pH will change the color to dark blue (4.6 - 7.4). Any product with a pH of more than 7.5 will turn the paper purple.

The pH pencil can be used in several ways. One way is to rub the pencil all over a small sheet of paper. Now you can dip the paper into the solution. It will turn yellow if the solution is acidic, or purple if the solution is alkaline.

The pH meter provides the most accurate method for measuring pH because it registers the exact pH of the product. It can also measure the pH of the acid mantle that coats the skin and hair.

Remember that products in the pH range of 4.5 - 5.5 will keep hair, skin and nails closest to their natural, healthy state. When using alkaline products, it is important to restore the acid balance once the service is complete. Keep in mind that in order for a product to have a pH rating or be tested for pH it must contain water and/or have the ability to dissolve in water. The chart below identifies general pH ranges for common professional hair, skin and nail products.

5

SHAMPOOS AND CONDITIONERS

Acid-Balanced Shampoo	4.5 -	5.5
Alkaline Shampoo	7.0 -	9.0
Acidifying Conditioner	2.2 -	5.5
Deep Penetrating Conditioner	3.5 -	5.5

PERMS AND RELAXERS

Acid Perm	6.9 -	7.2
Alkaline Perm	8.0 -	9.5
Relaxer	11.5 -	14.0
Neutralizer	3.0 -	7.0

COLORS AND LIGHTENERS

Oil Bleach	8.0 -	9.5
Powder Bleach	10.0 -	11.0
Tints	9.5 -	10.5
Hydrogen Peroxide	below 4.0	

FINISHING PRODUCTS

Mousse	5.5 -	6.0
Gel	4.5 -	5.5
Hair Spray	5.0 -	6.0

SKIN PRODUCTS

Cleanser	4.5 -	5.5
Toner	5.5 -	6.0
Moisturizer	5.5 -	6.0

NAIL PRODUCTS

Polish Remover	5.0 -	6.0
Cuticle Creme	5.5 -	6.0
Hand Lotion	4.5 -	5.5

ACTIVITY

Under the direction of your teacher, test various products you bring from home using nitrazine paper. Compare the results with those identified on the chart on the previous page.

Health Risks

Possible health effects of chemicals you work with depend on the following:

- The amount of the chemical in the product
- Its toxicity
- The length of time you are exposed
- How the chemical enters your body
- Your own individual sensitivity

Check each product's Material Safety Data Sheet (MSDS) for more information.

As a professional cosmetologist you will be using a variety of chemicals to improve the personal well-being of your clients. Your knowledge of the proper use of these chemicals will be necessary as you provide a safe and comfortable experience for client visits and for your personal health.

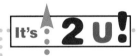

Build Your Critical Thinking Skills

In this chapter you have prepared yourself to meet the following Industry Standards for entry-level cosmetologists:

- Safely use a variety of salon products while providing client services

It's Up to You to know what to do. Using your training to this point, review the following case scenario and think through how you would handle the challenge.

You have just finished a consultation with your client and have determined that three months ago the client received a thioglycolate relaxer service. The client was not satisfied with the results and would like a service that would allow a straighter result. You feel that a sodium hydroxide product would be the best product for you to achieve the results the client expect. What would you do?

Chapter 6
SALON BUSINESS

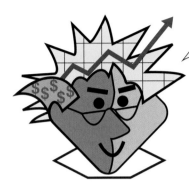

After studying this chapter you will be able to . . .

1. Establish short and long range personal goals within the beauty industry.

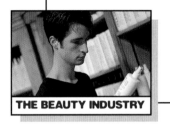

THE BEAUTY INDUSTRY

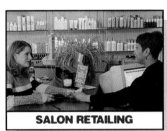

SALON RETAILING

5. Define the techniques used to recommend retail product sales to clients.

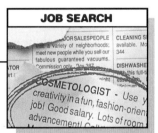

JOB SEARCH

2. Identify which job offer to accept by recognizing:
   • The steps necessary to search for a job
   • Questions to be asked during a job interview
   • Personal qualities that will be evaluated during the interview
   • Potential job benefits that an employer might offer.

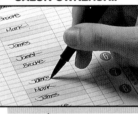

SALON OWNERSHIP

4. Describe salon ownership types, structure, operations and requirements for the practice of good business.

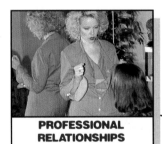

PROFESSIONAL RELATIONSHIPS

3. List the steps used to develop and maintain professional relationships, including building a clientele.

With this final chapter of Unit 1, you and I have come full circle. Doesn't it seem a long time ago that we first met and began "Salon Fundamentals" with Professional Development. Then we traveled through important theoretical considerations for our profession – Salon Ecology, Anatomy and Physiology, Electricity, Chemistry. Now we reach another significant part of your development as a professional, the business aspects of salon life.

Selecting the right salon environment for your employment will allow you to offer the best possible service and products to the clients you serve and will in turn allow you to feel proud of yourself and the profession you have chosen.

This chapter's VALUE probably leaps right out at you. It contains so many things you've been wondering about and wanting to know about your future: how to get that all-important first job, how to keep it, how to become a valued asset to both your clients and your salon team members. The BIG IDEA pulls all these areas together for your greatest personal, financial and professional good.

The ability to select the right salon and knowledge of salon business will ensure financial rewards and personal and professional growth and developement.

The PLAN I have for you here is a lengthy one, as you can see. Most of it, though, is so close to the heart of what you need to know that it should give you very little trouble. Let's get on with the business at hand, shall we?

THE BEAUTY INDUSTRY
What You Need to Know
Your Personal Goals

JOB SEARCH
Resumes
Job Interviews
Evaluating the Salon

PROFESSIONAL RELATIONSHIPS
Networking
Building a Clientele
The Stylist-Client Relationship
The Stylist-Staff Relationship
Performance Review

SALON OWNERSHIP
Self-Appraisal
Types of Salon Ownership
Requirements of a Salon
Getting the Right Advice
Space Requirements and Floor Plans
Borrowing Money
Rental Agreements
Types of Insurance
Taxes
Expenses and Income
Salon Philosophy, Policies and Procedures
Salon Operation

SALON RETAILING
Selling
Professional Products
Closing the Sale
Buyer Types
Follow Up
Effective Displays

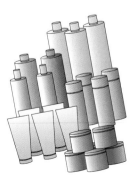

THE BEAUTY INDUSTRY

More than any time in its history, the cosmetology profession is growing and prospering. A new powerful energy and enthusiasm have elevated the cosmetology profession. Today the customer depends on and seeks out the advice of the expert stylist. The stylist is no longer a beauty "operator," but an artistic business professional, offering solutions and creativity on behalf of the client.

What You Need to Know

It takes more than styling talent to be successful in today's cosmetology world. You'll need to be knowledgeable in many areas of business, including communications, public relations and sales promotions. The areas in which you choose to develop your expertise will shape your career's future.

Your future will also be affected by today's constantly changing lifestyle. These changes have created an increasing demand for the services of the cosmetologist. Today's fast-paced lifestyle has resulted in an increased awareness of good grooming habits and the popularization of many new products. Several hair, skin, and nail care products have now become so important to our everyday life that they have actually become household names, such as mousse, gel, etc.

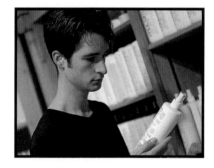

Another important reason for the popularization of specific products is "consumerism." That is, most people have become label readers. They regularly analyze the contents and quality of the products they purchase. They have also become more discriminating in their purchases. They have likes and dislikes and will not accept second best.

Because of these changes, there is an increasing demand for your advice. Manufacturers, distributors and industry organizations conduct and sponsor educational seminars, clinics and training programs designed to upgrade your technical and business skills and product knowledge on a regular basis. These educational events will give you a very important edge that will help you stay ahead in all aspects of the professional beauty business. Remember, the cosmetology industry changes quickly and so must you. Shared knowledge and creativity travel worldwide with a flick of a television switch or the click of a computer mouse.

At no other time in history has a career in the cosmetology field been more attractive or lucrative than today. The public continues to bestow well-earned respect, prestige and rewards on those who strive to be the best. Through the services you perform, you can take pride in your contributions to society and your unique artistic creations. You can be both a business person and an artist.

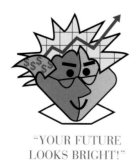

"YOUR FUTURE LOOKS BRIGHT!"

Your Personal Goals

Successful people in all professions create goals for themselves. A goal states and defines what path your career will take. You may want to own a salon...become a platform artist...teach in a school...or anything else that appeals to you. Your goals will motivate you on a daily, monthly and yearly basis. Listed below are four easy-to-follow guides that will help you determine your goals.

Establish a long-range goal. It identifies where you want your career to be in five years.

- Write it down.
- Discuss with someone that has accomplished a similar goal the obstacles that you might encounter.
- Make a commitment to yourself to dedicate your actions toward the goal.

Determine your short-range goals. They identify what you would like to achieve in the next year.

- Decide on immediate activities you can undertake to achieve this short-range goal. Examples would include job interviews, part-time work in a salon, etc.

Create a plan to achieve your goals.

- Be specific as you create a set of objectives and tasks. Examples would include continuing education, saving five dollars per week, etc.
- Consider your budget and include ways to support the plan financially.
- Include alternate plans.

Review your goals periodically and change them if they no longer reflect your chosen personal and professional life directions.

- This is where alternate plans come into play. You may need to save ten dollars per week or attend more seminars than you originally planned.

JOB SEARCH

Searching for a job can be an exciting and rewarding experience. As your search progresses, you'll be learning a lot about the inner workings of the industry and yourself. Remember, when searching for a job, do not compromise your goals.

Listed below are several methods you can use to find out about salons that are hiring personnel or interviewing for future positions:

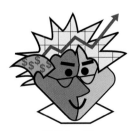

"Hiring Now. Apply Within"

1. Talk to stylists who work in the salons you admire. They might know of positions about to open up.

2. Check the classified section of your local newspaper. Many salons advertise there. The salon name may not be listed under the "Beauty Salons" section. Instead you may discover

an ad under "Hair Designer," "Professional Salon Stylist," "Makeup Artist," "Cosmetologist," or other special headings. The Sunday Classified Section generally has the widest range of employment opportunities.

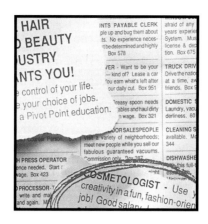

3. Talk to distributor sales consultants (from companies that sell hair, skin and nail care products to schools and salons) who may visit your school. Salons often inform these distributor consultants of their personnel needs.

4. Almost all cosmetology schools have job placement services for their graduating students. Refer to your school's bulletin board for job postings and ask your instructors to give you some ideas about seeking employment.

5. You may want to check with your city or state unemployment office for listings in the cosmetology field. While there, you can place your name on file and they will contact you with openings in the field.

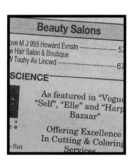

6. A very good idea is to canvass the area where you would like to work. Then make a list of those salons where you would like to begin employment. Call or visit the salons that impressed you most and ask if they are hiring new personnel.

7. You can also mail out resumes, attaching a cover letter to each, requesting the owner or manager to contact you for an interview if an opening becomes available.

Resumes

If you do decide to send a **resume**, be sure to develop one that describes your attributes in a brief, concise manner, including:

- Personal data (name, address, phone)
- Educational background (schools attended)
- Additional training (seminars attended, etc.)
- Previous employment (if applicable)
- Special skills or areas of expertise
- Any special awards or recognition

Also include:

- References (professional/personal)
- Interests (hobbies, skills)
- Most important: WHY you want to work in this particular salon

The big question when sending resumes is "What color paper should I use?" Most professionals recommend that you stay with white or a pale shade of beige, blue or gray. Important also is the stock (type and weight) of the paper and the legibility of the print. Professional resume writers recommend 10 - 11 pt. font size and 24 - 26 lb. classic laid or linen paper.

NOTE: Be sure to type your resume neatly.

There are professional business service offices that offer resume creation and writing at a very reasonable cost. You may want to use their services for printing your resume on professional paper stock or for assisting you in the creation of your resume. Always address your letter and resume to the owner or manager of the salon. If you don't know the owner's and/or manager's name, call and find out!

Even though you may have to write much of the same data on the application form, a resume can give the salon information about you that would not normally be asked on the application form. You have the option of including a photo of yourself with your resume. If you are applying for a position within a large salon and you know that many people complete the interview process, it might be good marketing to include your photo. The person interviewing you would appreciate having a visual reminder of who you are. Legally you are not required to supply a photo.

A **cover letter** is a necessity as a companion piece to your resume. The cover letter introduces you to the salon, offers a brief summary of why you would like to be employed at the salon and also provides a brief description of the qualities you feel you could bring to the salon. This letter should be neatly typed, contain a business letter format, the date, your address, salon address, greeting, closing and your signature.

	Name
	Address
	City, State, Zip
	Phone
OBJECTIVE:	A beginning job in hair design leading to a position as a platform artist.
EDUCATION:	**Pivot Point Beauty School**
	Chicago, Illinois
	Diploma in Cosmetology, 2000
	Professional training in all areas of hair artistry as well as skin care, nail care and personal and professional communications.
	Special Classes with John Doe and *People Skills* with Bob Wright.
	Chicago High School
	Chicago, Illinois
	Diploma in General Education, 1997
EXPERIENCE: 1995 - Present	Cashier - *Touhy & Western Standard* Chicago, Illinois Duties include maintaining inventory as well as operating electronic cash registers
AWARDS RECEIVED:	1st Place in Black Hair, 1st Place in Color and 3rd Place in Evening Makeup

Job Interviews

Your **first job interview** for a position as a stylist or a specialist in a salon may seem too far away to consider if you're just beginning your cosmetology course or make you nervous because you are about to graduate. Or perhaps, after months of study and practical experience, you're excited about obtaining a new job.

"I plan to put my best foot forward – not in my mouth!"

While interviews can be "nerve-wracking" for everyone, just remember to stay calm and be yourself. It won't take long for your skills, talents and positive attitude to outweigh your concerns. Proper preparation takes away most of the nervousness.

Personal Appearance

Before going to your interview, remember that your personal appearance and grooming habits are very noticeable. If you are neat and fashionably dressed...and if you have a contemporary hairstyle that flatters your face and physical features...if your skin looks healthy (makeup applied properly for females), you will begin the interview with a very good first impression. This initial impression will set the tone of your interview.

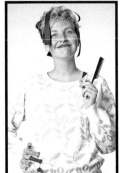

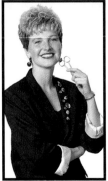

Inappropriate   **Appropriate**

Application

Before the interview begins, you may be asked to fill out an application for employment. Aside from standard information such as your name, address and telephone number, you will list where and when you graduated from cosmetology school, the date you completed your State Board of Cosmetology Examination and any additional educational training you may have had. If you have attended special classes, seminars or additional career-related training activities, list this information also.

Punctuality

Probably the first relationship you form with the prospective employer will be while applying for your job. The impression you make as a professional is your responsibility. You alone will have to promote yourself and your skills to the potential employer. An interviewer may intentionally schedule an appointment time that is early in the morning to determine your ability to be punctual. Be sure you arrive early for the appointment and that you have confirmed the exact location, parking availability and cost, if appropriate, and the approximate travel time you will need.

Technical and Communication Skills

The salon owner/manager will be interested in the skills and services you perform. Salons are always eager to have talented, capable staff members. The fact that you recently graduated from school can actually be an advantage since many salons will see you as having acquired no bad working habits.

Very often during an interview for a stylist's position (or other related position), you will be asked to demonstrate your skills to determine your level of technical expertise. The interviewer may do several things:

1. Ask you to demonstrate your skill level by bringing a model to cut, color or perm

2. Contact your school to get an appraisal from instructors

During the course of your conversation with the management or while demonstrating your skills, your interviewer will also be evaluating your communication skills and your ability to develop interpersonal relationships. Be as calm and professional during the interview and demonstration as you would be with a client.

Personal Qualities

Another area the interviewer will be evaluating is your personal qualities. The salon management may evaluate you on such qualities as your:

- Sincerity and honesty
- Motivation and enthusiasm toward the industry
- Understanding of the salon's goals
- Realistic career objectives
- Obvious desire to work

In the United States, illegal interview questions are those that discriminate on the basis of:
- age
- color
- race
- gender
- disability
- national origin
- religion or creed

- Ability to promote a new service or retail product
- Willingness to work as a member of the salon "team"
- Ability to organize and manage your time
- Educational and professional goals
- Ability to accept constructive criticism

Evaluating the Salon

Correctly evaluating your future work place is very important, for it is there you will be spending most of your days developing your career. To evaluate a salon in terms of its advantages and disadvantages, ask the owner/manager questions about the prospective job and consider some of the following criteria:

1. What is your impression of the salon management? Does the owner/manager appear to be someone who communicates with and encourages the members of the staff? Does he/she seem to be easy to talk to about goals and desires?

2. What services are performed there? Are the salon's products professional? Is the work performed of a high quality?

3. What does the salon charge for the services performed? Are the prices in line with the quality of the work done? Is the salon competitive with other salons in the area?

4. How large is the salon staff? Are you comfortable working with a group of people this size?

5. Which product line does the salon use and recommend to clients for use at home? Is it the same product line used on clients in the salon at the backbar?

6. What type of clientele does the salon have? (Students, business people, etc.)

7. Is the salon "growth-oriented?" What are its goals?

8. What is the salon's policy on advanced education for members of the staff?

9. What benefits does the salon offer its employees? (Medical insurance, retirement, paid holidays, educational advancement)

10. Does the salon have well-developed advertising and promotional programs to help bring in new clients?

11. What are the policies and procedures of the salon?

12. Who schedules clients? How?

13. What are the working conditions? (Will you be comfortable?)

14. What are the job responsibilities? (Will the job be a challenge?)

15. What will you be paid? (What are the advancement possibilities and benefits?)

If any of these questions remain unanswered after your initial interview, be sure to find out the answers during your final interview.

HINT: The size of the salon is probably the least important factor in deciding whether to accept a position. The physical size of a business is not an indication of its potential for growth or your potential to be successful. A small salon can be more successful in many ways (including financial) than a larger salon that is not working to its full potential.

Do not be overly influenced by the physical appearance or the busy activity that goes on inside a salon. Take time to evaluate each salon to make certain it will be a stimulating place to work. Determine if it is a professionally operated business that allows you to grow and achieve your goals. Spend enough time in the salon to get a feeling for the atmosphere and teamwork there.

BE PREPARED!

In the space provided below, write your answers to typical questions a salon interviewer might ask you:

How would your best friend describe your personal characteristics? _____

_____

What amount of time does it take you to apply oxidative color to a 1" (2.5 cm) regrowth area? _____

What amount of time does it take you to wrap a conventional perm on hair that is 5" (12.5 cm) long? _____

What would your instructor say is your strongest technical skill area? _____

What would your instructor say is your strongest professional characteristic in dealing with people?

_____

Job Benefits

Job benefits are a key factor that will determine whether you accept one job over another. **REMEMBER**, when viewing the potential of a job, the amount of money you'll get paid is not the most important issue. Often a job that pays less in salary is actually giving you more by providing you with costly benefits (extras) such as:

1. Salary and/or commission for services performed
2. Sales commission for retail products purchased by clients
3. Paid holidays, bonuses
4. Number of sick days allowed each year (paid or not)
5. Insurance benefits (health, accident, life)
6. Retirement plan

7.   Paid vacations

8.   Opportunities for travel

9.   Opportunity for advancement, new positions, responsibilities

10.   Educational seminars and events (Does salon share cost?)

11.   Ongoing salon educational programs and guest artist classes

12.   A motivating and comfortable workplace

13.   Length of lunch or dinner break and number of breaks during the day or evening

Tell your employer about any conflicts you may have with your work schedule during the interview. Before you accept employment with a salon, school or product manufacturer, etc., look at all the benefits offered. Determine which ones are important to you. Will you be happy without the benefits you want most?

Your New Job

In a salon, there are several approaches used to instruct new employees. Two of the most common approaches are:

1.   Many salons have a **general orientation program** to familiarize the new employee with the work habits and standards of the salon.   Most salons have Employee Handbooks, detailing such information. General orientation might also include a few days of technical training to familiarize you with techniques that are particular to your new salon position.

2.   Another approach has the new stylist assigned as an **assistant** or **apprentice** with an experienced stylist in the salon until she/he is totally familiar with salon procedures and practices. This method varies in length of time based on your skill level and expected expertise. Some salons prefer to offer a combination of assisting and assigning you new clients, which provides you an opportunity to build a clientele of your own.

Note: A combination of a general orientation program and assisting is also a common practice with new employees.

PROFESSIONAL RELATIONSHIPS

The beauty industry is multifaceted, drawing on a multitude of job descriptions, positions and career directions. Often it is assumed, incorrectly, that the person "behind the chair" is the only "important" part of the industry. Take a moment and think of all the professionals needed to make a stylist's day complete. Building solid professional relationships with other professionals is your foundation for the future. Your future is ready and waiting to unfold and your opportunities are virtually unlimited.

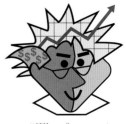

"The future is limitless!"

Networking

Professional relationships are based on open, honest, well-developed communication with everyone you meet during your career. Whether these people are clients, staff members, salon owners, managers or others you meet at seminars, trade shows or other industry-related programs...each can be important to your growth.

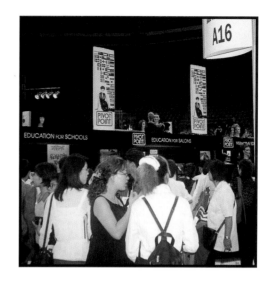

As these relationships grow, they reflect the strengths, creativity, dedication and tremendous effort of progressive, professional cosmetologists throughout the world. It is a rewarding challenge for everyone beginning a career to form professional relationships with fellow industry members.

The most important relationships you form at the beginning of your career are those that develop within the salon. Like all relationships, those in the salon begin with the first impression you create.

6

Building a Clientele

There are many techniques you can use to build a clientele. Some of the most effective techniques include the following:

Word of Mouth Advertising

Word of mouth advertising is probably the most effective way of building your clientele. Clients who are pleased with your services will recommend your services to their friends. Your expertise, your care with people, and your willingness to teach, all help bring clients and their friends into the salon.

Business Cards

If your salon has business cards printed with logo, name, address and phone number, ask the management if you can have cards printed with your name on them. Give these cards to current and potential clients. If the salon in which you are working does not provide cards, ask permission from the owner and consider supplying the cards yourself in an effort to build your business.

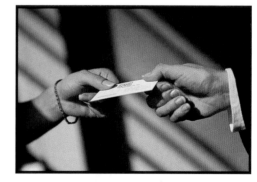

Referrals

Referrals are important because they increase your client base. If clients are telling their friends about you (referrals) and those friends are calling the salon and asking for you (requests), you're improving your reputation and income opportunities.

Rebooking

It sounds so simple, but one of the most effective ways to build your clientele is to ask clients to make a future appointment before they leave the salon. Taking the initiative to assist clients in maintaining regular appointments is one of the most effective tools for retaining a client base which builds success.

Promotional Literature

If the salon has printed promotional literature, such as flyers, newsletters or post cards, print your name on them, carry them with you and give them to people you meet. You'll be pleasantly surprised at the number of new clients you gain from this little extra effort.

Guest Appearances

If you enjoy speaking before an audience, you might try offering your services as a guest speaker or demonstrator. Civic groups, clubs, charities, high schools and college groups all enjoy hearing about the latest trends in fashion and style. They also like seeing the makeovers that you can present. Guest appearances can be an enjoy-

> **HINT:** If you perform at a fashion show or a civic organization, pass out your cards to interested members of the audience. These cards will refer new clients to you.

able experience and potentially develop a clientele that will ask for you by name. Be sure to check your area's regulating agency's rules governing doing demonstrations outside the salon.

Correspondence

Send thank you cards to every client after every appointment or call all new clients after their first visit to follow up. Send reminder notes one week before each appointment or call. With approval from the salon owner, send a birthday card to every client with a gift certificate for $5.00 off her next service or offer discounts on high ticket services, such as colors or makeovers. Send "I miss you" cards to clients who have not visited you in two months or longer.

Your Personal Touch

Spending a little extra time...sharing a styling tip...or suggesting a new style or product to your clients are all examples of your personal touch. If a client mentions a need for more time in the mornings, you might suggest an easier-to-care-for hairstyle. It is this personal touch that will keep your clients returning to you for future services.

IMPORTANT! You must continually be expanding your clientele. A certain percentage of your clients will leave the salon each year, so you need to be prepared to constantly keep your business growing.

The Stylist-Client Relationship

A solid pattern of communication with clients must be established on their first visit to the salon. If your clients feel that you are anxious to please them, they will develop a loyalty toward you. But first they must be convinced of your credibility and your abilities as a cosmetologist. To develop this credibility, you will need to establish a professional relationship with your clients. This stylist-client relationship is critical to your success as a cosmetologist and to the salon that employs you.

To communicate effectively with a client, you must first understand the individual. A large portion of this understanding will occur during your initial contact with the client. At that time you will conduct a client consultation, keeping in mind that the meeting will "set the tone" for the stylist-client relationship. During the client consultation, it is essential to determine the client's desires and needs and explain what might be best for overall appearance. You must learn how the client feels about making changes to his/her appearance and what service objectives he/she has in mind. Other information you will need to learn from the client regarding specific services is covered in detail in their respective chapters.

Keys to Successful Client Relationships

- Determine the client's needs.

- Clearly explain to the client what the "finished look" will be before beginning any service.

- Suggest alternative styles, if the client only wants to make a minor change, rather than a dramatic one. Further changes may be suggested later.

- Teach the client how to maintain the hairstyle, makeup application, nail care or other service at home.

- Provide the client with information on the correct product regimen to use at home and proper product application.

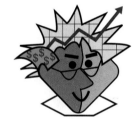

- Show the client pictures of new styles and suggest any additional services that would enhance the client's appearance. (Do not suggest to the client that he/she will look "just like" the photograph.)

"Do unto others as you would have them do unto you."

- Introduce change periodically so the client's appearance is both attractive and current.

- Accommodate the client whenever possible. If it is possible to adjust your appointment schedule for a client, do so (without inconveniencing other clients).

- Share new information about cosmetology and fashion with your clientele. It will generate excitement and enthusiasm for your services and for the salon.

- Treat your clients with the same respect and concern you would like them to exhibit toward you.

- Manage down time constructively by helping others, performing tasks around the salon and maintaining client base. Organize your work and prepare to have products and implements ready for each client. Serve clients promptly when they arrive. However, do not rush one client in order to serve the next. When making an appointment, be sure the time allotted for each person allows you to remain on schedule.

- Notify your clientele in advance if you plan to be absent for an appointment or on vacation and "re-book" (reschedule) their appointments with fellow stylists through the salon receptionist.

The Stylist-Staff Relationship

All successful businesses depend upon a strong "team" approach, involving all the members of its staff. This "team" concept revolves around several factors, some of which are listed below. See if you can think of some others.

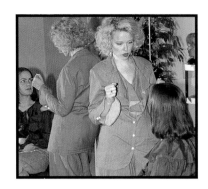

Common Goals

Each "team" member sets his/her personal goals for a day, month and year. Salons, research institutions, and manufacturers also set goals for themselves...such as financial, sales volume or educational goals. Teamwork flourishes when a blending of personal and business goals occurs.

Sharing Knowledge

As a member of the working staff, you are expected to share your knowledge and techniques with your fellow team members and other professionals. Sharing results in loyal, satisfied clients as well as in encouraging others to share with you. Should a special challenge or problem arise during your business day, you should consult with your fellow team members. As with the medical field, it is a sign of professionalism to consult with your colleagues about specialized or problem areas.

Because you are a team member, you should express your ideas, thoughts and feelings to create an open professional relationship with others. Dreams and aspirations, as well as frustrations and anger, may be expressed maturely with other members of the team. Problem situations will be quickly resolved through the application of good communication skills.

Helping Others

Although staff members have their own clientele to serve, sometimes you'll have extra time, so use it to help your co-workers. In return, they will help you when you need assistance. Perhaps the most important factor of teamwork cannot be taught. It is the all-important sense of togetherness and friendship that will hold your team together. The strong, positive, professional relationship that develops between you and other stylists in the salon will not be built overnight. Instead you must establish a rapport with each person and continue to work toward good communication, understanding and teamwork every day. The people you work with can become your friends and your professional associates.

Remember these valuable concepts used by successful business people in any industry.

1. Plan ahead
2. Create a professional image
3. Define your goals
4. Develop good professional relationships

The future is yours and the challenges you meet are the reflections of the goals you create.

Education + Skill + Confidence = SUCCESS!

NOTE: Good teamwork involves referrals. A client booked into a salon for a styling service might be referred to a specialist for skin care needs, or vice versa. In each case, the stylists reinforce the salon's concern for the client by suggesting treatments and services. Working as a team, you can provide each client with special care.

Performance Review

At regular intervals throughout your employment, the salon management will discuss your job performance with you. Called Performance Reviews, they have several common characteristics:

- Performance Reviews occur at predetermined intervals. It is important to do a self-appraisal prior to each performance review.

- You will be given suggestions to help you capitalize on your strong areas.

- You will receive constructive criticism about the areas where you could improve.

SALON OWNERSHIP

Perhaps your dream, maybe even one of your long-term goals, is to run your own salon. The successful salon owner, through ambition and hard work, can enjoy personal and financial security and the creative freedom to develop and build a lucrative business. Even if you have never thought of salon ownership or already know that you do not have a desire to own a salon, it will be beneficial for you to know the fundamental principles of various salon ownership models and operations. Understanding the inner workings of salons will create a foundation that will allow both you and the salon owner to meet goals together. This section of the chapter will explore how to begin the process of owning a salon.

Self-Appraisal

A salon owner does not have to be all things to all people. The stylist planning to open a salon should assess his/her own skills carefully to pinpoint any areas of weakness. Locating weaknesses allows the potential salon owner to hire employees for whom those same areas are strengths. Skills essential to a successful salon owner are:

1. The ability to recognize hair fashion trends and technical expertise (While the salon owner need not excel in every salon service performed, he or she MUST be able to recognize great color skills or perm techniques and hire staff accordingly.)

2. The ability to communicate with the public, not only in ordinary situations, but also in unusual or difficult instances

3. The ability to accept suggestions and criticism from clients and staff

4. The ability to exert self-control

5. The ability to manage the financial operations of a salon or to work with a professional bookkeeper or accountant to create a budget that predicts income and expenses

6. The ability to establish and adjust salon pricing in accordance with local economic factors

7. The knowledge to create business through promotion

8. The ability to set realistic business goals

9. The ability to organize a business plan into an executive summary, goals, market potential, marketing strategy, financial projection and exit plan

These skills can be learned and developed through study and hard work. The experience you gain working as a stylist in someone else's salon will provide you with invaluable opportunities to watch and learn. Poor or inexperienced management and/or poor bookkeeping systems have been the cause of failure for many salons. Many local colleges and universities, however, offer management and business training that can combine with your cosmetology education to help you become the owner of a successful salon.

Financial Status

Anyone thinking of opening a business must have money to invest. Few people have the thousands of dollars needed to equip and supply a salon. Therefore, you must prove you are a "good risk" before a bank or savings and loan will lend you money. Preparing a personal financial statement is the first step toward securing a loan.

Personal Financial Statement

A personal financial statement contains three basic elements. **The first is a list of all the property you OWN, your assets.** Assets include physical property, such as a house, car, recreational vehicle, antiques, jewelry, gold or silver, collections of valued goods, like stamps or coins, or any item for which you could receive payment. The best assets are cash-valued items, such as certificates of deposit, IRAs, life insurance policies, savings bonds, stocks/bonds, cash in money market, and checking and savings accounts. Together these are your TOTAL ASSETS.

Next is a list of all the money you OWE, your liabilities. Any outstanding loan balances on your assets (on a house or car), bills from credit cards or charge accounts, or student loans are liabilities. Together these are your TOTAL LIABILITIES.

The third and final figure, NET WORTH, is calculated by subtracting your liabilities from your assets. ASSETS minus LIABILITIES = NET WORTH

For example, if you had:	**$50,000 assets**
minus	**$30,000 liabilities**
You would have a:	**$20,000 NET WORTH**

In today's marketplace most banks loan only 10% of personal net worth. With a net worth of $20,000, for example, you could borrow approximately $2,000. A 5-stylist salon will cost on the average from $5,000 to $50,000, depending on location, improvements and equipment needed. It is possible to borrow money with a low personal net worth, but then you are categorized as a "high risk" and may have to pay interest rates 5 to 8 points higher than the usual rate.

As you can see, a future salon owner should begin accumulating cash or physical assets and paying off all liabilities from the day of graduation. Getting the help of a certified financial consultant is a step in the right direction. Some areas offer this service without charge. Your personal finances must be in order before you can go into business. Once you have determined your net worth and your ability to borrow money, you must have a plan. Now is the time to determine the kind of salon you want and can afford.

Types of Salon Ownership

There are four types of ownership:

1. **A sole proprietorship is a business owned by one person** who is in complete control of the business, receives all profits from the business and is responsible for all debts and losses.

2. **A partnership is a business owned by two or more persons.** All costs of opening, operating and maintaining the business are shared by the partners as agreed. Partnerships can be between persons with different management or styling skills. One may be an excellent designer while the other has management ability. This relationship builds on the strengths of each and avoids weaknesses. Caution: A partnership agreement should be legally written. The agreement should specify the rights and obligations of each partner. In the event that a partner decides to leave the partnership or sell his or her portion, there should be a written buy-out agreement. Verbal agreements lead to misunderstandings. A solidly based relationship between partners is essential for a partnership to work.

3. **A corporation** is a legal entity, separate from its shareholders, which is formed under legal guidelines. A corporation has a charter or articles of incorporation describing the purposes of the corporation and the structure of the company. **A corporation is actually owned by its shareholders.** The shareholders elect representatives known as the board of directors. The board of directors then appoints officers (such as the president, vice president and treasurer) to run the day-to-day business. Shareholders receive income based on the profits of the corporation. Corporations may be privately held by just a few stockholders or publicly held. If publicly held, stock of the corporation is owned by many people and is available for sale on one of the stock exchanges. As a general rule, stockholders are not liable for the corporation's debts or losses as long as the corporation is operated as a separate legal entity. Laws concerning liability or damage to persons or property as a result of a corporation's activities may be different according to where the corporation is formed and the place where it conducts its business. A lawyer and an accountant should be employed to ensure that the corporation is properly established and conducts its business in accordance with the local laws.

4. **A franchise** is more a form of operation than a form of ownership. **A franchise is simply an operating agreement in which a fee is paid to a parent corporation in exchange for fixtures, promotion, advertising, education and management techniques.** The owner of a franchise agreement can be a sole proprietor, partnership or corporation. Certain rules must be observed in the operation of a franchise. An initial purchase fee plus a monthly service charge is paid to the parent corporation. A franchise is an excellent way to share in the expertise of industry experts. However, simple policies about hours, products used, benefits for employees, salaries and even the color of the salon are decided by the parent corporation.

Requirements of a Salon

To begin the process of salon planning, you will need to research the following:

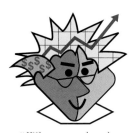

"What are the three most important factors to salon success? My real estate agent would say, location, location, location!"

1. **Location. The most important factor in opening a salon business is location.** What are the available locations in your area? You need to assess parking conditions, high-traffic activity (walk-by, drive-in or bus service), and rental fees per square foot.

2. **Market Need.** How many salons and stylists are there in the area? What are the cosmetology services offered, prices charged, types of potential clientele (age, income and social groups)? A ten-year forecast of the economic future of the community can usually be obtained from the local Chamber of Commerce or Economic Development Agency.

3. **Cost of Necessary Improvements.** Improvements include dollars that must be spent to meet a salon's unique plumbing and lighting requirements, such as shampoo bowls and color areas, and to upgrade electrical wiring, heating, air conditioning and so forth. A landlord will sometimes share in this expense. Salon equipment is a separate expense not included in improvements.

Getting the Right Advice

At this point any serious future salon owner will need the advice of some experts.

1. An **accountant** can tell you what a bank is likely to lend you, based on your net worth. An accountant is a financial advisor, not an expert on the beauty business. He or she is generally paid on a monthly or quarterly basis. The accountant's tasks would include:

   • Informing you about types of business ownership and their tax benefits and liabilities

   • Evaluating a rental agreement

   • Setting up a basic bookkeeping system, including periodic income statements to evaluate profit or loss

   • Recording and preparing tax payments to various government agencies

   • Representing you if you are audited by the Internal Revenue Service

2. An **insurance agent** will provide advice on insurance needed to safely open and operate a business. (See types of insurance in this chapter.) Insurance is a form of risk management. When you buy insurance, you are paying a fee to a company to assume your risk of loss. For example, car insurance is a set dollar amount of assumed risk on your car. The insurance company is betting you WON'T have an accident. You're betting your premium that you MIGHT have an accident. The rule of insurance is, "If you can easily afford to totally replace an item, don't insure it," UNLESS you could in some way be held responsible for personal injury if the item malfunctioned or if property for which you were responsible caused an accident. There are requirements that certain insurance, such as Workers Compensation, be carried to protect the consumer and the employee. As an owner, you must have this type of insurance. Select a reputable agent and company that offer the whole range of insurance policies needed by the salon. An agent is paid on a commission basis according to the policies of the company or companies represented.

3. A **lawyer** is an advisor on the legal obligations of business ownership, borrowing money, signing rental (lease) agreements and assuming tax responsibilities. You should employ a lawyer when documents are being signed or when establishing a type of ownership requiring a written agreement (a partnership or corporation). **You may also want to contact a lawyer prior to signing a purchase or rental agreement to determine the existence of any outstanding debt against the building or business.** Lawyers are normally paid on an hourly basis for all phone calls, in-person consultations or preparation of documents. Ask the rate before consulting with a lawyer.

COMPLIANCE

The salon owner's responsibilities also include being in compliance with all local, state/province and federal rules, regulations and laws. Examples include city zoning and building codes, city or county waste disposal rules, assigned state/province regulatory agency licensure regulations, the Internal Revenue Service, OSHA, and various acts such as ADA (Americans with Disabilities Act), which allows access and fair treatment in the business and educational environment to disabled persons. A lawyer is able to assist the salon owner to be in compliance with all regulations.

6

4. A **distributor sales consultant** representing a full-service, professional-only distribution (beauty supply) house is the link between the manufacturers of products and equipment and the salon. It can be beneficial to develop a strong relationship with one distributor. The full-service distributor will carry all products and equipment needed to open a salon. The distributor may have financing available, may help in salon design, may help find good salon locations, may aid in locating prospective employees and may provide in-salon education and large-scale educational seminars or workshops. The distributor sales consultant earns a commission on the dollar amount you purchase in supplies. However, he/she may be able to provide you with an efficient, cost-saving inventory control system that ensures a maximum return on every dollar invested in retail and professional-use products. If you don't make money, she/he won't make money. The distributor is a key professional relationship a salon owner must develop.

There are also discount and cash-and-carry beauty supply houses throughout the country that provide products or equipment with few or none of the above-mentioned services. In addition some manufacturers sell directly to salon owners. A salon owner must decide what is important to his/her salon operations when selecting a distributor.

Space Requirements and Floor Plans

In general, it takes 120 to 150 square feet per stylist to create an efficient working space. Square footage is obtained by multiplying the length of the location by its width. For example, a 15 by 30 foot space is a total of 450 square feet (15 x 30 = 450). A distributor sales consultant could help you design a sample salon layout based on three to four stylists working in a 450 square foot space. **Some regulating agencies have specific minimum space requirements for each stylist.** In this instance, the salon will be licensed to employ a maximum number of stylists working at one time. As the owner you could give more space per stylist, but you would need to be aware that your investment costs would rise, which may cost the salon more than is profitable. The ideal salon

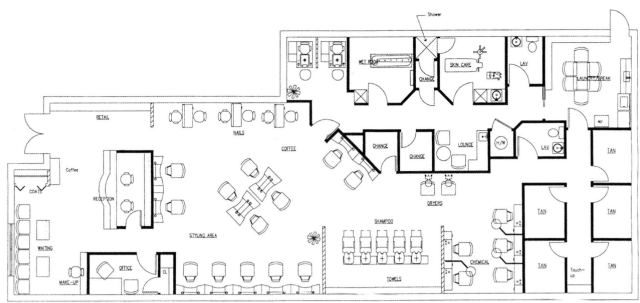

Image courtesy of Belvedere

arrangement has an efficient traffic pattern. The best design requires the fewest steps for the client and stylist to travel.

All salons require a reception area with seating and a desk for receiving clients, a dispensary, a restroom and other service areas such as shampoo and drying areas. In addition, many salons have a retail display and promotion area, a lounge, laundry and utility room.

Develop a floor plan for a proposed location before trying to determine any details on cost of equipment or interior decorating. If a location cannot be arranged with an efficient floor plan (with a minimum capital improvement cost), look at other locations. Salons can be installed with an investment from $1,000 up to $10,000 per stylist. Weigh the cost of installation for the salon you want. Sometimes a location is priced right, with good traffic and the type of clientele desired, but the cost of installation is too high. Examine many alternatives. Then work out the decorating details. Remember, this is YOUR salon. Make it one in which you'll enjoy working and one that will pay off.

Borrowing Money

After you have found a location, determined a suitable and affordable floor plan, determined the cost of fixtures and estimated the capital improvements necessary, you must determine how much money you will need to borrow. It is important to note that you should not sign a rental agreement until you have received your loan approval. Your accountant should advise you of the operating capital needed to open the salon and to pay the expenses of your business for at least six months. Generally, you must be willing to invest some of your own money in the salon for an institution to grant a loan. It is important to make all your loan payments on time to avoid default (failure to repay), since you will be granted future loans based on your ability and willingness to do so.

Rental Agreements

Upon obtaining a loan, you can enter into a rental agreement (called a lease). Normally a lease should extend for five years with an option for five more years, in order to avoid unexpected rent increases. It is unprofitable to install a salon for less than five years, due to the time needed for a new business to grow and flourish. You should negotiate for all or part of the capital improvements to be paid by the owner of the building or lessor. Such a request is reasonable because these improvements will stay in the building when you move out. **As the renter or lessee, you promise to pay rent and use the property according to the agreement.** It is common for salons to need extra water pipes, larger water heaters, more electric outlets, washer and dryer facilities, installation of shampoo bowls and large window areas. These special features will probably have to be paid for by the lessee (you). However, arrange for the maintenance or repairs on normal building equipment, such as furnace and air conditioner, to be the lessor's (owner's) responsibility.

A large portion of the expense of the salon is the rent. There are two kinds of rent:

1. **A fixed rent** is a set dollar amount paid each month to the lessor. A fixed rent allows you to predict your monthly expenses carefully.

2. **A variable rent** includes a set dollar amount paid per month PLUS a percentage of the total monthly income. Variable rents are common in malls and large shopping centers. However, with the small percentage of profit earned by an average salon, a variable rent could be a serious mistake. Have your accountant predict the results of a variable rent system before signing a lease.

Have a lawyer evaluate a tentative lease and make suggestions for change. You can negotiate changes in any lease. Remember, don't sign a lease unless you, your lawyer and your accountant are satisfied that it is fair and reasonable.

Types of Insurance

As stated previously, insurance is a form of risk management. It protects you from the financial difficulties that can follow unexpected loss of property, income and/or life. The following are types of insurance available to eliminate some of the risks of being in business.

- **Malpractice insurance is a policy that protects the salon owner from financial loss that can result from a stylist-employee's negligence while performing hair, nail and skin care services on salon clients.** A salon owner must insure each stylist in the salon. This insurance covers the cost of a lawsuit or settlement resulting from damage caused to a client during any service.

- **Property or premise insurance** is a policy that covers the actual salon equipment and physical location in case of natural disasters, fire, theft or burglary, or accidents occurring at the business. It covers replacement of lost items and carries a liability clause that will pay a claim if someone is injured on the premises.

- **Product liability insurance** is a recent addition to available insurance coverage. With the huge number of products found within the cosmetology industry, a need for protection has developed. Designed to offer protection in the case of product damage caused to a client's skin, hair or nails, through misuse or use, product liability insurance provides protection for a salon's financial and professional reputation.

- **Unemployment insurance** is required by federal law for all qualified employers. Employers pay into a central fund that offers compensation to laid off, displaced or otherwise eligible employees until suitable employment can be found and/or a designated amount of time has passed.

- **Worker's Compensation is a state-controlled insurance required by law.** This insurance is paid directly to the state on a quarterly basis to cover any expense resulting from an injury to an employee. If the employee is injured while working in the salon, all medical expenses are paid by the state, and the state provides the employee with a guaranteed income until the employee can return to work.

Taxes

The salon owner is responsible for withholding from an employee's income for payment of certain taxes and for paying these withholdings to the government. In the U.S., these include federal, state and local income taxes and social security tax. The salon owner also has a tax obligation to the employee. **For every dollar of social security tax paid by the employee, the salon owner must pay the same amount to the federal government. Social security is a planned savings/retirement fund for every worker in the United States.** Medicare is part of your social security tax and provides medical insurance coverage during retirement. In Canada , the salon owner is responsible for withholding Federal and Provincial tax, Employment Insurance (EI) and Canadian Pension Tax.

Internal Revenue Service (IRS) rules require you to register a daily log of all your tips, which is income. Keep a copy for yourself and submit a copy to your employer.

The salon owner must also provide an annual W-2 form for each employee. The W-2 form will indicate all taxes paid for the past year. It is important for all employees to verify that the salon owner is submitting taxes under the correct social security number so appropriate credit is given.

States have sales taxes on products and services. The salon owner is responsible for collecting and paying these monies to the state on a monthly or quarterly basis. A permit is required to collect taxes, and the payments are a permanent record of the salon's dollar volume. A salon owner must apply for a state sales tax permit before collecting tax on products or services sold.

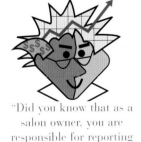

"Did you know that as a salon owner, you are responsible for reporting your employees' tips?"

Income Tax is paid on the profits (earnings) of a business. The Internal Revenue Service establishes criteria for reporting profit and loss.

Expenses and Income

In very basic terms, the financial success of a salon will be achieved when the salon's income is significantly greater than its operating expense. Income refers to all payments received from clients for services performed and home care products purchased.

Independent Contractor is an IRS term that can be applied to stylists who rent or lease styling stations from a building owner. Rental or leasing fees can vary, depending on urban or rural location. The building owner provides a location in which to work and pays the utilities. The stylist (lessee) provides all professional supplies, a telephone line and products for retail sale to clients.

In this system, the stylist is considered self-employed by the IRS. He/she must report his/her income quarterly to the government in the form of "self employment taxes." There are no benefits provided to the lessee by the salon owner, other than a place to work.

Operating Expense refers to all the costs incurred in running the salon each day. **If the salon's income is greater than the operating expense, the salon is operating at a profit. If the operating expense is greater than the income, the salon is operating at a loss.** The salon may operate at a loss, as clientele develops, during the first few weeks, months and even years it is open. Your accountant should help you take that fact into consideration when your initial financing is arranged.

If you make a profit, you pay a percentage of that profit to the federal, state and local governments. If you suffer a loss, you receive a tax credit (pay little or no tax). You can see that careful planning and control of expenses are essential.

6

Careful recordkeeping is required by law. It is wise to keep all records of your daily sales and service for 5 to 7 years. If you are audited by the IRS, these records are proof of your income. Failure to keep records is against the law in most areas.

The average cost of operating a business (by percentage of income) breaks down as follows:

INCOME – (minus) EXPENSES = (equal) PROFIT.

Compensation: 50 %
Salaries or commissions for yourself and your employees,
including payroll taxes

Rent: 12 %
Fixed or variable

Supplies: 5 %
Professional products used (consumption/consumable), retail products
sold and miscellaneous equipment and tools

Advertising: 3 %
Promotion of the salon

Utilities: 2 %
Water, electricity, gas, sanitation, phone

Insurance: 1.5 %
All types

Employee Benefits: 1.5 %
Education, paid vacations, pension plans or profit-sharing,
health insurance

Maintenance: 2 %
Repairs, laundry, cleaning and replacement of equipment

Cost of Doing Business: 2 %
Accounting, legal, licenses, subscriptions, professional dues, etc.

Services of Debt: 5%
Capital improvements, equipment and original loan expense

Depreciation: 3 %
An account established to save for replacement of equipment;
creates tax credit

Miscellaneous: 1 %
All other expenses

Total Operating Expense:	88 %

All the above expenses can be controlled. If your operating statement shows a particular expense that is too high, you can take steps to reduce costs. Expenses shown above may be higher or lower for your salon, depending on climate, size of community and region. Of course, increasing your profits in ways that have minimal effect on increasing your expenses will yield a higher net. Retail displays, for example, use existing space and require a one-time expense for the display unit. The only ongoing expenses are the costs of keeping the display well-stocked and, perhaps, retail commissions paid to your stylists and salon coordinator or receptionist on their retail product sales. Staff compensation is the largest ongoing salon expense.

Remember: **Income minus Expenses equal Profit.** The better you control your expenses, the faster you will pay off your debt and be able to see higher profits from the salon.

Salon Philosophy, Policies and Procedures

A salon should have a professional philosophy or standard of ethics. Creating a Policies and Procedures Handbook is the first step in developing these standards. It provides a set of rules for the owner and staff to work by and can be revised as needed. A salon handbook should thoroughly outline the salon owner's expectations of employees. Information contained in a salon handbook might include: job descriptions, educational and professional requirements, client-relations policies and employee-conduct guidelines, location of MSDS information, guidelines on dealing with client or staff disabilities, hours, prices, service standards, record-keeping policies, benefits, infection control standards, care of equipment, absence policy, complaint policy and causes for termination of employment.

A salon handbook should also inform the employee about what to expect from management. The employer is expected to provide a safe and pleasant working environment, reasonable working hours, equitable salary structure, products and supplies, and sanitation services. The employer should also provide a format, such as weekly or biweekly salon meetings, in which employees can offer suggestions and opinions and expect unbiased consideration to be given to any topic they might bring up. These provisions could be covered in the handbook as well.

Salon Operation

Now that you have explored the steps to opening a salon, it's time to consider important aspects of salon operation: hiring, compensation, pricing, advertising, retailing and receptionist duties.

Hiring

Hire employees who meet your standards of honesty and professionalism. You might consider conducting two to three interviews to determine if a stylist is the right candidate for employment in your salon.

The salon owner needs to apply for a Federal Employer Identification Number before hiring employees.

U.S. Federal Law states that you must determine if the employee is a legal citizen prior to final hiring by requesting proof of valid social security card, driver's license and/or birth certificate and completing what is called an I-9 form. A copy of the completed I-9 form, along with a photocopy of the supporting proof documents, should be placed in the employee's file.* After hiring, introduce the new employee to your entire staff and make him or her feel a part of your salon team.

*In Canada, a Social Insurance number is required as proof of ability to work.

Compensation

There are three common ways an employee can be paid.

1. A **commission structure** is based on a percentage of the dollar income the individual stylist creates by servicing clients. Perhaps the stylist does 10 cuts at $10 per cut in an eight-hour day. The total (or gross) income is $100. A percentage up to 50% is normally paid. At 50% the stylist receives $50 or $6.25 per hour wkrked. This pay structure is based on the number of clients and the amount of work done.

2. A **salary structure** is a compensation system that guarantees a set income on a weekly or monthly basis. This salary is similar to salaried positions in all professions. Salon owners like salaries because educational costs and employee benefits such as health insurance, pension plans, and paid vacations can be budgeted if the payroll is based on fixed salaries.

3. A **salary plus commission structure** guarantees a certain amount of money on a regular basis and allows additional payment based on the number of clients the stylist brings into the salon. This system gives the stylist a steady paycheck, while rewarding the stylist for building his/her clientele.

Pricing

Service prices should be determined by conducting a market survey before opening the salon. Price the services at a reasonable rate to fit the income range of the clients you want to attract. Create a profile of the clientele you hope will visit your salon and target them with your advertising. Determining what other salons are charging can be helpful. But remember, price is not the only reason clients select a particular salon. The community image of the salon, the quality of work performed, the personalities of the stylists, the ambiance and the salon location are major incentives for a client to return to your salon.

Advertising

Advertising tells the public about your salon – the services you perform, the quality of work you produce and any other reasons that clients should patronize your salon. **The best form of advertising is word of mouth.** Satisfied clients tell others about your salon, as do unsatisfied clients.

Advertising in the printed media can be very effective. Direct mail advertising involves sending postcards or flyers to prospective clients encouraging them to try your salon. Daily or weekly newspaper ads can create an image in the consumers' minds through the repetition of your name and logo. Magazines or periodicals that reach the types of clientele you are trying to attract can also be effective.

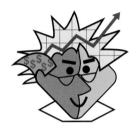

"One unhappy client will tell 10 people about the experience. Happy clients may only tell one person how happy they are with their style. Bad news travels fast and first!"

Television and radio ads can be effective but costly. Billboards, bus stop seats and public relations efforts, including holding styling shows or fund raising events for charity, can also promote your professional pursuits.

Involvement in community affairs, the chamber of commerce or service organizations can also promote your personal and professional image in the area. Be known as a worker. People will try your professional services if they like you and trust you as a person.

Plan a yearly advertising budget and stick to it. Alternate expensive forms of advertising with inexpensive methods. If one form of advertising works, repeat it. If something fails, drop it. Consider surveying your clients once a year for their opinions about your services, your community image and your advertising program.

Inventory and Product Control

Products are purchased by the salon owner and brought into the salon for use during client services and for retailing to the client. These products are referred to as inventory or stock in quantity. Inventory is generally identified by two categories, professional and retail. In order for the salon to operate at a profitable margin, it is important that a strong inventory system is in place that will allow close management of these valuable products. Proper inventory practices also indicate that emphasis must be placed on ensuring timely ordering of products. Not having a product available to perform a service or meet a purchasing need of a client is not good business practice.

Inventory control is a term applied to procedures used in the salon that will ensure that products are accounted for from the time they are brought into the salon until they are sold or used. In addition, inventory control guidelines are established to monitor the number of sales made of a specific product within an assigned time frame. Determinations on whether specific products should be continued as retail items are based on the number of "turnovers" or "turns", which means calculating the amount of time it takes to sell the product once it is on the shelf. It is not to an owner's business advantage to invest money in products that don't turn over in a timely fashion.

A salon owner should expect the stylists to sell products for home care to their clients. Setting a sales goal is essential to providing retail income to both the salon owner and the stylist. It is an industry-recommended goal that for each dollar in services a stylist performs on a client, that client should be purchasing a dollar in home-care products. A client who visits a salon for a cut every 6 weeks, at the average cost of $15.00, could easily spend another $15.00 on the retail products he or she will need for use at home. That same client, through careful product recommendations, may eventually spend more on retail products than on any salon services as she/he begins to purchase additional hair care products, skin care products and/or cosmetics.

Many salons pay a commission ranging from 8 to 15% of the stylist's total retail sales to the stylist. Some salon owners pay lower commission for lower dollar volume sales. A sliding scale creates the incentive to sell more. The salon owner is responsible for keeping an inventory of products for stylists to sell.

Receptionist Duties

In many cases the receptionist is the first person to greet the clients as they arrive. If the salon does not have a full-time receptionist, the salon owner usually appoints a stylist to serve in this capacity as needed or the stylists rotate throughout the day, meeting the needs of this area. In some cases, the receptionist also acts as the cashier, managing the operations of the cash register.

The primary duties of this very important position include:
1. Promote good will and client satisfaction
2. Schedule appointments in a fair and efficient way
3. Manage incoming and outgoing calls regarding appointments
4. Inform stylists of client arrival in the salon
5. Supervise the reception area to ensure organization and efficiency
6. Promote retail products and additional services to clients
7. Handle pressure and client complaints efficiently
8. Ensure client services are all paid and documented
9. Ensure messages are handled in order of priority and with efficiency
10. Work with stylists to ensure punctual schedules

Keeping client records easily accessible in a central location may be one of the receptionist's responsibilities.

A poor receptionist can ruin a salon's operations. Clients often judge the salon by how phone calls are handled and how they are treated as they arrive in the salon the first few minutes. It is crucial that the receptionist be cheerful and able to handle most situations. A great receptionist can make everyone's day go more smoothly and less stressfully.

Making Change

Cash operations are important to every business and the salon is no exception. The receptionist or assigned cashier needs to ensure accuracy and efficiency, providing the correct denomination of bills and coins for cash transactions and trouble-shooting during credit transactions. When giving change, always count back from the smaller denomination, usually coins, and move to the larger, usually bills.

"Over the next few weeks, be aware of how change is offered to you. Learn by listening and watching."

An example would be if the client's bill for services and products totals $32.97 and the client offers $35.00, the client would hear counted back "98, 99, 33, 34 and 35." This would indicate that you have offered the client change of three cents (to total $33) and then two singles (to total $35).

The most efficient method of offering change is to always give the client the fewest bills necessary to complete the transaction. Therefore, it is necessary that an adequate inventory of various bill and coin denominations is on hand. A client might say it is okay to receive twenty-five pennies because you are out of other coins, but in reality it is not good business, takes more time and is not as efficient.

Telephone Techniques

Your telephone answering technique creates the first impression a client will have of the salon. The telephone is used to make appointments, answer questions, receive messages, handle complaints and remind clients of future appointments. Because the telephone plays such an important role in the salon's business, it is imperative that anyone answering the phone is well trained and answering procedures are carefully planned. Telephone answering tips include:

1. Answer the phone within two rings.

2. Greet the client by saying:
   a. The salon name
   b. Your name
   c. How may I help you?

3. Listen carefully for:
   a. Client's name
   b. Service desired or other information (Ask client to repeat what was said if you cannot understand him/her.)

4. Book appointment and repeat back to client:
   a. Stylist requested
   b. Time and date of appointment

     c. Exact service to be done

     d. "Thank you for calling, (client's name)"

  5. If you cannot help the client personally:

     a. Ask the client, "Would you please hold?"

     b. Wait for a response (yes or no)

     c. Then place the line on HOLD and go get help

     d. Return to client within 1 minute

  6. If a message is being left, include:

     a. Date and time

     b. For whom the message is intended

     c. Name of caller

     d. Phone number of caller

     e. Exact message

     f. REPEAT BACK THE ENTIRE MESSAGE to caller

     g. Take the message to the person for whom it is intended

Note: Booking appointments can be done more effectively if the person answering the phone is aware of the stylists' skills, their speed, prices and availability.

Here are some additional phone tips:

- Do not talk to others in the salon while on the phone.

- Avoid sounding harsh, shrill or irritated.

- Use good grammar.

- Speak clearly, calmly and with enthusiasm.

- Be courteous, speak at a moderate pace and never interrupt the caller.

- Handle complaints tactfully by asking the client to come into the salon, so everything possible can be done to please her/him. If a client refuses, offer to compensate the client (according to salon policy) or ask the client, "What would make you happy?" Take a complaint very seriously. Just one unhappy client can directly affect your salon's reputation, the stylist's reputation and your future income.

- Always maintain self control.

- When informing clients of pricing, be exact. A client expects to pay a quoted price unless informed that a preliminary stylist-client consultation is required.

- Don't promise that a chemical service can be performed without hair analysis if an analysis is salon policy. Performing a chemical service on chemically damaged hair can result in even greater hair damage and can possibly result in a malpractice lawsuit against the salon and/or stylist.

- In a salon without a full-time receptionist, take turns answering the phone. Distribute new clients who don't request a particular stylist among all stylists with openings. Book others, and they will book you when they are answering the phone.

Remember, telephone techniques are tremendously important. Skillful handling turns a price inquiry phone call into a new client for your salon, soothes the ruffled feelings of a customer who might otherwise leave your clientele, and generally increases your salon's business.

Scheduling Appointments

The process of scheduling appointments is of primary importance within the operation of the salon. Generally appointments are scheduled according to the type of service and the speed of the stylist. Important information that is noted on the appointment book includes the following:

Stylist name	**Client name**
Scheduled service	**Date**
Appointment time	**Client phone number**

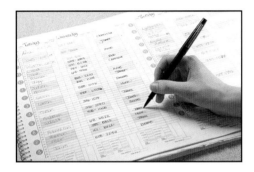

Frequently additional information is added to the appointment book by using codes that represent various types of clients. Codes used for identifying client types might include the following:

Walk-in clients might be represented by placing a "W" next to the client's name to indicate the client did not call ahead for an appointment.

Request clients could be indicated by placing an "R" next to the client's name to identify a specific stylist has been requested to perform the service. In an effort to serve the needs of the client, the salon could notify this client if the requested stylist is absent on the day of the scheduled appointment.

Transfer clients might be indicated by placing a "T" next to the client's name to indicate that this client is able to be transferred to another stylist. This code is very helpful if a stylist is running behind schedule or in the case of absence of the assigned stylist.

SALON RETAILING

Retailing in the salon – selling products for client home care – will help make you a successful stylist and will show your clients you are interested in their grooming needs. It is an ongoing process that requires effort and dedication, just as the services you learn to perform. Successful retailing in the salon requires you to look for new ways to interest your clients in the products you recommend.

Selling

Selling is the international pastime of exchanging service for product, money for expertise. This system of exchange is as old as human existence. Even in stone-age society, humans bartered to acquire daily needs. Bartering, which gradually became selling, represented a simple exchange for the essentials of life.

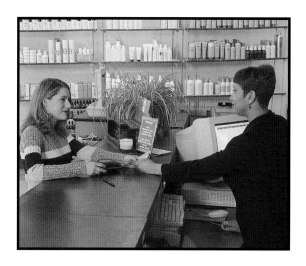

Today, selling combines psychology and sociology in a sophisticated system. Selling has become an important form of expression in society. The systems of exchanging are the same but the approach has become more subtle, more directed. **Successful selling could best be defined as the art of professional recommendation.**

In your daily communication you may be practicing recommendation without even knowing it. When you try to convince someone of the merits of an idea or your ability to get the job done, you are really asking them to believe in you. In the professional beauty industry, you take this a step further and begin to use confidence and expertise to recommend a product or service. You are, in effect, persuading someone else to trust and believe in your professionalism.

The keys to retail selling in a salon are remarkably similar to convincing others to like and believe in you. As a professional "recommender," you will be selling two important things:

1. Your artistic abilities, services, credibility and professionalism

2. Retail products, grooming aids and implements

Prescribing

When you begin working in a salon, you will be well trained in cutting and styling hair and will feel confident providing those and other related services to clients. Your clients will learn to trust and believe in you and your talents as a professional stylist and most will be very willing to listen to your recommendations.

Clients who come to you will want to learn how to take care of their hair, skin and nails at home between visits. A logical extension of your salon service is prescribing the kind of quality products for use at home that will complement your styling services. The term upselling refers to increasing the client's ticket by adding retail products as well as other salon services. Clients will appreciate your concern and will usually accept your recommendations of hair, skin and nail care retail products. Professional product recommendations will help you establish a clientele that will remain loyal to you and to the products you recommend. Retailing is part of a total professional concept, a complete approach to client service. Successful salons are those whose staff members are effectively prescribing their services and a quality line of retail products.

Knowledge & Confidence

To promote retail products effectively you must have confidence in yourself and the products you recommend. That confidence comes from thorough knowledge of each item and through first-hand experience with the product.

The more experienced you become while in school, the more successful you will be on the job. The next time someone comes in for a haircut, suggest something that will enhance the hair and benefit the client.

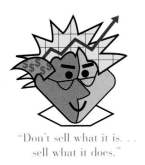

"Don't sell what it is. . . sell what it does."

Become an invaluable asset to any salon staff by:
- Listening to clients
- Recognizing their needs
- Offering sound advice
- Recommending the best products for home use
- Communicating professionally while performing services

Professional Products

It is your responsibility as a professional to familiarize yourself with the finest products for hair, skin and nails. Practice recommending products to your clients in school, and check with them periodically to be certain that the product is giving the expected results. Maintaining a binder that serves as a source of information about product ingredients, costs and promotions will assist you in remaining current with product information. Unless you are thoroughly familiar with a product, its uses and benefits, you will be unable to offer effective recommendations. It is necessary that you learn as much as possible about a line of products and try them yourself to become completely familiar with them. If you don't use and believe in products you're promoting, you'll have much more difficulty in being a success at getting others to try them!

Salons do have advantages over drugstores, department stores and supermarkets when retailing grooming aids. They have the opportunity to prove that a product works by demonstrating its use and effectiveness. Salons provide licensed professionals like you to give your recommendations about products that will most benefit the consumer. A salon will want to be certain that the products offered for retail are safe and that stylists do not overstate any warranty criteria. An in-depth knowledge of professional products begins with an understanding of their features and benefits.

Features and Benefits

Features of a product are its characteristics, which might include the size of the container, the aroma, or a specific ingredient. Benefits of a product are things that the product will do to enhance the appearance or improve the condition of the client's hair, skin or nails. When you begin working in a salon, study the features and benefits of all the retail products offered for sale. You'll soon discover this simple formula for success:

FEATURES + BENEFITS = INCENTIVE TO BUY

If features are presented in an appealing manner, benefits explained thoroughly, and both customized according to individual need, the client will most likely buy the product. Following are examples of features and benefits:

Features	Benefits
1. Size - bottle is small	1. Perfect for travelling
2. Ingredients - product contains protein	2. Reconditioning effect
3. Concentrated formula - small amount required	3. Economical purchase

6

One of the keys to successful prescribing is to customize the product's features and benefits to fit the needs of the client. In order to customize home care programs, you must first ask your clients questions to determine their needs, lifestyle, style desired and any hair and scalp problems they might have. Start with general questions like the following: (Your client's answers will give you additional direction.)

- Who recommended you to the salon?

- When did you have your last (perm, haircut, manicure, etc.)?

- What do you want from a (perm, haircut, permanent color, etc.)?

- What didn't you like about that (perm, haircut, permanent color, etc.)?

- Which (shampoo, conditioner, moisturizer, nail polish, etc.) works best for you? Why?

Involve the Client

Describe a product's features and benefits, and you will interest clients and gain their attention. The next step in successful recommendation is to let the client hold, smell or sample the product. The more the senses are used in examining a product, the more involved the client becomes with the product and the more personally he or she will identify with that item. It would be very difficult for a client to gain a feel-ing about the product if it were out of reach or behind glass. To effectively promote a product's benefits, you may wish to demonstrate the product for the client and make testers available to examine and try. With a skin care product, for example, you could give a "mini facial" and then have the client feel the effects on the skin's surface.

Personal referrals and recommendations of retail products provide your most effective advertising.

Suggest New Products

As new products are introduced in the salon, think of the clients who would benefit from their use. When those clients come in for a visit, present the products' features and benefits. Then suggest that they try the items at home. You are once again reinforcing your concern for your clients and your professionalism in the salon.

Your clients will return again and again to buy those items that they believe are best suited for them and this is the start of your successful repeat business! Having been "sold" on a product once and having used it and liked the results, clients will more than likely continue to buy products on their own initiative, leaving you time to teach new clients about home grooming care.

Closing the Sale

Just as important as presenting a product's features and benefits is the closing of the sale. If you are afraid to ask the client for a commitment after all your effort to present products, you have just wasted time!

You, as a salon stylist, cannot earn a retail commission or bonus unless you promote and conclude your professional recommendation of the retail items. Nor can you expect the professional services that you perform on clients, such as haircoloring or perms, to last and look attractive unless clients care for their hair at home with the right products.

The conclusion of a retail sale is something that you build up to from the beginning of the recommendation process. Your positive attitude, your knowledge of the product, your explanation of the product benefits and how it is to be used, and your customized treatment program for the client, all reinforce the fact that you expect the client to purchase the product.

The next time you make a retail purchase of some sort, listen to the salesperson's presentation. Evaluate it in terms of the features and benefits of the product.

State the price. If the client has an objection to the price of a retail product, that person is actually saying to you, "Prove to me that it's worth the investment."

If the product's features and benefits have been clearly and personally related to the client's needs, price will be less important. If a client does raise a price objection, you haven't presented the features and benefits thoroughly enough to convince them to make the purchase. By returning to the important points that have been missed in your presentation (such as personal need), you will give the doubtful client more reasons to buy the item. With the proper in-salon education, the client will plan to spend a certain amount of money each month on the right home hair-care products.

Buyer Types

Understanding different types of potential consumers and what motivates them to buy will help you in closing the sale.

Identify Buyers

- The **Ready Buyer** is open-minded and will take a chance on new products without hesitation. Be sure to keep this buyer aware of any new products the salon is offering.

- The **Logical Buyer** wants to know all the facts about a product, thinks carefully about buying without much regard for who else likes or uses the product. Explain to the logical buyer what a product will do, how it should be used, then supply him/her with available literature. Leave the client alone for a moment to make a decision.

- The **Emotional Buyer** bases purchases more on personal reasons than facts. Maybe the client's friend has a similar product. The emotional buyer is quite often an impulsive, spontaneous person who reacts to color of packaging or aroma of product. Describe how the product will improve cosmetic appearance, show results with proper use, and demonstrate the product's use for the customer. Make sure this buyer understands the benefits.

- The **Bargain Buyer** wants to save money at all costs and is not as interested in quality of product as price. Be sure to keep this buyer aware of any sale items or salon promotions offered. Don't push the client.

- The **Stubborn Buyer** puts up a struggle and has a strong desire to debate with you. Offer all the facts, describe results. Then, if the client still isn't convinced, send product literature home or offer a complimentary trial size if available.

These buyer types are only generalizations and can be found in several combinations. To effectively recommend products, you must believe in yourself and your professional ability to offer the proper treatments for your clients.

What Motivates Buyers

Each buyer is unique. However, all clients share similar motivations for buying, including need, desire to look good, profit or gain and impulse.

Needs are fairly easy to identify if you will observe and listen to your clients during each appointment.

Need is perhaps the easiest buyer motivation to recognize in the salon. For example, virtually everyone needs shampoo. Anti-dandruff shampoos, shampoos for color-treated hair, damaged hair, baby fine hair, dry or oily hair, all fill a need for your clientele.

Another need would be rinse to detangle the hair once it has been shampooed or a conditioner for damaged hair.

Creating need for a product means that you will be making clients aware of a product that will benefit them. By giving clients enough evidence that products are needed and will enhance their appearance, you convince the clients that they must have them.

Creating a need for a product in the mind of the client can be done through effective promotional displays in the salon, through client classes or individual consultations and analysis between the stylist and the client. If, for example, a client comes to you for a haircut, and through hair analysis you find that the hair shows a deficiency, you should identify the need to the client and recommend a conditioning product.

If clients are willing to care for their hair at home, you can write out customized formulas for them and recommend the necessary conditioning products. Follow these steps for successful recommendation.

1. Observe and listen

2. Identify/create the need

3. Recommend products

Salon services will last longer when the hair is properly cared for at home with the right products purchased at your recommendation.

Desire to look their best causes people to make retail purchases. Clients are very conscious of their appearance. They will welcome advice from you on how they can keep their hair and skin looking their best. Salons have a built-in market for skin treatment items and hair care products, such as conditioners and thinning-hair enhancement products. Clients who have experienced hair loss or aging of the skin require very little convincing to try a quality, professionally recommended series of products.

The next major category of buyer motivation is **Profit or Gain**. People like to believe that they make intelligent purchases, no matter what the items. If clients believe that they will benefit from using a particular type of product, they will make those purchases.

If clients need convincing a product is right for them, recommend that they try a small size of an item to see if it is effective for their needs. Once they have determined with the stylist that the product is beneficial, the stylist can then recommend a larger, more economical size of that item on the next visit.

Be careful not to prejudge the clients' ability to afford an item or their desire for a product. Even clients who have carefully budgeted their incomes will also appreciate information on more economical sizes of retail products and will feel complimented by your attention. If you have convinced your clients, they will plan for these retail purchases in advance.

Grooming aids lend themselves to **impulse buying**. Their retailers have created the need for these products through fashion magazines, television advertising and promotion. Salons have a built-in market of clients who want to be fashionable and attractive and who will respond to the need for new hair care and skin care products if the needs are effectively created through display and in-salon promotion. Statistics show that 45% to 65% of all purchases stem from impulse buying

Follow Up

Some clients simply forget how to use the products that you have recommended. To avoid confusion and to reinforce your recommendation of the home hair care program, you might take a product brochure and write instructions on the back regarding the frequency of use. Many salons have printed their own forms with their salon logo, name, address and phone number for additional product recommendations. The stylist or specialist merely fills in the client's name, the products recommended and any special instructions.

Benefits of written special instructions:

1. Reinforce the professionalism of your services and of the salon.

2. Clarify product use for clients so that they won't leave out an important step.

3. Remind clients to do the treatments, if they post the product recommendation form somewhere at home.

4. Help clients remember the products that have been suggested for their use.

5. Help the receptionist with retail recommendations before the client leaves the salon. Enable the stylist to select merchandise from the retail shelves for the client to purchase at the conclusion of the salon visit.

6. Offer referral opportunities. Clients often take product recommendation forms home and show them to their families, friends and neighbors. This sharing could create new clientele for the salon.

Keep in mind that recommending a product one time doesn't guarantee that the client will continue using that item. The record cards that you maintain on each client will help you to see when the last purchases were made and to judge whether the client will be needing additional products on his or her next visit to the salon.

It would be an excellent idea for you to examine the condition of each client's hair, skin or nails several weeks after you have sold them products. If the client has experienced any reactions or if there seems to be no appreciable change in their condition, you will want to change the recommendation for the client. If there have been no problems and even minor improvement, encourage the client to continue with the original program.

It is advised that you not only check the hair, skin and nail condition when a client returns for service appointments but also pay particular attention to seasonal weather changes and how these affect the client. A customized skin care program, for example, that suits a client perfectly during the warm summer months may not be adequate to protect the skin against the ravages of the cold winter. When necessary, revise your recommendations and explain why you are changing them.

Effective Displays

Appreciating the value of salon displays will be most helpful to your future as a professional stylist. When you begin working in a salon, you may be asked to help in the development and maintenance of salon displays. Promotional ideas do much more than brighten the area of the salon where your retail products are displayed. The following information will help you perform those duties in a professional and creative manner. Allocate adequate floor space for retail merchandise. Remember that the salon owner pays rent for every inch in the salon...even empty space! Don't let usable space stay empty; build a retail display to make that space pay! Display shelves for retail products, known as stock or stock inventory, should blend attractively with the salon decor but shouldn't disappear from sight because of their bland appearance. Use your imagination. Place displays in interesting areas of the salon.

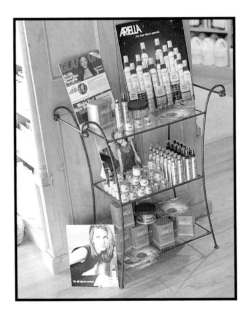
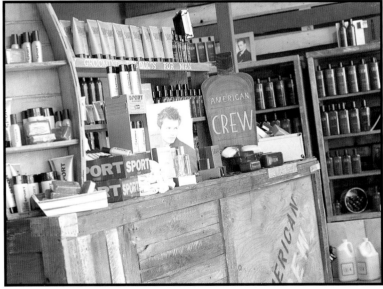
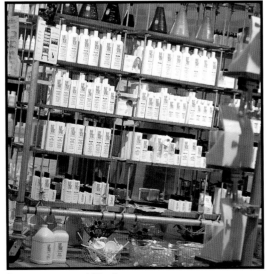
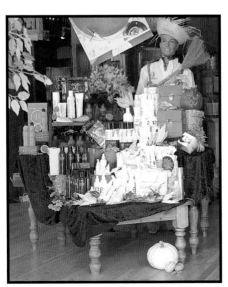

Images courtesy of The Space

Retail Display Guidelines

Organize Stock

- Display the products by category.

- Put top-selling products and sizes at eye level on the display. This saves time and allows client to shop on his/her own.

- Display product using island shelving (available on all sides) if possible. Utilize ends of island displays by placing shelving facing outward. This is called an "end cap" and is designed to catch the eye of the client as they enter the aisles.

- Rotate and rearrange the product to gain attention, prevent fading and ensure freshness of product.

- Place the latest shipment of same product in the back of the display when it arrives.

- Place displays in interesting areas, including high traffic areas, walls, windows, corners and work stations.

Price the Merchandise

- Price all retail products individually.

- Display price where a client can easily find it.

Ensure Quality Control

- Keep products on the edge of the shelves, facing the client. This creates easy access and high visibility of the product.

- Dust products daily and clean the shelves thoroughly at least once a week.

- Light the retail display area of the salon well.

Create Promotional Displays

- Use product identification cards below each product on the shelves.

- Display literature on each retail item near the retail shelves so that clients have additional information to read and take home.

Maintain Inventory Control

- Use an inventory control form so you can monitor what products are selling well. This also helps account for product sales and makes reordering easier.

- Ensure that ordering of products is timely and controlled.

- Keep sufficient quantity of stock on the shelves at all times.

Learn From The Display Experts

- The image of your retail area should attract a client's eye. View what other professional retailers are doing. Grocery stores, department stores and other specialty boutiques can give you great ideas on how their merchandising displays work for them.

6

As you reviewed earlier in this chapter, there has never been a time in history better than now to attain a career in the cosmetology field. A career as a professional cosmetologist will lead the way to many exciting opportunities and rewards. Your efforts to select the job best suited for you, establish career goals, maintain professional relationships and recommend products to clients will help put you on the path to success.

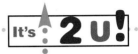

Build Your Critical Thinking Skills

In this chapter you have prepared yourself to meet the following Industry Standards for entry-level cosmetologists:

- Effectively market professional salon products
- Maintain business records on client development, income and expenses
- Efficiently manage product supply for salon use and retail sales

It's up to you to know what to do. Using your training to this point, review the following case scenarios and think through how you would handle each challenge.

1. You have just completed your very first haircut and thermal style client in the salon! Your client is very satisfied with the final results and you are just finishing your comments to her regarding how to care for her hair at home. As you walk your client to the front desk, you recommend that she purchase the mousse that you used when you styled her hair today. She is nodding her head in affirmation when, as you approach the retail area, you notice the shelf where the mousse sets is bare. It has completely sold out! What would you do?

2. The salon owner has just met with you during your first week on the job. He has suggested that you establish a goal of developing five new clients in the next two weeks. He has also challenged you to have these five clients be anyone other than your family, since you can already probably count on them coming in for a salon service. List your top 3 plans of action.

Chapter 7
TRICHOLOGY

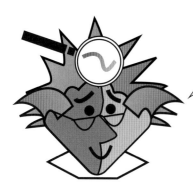

After studying this chapter you will be able to . . .

1. Define the theory of hair, including formation, growth, structure, behavior and color.

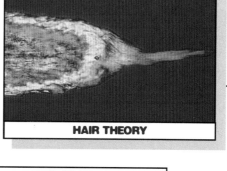

HAIR THEORY

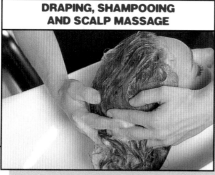

DRAPING, SHAMPOOING AND SCALP MASSAGE

3. Explain and demonstrate proper draping, shampooing and scalp massage services.

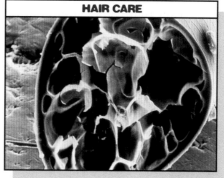

HAIR CARE

2. Recognize how to care for the hair by doing an evaluation for common hair disorders, including hair loss.

You're moving closer to your goal every minute. If you skim through its photos, this chapter probably looks more like what you expected in a cosmetology textbook. Isn't that a picture of a shampoo bowl right on this page? I bet your fingers are just itching to begin their skillful work in shampooing and scalp massage. This chapter on hair theory and care definitely holds a key for you into the world for which you've been waiting.

TRICHO (hair) + OLOGY (the study of) = TRICHOLOGY

You will be more successful with the services you perform if you know the composition, structure and behavior of hair, how to evaluate it for product selection and how to properly drape and shampoo the client and give a scalp massage. Clients may choose you specifically for the wonderful shampoo and massage you offer.

Nothing equals the security of being able to put yourself in good hands. The client who trusts a stylist can relax and enjoy the opening part of a hair care service. The VALUE your client perceives in your skill returns to you in customer loyalty.

The quality of your salon services depends on your knowledge of all phases of hair growth, of common hair and scalp disorders and of causes and treatments of hair loss as well as on your attentiveness and skill during the draping, shampoo and scalp massage.

My PLAN for you in this chapter is very straight forward. First you learn the essentials of hair theory and then of hair care. After that you begin to put this learning into practice through several simple procedures.

HAIR THEORY

Hair Bulb Formation
Hair Growth
Hair Structure and Behavior
Natural Hair Color

HAIR CARE

Hair Evaluation
Common Hair Conditions
Common Scalp Conditions
Hair Loss

DRAPING, SHAMPOOING AND SCALP MASSAGE

Draping Theory
Shampooing and Conditioning Theory
Scalp Massage Theory
Draping, Shampooing and Scalp
  Massage Essentials
Infection Control and Safety
Basic Draping, Shampooing and
  Conditioning
Basic Scalp Massage

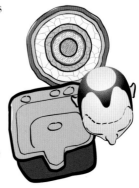

HAIR THEORY

Hair, you cut it and it grows again! It becomes damaged either by nature or improper care and it can be reconditioned. Its color can be changed and it can take on straight, wavy or curly shapes. **The main purposes of hair are protection from heat, cold and injury, as well as adornment.** But have you ever wondered what makes all this possible? The answers lie in the marvelous, mysterious biology of living matter or, for your purposes of study, *Trichology*, **the technical name for the study of hair.**

Living matter. What does it mean to say that something is alive? By definition, to say that matter has life means that it grows, it can reproduce, and it responds to stimulation. That is, it can act. It can react.

Is hair alive? Even though hair is primarily protein and protein is the basis for all living matter, **only the cells of the hair bulb are alive. The hair *fiber* or *strand* itself is not alive.**

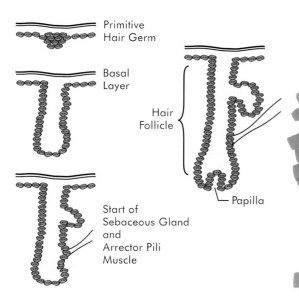

Primitive Hair Germ

Basal Layer

Hair Follicle

Start of Sebaceous Gland and Arrector Pili Muscle

Papilla

Hair Bulb Formation

To understand more about hair, you need to know how the hair bulb is formed. In fetal life, the hair follicle forms from a cluster of cells in the upper layer of skin, technically referred to as the *basal layer* of the *epidermis*. This cluster of cells, called the *primitive hair germ*, needs nourishment to grow into a fully developed hair follicle. To get nourishment, it works its way down into the lower (dermal) layer of the skin. As it does, the cell cluster pulls the upper layer down with it, creating a follicle or tube-like "pocket" called the root sheath, out of which the hair will grow.

The shape of this follicle will determine the shape (round, oval, elliptical, etc.) of the hair shaft as it grows from the follicle. Since the hair shaft actually grows out of the hair follicle, the diameter of the hair fiber will be the same as the diameter of the inside of the follicle.

Two Primary Parts of Hair
The **hair root** is the portion of hair that is inside the hair follicle *under* the skin's surface. The **hair fiber**, sometimes referred to as the *hair shaft* or *strand*, is the portion of the hair that extends above the skin's surface.

In straight or wavy hair, hair follicles are more or less vertical to the surface of the scalp, with a slight "tilt." The angle of the hair follicle determines the natural flow or wave pattern of the hair. **The follicle in straight or wavy hair is typically round or oval.**

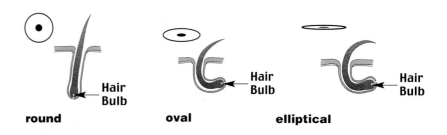

round — Hair Bulb

oval — Hair Bulb

elliptical — Hair Bulb

In hair that is curly/kinky, the hair follicles grow from the scalp at a much stronger angle. The follicle is almost parallel to the surface of the scalp. Furthermore, the hair bulb itself is nearly doubled back over the follicle in a growth shape resembling a golf club. **The hair follicle that produces a curly/kinky hair has a flattened, elliptical shape.**

Hair Growth

As this primitive hair germ continues its growth downward into the dermis and joins a small number of dermal cells, these cells eventually become the dermal **papilla. The papilla is filled with capillaries (small blood vessels) that supply nourishment to the cells around it, called germinal matrix cells.** The germinal matrix is the area of the bulb where cell division (mitosis) takes place. These germinal matrix cells produce the cells that ultimately *keratinize (harden)* and form the three major layers of the hair:

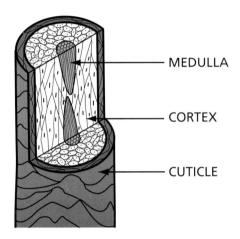

MEDULLA

CORTEX

CUTICLE

1. **Cuticle** - the outer covering of the hair shaft made up of overlapping layers of transparent scales

2. **Cortex** - the second layer consisting of unique protein structures (gives hair most of its pigment and strength [elasticity]

3. **Medulla** - the central core of the hair shaft, also called the pith or marrow (often absent in fine or very fine hair)

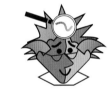

"Hair pulled out from the roots will grow again unless the papilla (origin of hair) is destroyed."

Attached to the side of the root sheath are bulges. These bulges are the beginnings of the sebaceous glands. **The sebaceous, or oil, glands produce sebum (oil) and send it up through the hair follicles to the surface of the skin to prevent the hair and skin from becoming too dry. Sebum mixes with the body's perspiration to form the "acid mantle." The acid mantle is important because it protects the cuticle, or outer covering, of the hair fiber and maintains the acid balance of hair and skin.**

The arrector pili muscle comes from cells in the dermis that attach to the follicle just below the sebaceous gland. This is the muscle that causes the hair to stand on end when a person is scared or cold. It also aids in the secretion of sebum from the sebaceous glands. The other end of the arrector pili muscle attaches to the dermis (or lower layer) just beneath the basal layer of the epidermis.

Cells Form Parts of the Hair

As cells begin their journey upward through the hair follicle, they are separated into specific types. In other words, some cells will become cuticle scales, others will make up the cortex and others will have the particular formation of medulla cells. The journey that began deep in the skin, then grew through the outer layers now becomes the visible hair fiber (shaft or strand). Another result of this process of traveling upward is keratinization. **Keratinization is a process whereby cells change their shape, dry out and form keratin protein. Once keratinized, the cells that form the hair fiber or strand are no longer alive.**

Amino Acids = Protein = Hair

Hair is made up primarily of protein, which is made from the linking together of amino acids. The cortex of the hair is made of chains that take the shape of a helix or coil. These amino acid chains coil around each other and become protofibrils. Protofibrils then twist around each other to become microfibrils. Microfibrils follow the same process and become macrofibrils that also spiral together. This process, when complete, forms the cortex of the hair. The cortex is then covered with the cuticle scales, which also contain protein. **This twisting gives hair the ability to stretch like a spring without breaking.**

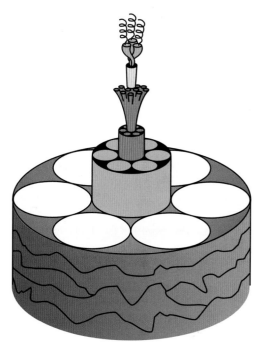

The prefix PROTO means first, the prefix MICRO means small and the prefix MACRO means large. Other examples would be prototype, microscope and macrobiotics.

Stages of Hair Growth

Genes determine the growing stages of the hair. There are three stages of hair growth:

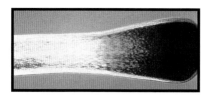

ANAGEN

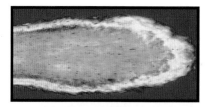

CATAGEN

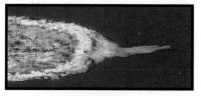

TELOGEN

1. The anagen or *active growing stage*, during which time each hair bulb has an attached root sheath. On the average 90 percent of a person's hair is in this stage which lasts from two to six years. Hair color is darker during the anagen stage.

2. The catagen, a *brief transitional stage*, when all cell division stops. This stage lasts only a few weeks.

3. The telogen or *resting stage*, when each hair bulb has no attached root sheath. At this time the hair falls out. On the average 10 to 15 percent of hair is in the resting stage, which generally lasts 3-4 months. Eventually, cell division is again stimulated, producing new hair, and the growth cycle starts again.

In humans, a mosaic pattern of hair growth occurs because each hair follicle has its own unique growing cycle. **Illness and lack of necessary vitamins and minerals can also affect hair and hair growth. In fact, anything that**

"In humans, the average rate of hair growth is 1/2" (1.25 cm) per month."

alters the physiological state of the body can affect the hair follicle and hair growth. Disease and medication can also affect hair growth by either stimulating the onset of the telogen phase or by causing the production of abnormal, brittle hairs. If a person has been ill or taking any medication, chemical services can damage hair that may be weak already.

Contrary to an old myth, hair does not grow after death. Hair never grows on palms, soles of feet, lips and eyelids.

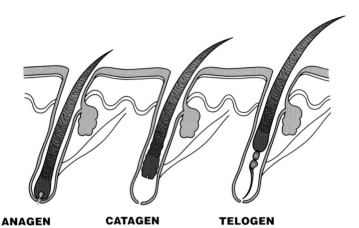

ANAGEN   CATAGEN   TELOGEN

Eyebrows and eyelashes are replaced every 4-5 months. Eyelashes are technically called cilia.

Hair Structure and Behavior

If all hair is made up primarily of protein, then why is everyone's hair so different? Why does a shampoo that works well on one person's hair not work well on another's?

The answer lies in the physical structure of hair. There are three factors that affect the behavior of hair.

1. The first factor is **heredity**. The genes that each person inherits from his/her parents will determine many things about the makeup of the hair, such as its color, shape and diameter.

2. The second factor is the **environment** or weather. If it's rainy or humid, hair will absorb moisture from the air. This extra moisture will alter some of the bonds that give hair its shape and, depending on the type of hair, it may become either limp or frizzy. On the other hand, wind may dry out the hair and sun may damage it. Both of these weather conditions—unusually wet or dry—can cause a need for products that either take excess moisture out of the hair or put more moisture back in.

3. The third factor is the **products** or **appliances** used on the hair. For example, shampoos, conditioners, hair dryers, curling irons, perms, relaxers and hair color all affect the structural organization of the hair.

To better understand the differences in peoples' hair, you will need to take a closer look at hair's structural organization. The following series of slides taken of hair magnified hundreds of times show differences in diameter of hair.

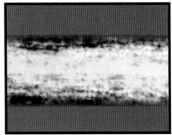

FINE

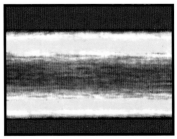

MEDIUM

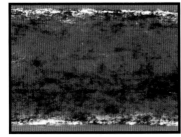

COARSE

In the next series, observe the difference between Caucasian hair, Asian hair and Afro-centric hair. Notice that the structural organization of hair as shown by diameter and amount of pigment are very different among the three races. Keep in mind that diameter and amount of pigment may vary within each race as well.

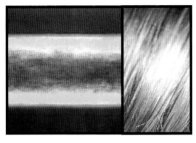

CAUCASIAN

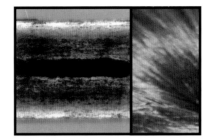

ASIAN

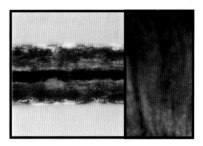

AFRO-CENTRIC

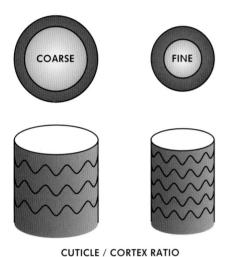

CUTICLE / CORTEX RATIO

One result of genetic coding is the diameter of the hair shaft. In the picture on the left, notice the cuticle of a cross-sectional view of fine hair. Next, notice the picture of coarse hair.

As you've already seen, the cuticle is the protective part of the hair shaft and is made up of a harder protein than the cortex. If the hair is fine, treatments will affect it differently than if it's coarse. Examples include how well the hair holds a set and how the hair takes a perm or relaxer. It's an exaggeration to say that fine hair is "all cuticle," but that is often how it behaves. In cross section, up to 40% of fine hair can be cuticle, compared with 10% or 12% in coarse hair. The diameter of coarse hair is much larger than fine hair.

The cuticle is a hard, resistant layer of protein compared with the soft, elastic quality of the cortex. If a particular hair is 90% cortex and 10% cuticle, then that hair behaves like the cortex. That means it has more elasticity and ability to be molded and reshaped. But if the cuticle (which is harder or firmer and not easily stretched) makes up 40% of the hair fiber, then that hair will behave more like the cuticle and be more resistant to perms, relaxers or holding a set.

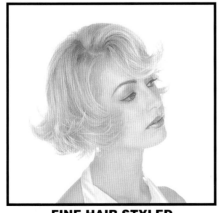

FINE HAIR STYLED

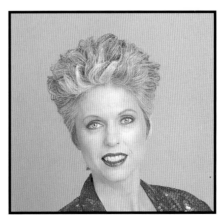

COARSE HAIR STYLED

Natural Hair Color

One of the most fascinating aspects of hair is how it gets its color. Many people know that a pigment (coloring matter) called chlorophyll gives plants their green color. Most people don't know that a pigment called melanin gives skin and hair their color. In the hair, melanin is found mainly in the cortex, the hair strand's second layer. Here is how the natural coloring process works:

1. Genes in the human body determine the number of melanocytes in the hair and the type of melanin they produce.

2. Melanin is produced by melanocytes, cells that exist among the dividing cells within the hair bulb.

3. Melanocytes that rest near the hair bulb's nourishment center, the dermal papilla, collect together and form bundles of a pigment protein complex called melanosomes.

4. The size, type and distribution of these melanosomes will determine the natural color of the hair.

In simple terms, melanin is formed by various melanocytes (melanin cells) that bundle together to create melanosomes (pigment protein complex).

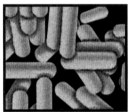 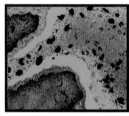 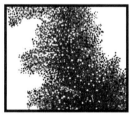

MELANOCYTES   **MELANOSOMES**   **MELANIN**

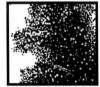

EUMELANIN   **PHEOMELANIN**

There are two types of melanin that create the large variety of hair colors, eumelanin and pheomelanin. Eumalinin is brown/black in color and pheomelanin is red in color. It is the amount and distribution of one or both of these melanins that influence the resulting hair color.

If the amount of pheomelanin is very concentrated and near the cuticle layer, the hair color will appear more red. People with very dark, black hair may even have melanin in the cuticle layer, while lighter hair has melanin only in the cortex. **When there is a total lack of pigmentation in the hair and skin, the resulting condition is called albinism. A person with this condition is called an albino.**

Gray hair is caused by reduced color pigment, melanin, in the cortex layer of the hair. Gray hair is sometimes referred to as mottled hair, indicating white spots scattered about in the hair shafts. Gray hair grows from the papilla with the gray color, not as some might believe, turning gray after it has protruded above the skin. The natural aging process in humans is the cause of graying hair. However, some serious illnesses or emotional conditions may cause the hair to turn gray. A hereditary condition occurring at birth may cause some to gray prematurely. This is usually a defect in pigment formation.

Melanin in the Skin

Melanin in both the skin and hair serves as protection from the sun's damaging rays. For instance, if skin is exposed to sunlight, more melanin is created and sent to the surface to protect these sensitive cells, resulting in more color, or what is commonly called a "suntan." Although skin color is passed on through the genes, races that originated closer to the equator developed a higher content of melanin in their skin to better protect it against the sun. The same is true for hair. For example, white hair, which lacks melanin, is at the greatest risk for sun damage and can turn yellow from too much exposure. Therefore, you should recommend products with sunscreen and encourage your clients to wear hats when they anticipate spending extended periods of time in the sun.

HAIR CARE

Now it's time to apply the science and "humanize" your newly gained knowledge. It is, after all, people you'll be dealing with in your career as a cosmetologist, not just knowledge. Each person you'll work with is unique. The condition of each person's hair will differ, at least slightly, from any other you may have seen before. Sometimes those differences will be dramatic. Hair in poor condition will not hold a style or show off your design talent. Before you pick up shears or a comb, you will need to evaluate your client's hair.

Hair Evaluation

Hair is a fiber, and like all natural fibers, hair has different characteristics. Becoming familiar with your client's hair prior to any service will allow you to support his/her individual hair needs.

1. **Determine your client's hair type and distribution**

Knowing whether your client's hair type is fine, medium, or coarse tells you what it can and cannot do on its own. You will usually determine your client's hair type by touch and visual examination. **The degree of coarseness or fineness in the hair fiber is referred to as texture.** The texture of coarse hair has the feel of wool, medium hair, the feel of cotton, and fine hair, the feel of silk. Other terms used to describe the feel of the hair include rough, wiry or soft. Once you know that, you're on your way to determining the particular cleansing and conditioning products that will best meet the hair's needs.

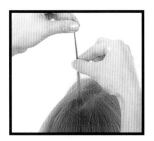

Visual examination will give you a lot of clues. You can usually see whether the hair is dry or oily but, when you suspect it's been chemically altered, confirm this with your client. Ask the client, "Is your hair currently permed or tinted? Relaxed?" These are key questions to determine which cleansing and conditioning products will work best.

A damaged or rough cuticle can cause hair to snag, look dull, or be hard to manage. You can test for cuticle damage by running your thumb and finger along a strand of hair against the direction of growth. The more "drag" you feel, the more damage you can assume. Additional visual examination would include determining hair density. **The density of the hair is judged by the number of active hair follicles per square inch on the scalp.** For instance, a person with a thick head of hair will have many more active hair follicles than a person with thin hair. Density is usually referred to as light, medium or heavy (sometimes as thin, medium or thick). Density of the hair influences the amount of hair that should be parted and wrapped around a perm rod, roller or curling iron. Heavy density requires smaller subsections than light hair to allow for absorption of styling and processing lotions. In addition, placing too much hair on a perm rod or roller weakens the expected curl. Larger subsections can be used for light density hair.

2. Determine your client's hair condition

Once you know the type of hair fiber with which you will be working, you need to know the condition of that fiber. The condition of the hair is usually determined by two key factors:

a. **Hair porosity, the amount of moisture able to be absorbed by hair.** Raised cuticles influence the amount of liquid that can penetrate the hair. *Resistant porosity* describes hair that is able to absorb the least amount of moisture, usually due to the closeness of the cuticle layers. Resistant porosity is also called "poor porosity." *Average porosity* describes hair with the normal ability to absorb moisture. Such hair is in good condition, suitable for most services. *Extreme porosity* describes hair that is damaged from chemical services, such as overprocessing or the environment. Hair with extreme porosity is not in good condition and would require treatments prior to chemical services. *Uneven porosity* is a combination of both porosities.

b. **Hair elasticity, the ability of hair to stretch and return to its original shape without breaking.** Elasticity is also referred to as resiliency. Additional descriptive words to use when discussing elasticity with your client include pliability, buoyancy and springiness. Hair with normal elasticity is lively, able to spring back and usually has a shiny appearance. **Normal dry hair is capable of being stretched about one-fifth of its length. Wet hair is able to be stretched 40% to 50% of its length.**

Test for Structural Strength

While visual examination for elasticity is not absolutely accurate, it can tell you a great deal. Just by looking at the hair and handling it, you'll make judgements about what it needs. You can also perform this test for elasticity. (Note that this test is intended for straight or wavy hair.)

- Remove a strand of hair from the side of the head above the ears.

- Hold it between your thumb and forefinger and, with your thumbnail and index finger of the other hand, run the distance of hair rapidly as you would curl a ribbon with scissors. This will create a series of small curls.

- Gently pull the hair taut for 10 seconds and release. If the hair completely, or almost completely, returns to the curl pattern, it is in good condition. If it returns only 50% or less, it is structurally weak and needs conditioning.

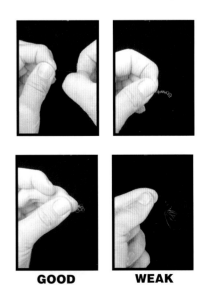

GOOD   WEAK

3. Consider the effects of your climate

Once you have thoroughly evaluated the fiber, it's important to consider the climate in which you live. Is your climate primarily dry or humid? Because the amount of moisture in the air governs the amount of moisture in the hair, predominant humidity makes a big difference in the way hair looks and feels and, thus, a difference in the shampoo and conditioners you'll use. In humid regions, where hair becomes heavy with moisture, curl retention is a challenge, and protein conditioning may be needed to balance the moisture intake. In dry climates, hair tends to be flyaway, so moisturizing and surface conditioning become very important to reduce static and soften the hair fiber.

The more information you can gain from the client, the easier it will be to achieve good results. You will want to give your client's hair whatever it needs to look, feel and behave beautifully, beginning with the right hair analysis and followed by proper shampooing and conditioning.

Common Hair Conditions

Each hair strand has about seven to twelve layers of cuticle scales. The cuticle layers protect the inside of the strand, which is called the cortex.

In healthy hair, the scales should lie flat along the cortex. The acid mantle lubricates the outermost layer of the cuticle and reduces friction. **Friction, as in combing and brushing, is one way in which the cuticle can be damaged.**

During your professional analysis of the hair fiber, a number of observations will alert you to possible problems you might encounter as you service the client's hair:

1. **Broken hair**. One of the most common causes of hair breakage is excessive stretching or traction. Hair subjected to excessive chemical processes, sun exposure and chlorine exposure may also exhibit breakage. The technical term for broken hair is **abraded hair**. One of the most common types of cuticle damage is called an **abraded cuticle. Abrasion can result from brushing or manipulating the hair while styling it, especially when it's still wet. Wet hair is more fragile than dry hair.** Rubber bands, tight hair clips and braids can actually break the cuticle. So can wrapping hair too tightly around a roller.

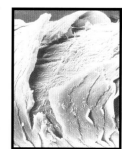

2. **Split ends. The technical terms for split ends are fragilitis crinium (frah-JIL-I-tas KRI-nee-um), brittle hair or trichoptilosis (tri-kop-ti-LOH-sis).** Split ends start as small cracks in the cuticle that deepen into the cortex. Eventually the hair is split entirely. Often there is no cuticle left in the region of a split and, if not cut off, the ends become frayed and unsightly. Split ends can be temporarily "sealed" by protein reconditioning. However, the process must be repeated frequently to keep the splits closed. In severe cases, it is advisable to cut off the split ends and reinforce the hair with a protein conditioner to prevent the freshly cut ends from splitting.

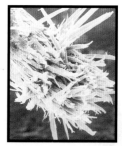

3. **Matting**. Excessive matting, called **pilica polonica** (**PIL**-i-ca **POL**-a-ni-ca), is characterized by a mass of hair strands tangled together in a mat that cannot be separated. The only remedy lies with a pair of shears. The cause of pilica polonica is usually excessive chemical hair lightening. In some cases, excessive friction can be the cause, as in repeated backcombing.

4. **Nodules**. **Trichorrhexis nodosa** (**TRIK**-o-rek-sis no-**DO**-sa), or knotted hair, **is characterized by the presence of lumps or swelling along the hair shaft**. These lumps are broken or partly broken places on the hair shaft. They can be caused by poorly performed chemical services, mechanical damage from curling irons or backcombing or by an inherited defect in the hair's keratin protein structure. Physical knotting of the hair (known as trichonodosis) results from friction of the scalp, as in vigorous towel drying or rubbing against a pillow.

5. **Canities** (ka-**NEESH**-eez). **Canities is the name given to grayness or whiteness of the hair.** Congenital canities occur at or before birth primarily in albinos and occasionally on people with normal hair. Acquired canities refers to the loss of pigment in the hair as a person ages (graying of hair) or an onset may happen in early adult life. Causes of acquired canities may be extended illness, nervous strain or heredity.

6. **Ringed hair**. When alternating bands of gray and dark hair exist, the conditon is referred to as ringed hair.

7. **Hypertrichosis** (hi-per-tri-**KOH**-sis) **describes an abnormal coverage of hair on areas of the body where normally only lanugo hair appears. Hypertrichosis is also referred to as hirsuties (hur-sue-SHEEZ) or superfluous hair.** Removal methods range from tweezing to electrolysis, depending on the amount of hair to be removed, location and client preference.

8. **Monilethrix** (mo-**NIL**-e-thriks). **Beads or nodes formed on the hair shaft is a condition referred to as Monilethrix.** Breaks in the hair occur between the beads or nodes. Treatments may be given to improve the hair condition.

Mechanical damage results from the incorrect use of styling tools. Some brushes can pull the hair and stretch it until it breaks or they can wear down and loosen the cuticle cells. **If a dryer is used too close to the hair or a hot curling iron is left on too long, the hair may become brittle and the cortex could possibly melt.**

Usually, if the cortex is damaged, the cuticle has been damaged, too. However, sometimes the hair is damaged inside with only barely noticeable damage to the cuticle scales. Compare the picture of a normal cortex with the picture of the melted cortex as seen below. Other examples of heat styling damage include blistering and fracturing of the hair fiber due to improper heat-styling or use of low quality styling appliances.

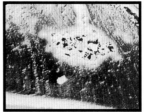 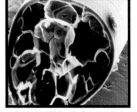

NORMAL CORTEX   **MELTED CORTEX**

Common Scalp Conditions

Listed below are the more common scalp disorders or diseases which you may come in contact with as a professional cosmetologist.

Disorder or Disease	Medical Term	Description	Treatment
Dandruff *Disorder*	Pityriasis (pit-i-REYE-ah-sis)	Chronic scalp condition with excessive flaking, which accumulates on the scalp or falls to the shoulders, as well as itchiness, tightness and irritation of the scalp	Frequent shampooing with an anti-dandruff shampoo containing either pyrithione zinc, selenium disulfide or ketoconazole
Dry Dandruff *Disorder*	Pityriasis capitis simplex (kah-PEYE-tis SIM-pleks)	Dry flakes attached to the scalp or on the hair which can appear translucent	
Greasy or waxy dandruff *Disorder*	Pityriasis steatoides (ste-a-TOY-dez)	Oily flakes combine with sebum which stick to the scalp in clusters and can appear yellowish in color	

Leading cause of dandruff is a naturally occuring microscopic fungus called Malassezia (mal-uh-SEEZ-ee-uh). The fungus feeds on the scalp's natural oils and creates by-products that cause irritation on the scalp. The body reacts to the irritation by accelerating the amount and rate of flaking of dead skin cells.

External Parasites

Be advised that the conditions listed on the chart below are contagious and require you to refer the client to a physician.

7

Disorder or Disease	Medical Term	Description	Treatment
Ringworm *Disease*	Tinea (TIN-ee-ah)	Red, circular patch of small blisters; caused by a vegetable parasite	Refer client to a physician
Ringworm of the Scalp *Disease*	Tinea capitis	Enlarged open hair follicles that are surrounded by clusters of red spots (papules); hair is likely to break in area infected; black spots may also be visible	Refer client to a physician
Honeycomb Ringworm *Disease*	Tinea favosa (fa-VO-sah) or Favus (FAY-vus)	Dry, yellow, encrusted areas on the scalp called scutula (SKUT-u-la); may have a peculiar odor; shiny pink or white scars may result	Refer client to a physician
Itch Mite *Disorder*	Scabies	Red and watery vesicles or pus-filled areas caused by an animal parasite (itch mite) burrowing under the skin.	Refer client to a physician
Head Lice *Disorder*	Pediculosis capitis (pe-dik-u-LOH-sis)	Infestation of head lice on the scalp causing itching and eventual infection	Refer client to a physician
Psoriasis *Disorder*	Psoriasis (soh-REYE-ah-sis)	Thick, crusty patches of red irritated scalp resulting from an autoimmune disease of the skin	Refer client to a physician

Hair Loss

As a salon professional, you are often the first person asked to respond to questions about hair loss. So knowing how to adequately address client concerns will greatly affect your client's well-being.

--Number of Hairs on Head

Red = 90,000	Brown = 110,000
Black = 108,000	Blonde = 140,000

There is an average of 1,000 hairs to a square inch on the average head.

Normal Hair Loss

Hair actually covers most of your body before you are born. Lanugo is the term assigned to this baby fine, silky hair, which is shed shortly after birth. Lanugo is replaced with vellus which covers most of the body including the head, and is often not visible to the naked eye. Vellus is short, fine, non-pigmented hair found more abundantly on women. Certain follicles are predetermined to produce long, thick pigmented hair, like normal scalp and eyebrow hair. This hair is referred to as terminal hair and replaces vellus hair around the time of puberty.

Everyone loses some hair every day. **Actually between 40 and 100 strands of hair is the average daily hair loss.** That's not as much as it sounds, considering that the average head has about 100,000 individual strands of hair.

Androgenetic Hair Loss

Alopecia, or excessive hair loss, may be caused by a fungal or bacterial infection or inflammatory disease of the scalp. This abnormal condition occurs in both men and women. If the scalp appears abnormal at all, do not attempt any services. Instead suggest that your client see a dermatologist. When there is no apparent scalp abnormality, hair loss may be caused by nutritional deficiency, drugs, emotional trauma and other physiological changes.

The most common form of alopecia is androgenetic alopecia, a combination of heredity, hormones and age that causes progressive shrinking, or miniaturization, of certain scalp follicles. This shrinking causes a shortening of the hair's growing cycle. Over time, as the active growth phase (anagen) becomes shorter, the resting phase (telogen) becomes longer. Eventually, there is no growth at all.

Recognizing Androgenetic Alopecia

In general, asking questions about family history will give a good indication of whether the hair loss is androgenetic or another type of alopecia. Ask your client if his/her parents or more distant relatives have hair loss, whether thinning has been gradual over several years or sudden or patchy. If the hair loss was sudden or patchy, advise your client to talk to a physician. If your client is a woman, ask her about crash diets, oral contraceptives, medications such as certain cardiovascular conditions, vitamin deficiencies, and thyroid disorders to rule out hair loss created by these factors.

Because hair length and thickness are determined by how long the hair is allowed to grow before entering the next resting and shedding phase, the hair-loss process is thus a gradual conversion of terminal hair follicles to vellus-like follicles.

The net result is an increasing number of short, thin hairs that are barely visible above the scalp surface, and eventually no more hair is produced out of these follicles. In addition, more follicles are in the resting phase at the same time. Consequently, there is less scalp coverage.

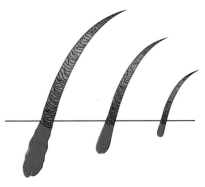

PROGRESSIVE MINIATURIZATION OF THE HAIR FOLLICLE

Despite the dramatic reduction in follicle size with androgenetic alopecia, the follicle is not altered in structure nor does the number of follicles change.

In men, androgenetic alopecia is known as male pattern baldness and frequently progresses to the familiar horseshoe-shaped fringe of hair. In women, it appears as a generalized thinning of the hair over the entire crown of the head. A significant difference between the genders is that most women exhibit scattered hair thinning. It is extremely rare for a woman to "go bald."

Women with androgenetic alopecia usually first notice a gradual thinning of their hair, mostly on top of their heads as their scalp becomes more visible. Over time, the hair on the sides may also become thinner. Women retain their frontal hairline, which may be straight or "M"-shaped.

In the area where the scalp shows the most, look for a large number of miniaturized follicles that are producing shorter, thinner, fewer hairs than the long ones. Unlike hairs that have been cut short and have a flat end, miniaturized hairs. Hold an index card near the scalp to help you see the miniaturized hairs. If you see a lot of miniaturized hairs, your client has androgenetic alopecia.

In addition to identifying miniaturized hairs by holding an index card close to the scalp, in the case of female clients, you may:

1. Part the hair in the middle of the scalp and look at the width of the part. A part that shows more scalp than normal indicates hair loss (a part on a normal head is very narrow).

2. Ask if the diameter of the ponytail has become smaller over the years (if applicable). A smaller diameter is one of the signs of androgenetic alopecia.

3. Ask your client if there are many hairs left on the brush after brushing once or if there are many hairs in the shower drain after shampooing. Check if your client has excessive shedding by simply running your hand through her hair. In general, anyone who has unusual, excessive shedding should see a doctor.

In the case of men, ask the client if the size of the bald spot has progressively increased over the years. In frontal balding, ask if the hairline has been progressively receding. With male clients, it is important to evaluate pattern separately from density because a man with a small pattern but a poor density may not respond to treatment as well as a man with a large area of hair loss and a fair density.

The degree of hair loss can be evaluated by rating pattern and density:
- Pattern refers to the shape and location of the area with hair loss.

- Density refers to how much hair is covering the scalp in the area of hair loss.

Note: Because women experience a single pattern of hair loss, only density needs to be evaluated.

DEGREES OF MALE-PATTERN BALDNESS

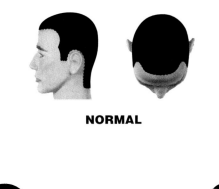

NORMAL

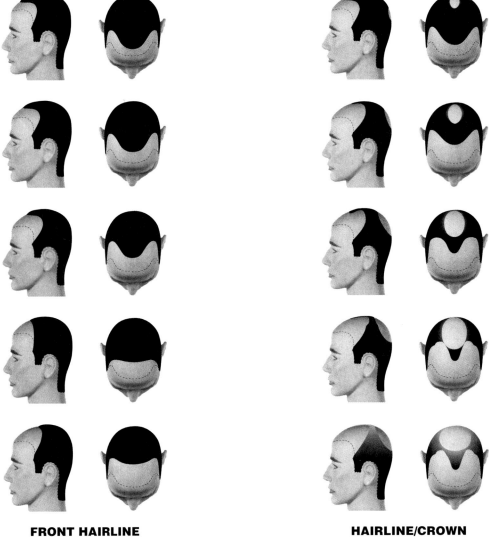

FRONT HAIRLINE   **HAIRLINE/CROWN**

Hair loss is identified according to various measurement systems. Each system identifies the pattern and density of the hair loss. Pattern refers to the shape and location of the hair loss, while density refers to how much hair covers the scalp in the area of the hair loss. These types of illustrations are often labeled so you can record and track your client's hair loss from one visit to another.

Other Types of Hair Loss

Postpartum Alopecia

Some women experience a "loss of hair" after having a baby. This temporary hair loss at the conclusion of pregnancy is called *postpartum alopecia*. The cause of this phenomenon is simple. During pregnancy, hair stays longer in the anagen cycle. Then, after childbirth, these hairs enter the telogen phase. Many women become concerned about this "sudden" loss of hair. But, actually, loss of hair is the result of the body's hormonal balance returning to its previous state. It isn't long until the amount of hair seems balanced again.

Alopecia Areata

Sudden loss of hair in round or irregular patches without display of an inflamed scalp is referred to as alopecia areata. This type of hair loss occurs in individuals who have no obvious skin disorder or serious disease. Alopecia areata is an autoimmune skin disease that is confined to a few areas and is often reversed in a few months, though recurrences may occur. The National Alopecia Areata Foundation estimates that 4 million men, women and children suffer from this type of hair loss.

Telogen Effluvium

Premature shedding of hair in the resting phase (telogen) can result from various causes such as childbirth, shock, drug intake, fever, etc. This premature shedding of hair during the resting phase is called telogen effluvium. Some women also experience sudden hair loss when they stop taking birth-control pills or if they follow a crash diet too low in protein. The hair loss is usually reversed once the condition is corrected.

Traction or Traumatic Alopecia

Hair loss due to repetitive traction on the hair by pulling or twisting is called traction or traumatic alopecia. **Traction** (excessive stretching or pulling) **alopecia** *may be caused by wearing tight chignons or pony tails, tight rollers, tight corn rows or excessive tension during brushing and combing, especially when hair is wet.* This hair loss is often caused by mechanical damage. However, it can also be caused by chemical damage, such as the excessive application of permanent wave solutions. This condition is usually reversed once the trauma has stopped.

Hair Loss Treatments

Treatment of Androgenetic Alopecia

Several products have been developed to treat androgenetic alopecia. If your client is working with a physician who has prescibed one of the treatments available to regrow hair and has requested assistance from you in applying product treatments, read and follow the manufacturer's directions.

Other hair loss treatments that your client might consider include:

1. FDA-approved products that regrow hair or prevent hair loss.

2. Products that provide an ideal environment for possible hair regrowth or loss prevention.

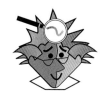

"The Food and Drug Administration (FDA) has ruled that products claiming hair regrowth or hair loss prevention cannot be marketed without prior FDA review and approval."

3. Surgical options are available mostly for men. Hair transplants, hair plugs and scalp reductions are performed by physicians or dermatologists. Several visits are necessary to achieve gradual results that allow periods of recuperation for the patient.

4. Wigs, toupees, hair additions or hair weaving are available as non-medical options. For additional information, refer to chapter entitled "Wigs and Hair Additions."

5. Cosmetic hair thickeners are products designed to volumize the hair. These products do not grow hair or put a halt to hair loss. They simply coat the hair, therefore giving it more body.

Whether you are dealing with hair loss, damaged or healthy hair, your goal remains the same: To leave your clients' hair in good, even better, condition following a service. Your knowledge of trichology will serve as the foundation for determining the right products to use and recommend for clients facing challenges with their hair. The extra effort you put forth will help win you a loyal clientele.

Hair loss today is often associated with cancer treatments. As a professional, it is important for you to know what resources are available to help your clients.

One of these resources, Look Good... Feel Better (LGFB) is a free, national, public-service program created from the concept that if a woman with cancer can be helped to look good, her improved self-esteem will help her approach her disease and treatment with greater confidence.

Look Good...Feel Better is offered through a national partnership of:

- The Cosmetic, Toiletry, and Fragrance Association (CTFA) Foundation - a charitable organization established and supported by the trade association that represents the U.S. cosmetics industry. The CTFA Foundation provides makeup, materials and financial support (through the cosmetic industry).

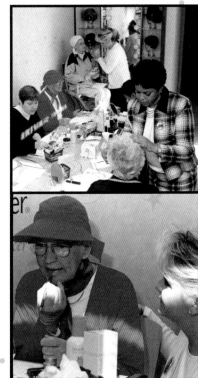

- The American Cancer Society (ACS), the nationwide, community-based, voluntary health organization dedicated to eliminating cancer as a major health problem. ACS administers the program nationwide and serves as the primary source of information to the public.

- The National Cosmetology Association (NCA) is a national organization of more than 45,000 hairstylists, wig experts, estheticians, makeup artists and nail technicians. NCA organizes and helps train the volunteer cosmetologists.

The three sponsoring partners work together to provide:

- Patient education, through group or individual sessions
- Free program materials, including videos and pamphlets
- Free makeup kits for patients in group workshops

For more information, go to: www.lookgoodfeelbetter.org
or call 1.800.395.LOOK

DRAPING, SHAMPOOING AND SCALP MASSAGE

Draping, shampooing and scalp massage are quite often the first service contacts you have with a client in the salon. Making this contact a delightful, memorable service experience can have enormous impact on building client loyalty to you and the salon.

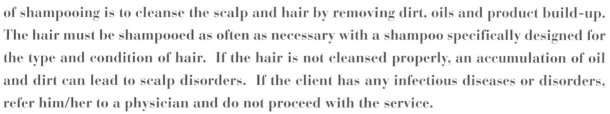

The safety, comfort and protection of the client's skin, hair and clothing are all part of the professional cosmetologist's responsibility and one of his/her foremost considerations.

Proper maintenance of the hair and scalp begins with a hygiene practice that many of you perform each and every day, shampooing. **The purpose of shampooing is to cleanse the scalp and hair by removing dirt, oils and product build-up. The hair must be shampooed as often as necessary with a shampoo specifically designed for the type and condition of hair. If the hair is not cleansed properly, an accumulation of oil and dirt can lead to scalp disorders. If the client has any infectious diseases or disorders, refer him/her to a physician and do not proceed with the service.**

Massage is a scientific method of manipulating the body by rubbing, pinching, tapping, kneading or stroking with the hands, fingers or an instrument. Massage dates back to antiquity and was used for health, beauty and medical reasons. Many believed that massage had beneficial qualities such as improving blood circulation, relieving headaches, reducing fat, diminishing fatigue, inducing sleep and preventing disease. Today, massage is not only a service in itself, but is included in other services such as shampooing, manicures and facials. This section of your chapter will focus on scalp massage offered alone or during a shampoo service. Your review of draping, shampooing and massage will begin with the important area of proper draping procedures.

"Did you know that in ancient times many superstitious people believed that the spirits protected their heads and that they might injure the spirits if they shampooed their hair? Shampooing the hair became a ceremonial practice performed once a year in honor of a god's or goddess' birthday."

Draping Theory

Draping is performed prior to hair care services, such as shampooing and scalp massage, to protect the client's skin and clothing. Prior to draping, ask the client to remove any jewelry (necklace, earrings, hair pins and eyeglasses) and store it in a safe place. For your protection and the protection of others in the service area, ensure that jewelry and other valuables, such as purses, are stored in a safe place and are not blocking traffic areas, where they could cause an accidental fall or injury.

Many regulating agencies require that shampoo capes used to drape the client during cosmetology services must be laundered in a solution capable of disinfecting the cape. Guidelines to protect the client also include making sure that the neck of the cape does not come in direct contact with the client's skin. Therefore, always use a neck strip and/or towel between the client's neck and the neckband of the cape. Use the following guidelines when determining proper procedures for draping:

- In general, a towel and plastic or waterproof cape is used for shampooing, wet hair cutting, wet styling and chemical services. The plastic cape protects the client and the client's clothing from becoming wet or damaged during these services.

- A neck strip is usually used to replace a towel following a shampoo service if a hair cutting service is going to be performed next. The neck strip is less bulky and will allow the hair to fall naturally. The neck strip is also used during dry hair cutting to help prevent loose hairs from embedding into the client's clothing.

- A cloth cape is usually used for dry styling or dry hair cutting services. The cloth cape is lighter weight and therefore more comfortable for the client and allows dry hair to slide to the floor more easily.

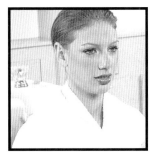
TOWEL

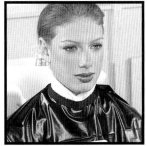
PLASTIC CAPE

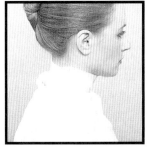
NECK STRIP

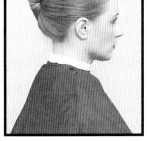
CLOTH CAPE

Shampooing and Conditioning Theory

The shampoo service is performed prior to most hair services except certain hair color or chemical straightening services. Since most hair colors are applied to dry hair, the hair is not shampooed unless it is extremely oily or dirty. However, in some instances color products require that color be applied to towel dried hair, following a shampoo service. Always read manufacturer's directions to be sure. For example, shampooing is not performed prior to chemical relaxing services since it could cause increased irritation, a burning sensation or actual burning once the chemical product is applied to the hair.

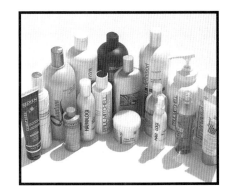

Understanding the pH (potential hydrogen) level of shampoos and conditioners will help you make the right selection for each hair type and condition. **For instance shampoos with a high ph level**

can make the hair dry and brittle, so for dry brittle hair, an acid-balanced shampoo would be recommended. Shampoos and conditioners are reviewed more in depth in the "Chemistry" chapter.

Water

Water (H$_2$0) is classified as soft or hard. **Soft water is generally preferred for shampooing. Soft water is rain water or water that has been chemically treated. Hard water contains minerals and does not allow the shampoo to lather freely. However, it can be softened by a chemical water softening process.** Knowing which type of water you are working with in the salon will enable you to make the proper choice of shampoo. For more information on water, refer to the "The Role of Water" on page 122 in the "Chemistry" chapter.

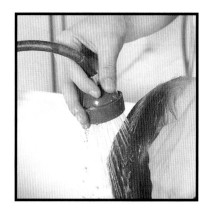

You always need to remember to **monitor the temperature of the water before applying the water stream to your client's scalp** and during the rinsing portion of the service. This can be done by holding the shampoo hose and positioning a finger in the water stream. In addition, make sure the amount of water pressure is moderate and not so forceful that it is uncomfortable for your client. Excess water pressure is a primary cause of water-spill accidents.

Sometimes water may be present on the floor in the shampoo area. **Always wipe up any water areas to prevent accidents that may occur if someone slips when crossing a wet traffic area in the school or salon.**

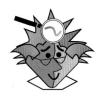

"Be careful not to drop the hose during the shampoo service. Many beginning cosmetologists have had this 'showering' experience!"

Brushing and Combing

Prior to the shampoo service, the hair should be brushed to remove tangles from the hair. Brushing also stimulates blood circulation to the scalp while removing dust, dirt and product build-up from the hair. Combing with a large-tooth comb or plastic brush with wide spacing is generally performed after a shampoo service to remove tangles from wet hair.

Usually brushes made from natural bristles are recommended, since they have many overlaying bristles that aid in cleaning the hair better than nylon bristles. **Keep in mind that brushing the hair prior to a chemical service or if any cuts or abrasions are evident is not recommended.** Since there are different ways to brush the hair, consider the following factors: Does the hair have extreme product build-up that makes it difficult to part the hair prior to brushing? Is the hair long or short? Is the hair naturally straight or curly? Under all circumstances, **you should begin brushing the hair from the ends first, then work toward the scalp.**

This will allow you to detangle the hair without adding additional stress or more tangles to the hair. Once the hair is free of tangles you can brush the hair thoroughly from the scalp to the ends.

Removing Tangles From Wet Hair

After the shampoo, tangles should be removed in a specific, methodical manner:

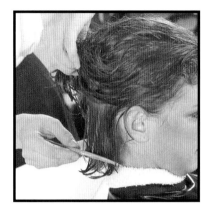

- Always start at the lowest point of the tangled area, in this photo the nape section. While lifting the weight of the tangled hair, release a section of hair with a large-tooth comb.

- Starting at the ends of the hair and progressing toward the scalp, comb downward through the hair. You may wish to hold the hair at the base to minimize discomfort while detangling. Keep in mind that chemically treated hair tends to tangle more easily than normal hair.

- Continue combing this section until all tangles are removed. To remove stubborn tangles, use short, gentle strokes.

- Part off another section immediately above the first section.

- Remove tangles in the same manner as before, starting at the ends. Comb through these two untangled sections and blend the hair together.

- Continue this procedure throughout the crown, sides and finally the top section.

In addition to knowing the importance of proper draping and shampooing, it will be key for you to understand the theory behind scalp massage and the relaxing and/or stimulating effects caused by this beneficial component of your client's shampoo experience.

Scalp Massage Theory

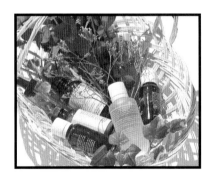

Scalp massage involves manipulations performed on the scalp to relax the muscles and stimulate blood circulation. Scalp treatments combine the benefit of massage with the use of products designed to improve the condition of the scalp. The relaxation experienced by the client during scalp massage is a "value-added" benefit that helps build client loyalty.

Although products such as essential oils, lotions or creams used in scalp treatments provide a specific benefit, these products may leave a residue on the hair. Plus the stimulation from the massage may cause scalp sensitivity for the client. For these reasons, you should avoid performing a scalp treatment immediately prior to a chemical service. Be guided by the condition of the client's hair and scalp, as well as manufacturer's directions.

When massaging the scalp, it is important to:

- Establish a soothing or stimulating 'rhythm' when performing the manipulations

- Maintain contact with the client throughout the manipulations to maintain a relaxing or stimulating experience

- Carry out manipulations with firm, controlled movements to maximize the full benefit of massage and gain your client's confidence

- Keep your nails at a moderate length to avoid scratching the scalp

Just as products vary, so will the manipulations you choose to use during the scalp massage. Customizing your own sequence of manipulations is another method you may use in creating client satisfaction and loyalty. Listed here are the basic massage manipulations and the effects they cause. As you review this area, be aware that effleurage, petrissage and tapotment are the three primary scalp manipulations, with petrissage being the most important. Petrissage stimulates the sebaceous glands, which produce natural oil (sebum). This oil is often lacking in the case of dry hair and scalp.

The Five Basic Manipulations of Massage

Manipulation	Movement	Effect
Effleurage (ef-**LOO**-rahzh)	Light, gliding strokes or circular motions made with the palms of the hands or pads of the fingertips; often used to begin and/or end a treatment; used on the face, neck and arms	Relaxing, soothing
Petrissage (**PAY**-tre-sahzh)	Light or heavy kneading and rolling of the muscles; performed by kneading muscles between the thumb and fingers or by pressing the palm of the hand firmly over the muscles, then grasping and squeezing with the heel of the hand and fingers; generally performed from the front of the head to the back; used on the face, arms, shoulders and upper back	Deep stimulation of muscles, nerves and skin glands; promotes the circulation of blood and lymph
Tapotment (tah-**POHT**-mant) or Percussion or Hacking	Light tapping or slapping movement applied with the fingers or partly flexed fingers; used on the arms, back and shoulders	Stimulates nerves, promotes muscle contraction; increases blood circulation
Friction (**FRIK**-shun)	Circular movement with no gliding used on the scalp or with a facial when less pressure is desired; applied with the fingertips or palms	Stimulates nerves; increases blood circulation
Vibration (vi-**BRAY**-shun)	Shaking movement; your arms shake as you touch the client with your fingertips or palms	Highly stimulating

7

Draping, Shampooing and Scalp Massage Essentials

There are many types of shampoos available and designed for specific hair types and conditions. Shampoos are designed for dry, oily, normal, color-treated and gray hair to name but a few. As a cosmetologist, making the proper selection will allow you to achieve the desired results. For shampoo ingredients, refer to the "Chemistry" chapter.

Hair conditioners and rinses are used on shampooed hair to condition, soften and make the hair tangle free for ease in combing. They are also used to restore the hair to its normal pH and remove soap residue. There are liquid rinses, thick creams and leave-in conditioners, all of which yield different effects. The liquid rinses and thick creams are applied and left in the hair anywhere from a few seconds to 10 minutes. The leave-in conditioners are left in the hair until the next shampoo. **Frequent use of cream rinses and conditioners can result in product build-up that can leave the hair dull and lifeless.** Clarifying shampoos are designed to remove this product build-up.

Draping, Shampoo and Scalp Massage Products

PRODUCT	FUNCTION
Shampoos	
All-purpose	Cleanse the hair without correcting any special condition
Acid-balanced (non-stripping)	Cleanse all hair types, especially lightened, color-treated or dry, brittle hair
Plain	Cleanse normal hair but not recommended for chemically treated or damaged hair
Soapless	Cleanse hair with either soft or hard water
Medicated	Prescribed by the client's doctor to treat scalp and hair problems and disorders; note: medicated shampoos may affect color-treated hair
Clarifying	Remove residue such as product build-up
Anti-dandruff	Control dandruff and other scalp conditions
Liquid Dry	Cleanse the scalp and hair for clients who are unable to receive a normal shampoo; effective in cleaning wigs and hairpieces
Powder Dry	Cleanse the hair of clients whose health prohibits them from receiving a wet shampoo service

PRODUCT	FUNCTION
Conditioning	Improve the tensile strength and porosity of the hair
Color	Enhance color-treated hair and tone non-color-treated hair temporarily; available in a variety of colors
Thinning Hair	Cleanse the hair without weighing it down

Rinses

PRODUCT	FUNCTION
Vinegar and Lemon (Acid)	Keep the cuticle compact, remove soap scum, return the hair to its pH balance and counteract the alkalinity present after a chemical service
Cream	Soften, add shine and smoothness to the hair while making the hair tangle-free for ease in combing
Anti-dandruff	Control dandruff and scalp conditions
Acid-balanced	Close the cuticle after a color service to prevent the color from fading
Acid	Remove soap scum
Color	Add temporary color to the hair, which lasts from shampoo to shampoo; for more information on color rinses, refer to nonoxidative colors in the Hair Coloring chapter

Conditioners

PRODUCT	FUNCTION
Instant	Coat the hair shaft and restore moisture to the hair
Normalizing	Close the cuticle after alkaline chemical services
Body Building	Displace excess moisture, providing more body to the hair; made from protein
Moisturizing	Add moisture to dry, brittle hair
Customized	Moisturize and build body

Scalp Treatments

PRODUCT	FUNCTION
Essential Oils	Provide invigorating, stimulating or soothing scents; allow fluid movement on the scalp
Scalp Toner	Adds a refreshing, stimulating feeling to the scalp; may have mild antiseptic properties and cleansing ability
Moisturizing Agent	Replenishes or restores moisture to dry scalp; formulated as creams, oils or lotions

7

Draping, Shampooing and Scalp Massage Implements and Supplies

IMPLEMENT/SUPPLIES	FUNCTION
Towels	Protect the client's skin and clothing; also used to dry the hair
Plastic Client Cape	Protects the client and his/her clothing during wet and/or chemical hair services
Cloth Client Cape	Protects the client and his/her clothing during dry hair cutting or styling
Neck Strip	Protects the client's skin
Natural-Bristle Hair Brush	Increases blood circulation to the scalp, removes dirt, debris and product build-up from the hair prior to the shampoo service
All-Purpose Comb	Detangles and combs the hair after the shampoo service
Plastic Cap	Covers hair to allow deeper penetration of conditioning treatment

Draping, Shampoo and Scalp Massage Equipment

EQUIPMENT	FUNCTION
Shampoo Chair	Allows client to sit or lay down during the shampoo service
Shampoo Bowl	Holds and drains water and product during a shampoo service
Shampoo Dispensary	Displays shampoos and conditioners
Towel Shelves or Cabinet	Store towels

Infection Control and Safety

Infection control and safety are essential while performing scalp massage services in order to protect the health and well-being of you and your client.

1. Do not brush the hair prior to a chemical service. If any cuts or abrasions are evident, a chemical service should not be recommended.

2. If shampoo gets into the client's eye, rinse immediately with tepid water. An eye wash cup (a cup that is held over the eye and is used to flush the eye with water) is recommended. If irritation persists, recommend that the client see a physician.

3. Disinfect shampoo bowl and implements as required by your regulating agency.

4. Discard contaminated and non-reusable materials (neck strip, cotton, etc.)

5. Wipe up any water-spill areas immediately.

6. Always test the temperature of the water prior to applying the water stream to your client's scalp. Continue to monitor the water temperature during rinsing by keeping one finger under the nozzle.

7. Ensure that the amount of water pressure is moderate to strong and not so forceful that it is uncomfortable for your client. Excess water pressure is a primary cause of water-spill accidents.

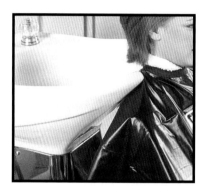

8. Decrease pressure during massage manipulations if client expresses sensitivity.

9. Keep the back of the cape on the outside of the chair during the shampoo service to prevent the water from running down the client's back and dampening the clothes.

10. Remember to detangle the hair thoroughly prior to and after the shampoo service.

CAPE OUTSIDE CHAIR

7

11. Wash your hands with antibacterial soap prior to the shampoo service.

12. Avoid giving a scalp massage:

   • When scalp abrasions or a serious scalp disorder are/is present

   • Immediately prior to the application of a chemical service, such as perming, relaxing, lightening or coloring

   • When the client has a history of high blood pressure or a heart condition; ask client to consult with physician before proceeding, since scalp massage may increase the circulation of the blood.

13. Wear gloves if required during a shampoo or scalp massage service; check with your area's regulating agency for guidelines.

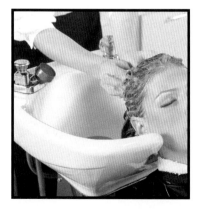

Basic Draping, Shampooing and Conditioning

Draping, shampooing and conditioning preparation and procedures vary based on the timing allowed for the service and each client's needs. For example, you may find it necessary to use a booster chair when shampooing a young child or, in some cases, it is recommended that elderly clients lean forward into the shampoo bowl rather than lean back for medical or comfort purposes.

There are several types of shampoo bowls and chairs available. Some bowls allow you to stand behind the client, which helps reduce back fatigue. Other units may have a hydraulic control that allows you to adjust the height of the chair or move it into a reclining position. Although the basic shampoo techniques remain the same, you will need to adjust your body position according to the type of shampoo bowl you are using and whether you are standing on the side or at the back of your client. Be guided by your instructor for variations and specific requirements.

Wet Hair Service Draping, Shampooing and Conditioning Preparation

The following is a list of draping and shampooing materials that are required for a wet hair service. Draping and shampooing for chemical services will be reviewed in the chapters covering those services. Assemble the following materials prior to draping, shampooing and conditioning your client:

- Towels
- Plastic cape
- Booster chair (if applicable)
- Shampoo, rinse or conditioning products

It is assumed in this procedure that you are moving directly from draping to shampooing. If there is a time lapse between draping and shampooing, it will be necessary for you to wash your hands again with antibacterial liquid soap prior to shampooing.

Wet Hair Service Draping, Shampooing and Conditioning Procedure

- Wash and sanitize hands
- Ask client to remove jewelry and glasses and secure in a safe place
- Clip client's hair out of the way
- Turn client's collar inward if applicable
- Place towel lengthwise over client's shoulders, cross ends in front
- Position plastic cape over towel and secure
- Examine the client's hair and scalp
- Position cape over shampoo chair
- Brush the hair
- Test the temperature and pressure of the water

- Wet the hair
- Apply shampoo
- Perform scalp massage manipulations
- Rinse thoroughly
- Repeat shampoo and rinse procedures if necessary
- Apply rinse or conditioner
- Rinse thoroughly
- Towel dry client's hair
- Detangle the hair

Wet Hair Service Draping, Shampooing and Conditioning• Standing in Back

1-2. **Wash and sanitize your hands.** **Ask client to remove jewelry and glasses and secure in a safe place. Clip client's hair out of the way** with a simple twist and clip placement. **Turn client's collar inward if applicable,** making sure that you are taking precaution not to damage client's clothing. **Place towel lengthwise over client's shoulders, and cross ends in front** to secure the towel.

3. **Position plastic cape over towel and secure,** being careful to not catch neck hair in the fastener. Adjust for client comfort. **Examine the client's hair and scalp** thoroughly. **Position cape on the outside of the shampoo chair.**

4. Begin at the hair ends and **brush the hair** to remove tangles.

5-7. **Test the temperature and pressure of the water** to be sure it is warm and comfortable for your client. **Wet your client's hair** thoroughly. Ensure that the hair and scalp are saturated with water. Cup your hand over the front hairline, ears and nape to protect your client from becoming wet.

8-9. **Apply shampoo** into your palm first, then into the hair, and work into lather.

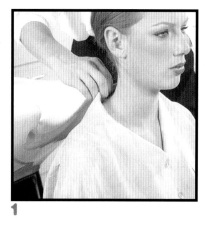
1

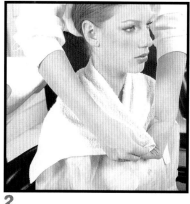
2

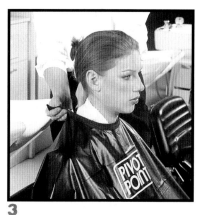
3

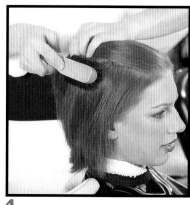
4

7

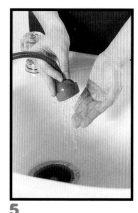
5

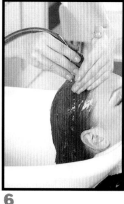
6

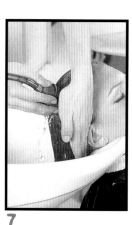
7

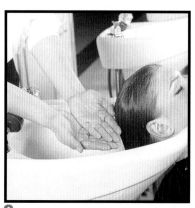
8

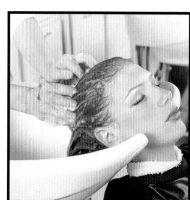
9

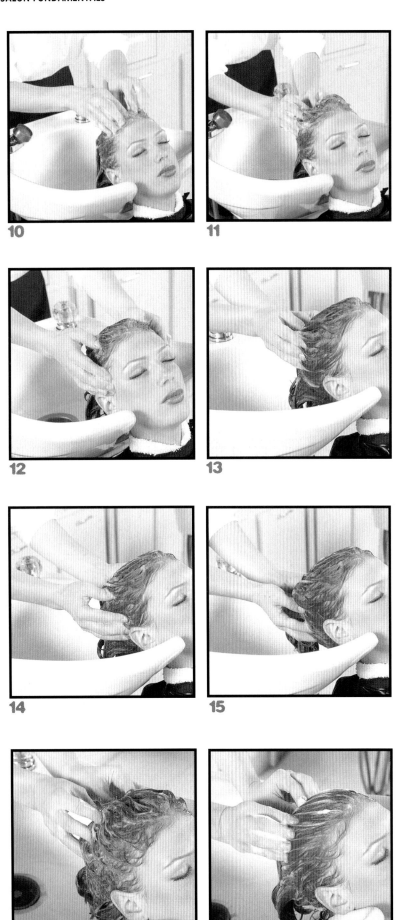

10

11

12

13

14

15

16

17

10-11. **Perform scalp massage manipulations,** starting at the front hairline. Use the cushions of your fingers, and circular or backward stroking (effleurage) manipulations. Maintain contact with the scalp and continue manipulations while you glide your hands gently toward the crown. Muscles affected during this time will be the frontalis (high on the forehead) and the aponeurosis (a-po-noo-**RO**-sis) (tendon connecting the frontalis and occipitalis). Repeat this and the following manipulations at least twice.

12-13. Glide back to the hairline and repeat the circular or backward stroking motion from the temporal area to the crown and then from in front of the ears to the crown. Maintain contact with the scalp while gliding.

14-15. Glide your hands behind the ear (auricular superior and posterior), and repeat effleurage manipulations up the back of the head (occipitalis). Use kneading (petrissage) movements at the nape area and work upward toward the crown, crossing over the occipitalis.

16-17. Massage the entire scalp area with attention to the hairline, crown and nape. Complete scalp massage manipulations. Remove excess shampoo.

18-19. **Rinse thoroughly,** protecting eyes, ears, etc. from spray and shampoo with your hand. When the spray is on, keep one finger curled over the edge of the nozzle so you can monitor any temperature changes in the water. Also keep in mind that the pressure of the water from the nozzle can range from a moderate to strong spray. Ensure that the spray is strong enough to rinse all the shampoo from the hair. Rinse the entire scalp area with additional attention at the nape. **Repeat the shampoo and rinse procedures if necessary.**

20. Apply rinse or conditioner. Work through the hair using gentle, stroking (effleurage) movements for 30-60 seconds. Follow manufacturer's directions for conditioning treatments that may need to be left on the hair for a longer period of time and may require a plastic cap and heat.

21-23. **Rinse thoroughly,** protecting sensitive areas from finishing rinse and/or water spray. Lift the hair and allow the water to run down the length of the strands. Squeeze excess water from the hair ends.

24. Towel dry client's hair with fresh towel. Wipe away any excess moisture from client's face

25. Detangle the hair, beginning at the nape to avoid tangling the hair. Comb outward from the ends of the hair and work toward the scalp.

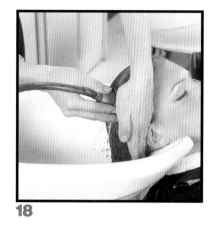
18

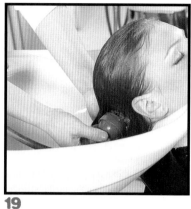
19

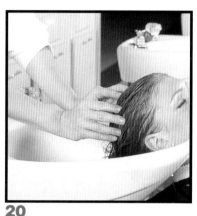
20

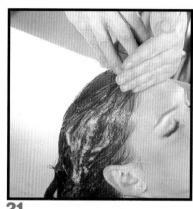
21

7

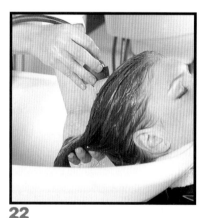
22

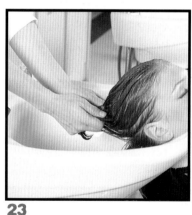
23

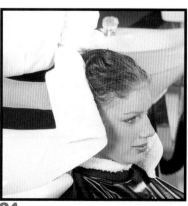
24

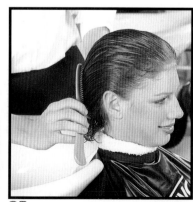
25

ALERT!

Never use firm massage manipulations when shampoo is to be followed by any kind of chemical service. In these instances, massage during shampoo should be very brief and very light. This light massage will help avoid the undesirable penetration of any chemicals into the skin, since deep massage can open pores into the dermis.

Optional Neck and Shoulder Massage

Before detangling the hair after the shampoo procedure, you may wish to perform this additional massage treatment:

- Place fingers over muscles near shoulder joints.
- Begin a combination of effleurage and petrissage manipulations to bottom of neck.
- Move fingers up the outside of the neck, back down toward spine and back up and out to shoulder muscle joints.
- Repeat.

Shampooing and Conditioning • Standing at the Side

Remember that shampooing and conditioning procedures basically remain the same, whether you are standing behind or at the side of your client. However, your body position will change and you may choose to include slightly varied scalp manipulations.

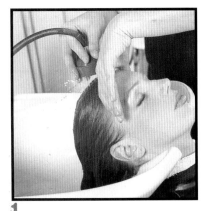
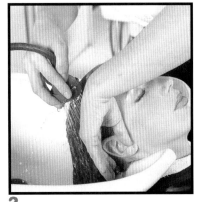

1

2

1-2. **Wet your client's hair** thoroughly. Protect your client's face, eyes and ears by positioning your hand along the hairline and cupping the ear. Monitor the water temperature with one finger positioned under the nozzle.

3-4. Perform scalp massage manipulations by using a circular motion with the cushions of your fingers from the front hairline to the crown. Perform petrissage manipulations with your thumbs. Work from the center front hairline to the crown. Then return to the front hairline, this time 1" (2.5 cm) away from the center, and repeat manipulations. Work toward each side.

5-6. Lift and support the head. Work from side to side in the nape using a stroking movement. Then use a scissoring movement throughout the entire head. Repeat a few times.

7-10. Rinse the hair thoroughly from the front hairline toward the crown and ends. Use one hand to lift and support the head. Cup your other hand over the nozzle and rinse to remove the shampoo at the nape. Use both hands to gently squeeze remaining water from the hair.

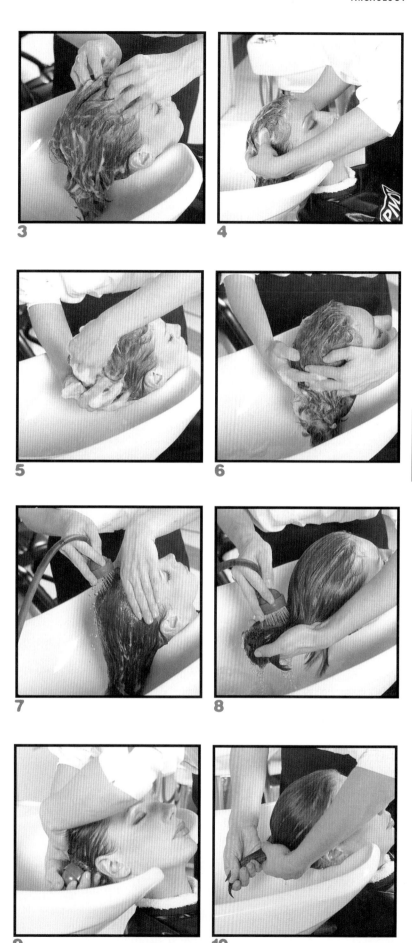

7

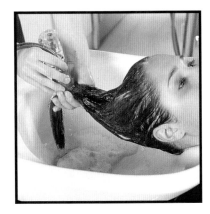 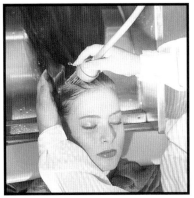

Long Hair Considerations

Long hair requires special considerations during shampooing and conditioning. Lift longer lengths upward while rinsing to remove the hair from the shampoo suds that have accumulated in the bowl. Shampoo bowls designed for long hair have extended basins that allow the hair to fall naturally, which prevents the hair from becoming tangled.

Wet Hair Service Draping, Shampooing and Conditioning Completion

- Clean shampoo service area before continuing with client; disinfect comb and brush following the entire service
- Ensure there is no water left standing in the shampoo service area
- Discuss the products you used on your client and proceed to the next service

Basic Scalp Massage

Basic scalp massage treatments involve scalp manipulations designed to relax your client's muscles and increase blood circulation. Treatments can vary according to the products and machines used. For instance, a dry scalp treatment may include a moisturizing scalp cream along with a scalp steamer or warm towels to help product penetration. Be sure to follow manufacturer's directions when using scalp treatment products.

Basic Scalp Massage Preparation

Assemble the following materials prior to providing a scalp massage service:

- Moisturizing agent, scalp toner or essential oils
- Towel
- Client Cape

Basic Scalp Massage Procedure

- Wash and sanitize hands
- Drape client for a wet hair service
- Detangle hair
- Apply scalp product
- Perform effleurage scalp manipulations
- Perform petrissage scalp manipulations
- Perform effleurage scalp manipulations

- Perform tapotment
- Rotate the scalp
- Conclude scalp massage
- Shampoo client's hair
- Rinse hair
- Dry hair or move to next service

Basic Scalp Massage

1. Wash and sanitize your hands. Seat the client in a comfortable chair. **Drape client for a wet hair service.**

2. Detangle the hair. Apply scalp product according to the treatment being performed and according to manufacturer's directions.

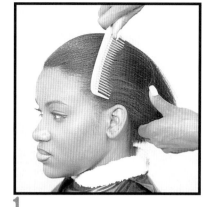
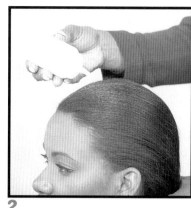

3. Perform effleurage scalp manipulations. Stand behind your client and begin the stroking manipulations at the front hairline (frontalis), gliding at approximately 1" (2.5 cm) intervals to the nape area. Return to the front hairline and repeat until all areas are covered.

4. Perform petrissage scalp manipulations. Starting at the front hairline, massage with a kneading action in a circular motion. Keep your fingers and thumbs spread out and firmly pressed to the scalp as you massage. Release your hands from the scalp only as you move to another part of the scalp. Begin the movements at the front of the head and finish in the nape.

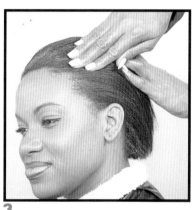
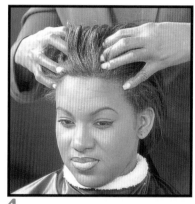

5-6. Perform effleurage scalp manipulations. Use lighter, circular manipulations as you move from the front hairline to the area above the ears at the crest (parietal) and then slowly returning to the top and repeating the manipulations. Cover the entire head. Then **perform tapotment.** Use the tips of your fingers and tap the scalp. Begin at the front hairline and work from side to side. Complete the tapotment technique at the nape. Customize your manipulations using a series of rotations with your thumbs, stroking movements with the palms of your hands or light strokes with the cushions of your fingers.

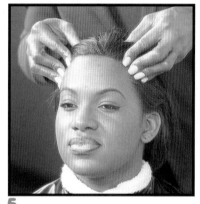
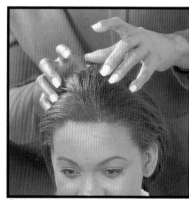

"You may choose to perform only a part of this complete scalp massage or you may want to develop your own special routine."

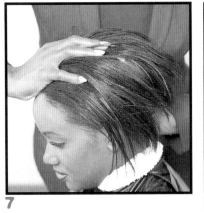

7

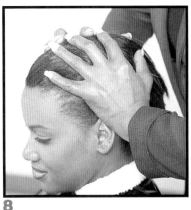

8

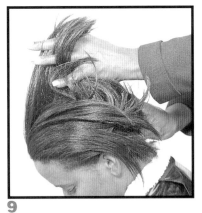

9

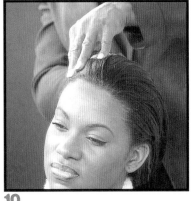

10

7-8. Use the palms of your hands and your fingers to **rotate the scalp** gently. Squeeze the head and release.

9-10. Conclude the scalp massage by using long, gentle effleurage strokes from the nape to the front hairline. Use a feather-like motion to remove hands from the scalp. Then use a light stroking motion from the front hairline to the nape. **Shampoo the client's hair** thoroughly, being careful to remove all scalp treatment product from the hair. **Rinse the hair** thoroughly and repeat shampoo and rinse if necessary. **Dry the hair or move on to the next service** scheduled for the client.

Basic Scalp Massage Completion

- Offer a rebook visit for your client. Discuss the next appropriate time to repeat this service based on the client's needs.

- Recommend appropriate retail products to your client.

- Clean your work area.

Aromatherapy for the Scalp

There is an increased awareness in salons across the world about how natural plant extracts can increase the benefits experienced during massage treatments. The term aromatherapy is used to describe the combination of our sense of smell and the use of plant extracts and their healing abilities. "Aroma" refers to the natural fragrance of plants and "therapy" means "cure". The therapeutic effects of aromatherapy are incorporated into many salon services including scalp treatments.

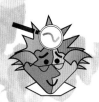

"Did you know that your sense of smell affects how you taste? When you have a stuffy nose from a cold, food tastes different or doesn't have a taste at all."

Essential oils and scalp products containing vitamins and plant extracts address many health and wellness concerns. Therapeutic effects include invigorating the scalp, encouraging renewed hair growth, relieving flaking associated with dryness or dandruff, increasing blood flow circulation and calming and soothing effect on the mind and body.

Aromatherapy expert, Blossom Kochar from India, shared the following list of recommended essential oils she uses in her custom recipes for the scalp. Note that essential oils should not be used directly on the skin, but blended with a base oil such as sweet almond oil or grapeseed oil. When blending oils, follow the recommended usage chart shown to the right.

RECOMMENDED USAGE	
ESSENTIAL OIL	**BASE OIL**
20 - 60 drops	3.5 fl oz (100ml)
7 - 25 drops	1 fl oz (25ml)
3 - 5 drops	1 tsp (5ml)

Pre-mixed scalp therapy oils, whether purchased from a manufacturer or mixed by you, can be applied directly to the scalp prior to manipulations. Essential oils can also be mixed with shampoo, which can then be applied to the scalp prior to the manipulations of a scalp treatment or incorporated into a shampoo service.

7

Normal Hair and Scalp

Rosemary
Chamomile

Oily Hair and Scalp

Patchouli
Cedarwood
Clary Sage

Dry Hair and Scalp

Ylang Ylang
Sandalwood
Lavender

Oily Dandruff

Lemon
Rosemary
Cedarwood
Thyme

Alopecia (Hair Loss)

Sandalwood
Bay
Lavender
Clary Sage
Rosemary

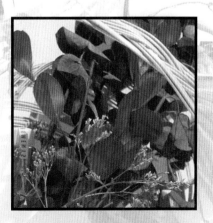

Your understanding of the structure, growth and condition of the hair, along with your application of basic draping, shampooing and scalp massage techniques will serve as the foundation of your client's first contact with your skill level. Strive to display your best ability as you proudly offer your expertise. Remember how powerful your "touch" can be to the client. As you move through the service, ask how you are doing. Be sensitive to your client's needs, making adjustments and recommendations for hair condition, water temperature and massage manipulations. You will soon be hearing these important words from your client, "I can't wait until my next visit!" or "My hair looks great when I leave, but I really come for the massage during the shampoo service!"

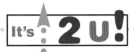

Build Your Critical Thinking Skills

In this chapter you have prepared yourself to meet the following Industry Standards for entry-level cosmetologists:

- Consult with clients to determine their needs and preferences as they relate to cosmetology services

- Provide hair related services in accordance with a client's needs or expectations

- Conduct services in a safe environment and take measures to prevent the spread of infectious and contagious disease

- Use a variety of salon products while providing client services

- Market professional salon products effectively

It's Up to You to know what to do. Using your training to this point, review the following case scenarios and think through how you would handle the challenge.

1. The client you have in your chair, Mrs. Brown, has been referred to you by one of your favorite clients, Mrs. James. When you performed a test for structural strength on Mrs. Brown's hair, the hair strand did not return to its curl pattern at all. Mrs. Brown would like to have a perm just like the one you gave Mrs. James last week. What would you do?

2. Several of your clients mention to you that the shampoo service they just received from your shampoo assistant was acceptable, but not as good as the service they receive from you. What do you do?

Chapter 8
DESIGN DECISIONS

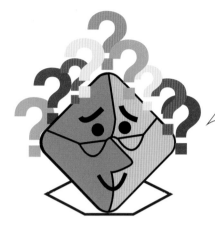

After studying this chapter you will be able to . . .

1. Identify proportions used when creating a design for the human body and face

DESIGN DECISION CONSIDERATIONS

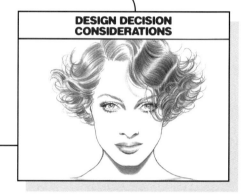

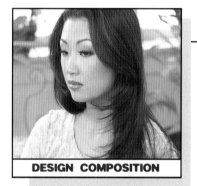

DESIGN COMPOSITION

3. Identify the design elements and principles used to compose designs

2. Recognize and analyze key areas to create and support the client's total image by using proper communication skills during the client consultation

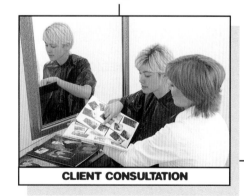

CLIENT CONSULTATION

8

Designs enrich almost every part of our lives. Wouldn't wallpaper be drab, wouldn't fabric be dull without design? Think of things you yourself have already designed – a valentine, a pinewood derby car, a flower garden, a holiday centerpiece, a scrapbook, a bedroom for a new baby, a web page . . . Design possibilities abound!

Design is even important in my life as a professor. I carefully design my lessons and all the chapters in your book. In this chapter you, too, will have the chance to see how important your design decisions can be to your career as a cosmetologist.

You will be the professional that clients depend on to help them make important decisions about their hair, fashion and makeup. Your role as an image-maker will prove to be very rewarding for both you and your client.

As an artist, a designer, you have great VALUE to offer your clients. You will not just be designing something *for* them. You might almost say you will be *designing them*, their hair, their face, their overall look. They will become the total image you help to create. That total image will flow from the BIG IDEA embedded in this chapter.

Design decisions are based on the considerations you make about proportion, results of the client consultation and your understanding of design composition.

You see that the BIG IDEA has three parts, Design Decision Considerations, Client Consultation and Design Composition. As you see in my plan for you, Design Decision Considerations involve your knowledge of the body and its proportions, Client Consultation your ability to communicate and Design Composition, your understanding of how to create exciting and successful hair and makeup styles. Refer to this chapter as you go through the other chapters in Unit 2.

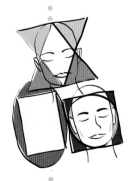

DESIGN DECISION CONSIDERATIONS
Proportion
Hair
Personality
Clothing
Lifestyle

CLIENT CONSULTATION
Communication

DESIGN COMPOSITION
Design Elements
Design Principles

DESIGN DECISION CONSIDERATIONS

In the past a famous celebrity could cause a rush to the salon. Almost everyone wanted that certain new haircut or color. Other fashion trends included particular skirt lengths, designer colors and shades of lipstick. Today when fashion experts are asked about the latest trend, the answer would have to be: "There is not one significant trend. There are many trend suggestions, but most consumers are choosing to wear what best suits their total image." Their personal choice includes decisions about clothes, makeup and hair. For this reason, most clients turn to their cosmetology professional for fashion and style recommendations Such recommendations are known as design decisions and need to be made after careful analysis and consultation with your clients. Sound design decisions begin with an understanding of proportion.

Proportion

What did Plato mean when he described beauty as existing in the proportion of things? Think of something beautiful-- a sunset, a melody, a person. All the parts flow into one breathtaking whole. No one certain feature or style produces beauty but rather the relationship or harmony created when all components come together into a total image. Why does a hairstyle, for example, look great on one client and terrible on another? Again the answer lies in the quote from Plato. It lies in the proportions. As a hair designer, you don't change a body or face shape, but you can use the hair to create good proportions between the hairstyle and the face and between the entire head and body.

Throughout history artists have drawn and sculpted the human body. They found out some golden rules about the ideal proportions between the body and the head, including the hairstyle. Today those proportions have created a standard that is taught in art classes all over the world.

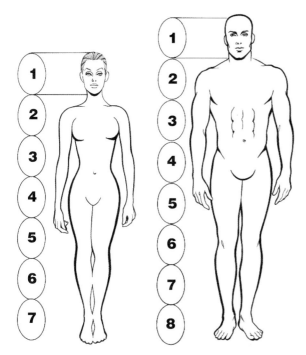

The Standard Proportion Between Head and Body

According to the standard most artists use, the head of a woman should be 1/7th of her overall body height, while the head of a man should be 1/8th of his overall body height. Therefore, when creating a hairstyle for your client, it is important to keep these proportions in mind. Note that hairstyles that are too large or too small for your client's stature will alter the illusion of their head to body proportions.

8

Body Shapes

In general there are three main body shapes that need to be considered. They are primarily divided by their height and bone structure and are referred to as tall and lanky, average and short and sturdy. Analyze your client's body shape at the beginning of the consultation. Have him/her stand in front of the mirror to see the overall body height and proportion.

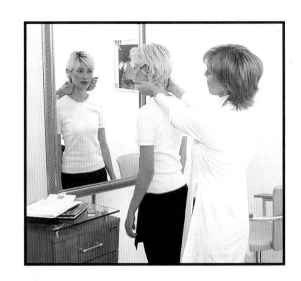

Tall and Lanky

Tall and lanky clients are people that have an overall elongated and narrow bone structure. Neither their hips nor their shoulders are dominant. They have long legs and arms and an unusually long neck. Due to their height, their heads seem to be small in proportion to their bodies. Women in this category would be approximately 5'10" (1.7 m) or taller and men would be approximately 6'1" (1.8 m) or taller.

Tall and lanky clients need volume and/or longer hair. Tall women's hair should touch the shoulders, at least in the back. Men should also have longer and fuller styles. In the examples below note the different illusions that are created by short, small hairstyles versus longer, fuller hairstyles.

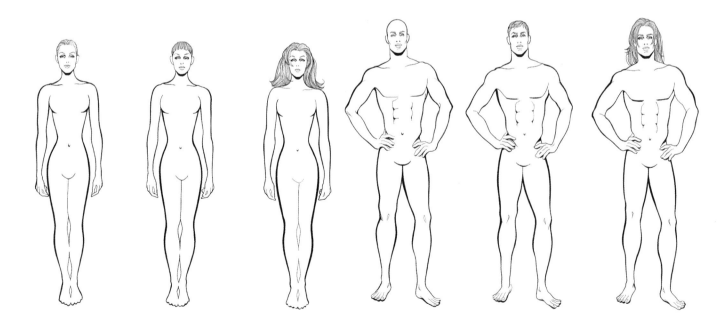

Average

Average clients are people with normal height, dominant shoulders and average hips. Their bodies usually have a good proportion. Women in this category are, in general, between 5'5" (1.6 m) to 5'9" (1.7 m) while men are usually between 5'7" (1.7 m) to 6'1" (1.8 m).

These clients can wear almost anything from fuller to close hairstyles and/or from short to long hair length. However, a hairstyle that is short with volume on top will make them look taller and a hairstyle that is long (shoulder length or longer) with volume at the bottom will make them look shorter.

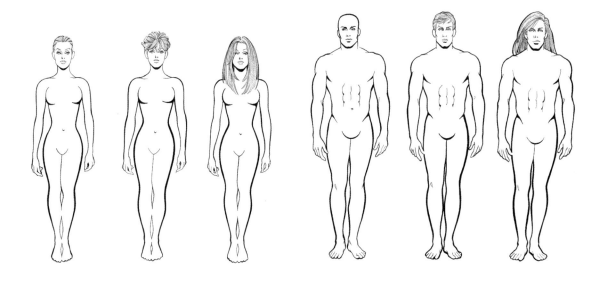

Short and Sturdy

Short and sturdy clients are shorter and have a heavy or robust bone structure. They often have wide shoulders and hips and short arms, legs and necks. Women in this category are generally 5'4" (1.6 m) or shorter, the men are 5'7" (1.7 m) or shorter. They need hairstyles with height and volume on the top. They should not wear any styles that touch the shoulders or have a lot of overall volume, since that would make them look shorter.

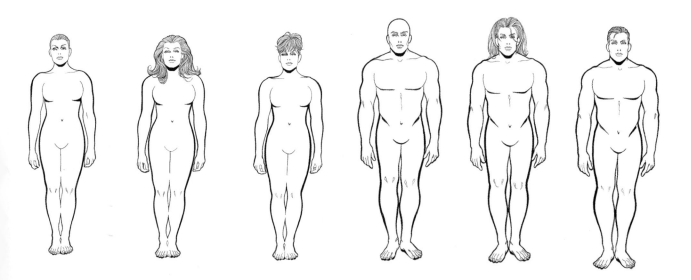

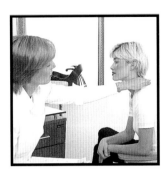

Neck

Besides the overall height and body proportion, there are also individual features that, if dominant, need to be considered separately. Very often the length of the neck reflects the overall body shape. A tall and lanky client will have a long neck while a short and sturdy client will have a short neck.

Clients with short necks should avoid volume at the neck. Long, wispy lengths are a good alternative since they visually elongate. Any outlining around the neckline should be narrow and elongated.

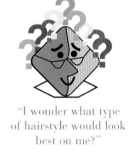

"I wonder what type of hairstyle would look best on me?"

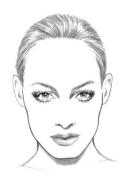
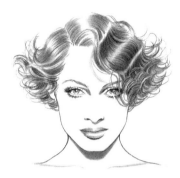

**SHORT NECK
KEEP HAIR CLOSE OR OFF THE FACE**

Long necks need mass and fullness around them. Longer, fuller hair at the perimeter is good for this characteristic. If the client likes shorter hair, choose a hairstyle that still shows hair along the neck from the front view. Leave the nape area longer and fuller. Cut a horizontal design line at the bottom to imply weight or fullness.

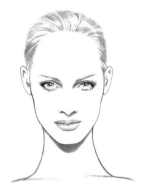
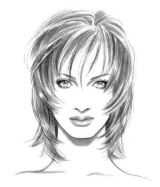
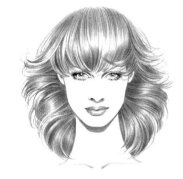

**LONG NECK
FRAME WITH HAIR**

Shoulders

As much as the neck reflects the overall body shape, so in most cases do the shoulders. A tall and lanky client will often have narrow shoulders, while a short and sturdy client will have wide shoulders.

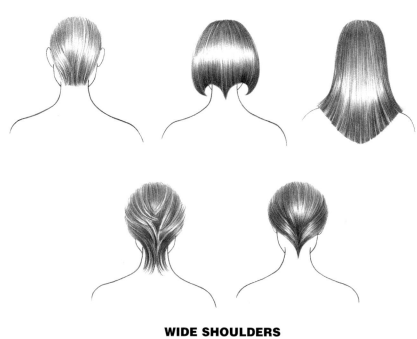

Wide shoulders need a hairstyle with a narrowing design line in the back. The design lines could be any lines that imply a narrow or a steep V shape. These lines give the illusion of narrowing the shoulders and stretching the body.

**WIDE SHOULDERS
ADD ELONGATION**

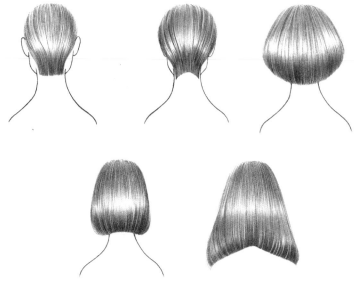

Narrow shoulders, however, need just the opposite. Hairstyles for narrow shoulders need design lines that imply horizontal lines or an A shape. Flat and wide, oval lines work as well. All of these lines need to be cut at low angles in order to add fullness and weight.

**NARROW SHOULDERS
ADD WIDTH**

Entire Body Shape

When considering the entire body shape, identify the widest area of the body. Visualizing the overall body silhouette, imagine the amount of volume needed for the hairstyle to bring this wide area of the body in proportion with the rest of the body. If the hair is too small for a large figure, the proportion will be unbalanced and the body will look even larger. A person with a petite body will easily become overpowered by a large hairstyle and, therefore, look even smaller.

**LARGE FIGURE
MORE HAIR**

**SMALL FIGURE
LESS HAIR**

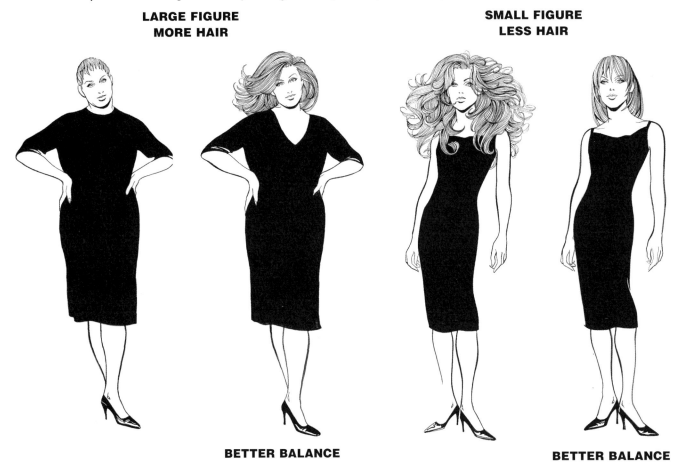

BETTER BALANCE

BETTER BALANCE

Face

Facial structure often reflects body structure. Many tall and lanky clients have elongated faces, while short clients often have wide faces. Any face can be beautiful if it is framed by the right hairstyle. To determine the most appropriate style, it is important to analyze the face using criteria such as bone structure, the hairline, and the widest and most dominant areas.

When determining your client's face shape, try to answer the following questions:

1. Is the face long and narrow or short and wide?
2. Is the shape of the face angular or rounded?
3. Which area of the face is most dominant?

Using these questions as a guide will easily and clearly determine which facial shape is present.

Most Common Facial Shapes

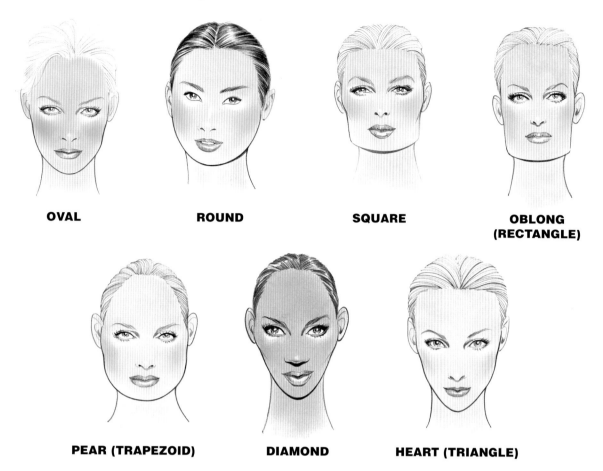

OVAL   **ROUND**   **SQUARE**   **OBLONG (RECTANGLE)**

PEAR (TRAPEZOID)   **DIAMOND**   **HEART (TRIANGLE)**

8

Three-Sectioning

Three-sectioning is an effective way to measure the proportions of the face. It is done by measuring the three sections of the face – section one: the front hairline to the middle of the eyebrows; section two: the middle of the eyebrows to the tip of the nose and section three: the tip of the nose to the tip of the chin. These sections are considered harmonious if they are equal. If there is more than 1/2" (1.25 cm) difference between any of these sections, they are not considered harmonious. Hairstyles and makeup can be used to create the illusion of balance. To measure the face using the three-sectioning technique, do the following:

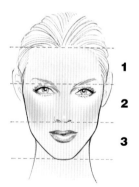

- Comb and pin all the hair out of the face
- Remove the client's glasses and jewelry
- Place client in front of a mirror
- Measure the three sections with a tape measure

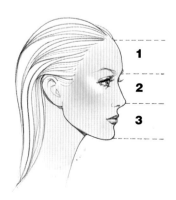

Oval Facial Shape

The oval face is rounded, long and narrow rather than wide and short. It has no dominant areas. Oval faces look very harmonious because they approximate even three-sectioning. Oval faces look good with almost any hairstyle, length or texture. Sometimes the oval facial shape lacks a focal point and can look plain. A stronger statement with the hairstyle may be used to create interest.

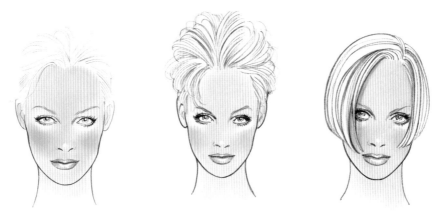

OVAL – MANY CHOICES

Round Facial Shape

The round face looks circular. It appears to be rather short and wide rather than long and narrow. Round faces have a low, round hairline and a short chin with a very rounded jaw line. These faces look very good with a geometric or linear hair style. When the face is well balanced, short and layered styles look very good. An asymmetrical hairstyle can also distract from the roundness of the face. Always add height and, when possible, cut long, wispy side areas to make the cheeks look narrow. Avoid volume at the sides since this would add even more width. Round faces shouldn't wear fringes–a few wisps of hair are better. Avoid curls since they emphasize the roundness of the face even more. If the client has naturally curly hair, create a very angular shape. Place the volume either below the jaw line or above the temple area.

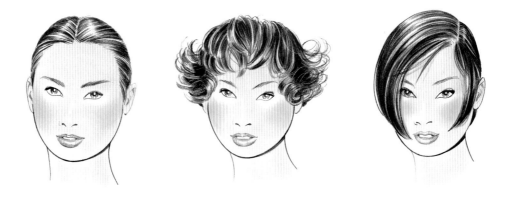

ROUND – AVOID WIDTH

Square Facial Shape

The square face is short and wide. It looks very angular with a lot of straight lines. For instance, the front hairline and jaw line are almost horizontal while the cheekbones protrude very little on the sides. The area most dominant on the square face is the jaw line. Square-shaped faces need height on top and narrowness on the sides. Shapes that elongate the face are preferable. Very short hair with height on top can look good on self-confident clients. For others, curly texture and wisps of hair around the face work well since this adds softness to the angular lines of the face. People with square faces generally shouldn't wear fringes or styles with width at the jaw line.

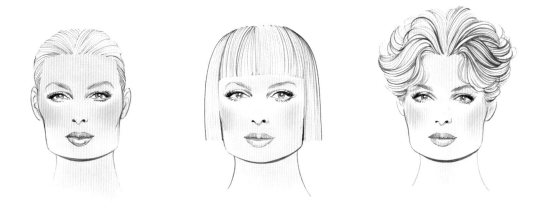

SQUARE – AVOID STRAIGHT LINES

Oblong Facial Shape

The oblong (rectangle) face is long, narrow and angular. The jaw line is wide and almost horizontal. The hairline on the oblong face is only slightly curved. The bone structure allows the sides to look vertical since the cheekbones barely protrude. In many cases one area of the face is longer, either the forehead, the chin or the middle portion. Oblong faces need softness and width and look good with longer and curly hair. Chin length hair with volume on the sides is also very flattering. A fringe can shorten the look of the oblong face. Women with oblong faces shouldn't wear extremely short hair, as it might look too masculine. Avoid adding any more height to the rectangular face. Also, avoid flat, long, straight hair that would make the face look even longer.

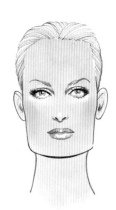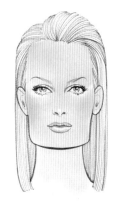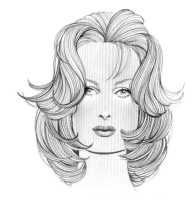

OBLONG – ADD SOFTNESS

Pear Facial Shape

The pear-shaped (trapezoid) face is most often elongated, with a forehead that is narrow and a jaw that is the widest area of the face. The pear-shaped face can wear graduated forms very well since these styles can push the volume up and above the jaw line into the narrow areas. If the hair is short, the volume should be placed at the upper crest area. If the client wears the hair long, it should reach past the jaw line. Curls and wispy hair can soften the angularity of the face. Also, long wispy side areas make the cheeks and jaw look more slender. In general the hair should be neither extremely short nor like a bob that ends at the jaw line.

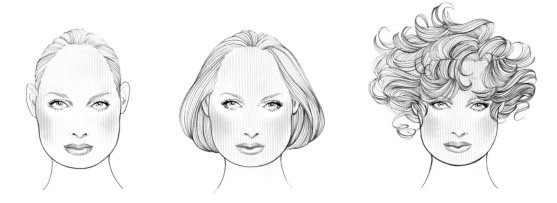

PEAR – ADD VOLUME ABOVE JAW LINE

Diamond Facial Shape

The diamond face is elongated and angular. Its widest area is at the cheekbones, while the forehead and chin are narrow. The diamond facial shape resembles the oval face, but looks harsher. Diamond-shaped faces need narrow sides and fullness at the chin. Bobs work very well for the diamond facial shape. Short hair also looks good on the diamond face shape as long as the nape lengths are kept longer and wispy so the hair can visually soften the pointed chin. The diamond-shaped face should avoid wearing height on top, volume at the sides, or a short cropped nape. Also, long, pointed side areas are not good since they emphasize the sharpness of the chin.

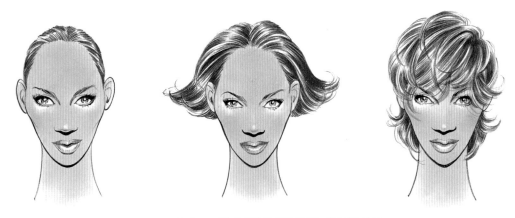

DIAMOND – REDUCE WIDTH AT SIDES

Heart Facial Shape

The heart-shaped (triangle) face is long. The heart face shape is angular and the chin area is sometimes elongated and pointed, while the forehead is wide. These faces look good with volume at the chin and no or little volume on top. Curls help to soften the features. If the hair is shorter, the nape still needs to stay full. Too much volume at the top of the hairstyle will make the face look even more triangular. Diagonal forward lines and long pointed side areas should be avoided. Short, cropped napes can make this face look too harsh.

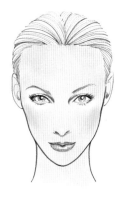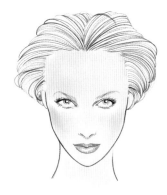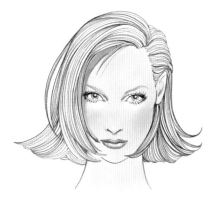

HEART – ADD VOLUME AT CHIN

When consulting with your client, it is important that you use terminology that expresses your knowledge without labeling the client. For example, instead of saying to a client that you find the client's facial shape to be pear-shaped, you should refer to fullness at the jaw and the narrow forehead area. In other words, the shape similarities are intended as a reference tool to aid in your understanding, not as a label for client consultation. The art of consultation includes finding the right words to encourage and support the client while making professional recommendations.

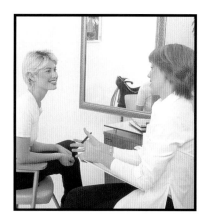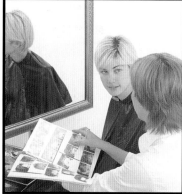

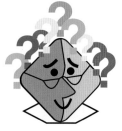

"Today individual beauty is much more appreciated, and any face shape can be considered beautiful as long as it is surrounded by the proper hairstyle."

FACE SHAPE		DO	DON'T
	Oval	Consider features to enhance Balance body proportions with style	Add too much height
	Round	Add height to the crown Add width below the jaw line or above temple Create angular shapes	Add a full fringe Add width on the sides Add equal fullness around the entire face
	Square	Sweep short hair up over ears Add soft texture to conceal square corners Begin side fullness at temples	Add solid lines at jaw line
	Oblong	Keep short hair equally full on top and above ears Add width at the sides Use a side part and diagonal fringe	Add height without width Style hair straight and flat
	Pear	Add width at the forehead (in short or medium styles) Let long hair cover the jaw line to conceal its width	Accentuate the pear shape with narrowness at the temples and width at the jaw line
	Diamond	Use a side part and diagonal fringe Add width at forehead and jaw line	Add width at cheekbones
	Heart	Add width at jaw line Leave fullness at the nape that can be seen from the front	Add width at forehead or cheekbones

Profile (outline of the face from the side)

Since your clients are viewed from various angles, it is important that their hairstyle complement their profile as well. The most notable features of the profile are the forehead, the nose and the chin. You may wish to give your clients a hand-held mirror to help them view their profile as you make recommendations. **There are three different types of profiles, straight, convex and concave.**

Straight Profile

A straight profile has a very slight outward curvature from the front hairline to the tip of the nose and from the tip of the nose to the chin. Straight profiles are considered to be the ideal and can be totally exposed.

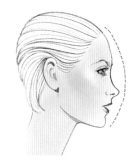

Convex Profile

A convex profile has a strong outward curvature resulting from either a protruding nose or a sloping forehead or chin. For the convex profile, it is advisable to create the illusion of a straight profile. Adding volume to the fringe area and the forehead will visually shorten the length of the nose. To balance a sloping chin, keep the shape of the hair tighter in the nape so the chin doesn't appear too small in comparison to the hair volume. With a bob, create a diagonal-forward perimeter line that points directly to the chin to make it appear larger. A receding chin on a male client can be camouflaged by a full beard and mustache.

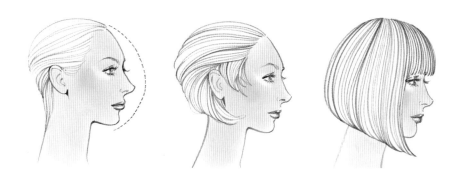

Concave Profile

A concave profile has an inward curve, which is most often the result of a dominant, protruding forehead and chin or a small nose. To compensate for the dominant chin, build fullness in the nape and avoid short nape lengths and diagonal forward lines, since this would cause the chin to stand out even more. To cover up a large forehead, cut fringes and style them with little volume. Moving the hair off and away from the face will compensate for the smaller nose.

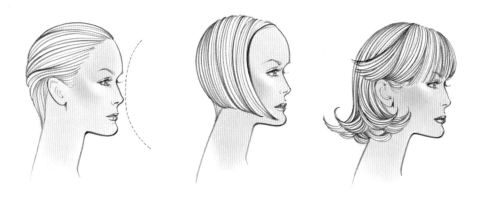

Special Considerations

Other areas that may need special consideration when determining proper proportions include a receding hairline, protruding ears and glasses.

Receding hairline

When a client has a receding hairline, avoid a side part directly in the center of the recession corner. Try to style the hair without any direct part and let it fall slightly forward to cover the receding area.

Protruding Ears

Large or protruding ears should be covered with longer hair or have more volume and fullness at the sides if the hair is short.

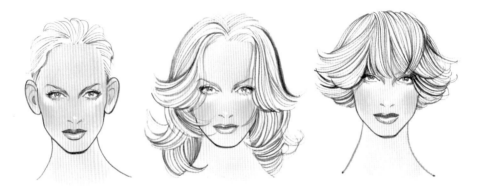

Glasses

A client who wears glasses may pose two different types of challenges. The first challenge involves the client asking you for advice on the type of frame shape to select. The other challenge is a client who needs a hairstyle adapted to the glasses already being worn. In general, the factors to consider when selecting a pair of glasses are similar to those for choosing a hairstyle: body shape, face shape, personality, clothing style and lifestyle.

Basic Guidelines for Selecting Glasses

- Select large glasses for a larger face and small glasses for a smaller face

- Determine if your client considers glasses to be a fashion accessory or a necessity. A client who views glasses as a fashion accessory may be happy with a pair that draws attention, through shape or color. A client who is not too happy about wearing glasses and sees them as a necessity will probably be more satisfied with a delicate frame in gold or silver or possibly unframed glasses.

- The shape of the frame can also be used to enhance or compensate for the shape of the face. A square-shaped pair of glasses can give a round face more interest while a round pair of glasses can soften a square face. A wide frame can add width to a narrow face, while a narrow frame makes a wide face look more slender.

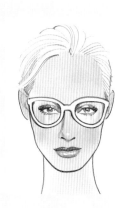 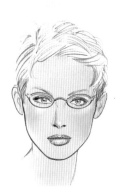 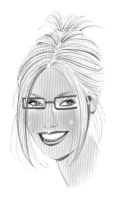 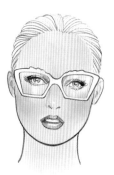 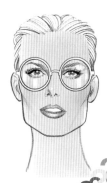

Keeping the goals that you wanted to achieve with the hair in mind along with the shape, size and color of glasses will result in helping the client achieve a total image.

"Glasses can influence the wearer's face almost as much as the appropriate hairstyle."

Hair

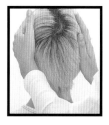

A cosmetologist could never make a design decision without analyzing his/her primary working material – the hair. It is important to determine several factors about the hair before deciding a particular style. These factors include color, texture, density, length, condition and growth pattern.

Hair Color

To be able to make the right design decision for your client's hair color, you will need to analyze his/her natural coloring. The right hair color can emphasize the natural skin tone or eye color and make the client look fresher and more radiant. The wrong hair color can cause the opposite effect.

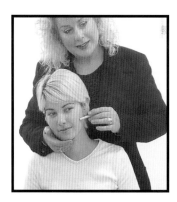 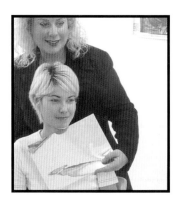 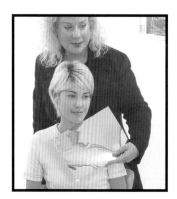

To determine which colors are most flattering for your clients, you first need to analyze the pigmentation of your client's hair, skin, eyes and lips. Use the following chart to determine whether your client's color scheme tends to be warm or cool and whether the intensity of those colors is mild or strong. Keep in mind that warm colors contain yellow, orange and/or red, and cool colors contain blue, green and/or violet. Place an X on the square that most closely identifies your client's natural color scheme and count the number of X's in each column. The totals will help you make the best hair color decisions (as well as makeup choices!) for your clients. Note that neutral colors tend to be balanced. Clients who have a neutral color scheme can look good in either warm or cool colors.

MILD   **STRONG**

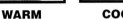

WARM   COOL   WARM   COOL

PIGMENTATION FACTORS	WARM		NEUTRAL	COOL	
	Mild	Strong		Mild	Strong
Hair Natural Hair Color					
Childhood Hair Color					
Skin Scalp					
Skin Behind the Ear					
Skin on the Face					
Cheek Color					
Freckles on Arms and Shoulders					
Shadows around the Eyes					
Eyes Eye Color					
Circle Around Iris					
Whites of Eyes					
Lips Natural Lip Color					
TOTAL					

The following images show the influence that colors have on the overall look of a client and whether they are chosen incorrectly or correctly. The first image shows the client without any makeup. Analyze the skin color, eye color and lips while you cover the other two images. After you determine into which category the client falls, look at the other two images and note the positive and negative effects that colors have on the total image. As you can see, the hair color as well as the makeup color should parallel the client's natural coloring and intensity in order to emphasize the natural beauty.

BEFORE

INAPPROPRIATE COLORING

APPROPRIATE COLORING

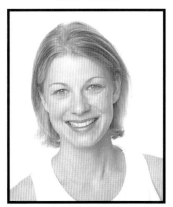

COOL MILD

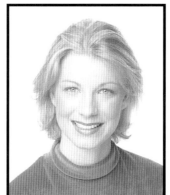

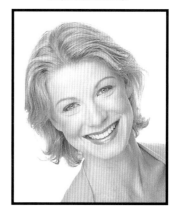

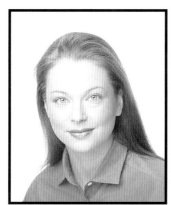

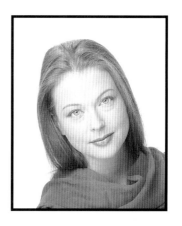

WARM MILD

8

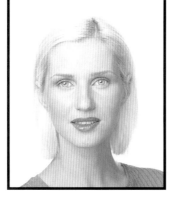

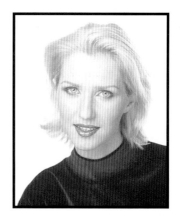

COOL STRONG

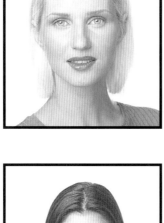

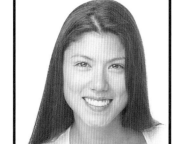

WARM STRONG

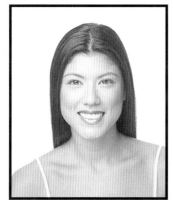

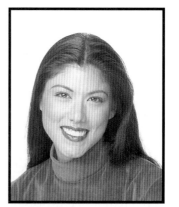

Hair Texture

Hair texture refers to the surface appearance or feel of the hair as well as the diameter of the hair strand itself. Texture can be described as either unactivated (having a smooth and unbroken surface) or activated (having a rough surface). It can also be described as fine, medium or coarse.

CUT

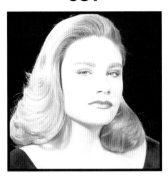

UNACTIVATED

CURL

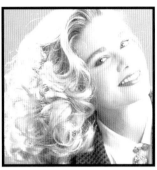

ACTIVATED

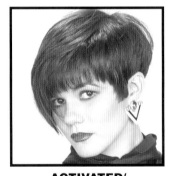

ACTIVATED/ UNACTIVATED

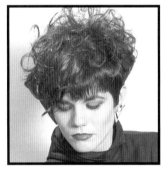

ACTIVATED

With unactivated styles you will find no hair ends exposed on the surface. The hair is often straight and cut as a blunt line. With activated styles you will see a rough surface and lots of movement. Activation is created either through curls or when the hair ends are exposed on the surface, such as with hair that is layered.

The surface appearance of the hair can be altered with a variety of salon services, such as cutting the hair blunt or in layers, perming, relaxing, as well as with different finishing techniques or products.

The texture of the hair itself (the hair's diameter) will determine which style will work best for your client. Hair with fine texture is usually easy to style but the hair collapses faster. Coarse hair is hard to style at first, but when done properly, the style lasts for a longer period of time. Curly, coarse hair tends to create a wider silhouette.

Hair Density

Density describes the amount of hair per square inch on the scalp and is usually referred to as light, medium or heavy (or thin, medium or thick). Hair density will determine the feasibility of certain hairstyles. For example, clients with light density generally won't have enough fullness for longer designs that go past the shoulders. Client's with heavy density hair generally won't look as good with curly perms or feel comfortable with upswept hair because of the additional weight. The amount of volume you are able to achieve in a hairstyle often depends on the density of the hair.

Another factor to consider with hair density is the use of styling products. Styling products offering manageability, lasting power and conditioning effects can all supplement varying degrees of hair density. The styling product label usually indicates appropriate usage and hold factor for various hair types. You may need to consider this hold factor when attempting to match the right product with the desired volume. For instance, thick hair may require a heavier styling product for better control. Thin density hair, on the other hand, may require a lighter styling product that won't weigh down the hair while providing volume and mobility.

Hair Length

A client's existing hair length might not be long enough to realize a chosen style immediately. It might be necessary to let some areas of the hair grow. Clients need to be informed about this delay to avoid disappointments.

Hair Condition

The condition of the hair, especially in relation to the client's history of chemical services is a very important consideration. The hair's present condition determines which additional chemical services can be performed without jeopardizing the integrity of the hair. It is important that the cosmetologist and client work together to achieve and maintain healthy hair. It is your responsibility to recommend appropriate chemical services and proper home care maintenance with the recommended products.

Growth Pattern

Every client has certain growth patterns in the hair. The natural growth pattern determines the angle and direction at which the hair grows out of the scalp. This angle and direction are usually very strong and can seldom be altered. For example, if the client's growth pattern directs the hair straight forward onto the face, it will be frustrating to try to wear it back and away from the face. As a professional cosmetologist you will need to consider a different alternative that is more practical for the client.

8

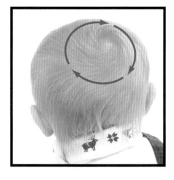 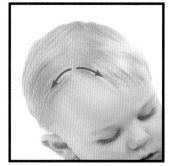 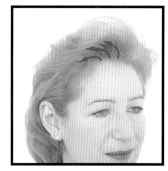

Personality

Many times certain looks or images are associated with certain personalities. Outgoing clients, for example, are usually seen as self-confident and loving. These clients attract the attention of others with their behaviors and actions as well as with their looks. On the other hand, shy clients may feel more uncomfortable if they draw too much attention to themselves. It is always important that the appearance of a client reflect the personality. A client's hair and clothing should not overpower the client as much as it should be neither overpowering nor understated.

"Personalities are often described with colorful words, such as bubbly, bright, dark or intense."

Identifying the client's personality from some key indicators is essential, especially for new clients when there hasn't been a chance to get to know them over a period of time. Through practice you will learn to read each person and to choose ways to build rapport that will make you more effective in your career.

Personality Type Indicators

Personality is defined as the outward reflection of inner thoughts, feelings, values and attitudes. Some initial gestures or comments that clients make may give you an indication of their personality type.

The first clues about a client's personality are often revealed at first glance. Good observation skills are necessary. Observe:

- How does the client enter the salon? Is it a grand entrance or does this particular client quietly enter the salon?
- How is the client's posture while sitting in the chair?
- Is this client relaxed and open?
- How is the client returning the handshake? Is it firm, or is it soft while trying to pull the hand away immediately?
- How is the client's voice while speaking?

Listen closely between the words! Is the volume high or low, is the speed fast or slow, is the tone warm and gentle or cool and firm? Adjust your body language and your speech to that of the client. A shy client will withdraw if you are too outgoing. If the client is outgoing and loud, you may have to be energized as well, otherwise you may have difficulty gaining the client's respect and confidence. Remember, it is not necessary to become a completely different person. You should just strive for a better fit or connection.

For your purposes as a stylist, personality types generally fall into two categories: outgoing or reserved. You should not use these indicators to put a label on your clients but rather to help you match their style and begin the process of building what will eventually be rapport with your clients. Listed below are some "quick indicators" for outgoing and reserved personality types.

Indicators of outgoing behaviors:	**Indicators of reserved behaviors:**
Friendly smile	Limited facial expressions
Twinkling eyes	Hesitant to make eye contact
Laughter	Controlled voice, no highs or lows
Introduce themselves	Wait for others to talk first
Speak before being spoken to	Wait for introduction; formal
Warmth	Arms folded across chest
Liking to hug and shake hands	Seem to be observant
Many gestures	Take time, moves slowly
Firm handshake	Soft handshake

Reserved clients will most likely want a hairstyle with a more natural color and one that doesn't draw too much attention. These clients generally prefer a functional style. Changing their hair will require you to have logical facts about why the change is needed. Reserved clients usually do not appreciate surprises and need some thinking time before possibly making the change at the next visit. Making sure that this client clearly understands what the look will be like and that it is what the client wants will avoid problems. This client will need facts clearly presented in order to understand why a change in the style could be positive. They are very often loyal clients once they have been satisfied with your work.

Outgoing clients care a lot whether other people like their looks, since they want to be liked and admired. Outgoing clients love to be the center of everyone's attention. Whatever is new and exciting, they want it and they can wear it. These clients are wonderful advertisements for every stylist, since they attract attention and can display all the cosmetologist's skills. Unfortunately, they often run late or decide, at the last minute, to get a new hair color that wasn't scheduled originally. They are certainly challenging customers, yet at the same time they allow the cosmetologist to express his/her creativity.

Clothing

The strongest, most convincing looks are the ones presented fully from head to toe. That is why clothing style is another important aspect to consider when designing the hair. You should always remember that the way your clients are dressed at the actual salon visit might not be the way the client normally dresses. Some clients don't dress up when they visit the salon. Other clients might be dressed more formally than usual due to plans they have after the visit. The best route for you to take is to ask the client a few questions about their clothing style to get the full picture. Internationally, designers and the fashion industry identify a few typical clothing styles. The six main styles are natural, romantic, dramatic, gamine, classic and casual.

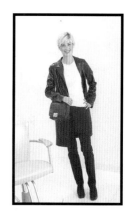

8

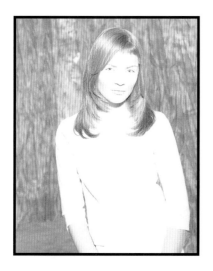

Natural

Clients in the natural category like to wear colors that are found in nature. Often their clothes are made from natural materials, such as flat leather shoes, string leather sandals, linen sneakers, and/or jewelry made out of natural materials such as stones or wood. Their hair needs to be low maintenance since most of these clients do not like to use a lot of styling products. They usually like their hair to look and feel healthy. Natural hair coloring products are very popular among these clients. They are often very conscious about the environment and animal testing when it comes to their choice of products.

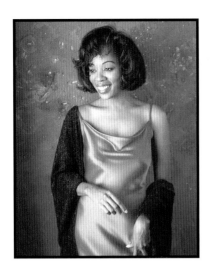

Romantic

Clients in the romantic category love silk, flower prints, lace, beads and pastel shades of color. They often shop at vintage stores to purchase accessories, such as shawls and very detailed, small jewelry. They often dress tone on tone. Soft and feminine hairstyles are good for these clients. They like curls, whether natural or permed, and soft hair colors, such as highlights of golden blonde, light brown and strawberry blonde.

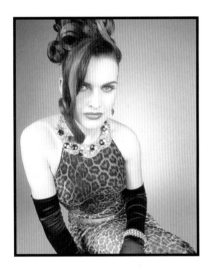

Dramatic

Clients in the dramatic category like anything out of the ordinary. They want to draw attention and make heads turn. They wear a lot of bold, strong colors and very dramatic shapes. They often wear large fashion jewelry and all kinds of extravagant accessories. If they have a bad hair day, they just wear a crazy hat. Even purses and shoes are extraordinary. These clients love crazy hair and hair colors. They seek out change and new ideas. Cosmetologists have the opportunity to practice their creativity with these clients. If a style is not dramatic enough, the client won't be happy and might not return.

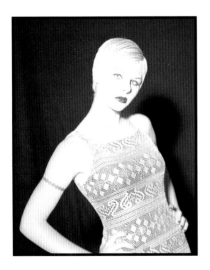

Gamine

Clients in the gamine category are playful and very feminine. They are very fashion-oriented and enjoy wearing the latest looks. They wear small jewelry, often geometric in shape. They have an eye for interesting detail. Their hair is usually short. Side parts are common.

Classic

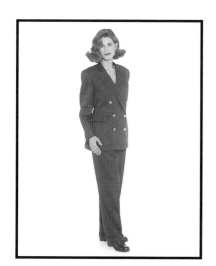

Clients in the classic category are very coordinated in their wardrobe. They wear classic colors, such as navy, black, white, cream, beige, brown and gray. Most things in their wardrobe can be combined with each other. Every piece of clothing is well chosen and usually exemplifies a design look. They have one favorite purse that goes with everything and they wear expensive, high quality shoes. Their jewelry is small but very valuable. Their hair always needs to be in good shape, with an appropriate shade of color. Sophisticated short hair is popular, along with classic bob styles. If the hair is long, it is often worn in a ponytail or in a bun. The hair color needs to be classic as well, for example thin highlights, natural reds, and various shades of brown. Hair is usually colored to brighten up the natural color or to cover gray.

Casual

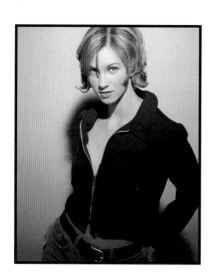

For clients in the casual category everything should be comfortable and/or low maintenance. Their wardrobe often doesn't include high heels, only flat and comfortable shoes and sneakers. Their purse is sometimes replaced by a backpack. They wear a lot of blue jeans, t-shirts and sweatshirts. Even for elegant events they will find a way to be practical and comfortable. Their hair has to be easy to style and maintain. Sometimes they like perms because it makes the hair easier to style. Often the hair is longer and pulled back into a loose ponytail.

Lifestyle

Considering your client's lifestyle when making a design decision is important since it will help determine a style's practicality. Factors that need to be considered are: job/career, hobbies (such as sports), family, time willing to spend on hair, skill or ability to care for hair and the money the client is willing to invest in the hair maintenance.

Job/Career

Consider what type of image the client's job requires. Since many clients spend most of their time at work, those requirements cannot be neglected. A client who runs the front desk in a five-star hotel will need a different look than someone working at a hospital, a farm, or a department store.

Hobbies

A lot of things clients like to do for fun, fitness or relaxation challenge their hair in a different way. For instance, a swimmer will have trouble with a flaming red hair color that will fade from excessive chlorine exposure, or a mountain climber will have trouble seeing if long hair layers fall in his/her face.

Family

Many clients find their partner's and/or family preferences important. Though some clients believe that their partner should like their choices despite any hairstyle, others may want to look pleasing to their partner. Asking how the client thinks about this issue will clear the question and avoid later disappointment. Whether or not your clients have young children may also influence the type of style they can wear. For them, a low maintenance style would probably be appreciated.

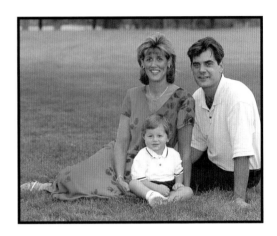

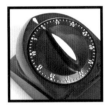

Time

The time a client is willing to spend on hair care gives a very fast indication of how elaborate the hairstyle can be. Client's wanting to only invest five minutes for daily hair care and styling need to know why their hair cannot look a particular way.

Skills

Even though clients may be willing to invest all the time and money necessary for a certain look, some clients may not have the necessary skills required to achieve it at home. That makes it your responsibility to give any support possible through perming, texturizing and explaining the proper tools or products to use and how to use them.

Money Investment

Finally, the question of the costs involved with the client's selected style needs to be made clear. The costs for the actual style change as well as its maintenance need to be discussed. If the client is aware of the whole picture ahead of time, the decision to make the style change will be favorable and you will have a satisfied, loyal client.

CLIENT CONSULTATION

Once you have gathered all the information necessary to make a proper design decision, it is important to communicate your recommendations. Creating a good client relationship is just as important and as much of an art as creating a unique new hairstyle.

Communication

Communication is often mistakenly considered what is said in words only. However, it is much more than that. Communication involves actions, gestures, tone of voice and speed. Earlier in this chapter you reviewed how to identify someone's personality pattern. Now you will analyze how to adapt the communication and consultation to different personalities. This skill will help to make your clients feel even more understood and put them at ease. Recognizing how people choose their words as well as voice volume, speed and tone will help you determine how to respond to them.

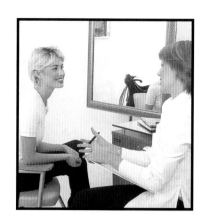

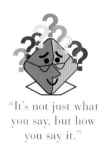

"It's not just what you say, but how you say it."

Adjusting your language and gestures to those of your client can avoid communication problems. This process of adjustment is known as building rapport.

For instance, an outgoing cosmetologist trying to establish rapport with a reserved client should try to relax and be less pushy, so as not to overwhelm the client. A reserved stylist, however, when confronted with an outgoing client needs to become more energized. Other factors that determine the success of a client consultation include time, environment and professional appearance.

Time

A consultation with a client will vary depending on the amount of time scheduled. Various salons have developed different ways to address this issue, such as:

- Some salons see a detailed consultation as a service by itself, which means that the client may be booked for an extra 30-60 minutes for the consultation only. There is an extra charge for this consultation and the client may be scheduled for the hair service immediately following the consultation or at some other future, scheduled time.

- Other salons schedule new customers for just fifteen minutes consultation time.

Environment

During a consultation the noise level from the environment or surroundings should be low for a more relaxed, intimate atmosphere. Choose the location for the consultation carefully. Natural lighting will help you identify the client's natural coloring and a full body mirror may also help when discussing the proportions between body and hairstyle.

Professional Appearance

Clients often see their cosmetologist as an image-maker. They observe and evaluate their stylist's look very carefully. Your appearance is immediately connected to the expectation the client has of your job performance. In other words, a cosmetologist exhibiting a poor image will be expected to have poor skills as well. A stylist exhibiting a professional image will create more interest and excitement from the client.

Once you've allocated the proper amount of time, seated your client in a pleasant environment and are sure you present a professional appearance, you will be able to proceed with the consultation in an efficient and trusting manner.

Keep in mind that there are five steps to a successful consultation, Greet, Ask, Agree, Deliver and Complete. Use the following chart as a guide when conducting a consultation with your clients.

FIVE STEPS TO CONSULTATION

Phase	How	Why	Material
Greeting 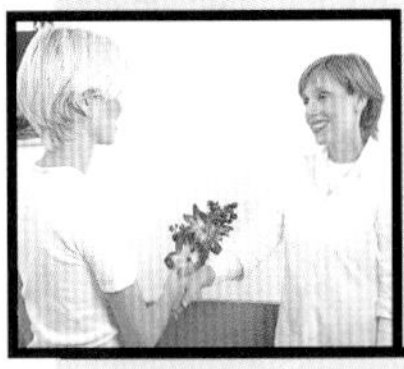	Welcome client; introduce with handshake; make eye contact with client	Break the ice; find out client's name; build rapport with client; get first clues on personality	Good appearance for positive first impression; friendly smile; good posture; strong handshake
Ask, Analyze, and Assess 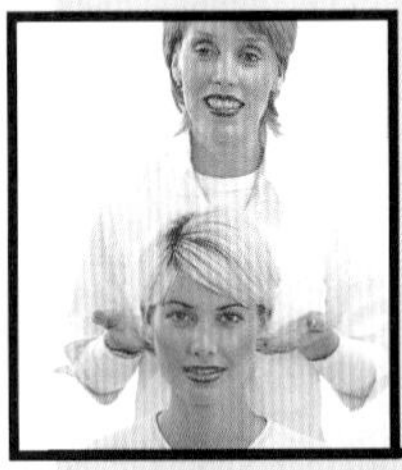	Ask questions about lifestyle, clothing style, personal likes and dislikes; analyze body height, face shape, hair, natural color scheme, personality	Discover clients needs to determine the design options; find out history of the hair and the client's previous experiences to determine service options	Consultation chart, (consultation computer system); hair style selector; color chart; comb; hand mirror; consultation skills, listening skills
Agree 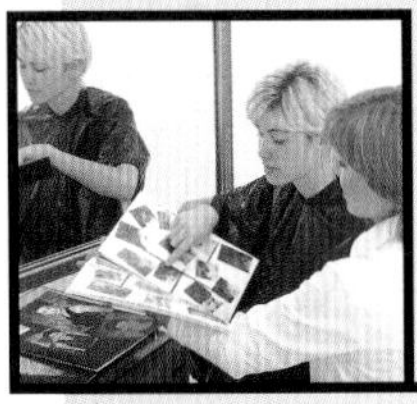	Summarize the design decisions; explain the services, the cost of upkeep and home care for the style; if any hesitation on client's side, return to Ask, Analyze and Assess	Gain client feedback on suggestions; ensure you're on the same page and have a true understanding about the style change; avoid disappointment for client or designer	Consultation chart, (consultation computer system); hair style selector; color chart; comb; hand mirror; consultation skills, listening skills
Deliver 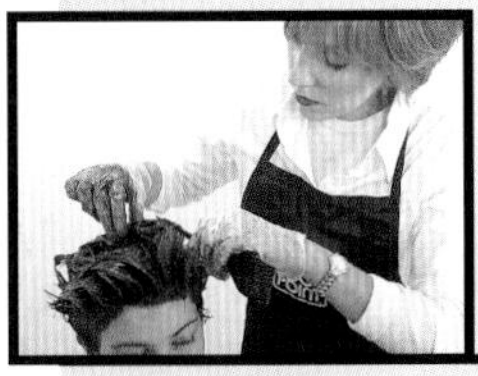	Ensure client's comfort during service; explain steps and actions that are taking place; commit to delivering the highest quality possible	Satisfy the customer's needs	Essential implements, products and equipment; service skills
Complete 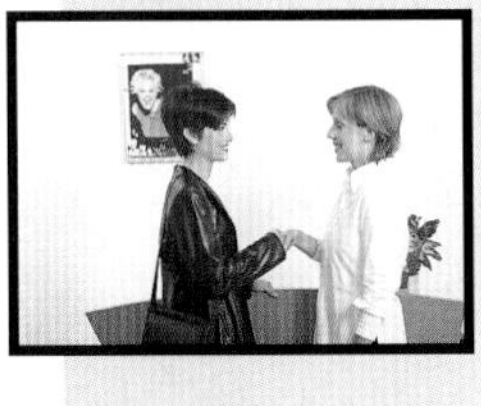	Gain feedback; ask questions; give styling tips; show and explain retail products; schedule next appointment; guide customer to front desk; give thanks and say goodbye	Ensure client is satisfied and understands how to keep up the style; enforce client/stylist relationship; encourage referrals for other customers	Good appearance; friendly smile; good posture; good handshake; appointment book; business cards

The success of a hairstyle depends on the satisfaction of your clients. Therefore, you want to make sure that you've understood their wishes and have communicated what you are able to do to satisfy those wishes. By building a trusting relationship with your clients and delivering excellent design results, you will establish a loyal customer base that will reward you with repeat business.

DESIGN COMPOSITION

It is often said that 80% of a hair designer's success is based on communication skills and ability to build rapport and 20% on technical skills. There is, however, an important link between these two sets of skills—design composition. Design composition is the coming together of all the individual elements of your intended design into one artistic whole.

Design Elements

Hair design follows the same basic artistic concepts as other art forms and applies them to the medium of hair. Every artist works with the three major design elements—form, texture and color. In creating a complete or finished design, whether in paint or with hair, not one of these elements can be ignored.

Form

Form, the first design element, describes the outline or silhouette of an object. A knowledge of lines is essential to the understanding of form. Lines create shapes to produce different forms and can be straight or curved.

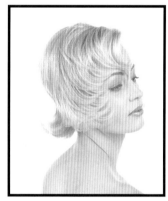
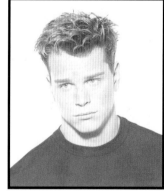

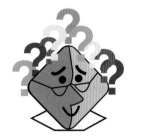

"Forms consist of shapes, which are created through lines."

Form needs to be viewed from a variety of different perspectives to get a real three-dimensional impression of the design. The form and size of a hairstyle should always complement the client's image and be in good proportion with his/her physical characteristics.

Terms to Know

 A **line** consists of a series of points that are connected with each other in a variety of directions.

 Angles are formed at the point where two lines meet.

 A **shape** is a two-dimensional figure consisting of points, lines and angles.

Line

Lines establish directions that lead the eye through a hairstyle and create visual illusions. Lines can be identified along the perimeter of a hairstyle as well as within the style itself. Lines are created by cutting, styling or chemical texturizing techniques.

Straight lines can be horizontal, vertical, diagonal left or diagonal right. Curved lines can be any part of a circle and can go in any direction

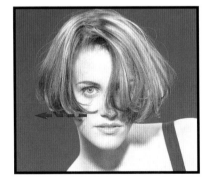

Horizontal Lines

- Are parallel to the horizon
- Add width
- Open a narrow face
- Add weight or bulk when cut into a shape

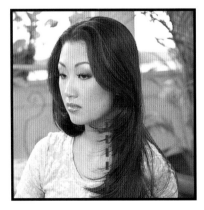

Vertical Lines

- Are at a right angle to the horizon
- Add the illusion of length
- Make a wide face look narrower
- Remove bulk when used in hair cutting

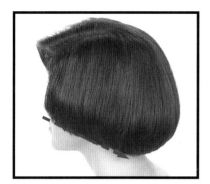

Diagonal Lines

- Lead the eye to a focal area
- Allow movement when used in hair cutting
- Diagonal forward lines move toward the face
- Diagonal back lines move away from the face

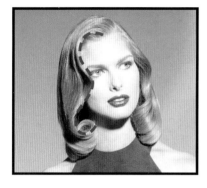

Curved Lines

- Softer than straight lines
- Soften angular faces
- Distract from hard features
- Allow blending when used in hair cutting
- Create the illusion of movement
- Moving in opposite directions, curved lines create wave patterns

Texture

As a design element, texture identifies the surface appearance of the hair, whether it is curly or straight, smooth or layered. Texture can be natural or created through a variety of services, such as a cut, perm, style or relaxer.

8

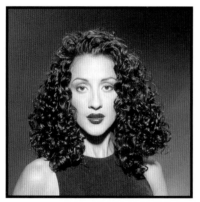

CURVILINEAR

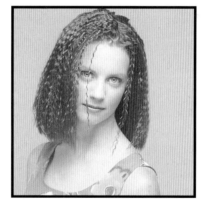

ANGULAR

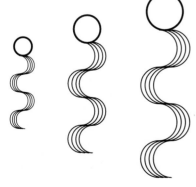

Texture speed describes the size of the actual texture pattern. Smaller patterns are called fast speeds and larger patterns are called slow speeds.

Different textures create a different character in a hairstyle. Generally, more than three textures within a design are not recommended since it may appear too busy.

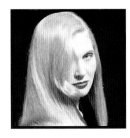

Smooth, shiny texture creates a very classic look.

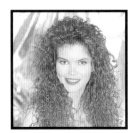

Texture with a lot of movement can be busy and unconventional.

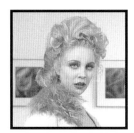

A contrast between two or three textures will create even more interest.

Color

Many designers consider color to be the most powerful design element of all, since it not only has an esthetic value in your design composition, it also has emotional value. In fact, studies about the influence of color, called color psychology, have proven the emotional effects of color. Color is even used in light therapy to give patients relief from certain discomforts.

"Feeling blue? Studies have shown that cool colors, such as violets, blues and greens, lower blood pressure and pulse rate and, in a sense, provide a "cooling" off effect. The opposite is true for warm colors."

The effects that different colors can have on a hairstyle are:

- Add depth
- Add dimension
- Add the illusion of more shine
- Add illusion of texture
- Draw attention to a special area

Warm Colors:

- Make you feel warm
- Attract the eye
- Are cheerful and exuberant

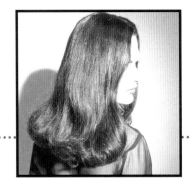

Cool Colors:

- Remind you of ice or coldness
- Are distant, quiet
- Can seem gloomy

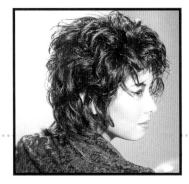

Light Colors:
- Soften the face
- Seem to come forward
- Add brightness

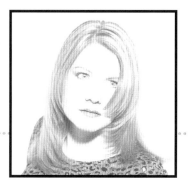

Dark Colors:
- Add harshness to the features
- Seem to recede
- Add depth

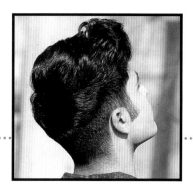

Design Principles

Understanding the design elements of form, texture and color and the way they influence hairstyles allows designers to explore different arrangement patterns that can be created with them. The patterns you follow when bringing the design elements into relationship with each other are called design principles. These design principles provide the artistic foundation on which cosmetologists create their works of art. Note that it is possible for one hairstyle to have different design principles for each design element. Here we've chosen the design element of color to demonstrate the various design principles.

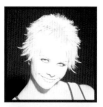

Repetition: A pattern in which an element is identical

Alternation: A pattern in which an element changes from one to another repeatedly

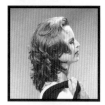

Progression: A pattern in which an element changes gradually in an ascending or descending scale

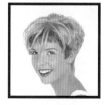

Contrast: A pattern in which an element has a relationship of opposites that create interest, variety and excitement

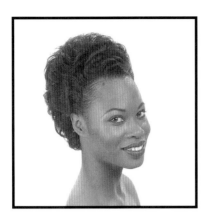

ACTIVITY:
Using the descriptions from the previous page, identify the design principles you see reflected in the form, texture and color of this image.

Form _____

Texture _____

Color _____

Balance

An important part of any design composition is the balance within the design. Balance is the state of equilibrium existing between contrasting, opposite or interacting elements. Without a sense of balance, or order, the eye travels aimlessly through a composition and eventually loses interest. Balance can be either symmetrical or asymmetrical.

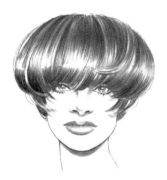
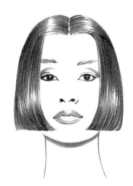

Symmetrical balance is created when weight is positioned equally on both sides of a center axis, creating a mirror image. The focus remains on the silhouette of the design.

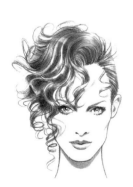
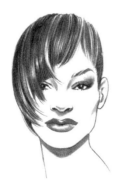

Asymmetrical balance is created when weight is positioned unequally from a center axis. However, visual balance can still be achieved even though the actual mass of the hair is off center.

Connecting the widest areas on either side of the head with an imaginary line creates a balance line. In a symmetrical design this balance line is usually horizontal. With asymmetry this balance line is diagonal.

Even an asymmetrical design needs to have healthy proportions between its larger and smaller parts. For instance, asymmetry in length should not exceed more than 1/3 of the face.

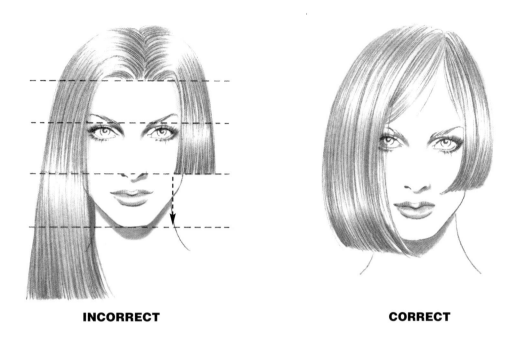

INCORRECT   **CORRECT**

Asymmetry in width should not exceed the distance from the tip of the nose to the side of the face.

8

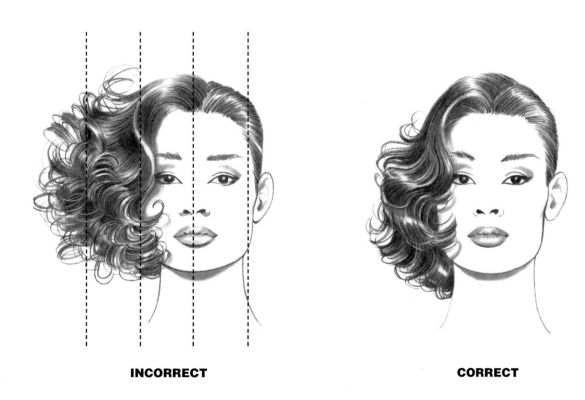

INCORRECT   **CORRECT**

This chapter gives you an introduction to the marvelous world of design. You've come a long way from your early paste and construction days toward the buzzing world of a busy salon. However, the same talent and educated eye you developed as you completed school projects and updates around your home will serve you now.

Your ability to make design decisions grows as you grow. You can already see that your design decisions will play an important role in your career as a cosmetologist. The following three factors will lead the way to client satisfaction:

- Identifying the proper design for a client using face and body proportions
- Communicating those decisions clearly
- Executing the style skillfully using design elements and principles

Your understanding of design will deepen and change as you mature as a person and as an artist. Throughout your career your designs may become more subtle or bolder, more original or more deeply rooted within classical traditions, yet they will never stray far from Plato's great insight: "Beauty lies in the proportion of things."

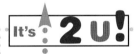

Build Your Critical Thinking Skills

In this chapter you have prepared yourself to meet the following Industry Standard for entry-level cosmetologists:

- Consult with clients to determine their needs and preferences

It's Up to You to know what to do. Using your training to this point, review the following case scenario and think through how you would handle the challenge.

You see a client for the first time and she asks you to recommend a haircut that would "look good on her" and that would best suit her busy lifestyle. You notice that she is a large-figured lady who is dressed conservatively. She has a round-shaped face and wears her hair long and straight. How would you go about making the right design decision for your client, what type of questions would you ask during the consultation and why?

Chapter 9
HAIRCUTTING

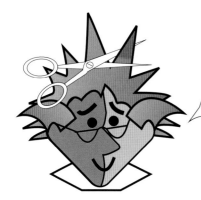

After studying this chapter you will be able to . . .

1. Identify the haircutting tools, areas of the head and fundamental cutting techniques you will use when cutting hair.

HAIRCUTTING PROCEDURES

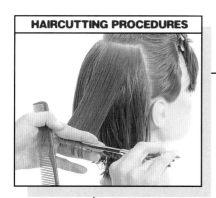

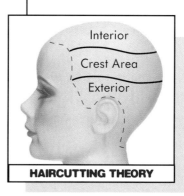

Interior
Crest Area
Exterior

HAIRCUTTING THEORY

2. Demonstrate proper procedures to achieve the basic haircuts.

9

Certain events mark milestones in life. A child's first birthday is often like that for parents and family. So is a first haircut. My parents have photos of me, their little Pivot, in the fateful chair, looking almost as handsome as I do now. They even saved a little lock of that hair. I wonder...Could that day have set me on my life path, have sparked an early interest in hair that has lasted me an entire lifetime? All I know for sure is that I still find haircutting very exciting and hope that after reviewing this chapter you will too.

Haircutting is one of the most valuable skills you can possess as a stylist. It will allow you to dramatically change a client's total look or offer subtle nuances to complement an existing image.

It's easy to talk about VALUE when value is so plain to see. As the number one requested service in all salons, haircutting is the bread and butter of your profession, wonderful and powerful in itself and the foundation of most other salon services.

Knowing and understanding the theory of haircutting along with the ability to perform haircutting procedures will allow you to develop a satisfied clientele and to successfully provide a foundation for other services.

My PLAN for you in this chapter is the height of simplicity. It aims to have you familiarize yourself with haircutting basics and then go in and practice, practice, practice. The more cuts you perform, the more confident you become and the more client satisfaction is guaranteed.

HAIRCUTTING THEORY

Form
Haircutting Essentials
Haircutting Fundamentals
Infection Control and Safety
Client Consultation

HAIRCUTTING PROCEDURES

Haircutting Procedures Overview
Solid Form Haircut
Solid Form Variation: Increase-Layered Front Hairline
Increase-Layered Form Haircut
Graduated Form Haircut
Uniformly Layered Form Haircut
Combination Form Haircut
Square Form Haircut
Overcomb Techniques
Fade Haircut

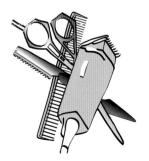

HAIRCUTTING THEORY

Throughout history, the length and/or shape of hair has fascinated and inspired people the world over. In biblical times, hair was equated with strength and virility, as in the story of Samson who lost his strength when his lengths were cut off. For reasons not fully understood, many ancient Egyptians shaved their heads. Some believe this act was for religious reasons, while others consider it was for sanitary purposes or as a relief from the burning Egyptian sun. In some cultures, such as the ancient Greeks, men and women resembled one another by wearing their hair long and naturally curly.

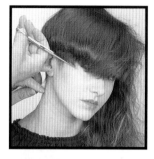 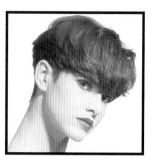
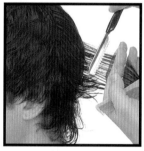 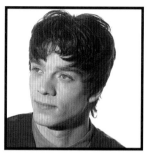

Whatever it's purpose, **haircutting can be defined as the artistic carving or removing of hair lengths with shears, taper shears, razors and/or clippers to create various forms and shapes.** Haircutting can stand alone as a salon service or serve as the foundation for a successful hairstyle and for other cosmetology services, such as a perm or color. Haircutting is also referred to as hair sculpting.

Today haircuts are designed to reflect your individual personality and personal sense of style. Throughout the years haircuts have been given names, with which you may be familiar, such as the Bob, the Wedge or the Shag. In this chapter you will learn to identify and create haircuts according to their structure or length arrangement, as opposed to a particular name. This will be explained in more detail as you continue through the chapter.

"Hair cutting dates back to antiquity and has always had significance in society. Shaving sets have been found that date back to 2000 B.C. and include bronze razors and tweezers, shaving mugs and combs."

It is crucial at this point in your education that the fundamentals of haircutting become second nature to you, since it is the foundation of all other hair services in the salon. After all, a primary part of your success will be your ability to perform a well-executed haircut. Without a good haircut, the desired style you and your client have in mind will be difficult to achieve and maintain.

Form

Almost everything that exists, whether created by nature or artificially, is composed of form, texture and color. Take a look around you and notice the different forms, textures and colors that make up everything you see. In this chapter you will focus on form, since it is the foundation of every haircut. You will learn more about texture and color in later chapters.

In haircutting, form is a three-dimensional representation of a shape. It has length, width and depth. A shape, on the other hand, consists of length and width only. Think of the difference, for example, between a circle cut out of paper (a shape) and a basketball (a form). Some common shapes include the triangle, square, rectangle, circle and oval. If these shapes were molded into sculptures, they would become forms since they would now have depth and would be three-dimensional. The length arrangement of a haircut (such as long to short or short to long) produces its form. You will learn more about shapes and forms, and how they relate to haircuts, later in this chapter.

Points, Lines and Angles

All forms and shapes are made up of points, lines and sometimes angles. A point is a dot or mark that, when extended, becomes a line. A line can be straight or curved and can move in any direction.

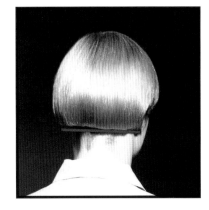

There are three basic straight lines, which are horizontal, vertical and diagonal.

Horizontal lines are parallel to the horizon and are considered stable or restful. These lines create a feeling of maximum weight or stability. Vertical lines, on the other hand, go straight up and down. These lines create a feeling of weightlessness or equilibrium, as with a standing human body.

Diagonal lines fall between horizontal and vertical. A diagonal left line slants toward the left and a diagonal right line slants toward the right. A diagonal forward line moves toward the face, while a diagonal back line moves away from the face. These lines create the illusion of movement and excitement.

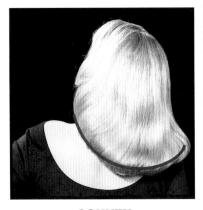

CONVEX

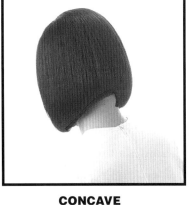

CONCAVE

There are two basic curved lines, which are concave and convex.

Concave lines curve inward, like the inside of a sphere, while convex lines curve outward, like the outside of a sphere. Both of these lines are combinations of a diagonal right and a diagonal left line, and therefore create a feeling of movement.

Angles are formed at the point where two lines join together or intersect. In haircutting, angles are used to create the shape and form of the haircut. The most common angles are 45° and 90°. A full circle consists of 360°, which (below) has been subdivided into 90° angles.

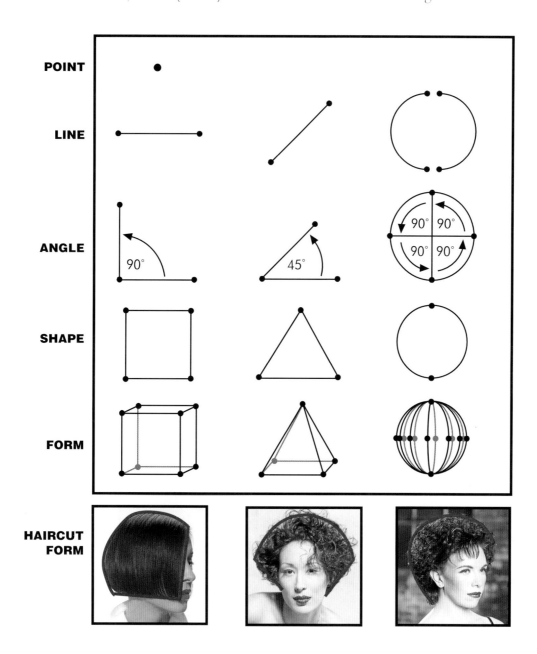

Structure

The structure of a haircut consists of the arrangement of lengths across the various curves of the head, such as shorter on top to longer at the bottom or nape. In this program, the structure or length arrangement of a haircut is identified and explained with a color-coded illustration called a structure graphic. The color-coding system will be explained further when you learn about the basic structures or forms of a haircut. There are two ways to analyze a haircut, which are natural fall and normal projection.

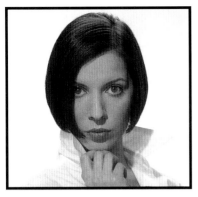

Natural Fall

Natural fall describes the hair as the lengths lay or fall naturally over the curve of the head. When identifying a haircut according to its natural fall, parts of the anatomy are used to describe where the lengths fall, such as at the chin, neck or shoulders.

Normal Projection

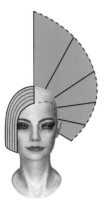

Another way to analyze the structure or length arrangement of a haircut is in normal projection. With normal projection, the hair is viewed abstractly as if it were sticking straight out from the various curves of the head. This view allows you to analyze the structure or length arrangement of the hair.

Two areas of the head are used to describe the length arrangement of a haircut. These two areas are divided by the crest (widest area of the head) and are known as the interior (above the crest) and the exterior (below the crest).

Texture

Texture refers not only to the diameter and feel of the hair, as you learned in the Trichology chapter, but to the hair's surface appearance as well. Texture can be described as unactivated (smooth) or activated (rough). In haircutting, texture is achieved by the cutting technique used. For example, with unactivated texture, the ends of the hair are not visible when viewed in natural fall. With activated texture, the ends of the hair are visible.

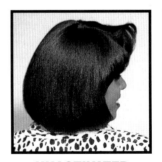
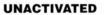
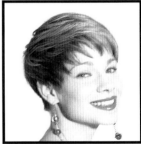

UNACTIVATED   **ACTIVATED**

Basic Haircuts

As mentioned earlier, in this program haircuts are identified according to their length arrangement or structure. The results of those structures, when viewed in natural fall, are called forms. These three-dimensional forms can also be viewed in two dimensions, as with a photograph, and can be identified according to their silhouette or shape. In this section you will learn about the basic forms used in haircutting. You will also see how the color-coded structure graphics are used to identify each form and how these forms relate to shapes. In addition, you will see what texture is created with each form.

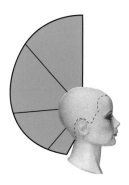
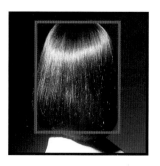

Solid Form

A solid form is also known as a one-length cut, bob, dutch boy, blunt cut or 0° angle cut

Structure: Shorter exterior progressing to longer interior

Shape: Rectangle or oval

Texture: Unactivated

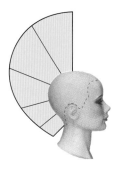
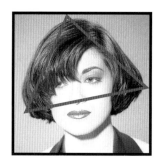

Graduated Form

A graduated form is also known as a wedge or 45° angle cut

Structure: Shorter exterior gradually progressing to longer interior

Shape: Triangle

Texture: Unactivated/Activated

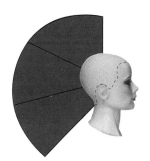
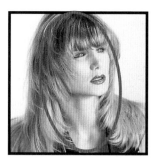

Increase-Layered Form

An increase-layered form is also known as a shag or 180° angle cut

Structure: Shorter interior progressing to longer exterior

Shape: Oval

Texture: Activated

9

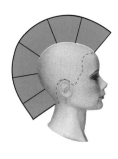
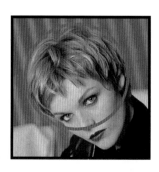

Uniformly Layered Form

A uniformly layered form is also known as a layered cut or 90° angle cut

Structure: Same length throughout

Shape: Circular

Texture: Activated

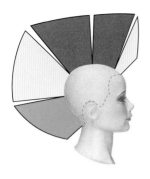
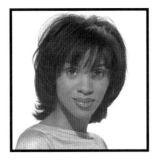

Combination Form

Structure: Two or more forms in any combination

Shape: Reflects forms chosen

Texture: Activated or a combination of activated and unactivated

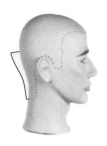
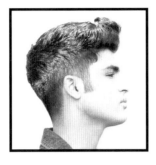

Gradation

Structure: Very short exterior gradually progressing to longer interior; similar to graduated form but shorter; fades and bald fades are very short forms of gradation

Shape: Rectangle or oval

Texture: Activated

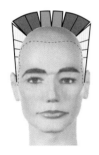
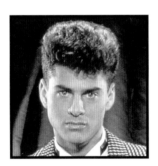

Square Combination Form

A square form is also known as a box cut.

Structure: Uniform at center top to increase layered at front and crown; gradated and uniform sides and back

Shape: Square/Rectangle

Texture: Activated

Haircutting Essentials

In order to perform a haircutting service, you will need a selection of implements (tools), products and equipment. In this program we've referred to these items as "essentials" and will be summarized for you later in this section in the form of charts called "Haircutting Essentials."

Cutting implements are the hand-held tools that you use. These tools must be disinfected after each use. Haircutting products are produced by many different manufacturers and are used to aid in the haircutting service. Haircutting equipment includes the furnishings and provisions necessary for a professional cutting service.

In this portion of the chapter, you will learn about the variety of tools you will need to cut hair. By becoming familiar with the cutting implements needed to perform a haircutting service, you will be better equipped to make the proper tool selection to achieve the desired results.

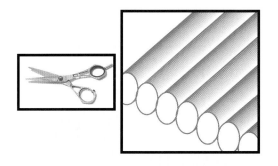

Shear

A shear creates a clean, blunt edge. By varying the position of the shear as you cut, you can create subtle variations in the hair.

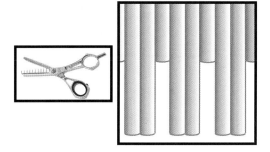

Taper Shear

A taper shear creates a distinct and regular alternation of shorter and longer lengths. More, closely spaced teeth will remove a greater amount of hair, while fewer, widely spaced teeth will remove less hair.

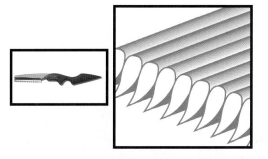

Razor

A razor creates tapering or an angle effect on the end of each strand, which produces a softer, somewhat diffused form line. This tapering may occur on the top or bottom of the strand, depending on the cutting technique you use.

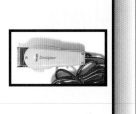
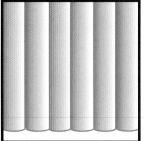

Clipper

A clipper can achieve a variety of effects, depending on the blade attachment (guard) used. For instance, it can be used to create clean, precise lines or a soft, broom-like effect. This tool generally cuts hair most quickly.

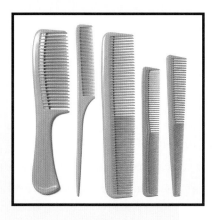

Combs

Combs are used to distribute and control the hair before and, sometimes, while cutting. The amount of space between the teeth of the comb is very important in determining which comb best suits your purpose. Generally, larger combs with wider spaces between the teeth are used to control larger amounts of hair, while smaller combs, often with a tapered shape, are used when cutting smaller sections of hair and very short hair.

9

Shears

Shears come in many different styles and lengths and are made from a variety of materials, ranging from porcelain to cobalt steel. The length and style of the shears you use are a matter of personal preference. Blade lengths range from as small as four inches (12.5 cm) to as long as 7.5 inches (18 cm). As a rule, short shears are used for more precision or detailed cutting, while longer shears are used for overcomb techniques and for cutting larger sections of hair. Shears are your primary tool for haircutting, so you will want to acquaint yourself with the different styles and lengths available in order to select the best one for you.

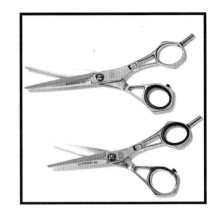

As with every implement, shears are an investment. Select a quality pair and care for them as you would any fine instrument. It is important that your shears be kept very sharp. To avoid dulling your blades prematurely, never cut anything but hair with your shears. Be sure to disinfect your shears before and after every service. Keep in mind that purchasing a quality shear and keeping it sharp and well maintained will help ensure that your tool will last longer.

Parts of the Shear

A pair of shears consists of a still or stationary blade, which is controlled by the finger grip, and the moveable or action blade, which is controlled by the thumb grip. The two blades are joined by the tension or hand screw. The thumb and finger grips may be even with each other or they may be offset. Some shears have a finger brace on which the small finger rests for comfort and balance. The finger rest may or may not be removable.

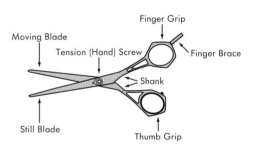

How to Hold the Shear and Comb

Being comfortable with your implements is the first step to overcoming any concerns you may have about haircutting, so it is important to learn how to hold them properly.

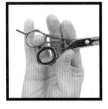

INSERT RING FINGER

Insert your ring or third finger into the finger grip to control the still blade.

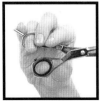

INSERT THUMB

Insert the tip of your thumb into the thumb grip to control the moveable blade. Note that placing more of your thumb into the thumb grip lessens the amount of control you have. Place your index and middle fingers on top of the shears for greater control. Rest your finger on the finger brace if your shear has one.

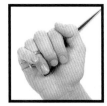

REMOVE THUMB AND PALM SHEAR

When cutting, it is sometimes necessary to hold the comb and shear in the same hand. To make this possible, without jeopardizing your client's safety, "palm" your shear by releasing the thumb grip and closing your palm over the shear.

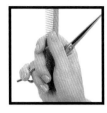

HOLD COMB

Hold the comb between your thumb and index finger of the same hand. Once the hair is distributed (combed), transfer the comb to the opposite hand for cutting.

"You don't need to be cutting hair in order to practice holding your shears and the correct cutting positions. Hold your shears in front of you now and try it. Remember, only your thumb moves when cutting!"

Cutting Positions

The cutting position you choose will depend on the area of the head on which you are working, the desired results and how comfortable the position is for you. Some common cutting positions include palm down, palm up (or out), palm to palm, on top of the fingers and under the fingers.

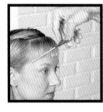

PALM DOWN

Position the palm of your cutting hand downward. This position is commonly used for cutting solid form lengths.

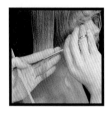

PALM UP

Position the palm of your cutting hand upward. This position is commonly used when cutting along diagonal lines.

9

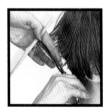

PALM TO PALM

When cutting graduated lengths, the hair is held away from the head. Position the palm of your cutting hand so that it faces the palm of your other hand.

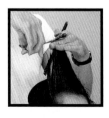

ON TOP OF THE FINGERS

In most cases you will cut under (inside) your fingers, as in the previous examples. However, when lifting the lengths on top of the head, you will need to cut the hair along the top of your fingers.

Taper Shears

Taper Shears, also known as thinning shears, are used for creating shorter lengths within the form or on the ends of the hair to reduce bulk and create mobility. One blade of the taper shear is straight and the other is notched (serrated). The purpose of the notch is to hold the hair. As the blade closes, only the hair held in the notches will be cut. The remaining hair will be pushed between the teeth and remain at the original length. The distance between the notches (teeth) of the taper shear blade will determine the amount of hair that will be cut and/or the degree of taper. Taper shears require disinfection. Follow manufacturer's directions and disinfection guidelines.

Parts of the Taper Shear

Taper shears have the same parts as shears, except instead of having two straight edge blades, taper shears have one straight edge blade and one notched blade. The notched blade has teeth that are spaced at different intervals. Taper shears are held the same way as shears.

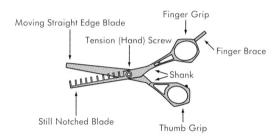

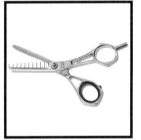
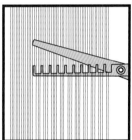

Taper 8 shears have teeth that are spaced 1/8" apart. Taper 8 shears are the best choice when a lightly tapered effect is desired, since it removes a minimal amount of hair within a parting.

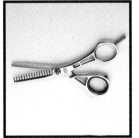
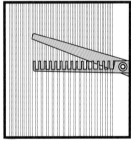

Taper 16 shears have teeth that are spaced 1/16" apart. Taper 16 shears are used to remove a medium amount of hair within a parting.

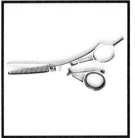
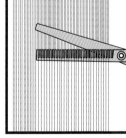

Taper 32 shears have teeth that are spaced 1/32" apart. Taper 32 shears are best for maximum hair removal and highly textured effects.

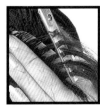

Channeling shears have wider notches that produce dramatic chunky effects. Channeling shears are primarily used for special effects such as extreme length variations and heavy fringes or notched perimeter lengths.

Razors

Although there are a variety of razors available to the professional hair designer, most razors consist of the same parts. However, razors have variations that suit different styles of cutting and levels of comfort. For example, some razors are foldable and some are not. Some include a guard, which is used over the blade for protection or for texturizing techniques. In addition, some razors have blades made from high-quality surgical steel, while others may have a soft, flexible steel blade. Some razor blades can be sharpened while most razors have disposable blades.

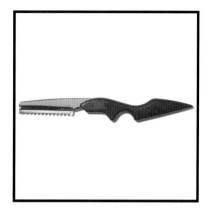
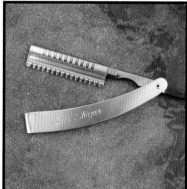

Parts of a Razor

The razor consists of a blade and, usually, a guard, which is used to protect you from coming in direct contact with the edge of the blade. The shank is used to hold the razor, while the handle, which is sometimes foldable, is used to rest your fingers. The tang is used to rest the little finger.

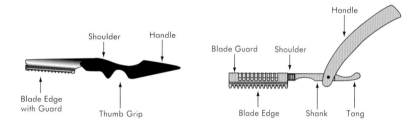

How to Hold the Razor

Depending on the type of razor, your level of comfort and the technique you are using, there are several ways in which you can hold the razor. Following is an example of how to hold a foldable razor and a non-foldable razor.

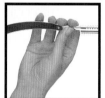

With a foldable razor, the handle is generally positioned straight out while you are cutting. Position your thumb at the bottom of the shank and position the rest of your fingers on top of the shank.

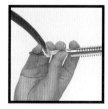
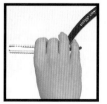

When cutting in tight areas, such as around the perimeter hairline, you may wish to rest your little finger on the tang.

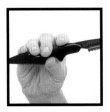

When working with a non-foldable razor, position your thumb in the thumb groove and position your remaining fingers on top of the razor. This hand position is good for texturizing techniques along a section of hair.

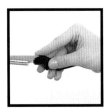

As an alternative, position your index finger on top of the razor while holding the razor with your thumb and remaining fingers. This hand position allows greater flexibility.

Important Safety Tips For Using a Razor

- Check with your area's regulating agency to determine whether or not you may remove nape or sideburn hair with the blade of a razor.
- Use the razor on damp to wet hair for the comfort of the client and ease in cutting.
- Use a guard when applicable.
- Disinfect your razor before and following every service using general disinfection guidelines.
- Read manufacturer's directions before attempting to change the blade of your razor.
- Replace the blade of your razor if it becomes dull.
- Use extreme caution when cutting around moles, scars and skin lesions.
- Discard used razor blades in a puncture-proof container.

Removing the Razor Blade

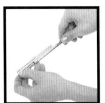
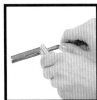

- Carefully remove the guard by tightly grasping the razor handle and shank with the cutting edge pointing upward, then carefully sliding the guard toward the end of the shank.
- Push the blade out using the guard. Place the flat side of the guard against the shank, with the razor blade positioned between the teeth of the guard.

Inserting a Razor Blade

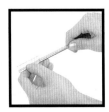
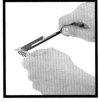

- Hold the razor handle and shank with the blade slot directed upward.
- Grasp the razor blade with the cutting edge pointing upward.
- Align the blade with the blade slot and insert the blade into the blade slot until it is secure.
- Position the outer edge of the blade between two teeth of the razor guard. Notice the teeth are locked into position in the blade slot. Maintain constant pressure and firmly push the blade into the full slot position.

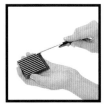

Razor Dispenser

Some razors come with a razor blade dispenser, which makes replacing razor blades safer and easier. Simply use the dispenser to slide on the new blade once the old one has been removed. Dispose of the old blade in a puncture-proof container.

Electric Clippers

Although electric clippers can be used to cut an entire head, they are generally used for creating specific effects in certain areas of the head. Some clippers come with attachments, called guards, which range from 1/8" (.30 cm) to 1" (2.5 cm). These guards enable you to consistently cut the hair at the same length as the size of the guard (i.e., a 1/8" guard will cut the hair 1/8" from the scalp). When extremely short lengths are desired, no guard is used. Another way to determine and vary the distance from the scalp while cutting is the clipper-over-comb technique. With this technique the clipper is positioned on top of the comb while cutting. Electric clippers are available with different blade sizes. Small clippers, known as trimmers or edgers, are used to outline and refine the hairline, beard, mustache and sideburn areas.

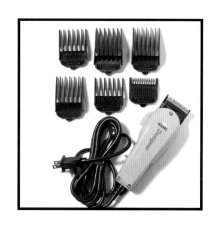

Parts of the Clipper

The stationary blade of a clipper, also called the heel, is similar in function to the stationary blade of the shear. The moveable blade moves in a side-to-side motion as it cuts the hair. The adustable blade lever is used to adjust the stationary blade. Some clippers have an electric cord, while others are charged on a power base.

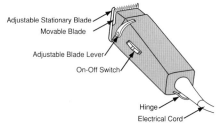

Adjustable Stationary Blade
Movable Blade
Adjustable Blade Lever
On-Off Switch
Hinge
Electrical Cord

9

A stiff-bristle clipper brush is used to clean the implement after each use. Remove the blades for cleaning. Do not clean the clipper while it is turned on. The detachable blade and heel should be kept disinfected. Clipper oil provides lubrication for the moving parts of the implement to keep them in good working condition, but should be used sparingly. Read manufacturer's directions for cleaning guidelines.

How to Hold the Clipper

The clipper can be held in a number of different ways, depending on the area of the head that is being cut, the line or angle at which you are cutting and your level of comfort.

ALERT!

Never use a clipper blade that has broken teeth and always align a new set of blades.

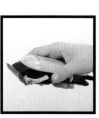
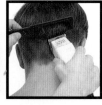

One way to hold a clipper is to position your palm over the clipper and position your thumb on the side of the clipper.

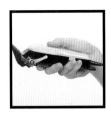
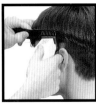

Another way is to position your thumb on top of the clipper, while positioning your remaining fingers underneath the clipper.

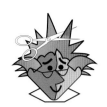

The following charts will help summarize what you've already learned about tools, while making you familiar with the products and equipment with which you will be working. The products you will use are available from a variety of manufacturers. Keep in mind that Material Safety Data Sheets (MSDS) for all products used in the salon must be available.

Haircutting Products

PRODUCT	FUNCTION
Cutting Lotion	Controls hair while cutting
Gel	Creates wet-look finishes
Mousse	Defines texture; creates light to firm hold on wet or dry hair
Pomade	Adds gloss and sheen to dry hair; creates texture separation; also referred to as polisher, glosser, lusterizer and brilliantine

Haircutting Implements/Supplies

IMPLEMENT/SUPPLIES	FUNCTION
Shear	Provides a clean, blunt edge or line
Taper Shear	Creates a distinct and regular alternation of shorter and longer lengths for mobility
Razor	Creates a tapered effect on the edge of each strand, which produces a softer, somewhat diffused line
Clipper	Creates clean precise lines or a soft, broom-like effect; various blade attachments (guards) allow the hair to be cut at various distances from the scalp
Trimmer	Used to outline the hairline, beard and sideburns
Cutting Comb	Parts and distributes the hair; primary comb for cutting and over-comb techniques
Large-Tooth Comb	Controls and distributes larger amounts of hair; also used for over-comb techniques

IMPLEMENT/SUPPLIES	FUNCTION
Taper/Barber Comb	Helps to cut short lengths and refine the perimeter when used against the skin
Towel	Protects client from getting wet during shampoo service
Plastic Cape	Protects client's clothing during the shampoo and haircutting service
Cloth Cape	Protects client's clothing during a dry haircutting service
Neck Strip	Protects client's skin from contact with the cape; replaces towel during the haircutting service
Spray Bottle	Holds water; used to keep the hair damp while cutting

Haircutting Equipment

EQUIPMENT	FUNCTION
Haircutting Station	Provides a place for tools to be displayed and organized
Hydraulic Chair	Provides proper back support for client during the haircutting service; adjustable
Wet Disinfectant Container	Holds solution for disinfecting implements
Shampoo Bowl	Supports client's neck and holds water and shampoo products during a shampoo service

Haircutting Fundamentals

By developing your technical skills and following a systematic procedure, you will experience accuracy and consistency in all your work. The following haircutting techniques are presented in the order or sequence in which you will perform any given haircut. These techniques consist of sectioning, head position, parting, distribution, projection angle, finger and shear position and design line. Other techniques with which you'll need to be familiar in order to be proficient at haircutting include crosschecking, texturizing, outlining and special grooming. However, prior to learning about any of these techniques, you will need to be familiar with the areas of the head.

Areas of the head

The most common areas, or reference points, of the head are the crest (parietal), interior, exterior, front, back, sides, nape, crown, occipital, apex, fringe and perimeter. As mentioned earlier, the crest is the widest area of the head. The area above the crest is referred to as the interior and the area below the crest is the exterior. The front and back are divided vertically from ear to ear. The side is the area in front and on top of the ear. The apex refers to the top or highest point of the head. In the back of the head, right below the crest area, is a bone that protrudes from the head. This bone is known as the occipital. Below the occipital is the nape, while above the occipital is the crown. The front area of the interior is referred to as the fringe (bangs). The area all around the hairline is referred to as the perimeter.

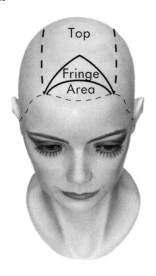
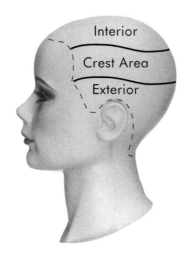
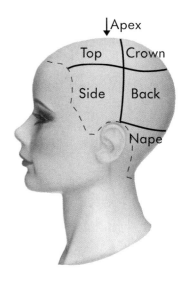

Sectioning

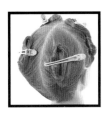

Every successful haircut begins with sectioning. Sectioning involves dividing the head into workable areas for the purpose of control. The most common sectioning pattern divides the hair into four sections: the front hairline to the nape and ear to ear. The number of sections and the type of sectioning pattern you choose depends on the type of haircut you will be creating.

Head Position

The position of the client's head during the haircut will greatly influence the final results. The most common head positions are upright, forward or tilted to either side.

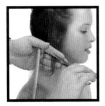

When cutting the hair in an upright head position, the most natural, pure result of the line is achieved.

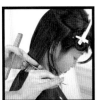

When cutting the hair in a forward head position, the neck is stretched. When the head is returned to an upright position, a slight under-bevel (ends are turned under) effect is achieved. This under-bevel occurs because the hair in the nape is now shorter than the surface lengths resulting in an inclination or a slight graduated effect.

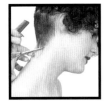

To refine the perimeter hairline, the head is generally tilted to allow for your comfort and ease in seeing and cutting in this area.

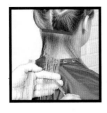

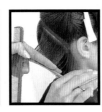

Parting

Partings are lines that subdivide sections of hair in order to separate, distribute and control the hair while cutting. Generally, the parting pattern will be parallel to the design line, which is the guideline used

270

while cutting. The most common parting lines are horizontal, vertical, diagonal back, diagonal forward, concave and convex. For maximum ease, efficiency and precision when making partings, the hair is combed in the direction that the parting will be made.

Distribution

Distribution is the direction the hair is combed in relation to the parting. The four types of distribution are natural, perpendicular, shifted and directional.

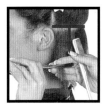

Natural Distribution

Natural distribution is the direction the hair assumes as it falls naturally from the head due to gravity. Natural distribution is used from horizontal, diagonal, concave and convex lines and is primarily used to cut solid forms.

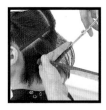

Perpendicular Distribution

With perpendicular distribution, the hair is combed at a 90° angle from its parting. This type of distribution can be used from any line and is primarily used to cut graduated and layered forms. Keep in mind that perpendicular lines intersect to form a 90° angle.

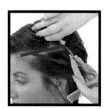

Shifted Distribution

When the hair is combed out of natural distribution in any direction except perpendicular to its parting, it is known as shifted distribution or overdirection. Shifted distribution can be used when cutting most forms except solid form. It is generally used for exaggerated length increases and blending between different areas of the head.

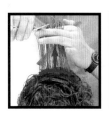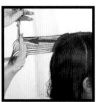

Directional Distribution

With directional distribution the hair is distributed vertically, or straight up from the head, and horizontally, or straight out from the head. Directional distribution results in length increases due to the curve of the head.

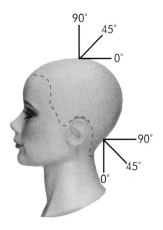

Projection

Projection, also known as elevation, is the angle at which the hair is held in relation to the curve of the head prior to cutting. The most common projection angles used in haircutting are 0°, 45° and 90°. Angles between 0° and 30° are considered to be low projection, between 30° and 60° medium projection and between 60° and 90° high projection. Projecting below 90° produces weight. Projection angles 90° and above begin to layer the hair.

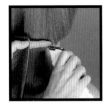

Natural fall is the natural position hair assumes due to gravity.

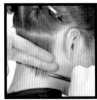

With **0°** the hair is held flat to the surface of the head while cutting.

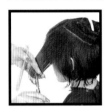

With **45°** the hair is held halfway between 0° and 90° while cutting.

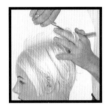

With **90°** the hair is held straight out from the curve of the head while cutting.

Finger and Shear Position

Finger and shear position refers to the position of the fingers and shear relative to the parting. The two basic types of finger and shear position are parallel and nonparallel.

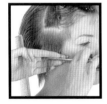

With a parallel finger and shear position, the fingers are positioned at an equal distance away from the parting. Cutting in this manner will result in the purest reflection of the chosen line.

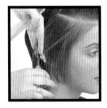

With a nonparallel finger and shear position, the fingers are positioned unequally away from the parting. Nonparallel cutting is generally used to blend between contrasting lengths and to create exaggerated length increases.

Design Line

A design line is the artistic guideline used while cutting. Any line, such as horizontal, vertical or diagonal, can be used to create a design line. The two types of design lines are stationary and mobile.

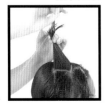

A stationary design line is a stable guide to where all lengths are directed. This design line is generally used to cut solid and increase-layered forms and to achieve a weight area (concentration of lengths) in graduated forms.

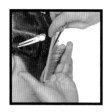

A mobile or traveling design line is a moveable guide that consists of a small amount of previously cut hair, which is used as a length guide to cut subsequent partings. A mobile design line is used to cut graduated, layered and square forms.

Crosschecking

Crosschecking is used to check a haircut for balance and accuracy. This technique is performed by using the opposite parting pattern that was used to cut the hair. For example, if you've cut the hair horizontally, you will crosscheck it vertically. In addition to crosschecking your haircut after the service, you may wish to crosscheck it periodically throughout the haircut in order to monitor yourself and avoid mistakes.

Texturizing

Texturizing, which is sometimes referred to as thinning, involves cutting shorter lengths within the form to reduce bulk and create support, closeness, fullness, mobility and visual texture in the haircut without shortening the length or removing weight. Texturizing can be done with a razor, shear or taper shear to create various results, depending on the type of tool you use and the position of the tool in relation to the hair. For instance, when thinning the hair with the razor, positioning the blade flatter and reducing the pressure applied will decrease the amount of hair removed. As mentioned earlier, when you use the razor, the hair should be damp to wet. On the other hand, the hair may be damp to dry when shears or taper shears are used. Generally there are three areas of the strand where texturizing techniques are performed, which are the base, midstrand and ends. In addition to cutting with taper shears, texturizing techniques include razor etching, slithering and razor rotation.

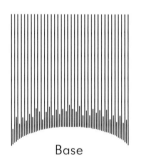

Base

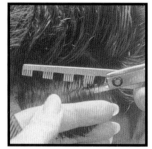

Base Texturizing

Base texturizing, which is performed between the scalp up to 1" (2.5 cm) away from the scalp, creates expansion and fullness. This technique removes weight at the base area, allowing the hair to lift away from the head. The shorter lengths support the longer lengths to encourage natural texture and movement.

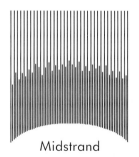

Midstrand

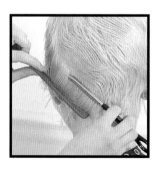

Midstrand Texturizing

Midstrand texturizing, which is performed between the end of the base area up to 1" (2.5 cm) before the ends, reduces bulk and weight. The shorter lengths support the longer lengths to create fullness or a contoured effect.

9

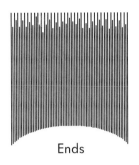

Ends

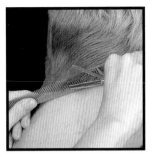

End Texturizing

End texturizing, which is performed on the ends of the hair, reduces bulk and weight to allow for mobility. End texturizing also softens the ends and helps to blend weight lines.

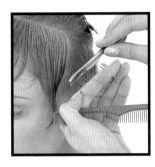

Razor Etching

Razor etching, which is used to reduce weight or remove length, is a technique in which the ends of the hair are carved into with a razor using a back-and-forth motion. The blade may be positioned at the side of a hair section, parallel to the fingers, or at the top of a section, perpendicular to the fingers.

Slithering

Slithering, which is also referred to as effilating, is a technique in which the shear is opened and closed rhythmically while moving upward from the ends. **Slithering removes bulk and creates mobility.**

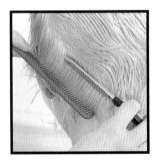

Razor Rotation

Razor rotation is performed by rotating the razor and comb along the hair strand to remove weight. This technique is used for blending and creating close-fitting contours. **The hair should be damp when performing razor rotation in order to avoid client discomfort.**

Texturizing Considerations

Before doing any of these texturizing techniques, always consider the hair's natural texture in order to determine where on the hair strand to perform the technique. For instance, **fine hair can be texturized closer to the scalp than coarse hair, since fine texture needs the extra support of the shorter lengths underneath in order to achieve a fuller-looking effect. When coarse hair is texturized too close to the scalp, the shorter lengths will "poke through" the surface hair, creating an uneven, spiked effect.**

As a general rule, **coarse hair should be texturized at least 1.5" (3.75 cm) away from the scalp. Medium hair should be texturized 1" (2.5 cm) away from the scalp, and fine hair can be texturized as close as 1/2" (1.25 cm) from the scalp. Keep in mind, however, that a very light stroke must be used to avoid a chunky texturized effect.**

Very curly hair requires some special considerations. Although it is generally recommended to texturize the hair while it is damp, very curly hair should be texturized while it is dry to allow for more control and the shrinkage factor. An emollient-based product may be applied to the scalp hair prior to texturizing for further ease while cutting.

As a professional stylist, you will need to determine which types of texturizing techniques and the amount of texturizing needed for each client according to hair type and desired results. Texturizing should be done where the most bulk exists. When in doubt, remember that it's always better to remove less hair than too much. **Never thin the very ends of the hair, or anywhere around the hairline.** Such thinning creates short, uneven hairs in areas that are difficult to control.

Outlining

Outlining the hair is a cutting technique used to define the perimeter hairline. A shear, razor or clipper can be used for this technique. Personalizing the nape is a very crucial step in completing a hair cut. Be sure to analyze and follow the natural growth pattern when outlining the nape hairline.

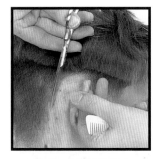

The tips of a shear may be used to outline the entire hairline, including the sideburns, ears and nape. Generally the tips of the shear are used first to create the outline. Then a clipper or razor is used to cut the hair beyond the outlined area. Remember that some local laws prohibit the use of a razor on the skin. Check with your regulating agency's rules.

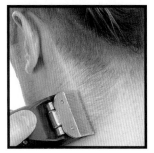

A clipper may also be used for outlining. The clipper blade is placed against the skin and the hair is cut section by section.

9

Special Grooming

Special grooming for men includes trimming eyebrows, ears and nose hair. Beards, goatees and mustaches are also part of the grooming and outlining process. Once the design is decided upon, any tool can be used to achieve the desired effect. Generally, overcomb techniques are used to groom the eyebrows and trim the beard or mustache.

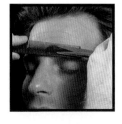

The shear-over-comb technique (controlling the hair with a comb, then cutting the lengths protruding from the comb) is generally used to cut eyebrow hair that has grown too long.

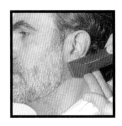

A trimmer can be used to maintain the shape of a beard or mustache.

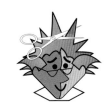

"In ancient times, pulling one's beard or shaving it without permission was punishable by law!"

Other Fundamental Considerations

When performing any of the techniques described in this chapter, it is important to consider the client's natural growth patterns to determine which haircut will work best as well as to personalize that cut through fringe and/or nape variations.

Fringe and Nape Variations

The fringe is the hair that partially or completely covers the forehead in a hairstyle. The nape is the hair that covers the area at the back of the neck. It is important to adapt the fringe to the shape and features of your client's face and to the haircut, as well as to consider the length and width of your client's neck when determining the right nape design. While your design options are virtually limitless, here are a few examples:

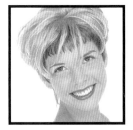

A solid fringe can frame the eyes.

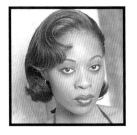

A longer fringe can be swept to the side to expose the forehead.

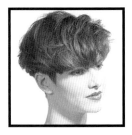
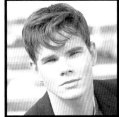

A layered fringe area adds texture, fullness and height.

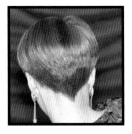
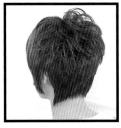

Nape variations can be customized according to your client's growth patterns and desired results. Refer to the "Design Decisions" chapter for further guidelines.

276

Growth Patterns

In addition to considering the hair's texture, it is important to determine other critical design elements before you begin cutting. For instance, the hair in each area of the scalp is likely to grow differently. You will need to adapt your cutting techniques to accommodate each of these areas.

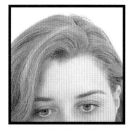

WIDOW'S PEAK

Prominent hair growth pattern that forms from a point at the front hairline and curves to one side. Leave fringe area longer to avoid spiking (sticking straight up) effect.

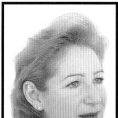

COWLICK

Usually found in straight or wavy hair at the front hairline or crown; represented by strong growth pattern that moves to the right or left. Cut the hair following the same direction it naturally grows and falls; allow additional length in this area to avoid spiking.

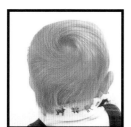

WHORL

Strong circular directional growth on either side of the nape or crown. Allow additional length so the hair will remain flat, or cut the hair very close to the scalp to avoid spiking.

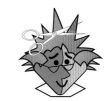

"A whorl is defined as anything that circles or turns on or around something else. A person can be identified by the whorls of his/her fingerprints!"

9

Infection Control and Safety

The following is a list of safety precautions you must follow prior to and during a haircutting service.

- Practice infection control guidelines.

- Wash and sanitize hands.

- Protect the client and his/her clothing with proper draping procedures. Refer to the "Draping" portion of the "Trichology" chapter.

- Check the scalp for any diseases or disorders. If any are evident, refer the client to a physician and do not proceed with the service.

- Disinfect and sanitize all implements after each use.

- Discard disposable razor blades after each individual use and place in a puncture-proof container.

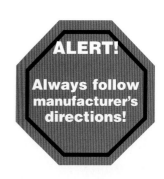

ALERT!

Always follow manufacturer's directions!

Client Consultation

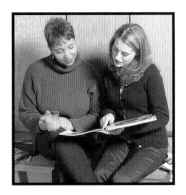

As with all hair services, consulting with your client prior to the actual service will ensure predictable results and will help you avoid any misunderstandings that may arise. To ensure client comfort, you should perform your consultation in a private area. Use photos and magazines while communicating with your client to clarify your design intentions.

To help you remember the important steps in the consultation process, remember: Great Artists Always Draw Creatively, and use the first letter of each word for each of the five steps: G for Greet, A for Ask, Analyze and Assess, A for Agree, D for Deliver and C for Complete.

Greet

- Meet and greet the client with a firm handshake and a pleasant voice.
- Communicate with the client to build rapport and develop a relationship with him/her.

Ask, Analyze and Assess

- Ask questions to discover client needs. For example, ask questions such as "Why would you like your haircut today?" Some responses may include, "I'd like a more trendy look," or "I'd like it shorter since I don't have time to take care of it." You might also want to ask "What haven't you liked about your previous haircuts?" This will, hopefully, bring out any areas of concern that the client might have.

- Ask questions about his/her lifestyle, such as "Do you have a lot of time to spend on your hair?" Remember, if he/she is leading a hectic lifestyle, you probably won't want to perform a haircut that will require a high degree of maintenance.

- Ask key questions, such as "Would you like layers in your hair?" or "Would you like your ears or neck exposed?"

- Analyze your client's face and body shape, physical features, hair and scalp. Refer to "Body and Face Shapes" in the "Design Decision" chapter for further guidelines.

- Assess the facts and thoroughly think through your recommendations.

Agree

- Explain your recommended solutions and the price for today's service(s) as well as for future services.
- Gain feedback and approval on your recommendations from the client.
- Return to "Ask, Analyze and Assess" if your client is hesitant with your recommendations.

Deliver

- Ensure client protection by draping the client with a towel and plastic cape during the shampoo process. Replace the towel with a neck strip during the actual haircut.
- Ensure client comfort during the service.

- Stay focused on delivering the service to the best of your ability.
- Teach the client how to perform at-home hair care maintenance.

Complete

- Request satisfaction feedback from your client.
- Escort client to the retail area and show at least two products you used.
- Recommend products to maintain appearance and condition of your client's hair.
- Invite your client to make a purchase.
- Suggest a future appointment time for your client's next visit.
- Offer appreciation to your client for visiting the school or salon.
- Record recommended products on the client record card for future visits.
- Complete client record card.

Children as Clients

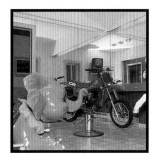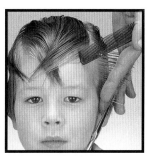

Do you remember your first haircut? Perhaps your parents have reminded you of this first experience. Although many children pose no challenge when performing a haircut, some children need to be treated more carefully to help alleviate their fears and concerns. You can help offer reassurance to a timid child by taking a few simple steps prior to and during a professional hair service.

- In the reception area, kneel down and make eye contact with the child or sit down next to the child.
- Introduce yourself and, if the child is very young, explain what is about to take place. Use fun language when explaining the process. For example, talk about the "ride" in the chair when you pump it up and that you have a cape that he or she can wear, just like the super heroes wear!
- If the parent and child allow you, take a young child by the hand as you lead him/her to your station.
- While performing the service, maintain continual eye and voice contact. Keep the child informed of everything you are doing. Also use firm contact with the head and hair to instill confidence.
- Keep in mind that many young children do not know the difference between left and right. You might try putting different color hair clips on their shoelaces and refer to them when you need the child to move his/her head in a certain direction.
- To keep a child from squirming, offer a reward, such as a balloon, if he/she cooperates. You may also indicate that squirming may cause you to cut yourself. Do not, however, tell a child that you might cut him/her.
- If an older child or teenager comes into the salon without a parent and requests a style, it is recommended to call the parent first and get permission.

9

HAIRCUTTING PROCEDURES

Once you understand the *theory* behind cutting hair, you are ready to use your knowledge and *apply* it to the medium of hair. Fortunately your mannequins won't complain, so practice, practice, practice. Someday soon you will be creating beautiful haircuts on your clients.

Haircutting Procedures Overview

The following forms will be demonstrated in each procedure following this section of the "Haircutting" chapter. By understanding these forms, you will be able to create an endless array of haircuts for your clients. Keep in mind that techniques and forms can be combined within a haircut for a variety of results.

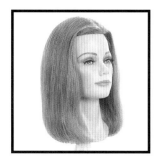 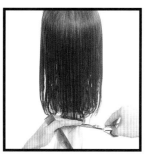

Solid Form
NATURAL FALL
0° PROJECTION

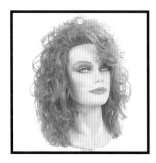 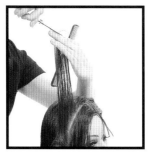

Increase-Layered Form
DIRECTIONAL DISTRIBUTION
NONPARALLEL FINGER/SHEAR POSITION

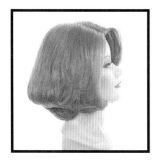 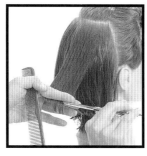

Graduated Form
PERPENDICULAR DISTRIBUTION
MEDIUM PROJECTION

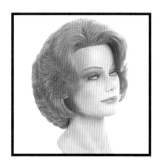 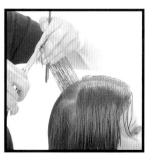

Uniformly Layered Form

PERPENDICULAR DISTRIBUTION

90° PROJECTION

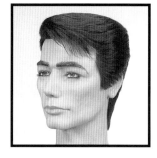 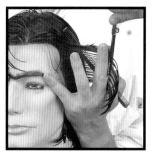

Square Form

DIRECTIONAL DISTRIBUTION

PARALLEL FINGER/SHEAR POSITION

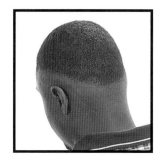 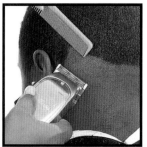

Fade

CLIPPER-OVER-COMB

9

Solid Form Haircut

Solid form haircuts have a totally smooth cut texture, which is achieved by cutting the hair in natural fall with 0° projection. Generally, any parting pattern, except vertical can be used to cut the solid form, while the finger/shear position and design line parallel the parting pattern.

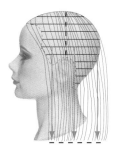 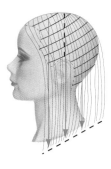 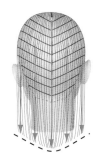

This solid form haircut will be cut horizontally. The structure graphic shows the length arrangement of the solid form, which consists of shorter exterior lengths progressing to longer interior lengths. Natural distribution, horizontal partings and a parallel finger/shear position are used throughout.

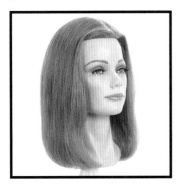 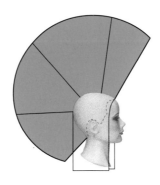 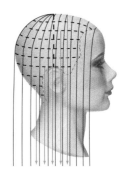

Solid Form Preparation

As with any professional service, it is important to have your area, products, implements and equipment in proper order. Before performing a solid form haircut service, be sure to satisfy the following points:

- Clean cutting station with disinfectant
- Arrange implements/supplies, including shears, razor with guards and disposable blades, cutting combs, sectioning clips and spray bottle
- Wash your hands with antibacterial soap
- Perform analysis of hair and scalp
- Ask the client to remove jewelry and store in a secure place
- Drape client for a wet service
- Shampoo and condition client's hair
- Replace client's towel with neck strip

Solid Form Procedure

- Subdivide hair into four sections
- Position head upright
- Create a horizontal parting at the nape, across both back sections
- Use natural distribution
- Position fingers/shear parallel to parting
- Cut a horizontal stationary design line
- Work upward using horizontal partings, natural distribution and no projection
- Distribute hair naturally at crown area
- Complete back
- Create a horizontal parting at side and extend to back

- Distribute hair in natural fall
- Position fingers/shear parallel to part
- Cut horizontal line
- Continue upward
- Complete side
- Release and cut first parting on opposite side
- Check for balance
- Work upward using horizontal partings, natural distribution and no projection
- Complete side
- Crosscheck

Solid Form Haircut

1-3. **Subdivide the hair into four basic sections**, from the center front hairline to the center nape, and from ear to ear.

4-5. **Position the client's head upright. Create a horizontal parting at the nape, across both back sections,** using the wide teeth of the comb. **Use natural distribution** and **position your fingers and shear parallel to the horizontal parting. Cut a horizontal stationary design line** using minimal tension. The size of the parting is determined by the density of the hair.

6-7. Work upward using horizontal partings, natural distribution and no projection.

8-9. Distribute the hair naturally at the crown area and **complete the back. Make sure the back is balanced before you proceed to the sides.**

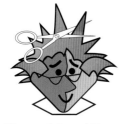

"To avoid Carpal Tunnel Syndrome, caused by repetitive movement of the wrist and fingers, take some preventative measures as outlined in the 'Ergonomic' section of the 'Professional Development' chapter."

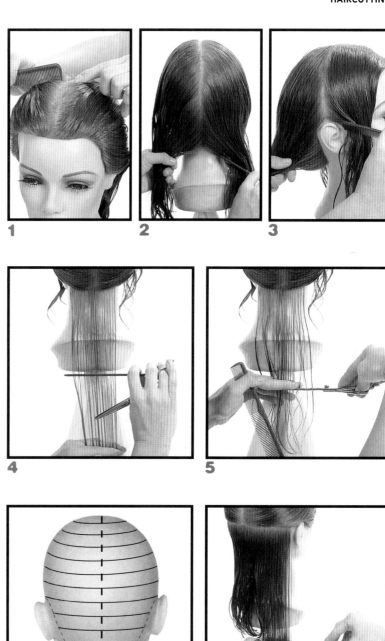

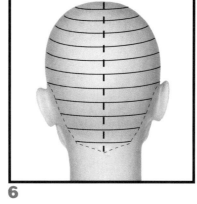

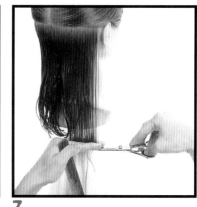

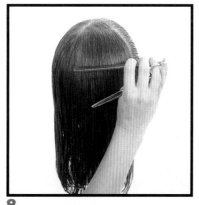

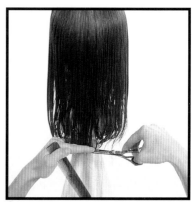

9

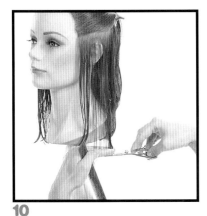

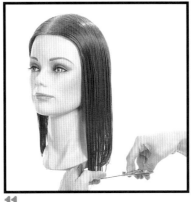

10

11

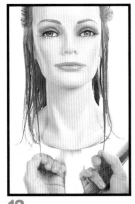

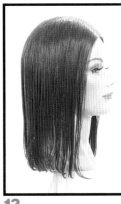

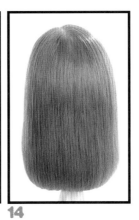

12

13

14

10-11. Create a horizontal parting at the side that extends to the back. This will ensure blending and a continuous horizontal line. **Distribute the hair in natural fall. Position your fingers and shear parallel to the part** and **cut a horizontal line. Continue upward** using natural distribution and no projection. Cut parallel to the horizontal parting. **Complete side.**

12-14. Release and cut the first parting on the opposite side. Check for balance with the opposite side. **Work upward using horizontal partings, natural distribution and no projection. Complete side. Crosscheck.** Sweep up hair after completing the haircut. Refer to the "Hair Styling" chapter for finishing techniques on this form.

Solid Form Completion

- Offer a rebook visit to your client
- Recommend retail products to your client
- Discard non-reusable material, disinfect implements and arrange work station in proper order
- Wash your hands with antibacterial soap

Solid Form Variation: Increase-Layered Front Hairline

Conversion layering, which is shown on this variation, is a common cutting technique used to create increase-layered forms. With this technique each parting is converged to a stationary design line opposite the area of the desired length increase. The farther the hair travels to reach the stationary design line, the longer the result. Perpendicular distribution from vertical and pivotal partings and either a parallel or nonparallel finger position may be used to cut increase layers around the fringe. Generally, standing opposite the desired length increase and directing the lengths toward you will help maintain a constant projection angle of the stationary design line.

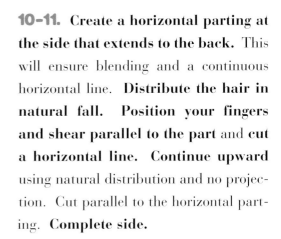

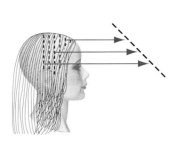

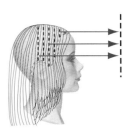

284

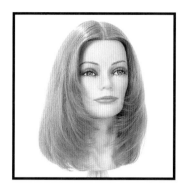

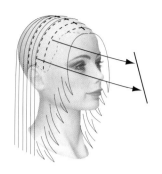

In this procedure. a few softened layers are achieved along the front hairline of the solid form haircut by using a stationary design line and the conversion layering technique. A nonparallel finger position is used along vertical partings.

Solid Form Variation:
Increase-Layered Front Hairline

1-2. Subdivide the hair from the center front hairline to the crown. Position the head in an upright position. Take a small 1/4 inch (.75 cm) section at the center front hairline. Establish a length guide. Release the perimeter hairline. Distribute the hair forward and use a nonparallel finger position. Position the razor parallel to the outside of your fingers, with your knuckles facing the head. Use the etching technique as you cut downward from the top of the parting. Work to the bottom of the parting to establish the stationary design line.

3-4. Repeat the same procedure on the opposite side. Note that the nonparallel finger position will create an exaggerated length increase while maintaining perimeter length.

5-6. Take vertical partings and distribute the hair forward using the conversion layering technique. Use a nonparallel finger position and the etching technique. Work toward the back until the lengths no longer reach. Then repeat on the opposite side. Sweep up hair after completing the haircut. Refer to the "Hair Styling" chapter for finishing techniques on this variation.

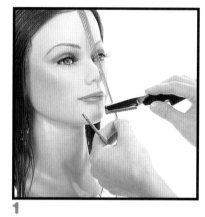

1

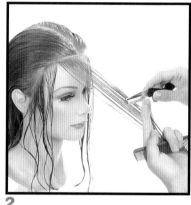

2

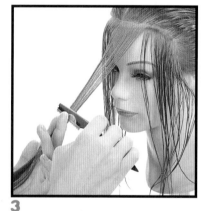

3

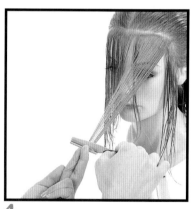

4

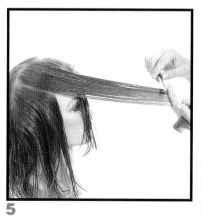

5

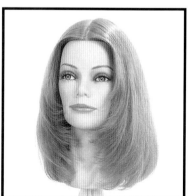

6

9

Increase-Layered Form Haircut

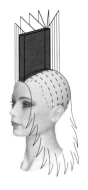
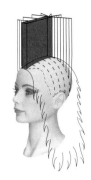

As you've already learned, increase-layered forms have an activated cut texture that can be achieved using a stationary design line and the conversion layering technique. However, another way to achieve an increase-layered form is with directional distribution and a mobile design line. With directional distribution the hair is distributed straight up or out from the various curves of the head. Directional distribution automatically results in a length increase due to the curves of the head. A parallel or nonparallel finger position may be used from any parting.

This increase-layered form has been finished with a scrunching technique to further accentuate the activated cut texture. You will learn more about this finishing technique in the "Hair Styling" chapter. The structure graphic shows shorter interior lengths progressing to longer exterior lengths. A nonparallel finger/shear position is used from vertical and pivotal partings to create a length increase while preserving perimeter lengths.

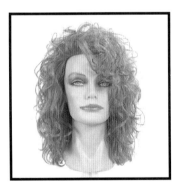
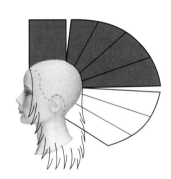
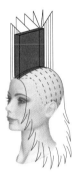

Increase-Layered Form Preparation

As with any professional service, it is important to have your area, products, implements and equipment in proper order. Before performing an increase-layered form haircut service, be sure to satisfy the following points:

- Clean cutting station with disinfectant
- Arrange implement/supplies including shears, cutting combs and spray bottle
- Wash your hands with antibacterial soap
- Perform analysis of hair and scalp
- Ask the client to remove jewelry and store in a secure place
- Drape the client for a wet service
- Shampoo and condition the hair
- Replace client's towel with a neck strip

Increase-Layered Form Procedure

- Subdivide hair from hairline to nape
- Position head upright
- Create small center section
- Establish length guide
- Distribute hair straight up from center section
- Position fingers and shear parallel to floor
- Cut hair from front to crown
- Take parting at front hairline, from center top to outside corner of eye
- Distribute hair straight up

- Use nonparallel finger position
- Cut hair using center parting as length guide
- Use portion of previous parting as mobile design line
- Work toward center back using vertical and pivotal partings, directional distribution and nonparallel finger position
- Repeat same cutting procedures on opposite side
- Crosscheck

Increase-Layered Form Haircut

1-3. **Subdivide the hair from the center front hairline to the nape. Position the head in an upright position. Create a small center section,** approximately 1/4" (.75 cm) wide, from the front hairline to the crown. **Establish a length guide** by using a portion of hair from the front hairline. Then **distribute the hair straight up from the center section. Position your fingers and shear parallel to floor** and **cut the hair from the front to the crown.**

4-5. **Take a parting at the front hairline, from the center top to the outside corner of the eye. Distribute the hair straight up** using directional distribution. **Use a nonparallel finger position** and **cut the hair using the center parting as a length guide.**

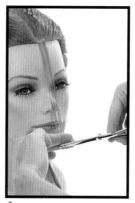

1

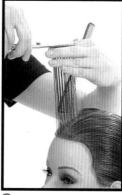

2

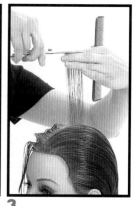

3

9

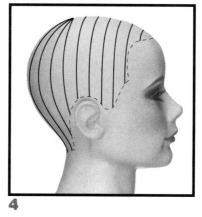

4

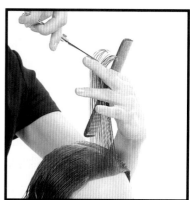

5

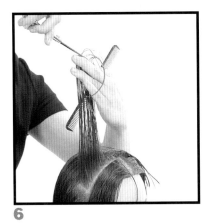

6

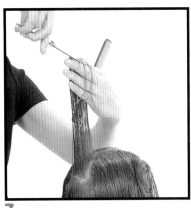

7

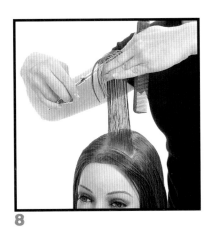

8

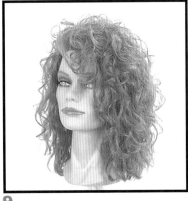

9

6-7. Use a portion of the previous parting as a mobile design line. Work toward the center back using vertical and pivotal partings, directional distribution and a nonparallel finger position. (Note that the perimeter lengths may not reach due to the previous cut on mannequin.)

8-9. Repeat the same cutting procedures on the opposite side. Note that on one side your fingers angle toward the center guide while on the opposite side they angle away from the center guide. **Crosscheck.** Sweep up hair after completing the haircut. Refer to the "Hair Styling" chapter for finishing techniques on this form.

Increase-Layered Form Completion

- Offer rebook visit to your client
- Recommend retail products to your client
- Discard non-reusable materials, disinfect implements and arrange work station in proper order
- Wash your hands with antibacterial soap

Graduated Form Haircut

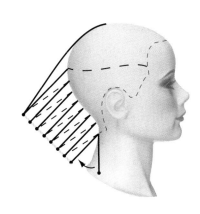

Graduated form haircuts have a combination of activated and unactivated cut texture achieved by projecting (lifting) the hair and using mobile and stationary design lines. The line that visually separates the two textures is known as the ridge line. Although any parting pattern, distribution and finger/shear position may be used to achieve this form, keep the following guidelines in mind:

- Use perpendicular distribution and projection from horizontal partings
- Use perpendicular distribution from diagonal partings with or without projection
- Use a nonparallel finger position when working from vertical partings in the nape

Generally, graduated forms are cut from the perimeter upward. The first section that is projected will determine the progression of lengths, which establishes the line of inclination. The line of inclination refers to the line created between the initial design line and the next projected section. An extension of the imaginary line guides you in the development of the form, as all subsequent sections travel to this line.

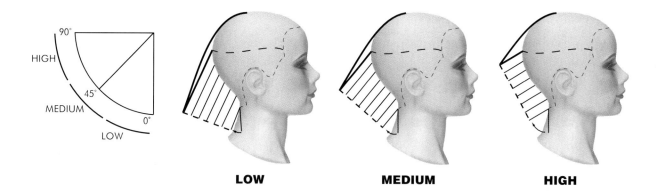

LOW   **MEDIUM**   **HIGH**

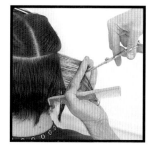

The three lines of inclination are low, medium and high. Keep in mind that the higher the projection angle, the steeper the line of inclination.

When using a vertical parting pattern to cut graduated forms, the angle of your fingers determines the line of inclination.

This procedure features a medium graduated form haircut. The structure graphic shows shorter exterior lengths progressing to longer interior lengths. A mobile design line and a medium projection angle are used in the exterior to create a medium line of inclination. A stationary design line is used in the interior. Natural expansion and a weight corner occur where the two textures meet. Horizontal partings are used in the back and slight diagonal forward partings are used at the front and sides.

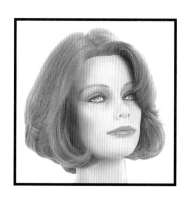

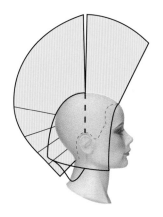

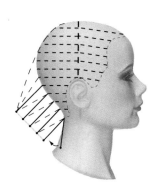

Graduated Form Preparation

As with any professional service, it is important to have your area, products, implements and equipment in proper order. Before performing a graduated form haircut service, be sure to satisfy the following points:

- Clean cutting station with disinfectant
- Arrange implements/supplies including shears, cutting combs, sectioning clips and spray bottle
- Wash your hands with antibacterial soap
- Perform analysis of hair and scalp
- Ask the client to remove jewelry and store in secure place
- Drape your client for a wet service
- Shampoo and condition the hair
- Replace towel with neck strip

Graduated Form Procedure

- Section hair into four sections
- Position head upright
- Take horizontal parting at nape
- Use perpendicular distribution and one-finger projection
- Position fingers/shear parallel to part
- Cut from center to one side, then other establish mobile design line
- Continue to cut upward, using horizontal partings and a mobile design line
- Use perpendicular distribution and a medium projection angle
- Use last projected section at crest area as stationary design line for remaining back lengths
- Take slight diagonal forward partings at sides
- Use perpendicular distribution and same projection as back
- Cut parallel to parting
- Continue to center top
- Complete side
- Cut first parting on opposite side
- Check the balance
- Complete this side using same procedures
- Crosscheck

Graduated Form Haircut

1-2. Section the hair into four basic sections. Position the head upright. Take a horizontal parting at the nape across both sections. Use perpendicular distribution and one-finger projection (lifting the hair as high as the width of your finger). Position your fingers/shear parallel to the part. Cut from the center to one side, then the other to establish the mobile design line. Note that a palm-to-palm hand position is used to cut this form.

3-4. Continue to cut upward using horizontal partings and a mobile design line. Use perpendicular distribution and a medium projection angle from each parting. Position your fingers parallel to the parting and cut from the center to one side, then the other. Note that a medium line of inclination is now established.

5-6. Use the last projected section at the crest area as a stationary design line for the remaining back lengths. Note that this will create a weight area. At the crown area, be sure to distribute the hair as it naturally grows.

7-8. Take slight diagonal forward partings at the sides. Extend the partings to the back to ensure blending. Use perpendicular distribution and the same projection angle as the back. Cut parallel to the parting.

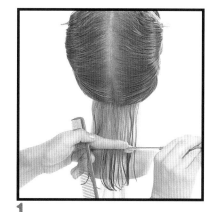

1

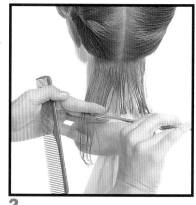

2

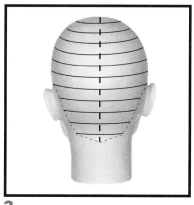

3

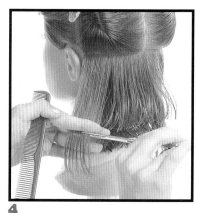

4

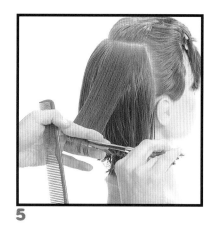

5

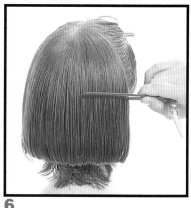

6

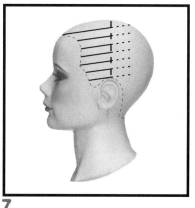

7

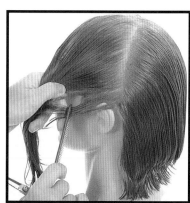

8

9

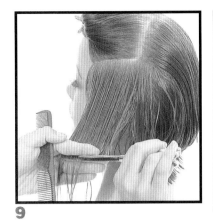
9

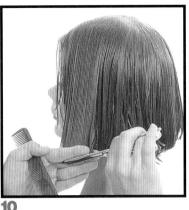
10

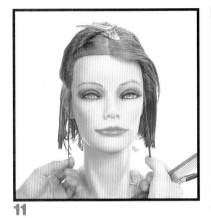
11

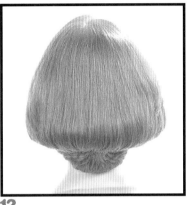
12

9-10. Continue to the center top using the same procedures to **complete this side.**

11-12. Cut the first parting on the **opposite side** and **check the balance.** Then **complete this side using the same cutting procedures. Cross-check.** Sweep up hair after completing the haircut. Refer to the "Hair Styling" chapter for finishing techniques on this form.

Graduated Form Completion

- Offer a rebook visit to your client
- Recommend retail products to your client
- Discard non-reusable materials, disinfect implements and arrange work station in proper order
- Wash your hands with antibacterial soap

Uniformly Layered Form Haircut

The uniformly layered form has a totally activated texture. A consistent 90° projection angle and a parallel finger/shear position are used along the curves of the head to achieve this form. Perpendicular distribution from any parting pattern and a mobile design line are used to cut the uniformly layered form.

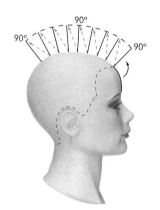
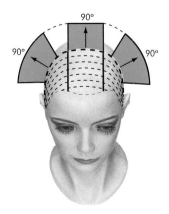
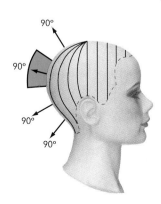

The structure graphic for this uniformly layered procedure shows equal lengths throughout. The head is subdivided into five sections. Horizontal, vertical and pivotal partings are used.

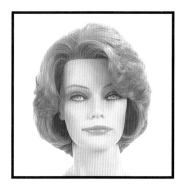 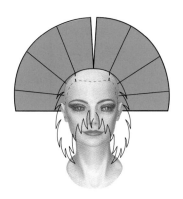 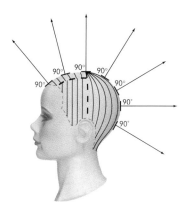

Uniformly Layered Form Preparation

As with any professional service, it is important to have your area, products, implements and equipment in proper order. Before performing a uniformly layered form haircut service, be sure to satisfy the following points:

- Clean cutting station with disinfectant
- Arrange implements/supplies including shears, cutting combs, sectioning clips and spray bottle
- Wash your hands with antibacterial soap
- Perform analysis of hair and scalp
- Ask the client to remove jewelry and store in secure place
- Drape your client for a wet service
- Shampoo and condition the hair
- Replace towel with neck strip

Uniformly Layered Form Procedure

- Subdivide hair into five sections
- Position head upright
- Establish length guide at center front hairline
- Begin with center top section
- Take horizontal parting at the front hairline
- Use perpendicular distribution, 90° projection
- Position fingers parallel to head
- Cut parallel to fingers to establish mobile design line
- Take next parting, use perpendicular distribution, 90° projection
- Cut parallel to head

- Work toward back of top section
- Complete top section
- Cut side using top section as length guide
- Use vertical partings, perpendicular distribution and 90° projection
- Position fingers parallel to head, cut parallel to fingers
- Use top and side section as length guide to cut back
- Use pivotal partings, perpendicular distribution and 90° projection
- Complete other side and back section using same cutting procedures
- Crosscheck

9

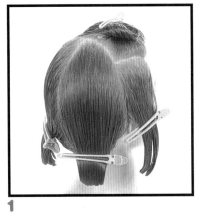

1

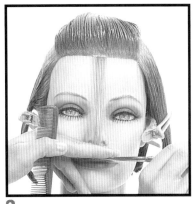

2

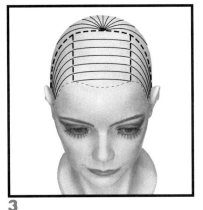

3

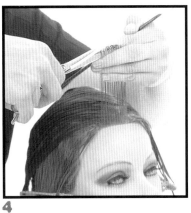

4

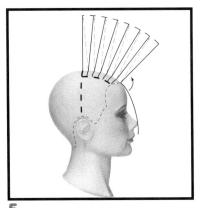

5

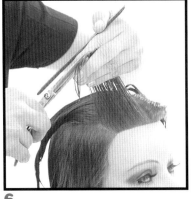

6

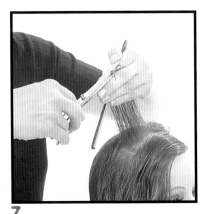

7

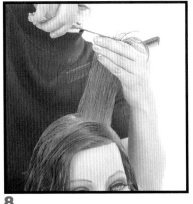

8

Uniformly Layered Form Hairut

1-2. Subdivide the hair into five sections. Subdivide the front from the back. Then section the back in half. Subdivide the top and sides. **Position the head upright. Establish a length guide at the center front hairline.**

3-4. Begin with the center top section. Take a horizontal parting at the front hairline. Use perpendicular distribution and a 90° projection angle from the curve of the head. **Position your fingers parallel to the head** and **cut parallel to your fingers.** Cut from the center to either side to **establish the mobile design line.**

5-6. Take the next parting and use a portion of the previously cut section as a length guide. Continue to **use perpendicular distribution and 90° projection. Cut parallel to the head.**

7-8. As you **work toward the back of the top section**, be sure to maintain a 90° projection angle from the various curves of the head. **Complete the top section.**

9-12. Cut the side using the top section as a length guide. Use vertical partings, perpendicular distribution and 90° projection. Position your fingers parallel to the head and cut parallel to your fingers. Be sure to maintain a 90° projection angle as you cut along the various curves of the head. Complete this side.

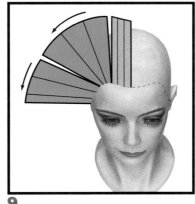

9

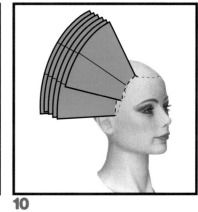

10

13-14. Use the top and side sections as a length guide to cut the back. Use pivotal partings, perpendicular distribution and 90° projection as you cut parallel to your fingers. Work from the top to the bottom of each parting as you work toward the center back. **Complete the other side and back using the same cutting procedures.**

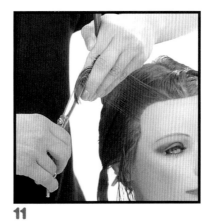

11

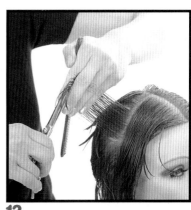

12

15-16. Note that an alternate hand position may be used at the nape as you blend the lengths to the previous haircut. **Crosscheck.** Sweep up hair after completing the haircut. Refer to the "Hair Styling" chapter for finishing techniques on this form.

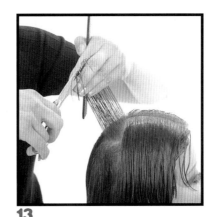

13

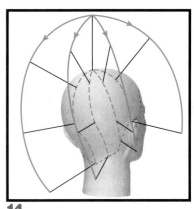

14

Uniformly Layered Form Completion

- Offer a rebook visit to your client

- Recommend retail products to your client

- Discard non-reusable materials, disinfect implements and arrange work station in proper order

- Wash your hands with antibacterial soap

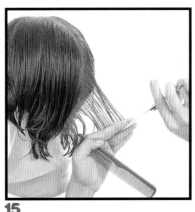

15

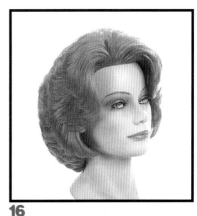

16

Combination Form Haircut

Combination forms consist of two or more forms. Some examples include increase layers over graduated lengths or uniform layers over graduated lengths. When cutting combination forms, follow the same cutting techniques used for each particular form.

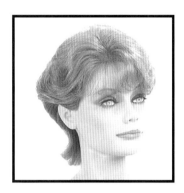 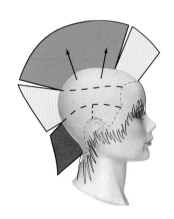 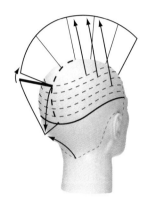

This procedure features a combination of uniform, graduated and increase-layered forms, as can be seen in the structure graphic. Three sections are used. A combination of curved lines (concave and convex) is created below the crest area and the remaining hair is subdivided in half. The nape lengths are converged to the curved line and cut parallel to it. The lengths above the curve are graduated to create a weight area along the curved line. To reduce some of the weight along the weight area and to achieve softened layers, the interior is cut using the conversion layering technique. Finally, the form is personalized using texturizing techniques.

Combination Form Preparation

As with any professional service, it is important to have your area, products, implements and equipment in proper order. Before performing a combination form haircut service, be sure to satisfy the following points:

- Clean cutting station with disinfectant
- Arrange implements/supplies including shears, taper shears, razor with guard and disposable blades, cutting combs, sectioning clips and spray bottle
- Wash your hands with antibacterial soap
- Perform analysis of hair and scalp
- Ask the client to remove jewelry and store in secure place
- Drape your client for a wet service
- Shampoo and condition the hair
- Replace towel with neck strip

Combination Form Procedure

- Subdivide top in half
- Part out curved section around head
- Balance curve on both sides
- Begin center back
- Direct all lengths from perimeter hairline upward to curved line
- Use perpendicular distribution and medium projection
- Cut parallel to parting
- Work from center to behind each ear
- Use diagonal forward partings at sides, below curved line
- Distribute hair to shortest lengths behind the ear
- Cut parallel to diagonal partings
- Use first parting as stationary design line
- Repeat techniques on opposite side
- Take curved partings above curved line
- Use shortest lengths and same projection angle from previous section as length guide

- Use perpendicular distribution and cut parallel to parting
- Use first parting as stationary design line for subsequent partings
- Work to top of each section
- Release thin center section from front hairline to weight area
- Use weight line from back section as length guide
- Project hair at 90°
- Cut parallel to parting
- Take partings parallel to center guide
- Use conversion layering technique
- Crosscheck
- Personalize fringe and perimeter hairline using razor etching technique
- Use taper shear to create end mobility in interior
- Use razor rotation in nape
- Crosscheck

Combination Form Haircut

1-2. Subdivide the top in half. Part out a curved line around the head, below the crest area. Balance the curve on both sides. Note that the resulting curved lines are concave and convex.

3-4. Begin at the center back. Direct all the lengths from the perimeter hairline upward to the curved line. Use perpendicular distribution and a medium projection angle from the curved parting and **cut parallel to the parting. Work from the center to behind each ear** using the same procedure. Be sure to cut parallel to the curved parting. Note that an increase of lengths occurs toward the hairline.

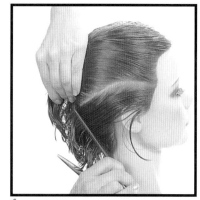
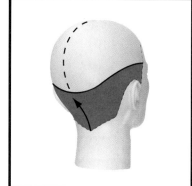
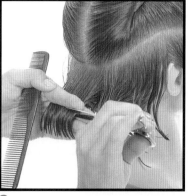
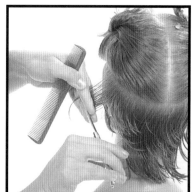

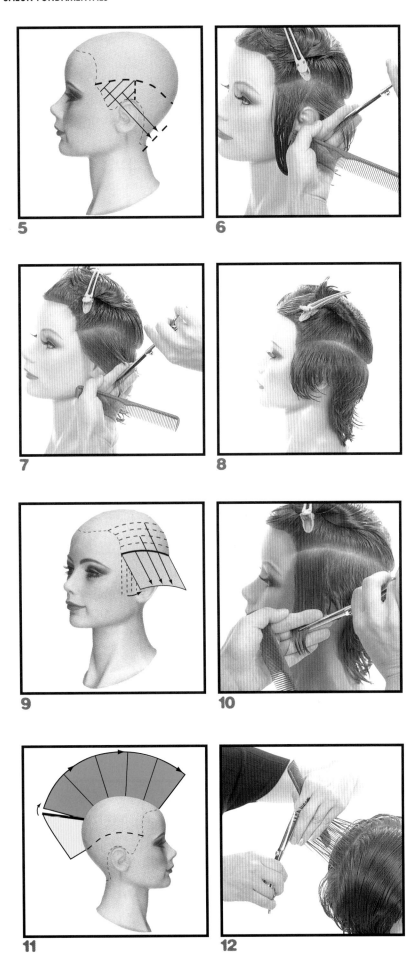

5 **6** **7** **8** **9** **10** **11** **12**

5-8. Use diagonal forward partings at the sides, below the curved line. Distribute the hair to the shortest lengths behind the ear and cut parallel to the diagonal partings. Use the first parting as a stationary design line for the subsequent partings. Repeat technique on the opposite side. Note the increase of lengths from the shortest over the ear to longer toward the face. Also note the resulting curved line and how the nape lengths conform to the curve of the head.

9-10. Take curved partings above the curved line. Use the shortest lengths and the same projection angle from the previously cut sections as a length guide. Use perpendicular distribution and cut parallel to the parting to create graduated lengths. Use the first parting as a stationary design line for subsequent partings. Work up to the top of each section.

11-12. Release a thin center section from the front hairline to the weight area. Use the weight line from the back section as a length guide. Project the hair in this center section at 90° and cut parallel to the parting to create uniformly layered lengths.

13-14. Then **take partings parallel to the center guide**. Use the center guide as a stationary design line. Distribute the partings to the stationary design line and **use the conversion layering technique** to create increase-layered lengths. **Crosscheck.**

15-16. **Personalize the fringe and perimeter hairline using the razor etching technique** to create softer end texture and a wispy effect. **Use the taper shear to create end mobility in the interior.** Position the taper shear about 1" (2.5 cm) from the ends to reduce weight.

17-18. Use the **razor rotation technique in the nape** to remove bulk and create closeness. Work from one side to the other and repeat in the opposite direction. **Crosscheck.** Sweep up hair after completing the haircut. Refer to the "Hair Styling" chapter for finishing techniques on this form.

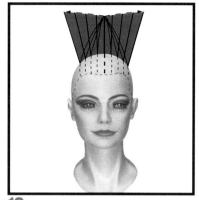

13

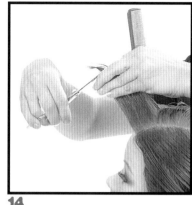

14

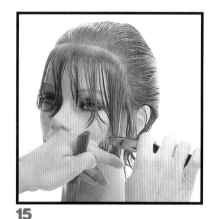

15

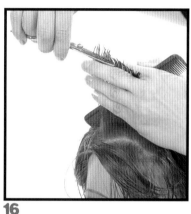

16

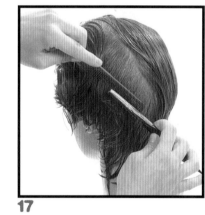

17

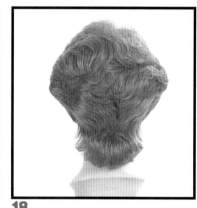

18

9

Combination Form Completion

- Offer a rebook visit to your client
- Recommend retail products to your client
- Discard non-reusable materials, disinfect implements and arrange work station in proper order
- Wash your hands with antibacterial soap

Curly Hair Considerations

The cutting techniques that you have just learned can be applied to straight or curly hair. However, prior to cutting curly hair, consider how the hair will be worn naturally. Also consider that curly hair looks longer when wet, so you will need to take into consideration the shrinkage factor as it dries.

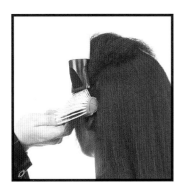 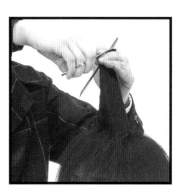 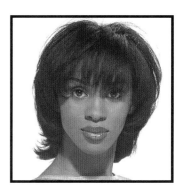

If the hair will be worn straight, you may wish to shampoo, air form (blow dry) and/or thermal press the hair straight first prior to cutting. (Refer to the "Hair Styling" chapter for more information.) By straightening the hair first, you will see how long the hair actually is and be able to cut the hair accordingly.

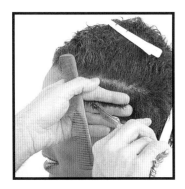 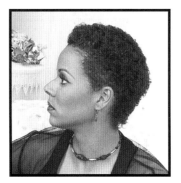

If the hair will be worn naturally curly, you may first wish to shampoo and towel dry the hair thoroughly. Towel drying the hair thoroughly will allow you to observe the natural curl formation and response of the hair while cutting. Cutting the hair damp instead of wet reduces the amount of stretching. Cutting hair that is partly wet and partly dry will create an uneven effect.

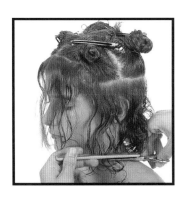 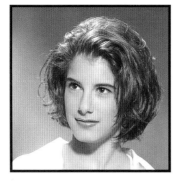

Consider the shrinkage factor while cutting curly hair. Stretching or applying tension to curly hair while cutting may result in shorter lengths than anticipated. In some cases, you may wish to use a comb (instead of your fingers) to control curly hair while cutting. The comb allows for minimal tension on the hair, which will allow you to view how the hair will fall naturally.

Square Form Haircut

Square forms consist of a combination of forms and have an activated surface texture. Square forms can be achieved with directional distribution. As you've already learned, with directional distribution the hair is distributed straight up or straight out from the curve of the head, resulting in a combination of forms. Although any parting pattern may be used, generally horizontal partings are used at the top while vertical partings are used at the sides and back. A mobile design line is used to cut the square form.

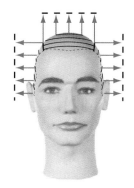
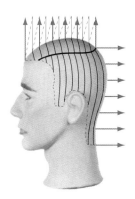

For this procedure, a men's medium square form is achieved with directional distribution as is shown on the structure graphic. A horizontal parting pattern is used in the three top sections and a vertical parting pattern is used in the three remaining sections.

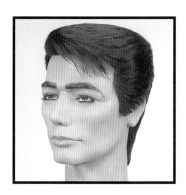
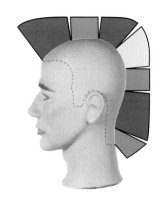
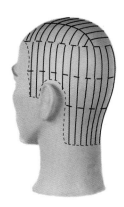

Square Form Preparation

As with any professional service, it is important to have your area, products, implements and equipment in proper order. Before performing a square form haircut service, be sure to satisfy the following points:

- Clean cutting station with disinfectant
- Arrange implements/supplies including shears, taper shears, razor with guard and disposable blades, cutting combs, sectioning clips and spray bottle
- Wash your hands with antibacterial soap
- Perform analysis of hair and scalp
- Ask the client to remove jewelry and store in secure place
- Drape your client for a wet service
- Shampoo and condition the hair
- Replace towel with neck strip

Square Form Procedure

- Begin with center top section
- Position head upright
- Take horizontal partings at front hairline
- Establish mobile length guide
- Take next parting
- Distribute hair straight up
- Position fingers horizontally
- Cut parallel to fingers
- Work from front to crown using directional distribution
- Repeat with next section
- Complete last top section
- Distribute hair straight out at sides and back
- Use vertical partings

- Position fingers and shear perpendicular to floor
- Cut parallel to fingers
- Work from front hairline to center back, using top and previously cut section as length guide
- Complete one side, then other
- Work from one side to other side in the next lower section and repeat techniques
- In the nape, repeat same techniques as you work from one side to other side
- Crosscheck
- Personalize perimeter hairline
- Texturize ends with taper shear

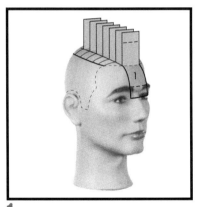

1

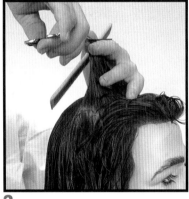

2

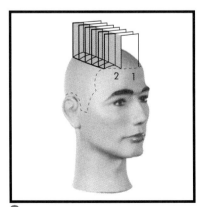

3

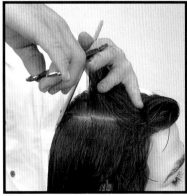

4

Square Form Haircut

1-4. Begin with a center top section. Position the head upright. Take a horizontal parting at the front hairline. Establish mobile length guide. Then take the next parting. Distribute the hair straight up and position your fingers horizontally. Cut parallel to your fingers. Work from the front to the crown using directional distribution. Repeat with the next section.

5-6. **Complete the last top section** using horizontal partings and directional distribution.

7-8. **Distribute the hair straight out at the sides and back from vertical partings. Position your fingers and shear vertically (perpendicular to the floor). Cut parallel to your fingers.** Work from the front hairline to the center back using a portion of the top section and the previously cut section as a length guide. Complete one side, then the other.

9-10. **Work from one side to the other side in the next lower section and repeat techniques.** Use directional distribution from vertical partings. Position your fingers vertically and cut parallel to your fingers. **In the nape, repeat the same techniques as you work from one side to the other side** to complete the cut. **Crosscheck.**

11-13. **Personalize the perimeter hairline** with a horizontal design line. Use diagonal partings behind the ear to blend the sides with the back.

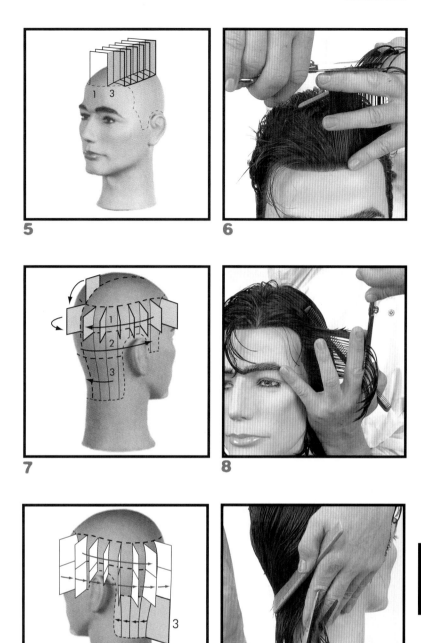

5

6

7

8

9

10

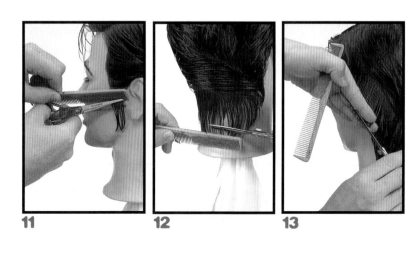

11

12

13

9

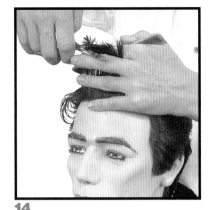

14

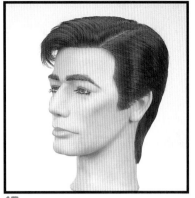

15

14-15. Then **texturize the ends** throughout with a taper shear to reduce bulk and increase mobility. Use the same parting pattern that was used to create the cut. Sweep up hair after completing the haircut.

Square Form Completion

- Offer a rebook visit to your client
- Recommend retail products to your client
- Discard non-reusable materials, disinfect implements and arrange work station in proper order
- Wash your hands with antibacterial soap

Overcomb Techniques

Generally overcomb techniques are used to cut very short exterior lengths, which often progress to longer lengths toward the crown. Overcomb techniques are performed with a comb and cutting tool, such as a shear, taper shear or clipper. The comb and tool are used simultaneously to cut the form. The comb controls the hair, while the tool cuts the hair that extends beyond the comb.

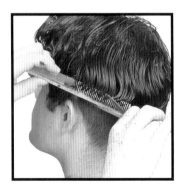

Shear-Over-Comb Technique

With the shear-over-comb technique (whether a straight shear or taper shear), both tools move upward in unison. The shear is positioned parallel to the comb. The comb controls the hair while the shear is opened and closed repeatedly. This technique is performed as many times as necessary to complete the form.

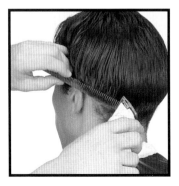

Clipper-Over-Comb Technique

With the clipper-over-comb technique, the hair is directed up and held in position with the comb. The clipper is positioned on top of the comb, which can be positioned horizontally, vertically or diagonally. The clipper-over-comb technique allows you to remove hair lengths very close to the scalp or to create square forms, such as the flat top.

Comb Control

Various comb sizes and shapes can be used to control the hair while cutting. A large comb is used to quickly remove lengths. A cutting comb is used to cut shorter lengths, while the taper comb is used to define design lines and to refine the perimeter. The angle at which the comb is held and the distance between the comb and the scalp determines the amount of hair to be cut. The higher the angle of the comb, the greater the amount of transparency or visibility of the scalp that will be achieved.

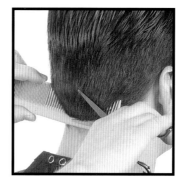
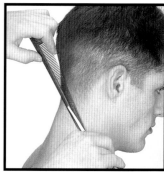

Fade Haircut

A fade incorporates gradation and consists of extremely short lengths in the exterior progressing to longer interior lengths. The bald fade is cut with the clipper positioned directly on the skin as well as with the clipper-over-comb techniques. The lever switch on the clipper is used to vary the distance of the clipper from the scalp. The fade can also be performed with clipper-over-comb or shear-over-comb techniques.

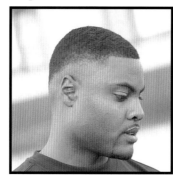
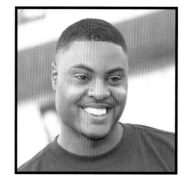

Fade Preparation

As with any professional service, it is important to have your area, products, implements and equipment in proper order. Before performing a fade clipper cut service, be sure to satisfy the following points:

* Clean cutting station with disinfectant.
* Arrange implements/supplies including clipper with guard attachments, shears and cutting combs
* Wash your hands with antibacterial soap
* Perform analysis of hair and scalp
* Ask the client to remove jewelry and store in a secure place.
* Drape your client for a dry haircut service.

Fade Procedure

- Begin at center back and work from hairline upward
- Use clipper, without a guard, against skin to cut very short lengths in level one
- Work from back to side
- Complete other side
- Balance line around head
- Attach small guard to clipper
- Cut level two

- Work from center to either side to complete second level
- Attach larger guard to clipper
- Cut level three
- Work up back and sides
- Work from front hairline to crown
- Remove guard
- Blend each level
- Texturize ends by cutting into hair with tips of shear
- Outline perimeter

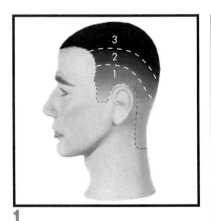

1

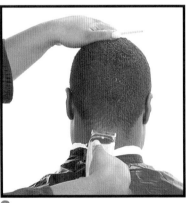

2

Fade Haircut

1-2. The fade is cut in three levels for a smooth transition from the shortest perimeter lengths to the longest interior lengths. **Begin at the center back and work from the hairline upward. Use the clipper, without a guard, against the skin to cut very short lengths in level one.**

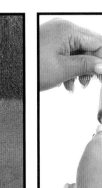

3

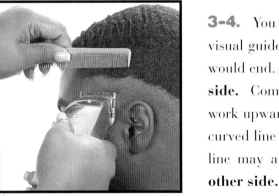

4

3-4. You may position the comb as a visual guide to determine where the fade would end. **Work from the back to the side.** Comb the hair downward as you work upward in each section. Although a curved line is established here, a straight line may also be used. **Complete the other side.**

5-6. Be sure to **balance the line around the head.** The first level is now complete. Note that although the shortest lengths in this haircut are at the temple area, generally the eyebrow is used as a guide for the shortest lengths. Let your client's facial features and personal desire be your guide.

7-8. **Attach small guard to the clipper. Cut level two.** Work upward approximately 1" (2.5 cm) from the shortest lengths and arc the clipper away from the scalp. Arcing away from the scalp will allow you to leave the lengths longer, which will blend into the longest lengths. **Work from the center to either side to complete the second level.**

9-10. **Attach a larger guard to the clipper.** Work upward from level 2. **Cut level three. Work up the back and sides. Then work from the front hairline to the crown.**

11-12. **Remove the guard.** Stretch the skin and cut the lengths very close to the scalp. Stretching the skin allows you to work around the various growth patterns. Work from the back to one side in level one then complete the other side.

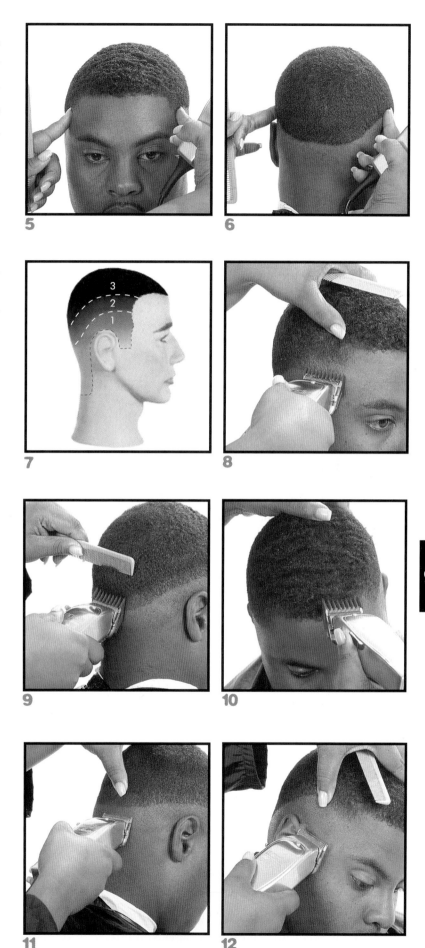

9

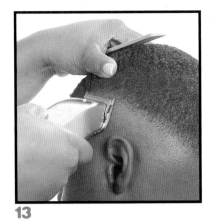
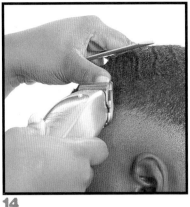

13

14

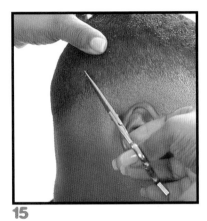
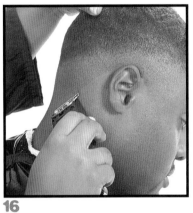

15

16

13-14. Arc the clipper away from the scalp as your further refine and **blend each level.**

15-16. To further blend the levels, **texturize the ends** by cutting into the hair with the tips of the shear positioned vertically or diagonally. Then use the clipper or trimmer to **outline the perimeter.** Use a neck brush to remove loose hair from the client's neck.

Fade Completion

- Offer a rebook visit to your client
- Recommend retail products to your client
- Discard non-reusable materials, disinfect implements, oil your clippers and arrange work station in proper order
- Wash hands with antibacterial soap

The theory and procedures you learned in this chapter will form the basis for advanced work in the ever-growing field of haircutting. Your future awaits as you practice to gain mastery.

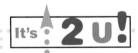

It's **2 U!**

Build Your Critical Thinking Skills

In this chapter you have prepared yourself to meet the following Industry Standards for entry-level cosmetologists:

- Consult with clients to determine their needs and preferences
- Provide a haircut in accordance with a client's needs or expectations

It's Up to You to know what to do. Using your training to this point, review the following case scenario and think through how you would handle each challenge.

A client comes in an tells you she wants a short haircut. Without a consultation, you tell the client no problem and immediately begin to cut her hair. The salon manager asks you to step to the back room for a moment. Once away from the client, the manager states you have not performed a thorough consultation. What have you missed and how would you now approach your client to get the information you need?

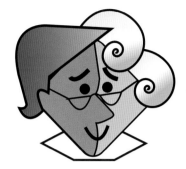

Chapter 10
HAIRSTYLING

After studying this chapter you will be able to . . .

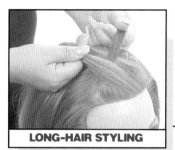

LONG-HAIR STYLING

1. **Recognize and identify the primary considerations and fundamentals of hairstyling theory.**

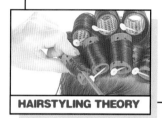

HAIRSTYLING THEORY

4. **Explain and demonstrate long-hair styling.**

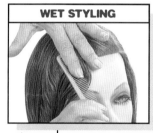

WET STYLING

3. **Explain and demonstrate wet styling.**

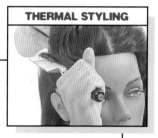

THERMAL STYLING

2. **Explain and demonstrate thermal styling.**

10

"Style! You've got style!" Don't most of us wish to be a bit more stylish than we are? Just what makes up personal style? We know at least that it is a distinctive and characteristic manner of thinking, speaking, moving, behaving and dressing that sets a person apart. In this chapter you get to explore the contribution that hairstyles make to a person's overall sense of style. Hairstyling allows the artist in you to mesh with a client's wishes, dreams and sense of style to create an overall, day-to-day image or an image for those precious, once-in-a-lifetime occasions. By the way, what hairstyle would you choose if you had the chance to meet me in person?

Hairstyling is the heart of your craft. The reward any artist feels at the moment of accomplishment can be yours when your fingers "finish" an exciting and successful design for a client.

True artists need outlets for expression almost as much as they need air. That is why this chapter has such personal VALUE for you as an artist. It teaches you the foundations of many creative ways to style hair. As you begin to master the procedures in this chapter, your own artistic sense will begin to suggest new possibilities for your future work with clients. As with any artist, you are constantly working on two fronts, the improvement of technique and the sharpening of vision. The BIG IDEA in this chapter unites both.

Form and texture combine with direction and movement to create hairstyles.

As always, BIG IDEAS start with small steps. No one becomes an artist overnight. Not even I, your Professor P, did that. I had to carefully work my way through all the procedures in the PLAN I now have for you, repeating each one over and over to gain confidence and finally mastery. I know you can do the same!

HAIRSTYLING THEORY

Primary Hairstyling Considerations
Hairstyling Fundamentals
Hairstyling Essentials
Infection Control & Safety
Client Consultation

THERMAL STYLING

Thermal Styling Theory
Infection Control & Safety
Thermal Styling Procedure Overview
Air Forming Solid Form
Scrunching Layered Form
Air Forming Graduated Form: Round Brush
Air Forming Layered Form: Round Brush
Air Forming Combination Form: 9-Row Brush
Air Forming Combination Form: Round Brush/Curling Iron
Pressing and Curling
Press and Curl Variation: No Part

WET STYLING

Fingerwaves
Pincurls
Skip Waves
Rollers
Wet Styling Procedure Overview
Fingerwaves and Flat Pincurls
Straight Volume Rollers and Pincurls
Curvature Volume Rollers and Pincurls

LONG HAIRSTYLING

Long Hair Fundamental
Long-Hair Styling Procedures
Three-Strand Overbraid
Three-Strand Underbraid
French Twist

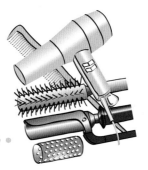

HAIRSTYLING THEORY

Throughout history, various hairstyles have influenced and, in some cases, inspired fashion and design for an entire society. For an individual, as well, a particular hairstyle may become that person's most identifiable or describable characteristic. As an aspiring cosmetologist, you are becoming aware that offering professional hair services to your clients can be a very exciting and competitive task. Most clients who sit in your chair want to be dazzled by your creative abilities. It is your challenge, as a professional, to understand the individual needs of each client based on age, personality and lifestyle and then use that to work with the natural or artificial texture and patterns of the hair.

Hairstyling is the art of dressing and arranging hair to create temporary changes in the form and texture of the finished hairstyle. Hairstyling can 'make or break' the success of the other services you perform in the salon. You may create a technically perfect haircut or a great perm, but if you are not able to 'finish' the design successfully, your client may not appreciate your initial skills. Offering a variety of styling options builds client loyalty and satisfaction.

You'll need to develop a repertoire of hairstyling skills to serve your clients well. This chapter is subdivided into the three major areas of hairstyling. All three, wet styling, thermal styling and long-hair styling, are interrelated and important for you to understand.

Altering texture or adding volume can change the entire feeling of a design. Mastery of the components of movement and direction, along with balance and proportion, will serve you well in any design service that you perform.

Thermal styling, which uses blow dryers, brushes and curling irons, has become the most popular styling method today. It requires minimal time and clients are able to closely duplicate results at home.

10

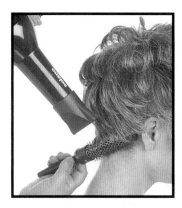
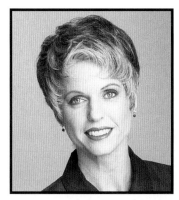
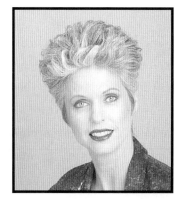

Wet styling includes molding, classic fingerwaving and setting the hair with rollers and pincurls to create long-lasting hairstyles.

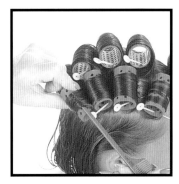 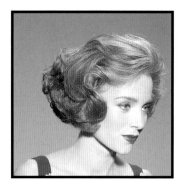 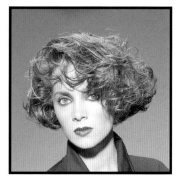

Long-hair styles are most often requested for formal occasions, such as weddings or proms. The hairstyling techniques that you use will vary according to the client, her hair and the reason she has come to the salon.

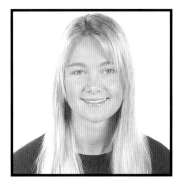 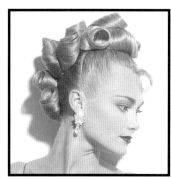 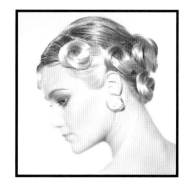

Primary Hairstyling Considerations

Just as a dress designer must consider the lines of a garment as well as the texture and drape of the fabric before creating the pattern, there are primary considerations for you as a hairstylist. These primary considerations include form, texture, direction and movement. Hairstyling offers you the options of changing the form or shape of your client's hair as well as its texture or surface pattern, direction and movement.

Form

As you know from the "Haircutting" chapter, the form of a haircut is the three-dimensional result of the specific arrangement of lengths across the curve of the head. Generally, we analyze the form of a haircut in a 'basic' finish. Hairstyling offers you the options of changing the form or shape of the design as well as the texture and direction. As volume and texture are added, weight may shift within the form. The space around the head is filled in a new way, giving the appearance of a different shape or silhouette. To analyze the form of a hairstyle, look for these qualities:

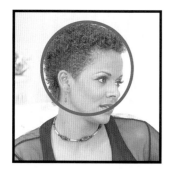

More or less equal length and width in the overall style. The rounded or spheroid shape or form is the result of relatively equal volume throughout the design.

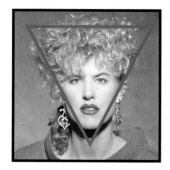

More width than length evident in the shape or form. This style is the result of more volume at the sides. Sometimes this form can appear triangular and is sometimes called oblate.

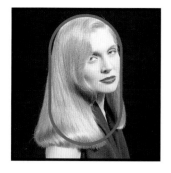

More length than width evident in the shape or form. Volume at the top can create an elongated effect or this may be due to length at which the hair falls. May create an oval or prolate effect.

When designing a hairstyle, you must be aware that you can dramatically alter the form with the addition of volume and texture. In some cases, the resulting form will look completely different than the sculpted form. In the case of long-hair styling, the final design will bear little or no resemblance to the shape or form of the haircut.

In this example, long uniform layers over a solid form, the perimeter weight is quite evident and the length of the layers avoids any impression of volume. Setting the hair on very small rollers (or even a small-barreled thermal iron) will cause the lengths to shrink up and appear much shorter. Back-combing accentuates interior volume. The finished result is quite round.

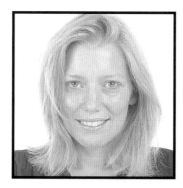 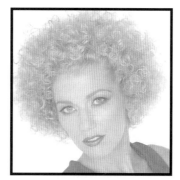

Texture

The addition of temporary texture through hairstyling services alters the surface appearance of the design and can also create changes in the shape. Adding texture to the hair may result in some degree of length reduction. The term texture character refers to the shape or pattern of the texture. These patterns include waves, curls, spiral curls, crimped texture or any combination.

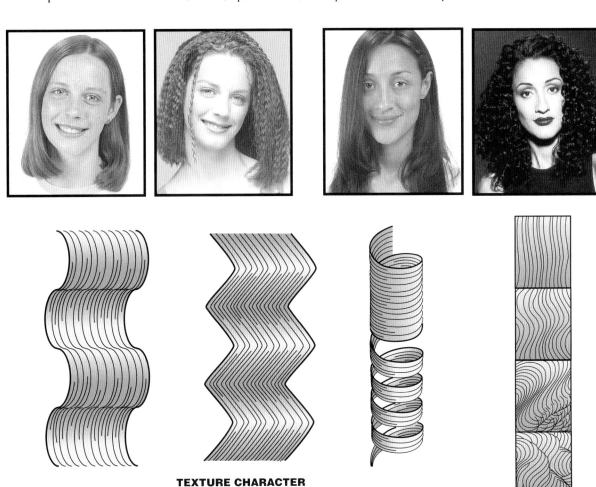

TEXTURE CHARACTER

Texture can also be identified by the 'speed' of the texture pattern. The speed of the texture will be closely related to the diameter of the tool used. Observe the difference between:

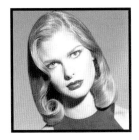

A long, slow wave...

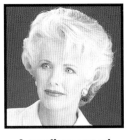

A medium-speed curl pattern...

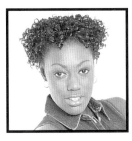

And a fast-speed curl pattern.

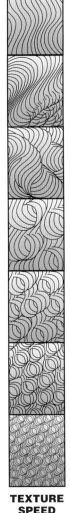

TEXTURE SPEED

Direction

You'll also need to analyze the direction or directional emphasis of every hairstyle you create. The hair can be directed toward or away from the face. It can be directed back in one area and forward in other. In long-hair styling, the placement of volume can create an upward or downward directional emphasis.

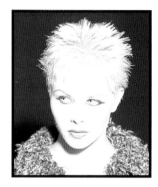 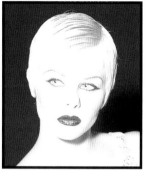 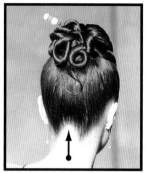 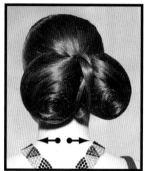

Movement

Movement is closely related to direction. If you let your eye glance over a hairstyle, you'll find that it will 'follow' certain parts of the style more readily. Those areas will have more distinct movements for the eye to look at and move along with. Movement is generally classified as straight or curved. Movements may blend with each other, move toward each other or move away from each other.

Motion begins at a single point. A point extends to become a line and multiple lines create movement. It is the pattern in which the hair is combed, or the distribution, that creates this movement. Distribution is classified as either parallel or radial.

 Lines that extend from multiple points and travel at an equal distance from each other are called parallel. Hair combed in this pattern is called parallel distribution. Parallel distribution may be curved or straight.

 Lines that radiate outward from a single point, like the spokes of a wheel, are called radial. These lines may begin as straight lines and then become curved.

  Parallel and radial curved lines are identified as moving clockwise or counterclockwise.

An artistic combination of form, texture, direction and movement creates the beautiful effects that are the hallmarks of good hairstyling.

Hairstyling Fundamentals

Whether you are air forming and iron curling the hair or setting wet hair on rollers, the fundamentals are basically the same! The physical actions vary, but the principles behind controlling the hair remain the same. Thorough knowledge will ensure the best hairstyling results for you and your client.

The essence of any hairstyle is in creating the desired direction and movement, combined with various degrees of volume and closeness. In order to achieve these goals, you need to understand the importance of distributing or molding the hair, as well as sectioning and parting, prior to the application of a roller, pincurl, round brush or thermal iron. These preliminary tactics will help ensure your styling results.

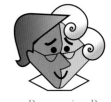

"Proper Preparation Prevents Poor Performance!"

Distribution and Molding

To achieve the desired directions and movements in the hairstyle, you will need to distribute or comb the hair into a basic 'pattern,' which reflects the style you and your client have agreed upon. The design may or may not include a part.

Parts

Whether a part is related to the client's natural growth pattern or is a distinct element of your design plan, correctly placed parts will enhance the appearance of your client's hairstyle. Consider your client's facial shape, growth directions and hair texture along with the result you are trying to achieve.

As a general rule, center parts work well with an oval face shape, and not with a round, square or long, thin facial shape. A center part on a round or square face will only accentuate the roundness or squareness; on a long face, a center part will emphasize the length.

Because the oval shape is generally recognized as the "ideal" face shape, the correct parting on a round or square face can be used to create the illusion of ovalness. To accomplish this, begin the part off center and slant it down and away from the center of the head. For a long, thin face shape, the illusion of width can be created by forming a part low on the side of the head and combing the hair across the top.

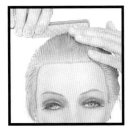 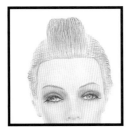

Molding or shaping is the process of combing wet hair into the desired position. These molded movements can be further subdivided into shapes. In this example, the hair is distributed back off the face using parallel distribution. The hair is then sectioned to create a rectangular shape.

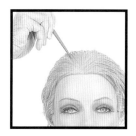
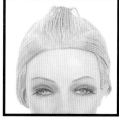

Here radial distribution is used to determine the position for a triangular shape. Parallel distribution is then used to distribute the hair within the triangle.

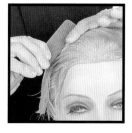
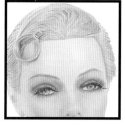

Radial distribution and a counterclockwise direction are used to mold this circular movement.

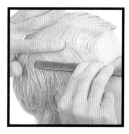
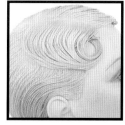

Curved, parallel distribution is used in this example to create an oblong shape.

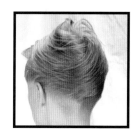

Hair Wrapping
Molding or wrapping the hair around the head so the finished hair style takes on the shape of the head.

Sectioning

After the hair is molded into the lines of the style, you will either let it dry or set it with tools. Before beginning to set the hair, you'll need to subdivide the head into major areas or sections. Sectioning the hair into workable areas allows you to have better control of the hair and to more carefully plan your design. Sections that you are not working on are pinned or clipped out of the way until you are ready to work with them. Note that sections may or may not relate to molded patterns. Therefore, larger sections may be molded and then subdivided into subsections. The process of sectioning is related to the intended design and the shape of the client's head. It also takes natural growth patterns into consideration. Sections will very often take the form of geometric shapes. Some of the geometric shapes that might be used to section the head into workable areas are: circles (or parts of a circle), oblongs, rectangles, squares, triangles and trapezoids.

Some shapes dictate that specific distribution patterns be used. For instance, a circle requires the use of radial distribution. Oblongs are created using parallel curved distribution. Triangles and squares, on the other hand, can be used with radial or parallel distribution. It is important to remember that an entire design or hairstyle will always be composed of some combination of shapes. How you choose to fit the 'pieces of the puzzle' together will determine how well the finished style works.

10

Straight Shapes

The most common straight shapes are the square, rectangle and triangle. With a square, the hair is usually distributed evenly (radially) from the center of the shape. This shape is often subsectioned into four triangles. This distribution pattern disperses the hair evenly, from the center of the shape to cover an area, such as the top of the head.

Rectangular shapes are used to move the hair in one direction, generally away from the face. Triangular shapes have radial or parallel distribution. Trapezoid shapes have parallel distribution

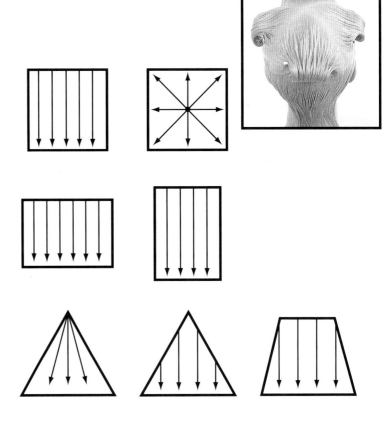

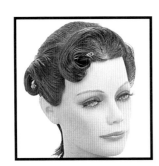

Curved Shapes

Curved shapes or sections include circles, ovals and oblongs. A circle features equal movement on either side of a central point. An oval features an off-center point with unequal movement on either side of the point. An oblong is an elongated, curved shape used in hair design that has an open end and a closed end. A single oblong creates a "C"-shaped movement. When two oblongs alternate, they create an "S"-shaped movement or a wave. Any of these curvature shapes can be distributed to move in either a clockwise or counterclockwise direction.

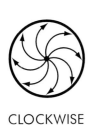

CLOCKWISE

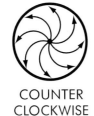

COUNTER CLOCKWISE

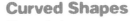

Once straight or curved sections have been sectioned, the hair is set with rollers or pincurls to produce the final desired result. The same basic sectioning principles apply when thermal styling and iron curling the hair. In the case of fingerwaves, the carefully molded movements provide the final result.

Partings

Partings are lines that subdivide shapes or sections to help distribute and control the hair. These subsections are often called bases and, generally, are the areas of hair on which you will apply the various tools and techniques.

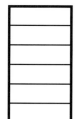

Horizontal partings within this rectangle shape create rectangle bases.

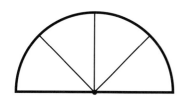

Radial partings within this circular shape create triangle-shaped bases.

Later on in the chapter you will learn about base control, which will help you to understand just how important clean, accurate partings are to the art of hairstyling.

Components of a Curl

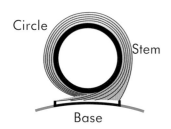

Defined curls and waves are achieved in hairstyling by using rollers, pincurls, thermal irons and/or round brushes. The diameter of the curl will be determined by the diameter of the tool or pincurl. The three components of each curl, which you will look at now, are basically the same, regardless of the tool or technique used. They are the base, the stem and the circle. The stem is also called arc.

Components of a Roller, Thermal-Iron or Round-Brush Curl

In this section of the chapter you will learn about the curl's three components (base, stem, circle) in relation to rollers, thermal irons and round brushes. (Pincurls will be discussed in the "Wet Styling" portion of this chapter.) **The curl base is the area between partings within a shape or, in other words, the section of hair on which the roller, thermal iron or round brush is placed.** Partings will generally be straight when working with these tools.

The stem is the hair between the scalp and the first turn of the hair around the roller, thermal iron or round brush. The stem determines the amount of movement of the section of hair. Longer stems create more movement and shorter stems create more base strength and less movement.

The circle of a curl is the hair that is positioned around the roller, thermal iron or round brush. It determines the size of the curl. The diameter of the tool you choose will determine the size of the circle.

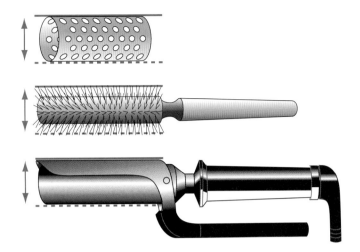

Base Controls for Hairstyling

The base is the area between straight or curved partings within a shape. Whether the hair is wet set (using rollers or pincurls) or thermal styled, the size of the base in relation to the tool or curl being used and the position of the tool or curl in relation to the base will determine the final results of the hairstyle. The combination of the size of the base and the position of the curl in relation to the base is called base control.

The base control used within a hairstyle affects the amount of volume (lift, fullness, mass) or closeness (flatness) achieved. You will determine the degree of volume or closeness desired during your consultation with your client. Some hairstyles will require areas of hollowness or depression, known as indentation, between areas of volume.

In summary, base size and base position determine closeness, volume or indentation in a hairstyle. Base controls used for rollers, round brushes and thermal styling are reviewed in this chapter. The tools with which you choose to work will be determined by the desired results, your client's hair and personal preferences.

Base Size

The diameter and length of the tool usually determine the size of the base to use. Base size (width) is measured according to the diameter of the tool, which is the outside measurement across the end of the tool. The most commonly used base sizes are 1 diameter (1x), 1.5 diameters (1.5x) and 2 diameters (2x).

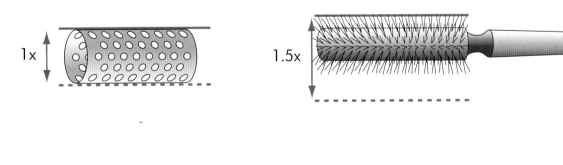

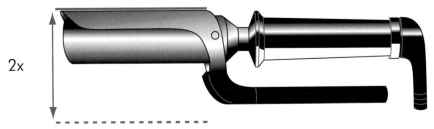

- One diameter means that the width of the section is exactly the same as the diameter of the tool being used. This size is also referred to as equal or full diameter. Note that the length of the section should be equivalent to the length of the tool.

- A 1.5 diameter section indicates the width of the section is one and one half times the width of the tool being used for placement. Notice, however, that the length of the section is still equivalent to the length of the tool being used.

- A two-diameter section indicates that the width of the section is equal to two times the diameter of the tool. The length of the base is still influenced by the length of the tool being used.

Tool Position

The base controls that are used in hairstyling are the same, regardless of the technique or tool being used (rollers, pincurls or thermal irons). They are:

On Base (Full Base): The tool or curl is centered between the top and bottom partings of the base. This base control will result in the most volume and the strongest base strength. The base is equal to the length and diameter of the roller or tool being used. The hair is held at 45° above the center of the base, then rolled to the center of the base.

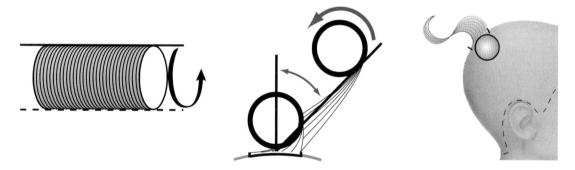

Half-Off Base (Half Base): The tool or curl sits directly on the bottom parting of the base, with half the curl on the base and half the curl off the base. The resulting curl has less base strength and less volume (lift) than an on-base curl. The hair is held at 90° from the center of the base and is rolled to sit on the bottom parting.

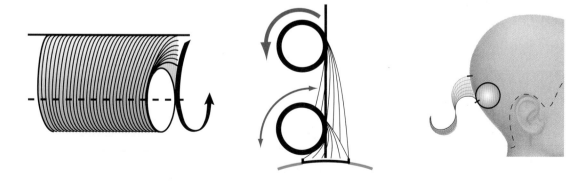

Off Base: The tool or curl sits below the bottom parting of the base, creating minimum base strength and the least volume or lift. The hair is held at 45° below the center of the base and rolled to sit below the bottom parting.

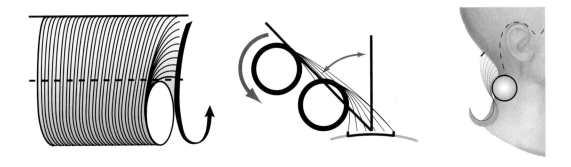

Underdirected: The tool or curl sits in the lower portion of the base, but not on or below the parting. The size of the base must be at least one and one half times the diameter of the tool or curl. The base control results in reduced volume and base strength. The hair is held at 90° from the center of the base and rolled to sit in the lower portion of the base.

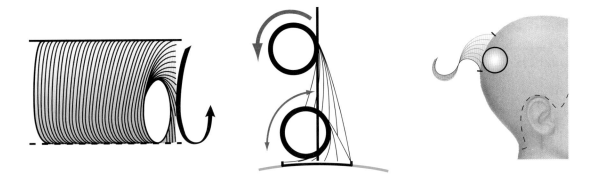

Overdirected (Volume Base): The tool or curl sits in the upper portion of the base, but not on or above the parting. The size of the base must be at least one and one half times the diameter of the tool or curl. This base control results in exaggerated directional movement and volume or lift, with less strength at the base. The hair is held at 45° above the center of the base and rolled to sit in the upper portion of the base.

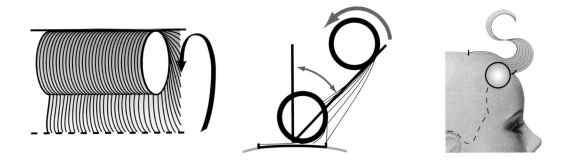

This chart will help you to remember the base controls used in hairstyling. Remember that these general guidelines are the same for rollers, round brushes, thermal irons and pincurls.

BASE CONTROL–VOLUME	DESCRIPTION	EFFECT
On Base (Full Base)	Roller or tool sits completely on the base	Maximum volume; maximum base strength
Half-Off Base (Half Base)	Roller or tool sits half-off or half-on the base	Less volume; less base strength
Off Base	Roller or tool sits completely off the base	Least volume; least base strength
Underdirected	Roller or tool sits within the base close to the bottom parting	Reduced volume; reduced base strength
Overdirected (Volume Base)	Roller or tool sits within the base close to the top of the parting	Exaggerated direction and volume; reduced base strength

Base Control–Indentation

With indentation the position of the tool and the size of the base influence the amount of hollow space or flatness (closeness) achieved. Tool position also influences the strength of the base and the mobility of the curl. The indentation roller placement is most widely used in creating a flip effect. However, the many assorted needs of the indentation base position will become more evident as you progress in creative hairstyling.

VOLUME BASE CONTROL OPTIONS	
Tool Position	**Base Size**
On base	1x
Half-off base	1x, 1.5x, 2x
Off base	1x, 1.5x, 2x
Underdirected	1.5x, 2x
Overdirected	1x, 2x

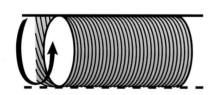
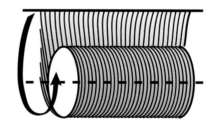
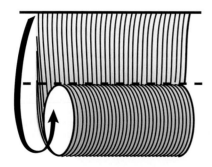
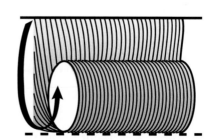

10

BASE CONTROL – INDENTATION	DESCRIPTION	EFFECT
On base – indentation	Roller or tool sits completely on its base, rolled in an upward direction	Maximum base strength and volume
Half-off base – indentation	Roller or tool sits half on and half off its base, rolled in an upward direction	Medium base strength, allowing more curl mobility
Off base – indentation	Roller or tool sits completely off its base, rolled in an upward direction	Minimum base strength, maximum curl mobility
Underdirected – indentation	Roller or tool sits within the base close to the bottom of the parting, rolled in an upward direction	Medium base strength, strong curl flare

INDENTATION BASE CONTROL OPTIONS	
Tool Position	**Base Size**
On base	1x
Half-off base	1x, 1.5x, 2x
Off base	1x, 1.5x, 2x
Underdirected	1.5x, 2x

Note that there is not an overdirected indentation base control.

Finishing the Hairstyle

Whether rollers, pincurls or thermal styling have been used to change the texture, direction and movement of the hair, the techniques you use to finish the style will be very similar. This finishing phase of hairstyling is often referred to as the 'combout' of the style. At this point, you will address any areas of the design that require blending. You'll also create support, add volume and refine the form while adding any embellishments.

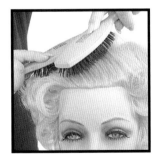

Relaxing the Set

Whether the hair is set on rollers, in pincurls or with a thermal iron, you will need to relax the hair in order to integrate the set and blend the partings. Relaxing the set is done by using one or two cushion brushes and brushing all the way to the scalp to integrate the bases. You will want to work within the lines of the set and also against the lines to ensure that the set is completely relaxed while simultaneously softening the texture of the hair.

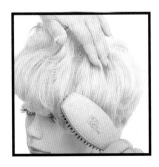

Re-establishing the Lines of the Design

Once you have relaxed the set, you'll need to re-establish the lines of the set pattern and finished hairstyle. To do this you will use a cushion brush to retrace the lines of the set, following each movement with the other hand. Note that the lines may be somewhat over-emphasized at this point in the process.

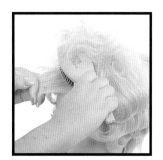

Backbrushing and backcombing

Backbrushing and backcombing techniques are used to add volume to the hairstyle and further connect the shapes within the set, while adding longevity to the style. These techniques use a comb or brush to systematically push the shorter lengths toward the base to create a cushion effect. In addition to following the movements of the set, you will want to use the base control of the set as a guide to determine how much volume you need to create in a specific area of the hairstyle.

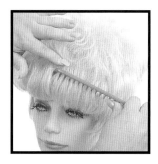

Refine the Lines and Texture

To refine the line and texture you will use a brush or comb to create the desired textural effects. Emphasize the movements of the hairstyle without exaggeration. Refining can be the final step of the process if you and your client are pleased.

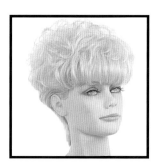

Detailing

Smaller, more refined touches, such as pleated textures or creative 'piecing' of the hair, for a more personalized hairstyle are known as detailing. At this point you can really emphasize your client's personal style. Detailing requires a light touch and a certain amount of restraint on your part. Too much 'detail' can overwhelm the integrity of the design, resulting in a fussy or overworked hairstyle.

Hairstyling Essentials

In order to achieve the styling effects desired, you need to be familiar with the implements/supplies, products and equipment used during hairstyling services. The following charts identify these styling essentials and equipment and define their basic functions. Styling products are also called liquid tools since they are essential to achieving lasting styles.

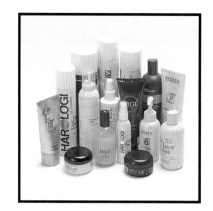

Hairstyling Implements/Supplies

IMPLEMENT/SUPPLIES	FUNCTION
Combs	
All purpose Styling Comb (Molding or Cutting Comb)	Parts and distributes the hair; accurately measures if comb is calibrated; closely set teeth create a smooth surface; wider spaced teeth separate and arrange hair
Tail Comb	Sections, parts and distributes the hair

10

IMPLEMENT/SUPPLIES	FUNCTION
Master Sketcher Comb	Detangles and backcombs hair
Rake comb	Detangles; styles curly hair; defines texture
Lifter	Details; lifts; backcombs
Brushes	
Vent Brush	Achieves lift or volume when air forming smoother textures or creating directional emphasis
7 or 9-row Air Forming Brush	Smoothes wavy or curly textures; adds directional emphasis when air forming
Round Brushes (various diameters)	Impart varying degrees of curved or curled texture and volume
Cushion Brush	Relaxes sets; backbrushes; dry molds, styles or refines the form
Rollers, Pins And Clips	
Cylindrical Rollers	Create uniform curl formation/diameter across width of base; used in straight-shape roller setting
Conical or Cone-Shaped Rollers	Create progression of curl diameter from narrow end of base toward wide end; Used in curvature-shape roller setting
Picks	Secure rollers in place while hair dries; also secure perm rods
Single-Prong Clips	Secure pincurls
Double-Prong Clips	Secure molded shapes/sectioning; also secure rollers if picks are not used
Bobby Pins	Secure hair in place for finished style, especially in long hair designs
Hair Pins	Secure hair in place for finished style, especially in long hair designs
Long-Hair Pins	Define textural detail and movement
Wave or Styling Clamp	Keeps fingerwaves in place
Thermal Styling	
Blow Dryer	Air forms in combination with various tools to create directional and textural changes
Thermal Irons	Add curled or waved texture to the hair
Hot Brush/Comb	Dries hair while creating waves or curls
Pressing Comb	Straightens overly curly hair

Hairstyling Products

PRODUCTS	FUNCTION
Gel	Creates maximum control and support of the hair especially for wet setting; varying strengths available
Mousse	Supports volume and movement; foam consistency, may or may not contain conditioners
Styling lotion	Supports volume and movement; liquid consistency
Spray Gel	Supports volume and movement; firmer hold than lotion, liquid consistency
Non-Aerosol Hairspray	Holds finished style in place, liquid dispensed through pump
Aerosol Hairspray	Holds finished style in place, available in a variety of strengths; liquid dispensed through compressed gas and spray
Pomade	Adds shine and texture definition; adds weight to the hair
Pressing Oil	Prepares and protects hair during pressing service; helps prevent scorching and breakage; conditions and adds shine; use less pressing oil to avoid smoke or burning; helps hair stay pressed longer

Hairstyling Equipment

EQUIPMENT	FUNCTION
Hairstyling Station	Provides a place for tools to be displayed and organized
Hydraulic Chair	Provides proper back support for client during the service; adjustable
Wet Disinfectant Container	Holds solution for disinfecting implements
Shampoo Bowl	Supports client's neck and holds water and shampoo products during a shampoo service

Infection Control and Safety

Following is a list of safety precautions you should follow prior to and during a hairstyling service. Additional precautions are listed in the categories of thermal hairstyling.

- Practice infection control guidelines.
- Wash and sanitize hands with liquid antibacterial soap.
- Check the air-intake area on the blow dryer to ensure it is free from debris before beginning the air-forming procedure.

- Check the scalp for any diseases or disorders. If any are evident, refer the client to a physician and do not proceed with the service.

- Make sure that client does not have sensitivities to any styling products that will be used during the service, such as mousse or gel.

- If the client will be placed under a hair dryer, be sure to check it occasionally to see if the client is comfortable and not being adversely effected by the heat. This is especially important when working with elderly clients who may be more sensitive to the higher temperatures.

- Try to avoid excessive amounts of styling products on the scalp, which might cause irritation.

- Avoid using excess tension on the hair and scalp when back-combing or backbrushing. This may be uncomfortable for your client and may unduly stress the hair.

- Be gentle when removing backcombing or backbrushing prior to shampooing the hair. Use caution when detangling the hair.

- Disinfect and sanitize all implements after each use.

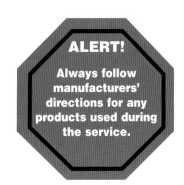

ALERT! Always follow manufacturers' directions for any products used during the service.

Draping Procedures for a Hairstyling Service

Generally a plastic cape is used during the shampooing, conditioning, and wet styling phases of a service to protect the client's skin and clothing. A neck strip is often substituted for the towel during the cutting phase, to allow for natural hair fall. A styling cape of lighter weight may be selected during the dry styling phases of the service. Refer to the "Trichology" chapter for details on the proper draping procedures.

Client Consultation

All hair services require that you consult with your client prior to the service to ensure predictable results that meet both your client's and your own expectations. When consulting for hairstyling services, remember that many clients have booked this appointment in preparation to attend a special event, so there may be some emotional attachment to the expectations. A mother-of-the-bride might be especially nervous, so make sure that you reach a clear agreement of the service to be performed. Use photos and magazines to facilitate the dialogue between you and your client. Remember to concentrate on changes that can be made in the form, texture, direction and movement of the design. If possible, show your client styling options that were created on the same or similar haircut as the one she has.

You can also teach your client some styling basics. Knowing some options she can do at home will increase the longevity and enjoyment of her haircut.

To help you to remember the important steps in the consultation process, remember: Great Artists Always Draw Creatively, and use the first letter of each word for each of the five steps: G for Greet, A for Ask, Analyze and Assess, A for Agree, D for Deliver and C for Complete.

Greet

- Meet and greet the client with a smile, a firm handshake and pleasant voice.
- Communicate with the client to help build rapport and develop a relationship.

Ask, Analyze and Assess

- Ask questions to discover your client's need. You might ask questions such as: "Why do you want your hair styled today?" Answers might be, "I have an important business dinner to attend this evening.," or " My cousin is getting married and I'm a bridesmaid," or "I love this haircut but I could use some new styling ideas."

- Ask if the client has any particular ideas about the hairstyle. She may not feel comfortable or attractive with her hair swept back off her face, or up and off her neck. Get as much information as you need to find out what your client really wants.

- Many hairstyling appointments are pre-booked with a special date or occasion in mind, so you can determine time constraints ahead of time. Determine whether your client will need a wet set, a thermal style or a long-hair style. Once this is determined, you can appropriately book the next appointment, allowing the correct amount of time.

- Ask questions to determine the amount of volume and curl texture the client desires. These are two areas of hairstyling that can easily be miscommunicated between the client and the stylist. Make sure you understand your client's specific desires.

- Analyze your client's face and body shape, physical features, hair and scalp. Refer to "Body and Face Shapes" in the "Design Decision" chapter for further guidelines.

- Assess the facts and thoroughly think through your recommendations.

Agree

- Explain your styling recommendations and clarify the price for today's service(s) as well as for any future styling appointments.
- Gain feedback and approval on your recommendations from the client.
- Return to "Ask, Analyze and Assess" if your client is hesitant with your recommendations.

Deliver

- Ensure your client's protection by using the proper draping procedures.
- Ensure client comfort during the service.
- Stay focused on delivering the service to the best of your ability.
- Teach your client about any special maintenance of the new hairstyle.

Complete

- Request satisfaction feedback from your client.
- Recommend products to maintain appearance and condition of your client's hair.
- Ask your client for referrals for future services.
- Suggest a future appointment time for your client's next visit.
- Offer appreciation to your client for visiting the school or salon.

10

THERMAL STYLING

Many hairstyles can be created using thermal styling techniques, such as blow drying or iron curling. Thermal styling is especially effective for looks that are more casual, less 'dressed' or simply softer looking than traditional wet set designs.

Thermal styling is the technique of drying and/or styling hair by using a hand-held dryer while simultaneously using your fingers, a variety of brushes, pressing comb and/or a thermal curling iron. Thermal means relating to or caused by heat. It is important to remember that heat is a form of energy that needs to be treated with great care, especially when used on hair.

Efficiency and creativity go hand in hand with thermal styling, since thermal styling generally allows the client a shorter appointment time. As mentioned earlier, with the right tools and knowledge, clients can often work very well with these types of styles on their own. Blow dryers, thermal irons, thermal combs and thermal brushes are the thermal implements available to the cosmetologist. Using these implements in conjunction with a variety of styling brushes and combs, you can achieve any number of creative and practical design solutions.

Thermal Styling Theory

How does thermal styling really work to create what is sometimes called 'quick service' hairstyling options? As you remember from the "Trichology" chapter, hair is composed predominantly of proteins connected by both physical and chemical bonds. Many of the physical bonds are hydrogen bonds that are easily affected and broken by both water and heat. When the hydrogen bonds of the hair are weakened (broken down), the protein chains are able to shift, accepting a new position, but only temporarily. After blow drying or thermal curling, the bonds are reformed in the new configuration as the hair cools. For this reason it is necessary to allow the hair to cool completely prior to brushing or combing.

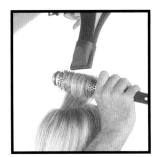
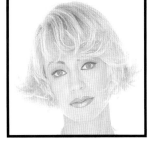
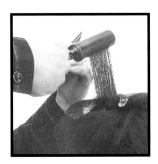
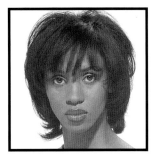

If the hair is stretched while it is still warm (and the bonds are in a weakened state), the curl pattern will not hold. Water will also break the new pattern. Rain, humidity and shampooing will all cause the hair to return to its original shape and curl configuration. Since heat and water can change the hair's curl pattern, thermal-styling services are considered to be only temporary.

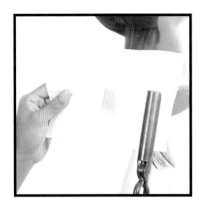

It is of the utmost importance when thermal styling, that you protect the hair from excessive heat. Most thermal styling tools are manufactured so that the temperature is maintained at a level that is safe for the hair. **When working with stove-heated thermal irons, you'll need to check the temperature by testing the iron on a piece of white paper towel.** If the paper towel scorches after about five seconds, you will need to let the iron cool somewhat prior to using it on the hair.

There are also many styling products available to the cosmetologist (and the client) that are formulated to prepare the hair for and protect it from the heat of thermal styling tools. Using these products sparingly will ensure good results while maintaining the condition and integrity of the hair.

Air Forming

The term air forming, also called blow drying, refers to the process of drying the hair and styling it simultaneously to create a new form. Blow dryers and their attachments are used to air form wet hair while using brushes, combs and your fingers to create temporary direction and texture changes.

Blow dryers are available in different sizes and shapes and also vary in the amount of wattage (generally from 1,000 watts to 1,800 watts). A blow dryer consists of a (slotted) nozzle, heating element, a small motor (or fan), temperature and air flow controls and, of course, a handle.

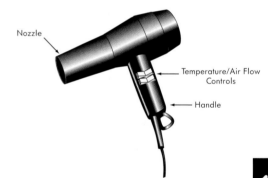

Nozzle

Temperature/Air Flow Controls

Handle

Blow dryer attachments that fit on the nozzle of the unit include concentrators and diffusers. Concentrators focus the air flow to a small area, which allows you to control the air flow and heat specifically.

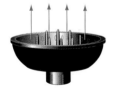

Diffusers spread a gentle air flow over a larger area and are generally used for freeform drying techniques such as scrunching. Temperature controls on the blow dryer provide a cool to hot setting, allowing for client comfort and style control.

To Properly Hold the Blow Dryer:

Loop the electric cord over the wrist when holding the blow dryer. This will allow the cord to travel in the same direction as the blow dryer and will also prevent the cord from hitting the client or trailing on the floor.

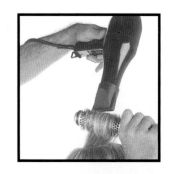

Air Forming Guidelines

- Always use a heat-protective styling lotion or other styling product before any heat-styling process to reduce friction and form a clear, protective barrier against mechanical damage or the drying effects of heat. Excessive blow drying can cause hair to lose elasticity or create split ends and an overall drying effect.

- Remove approximately 90% of the water before styling. Towel blot hair to eliminate excess water, then use the blowdryer. You'll save both time and energy. Hair that is too wet will not effectively transfer heat. Also, because water keeps the hydrogen bonds in a softened state, styling with heat at this overly wet stage is less effective.

- Dry the hair on the high setting, move to the medium setting for styling and set style with cool air. A progressive decrease in temperature helps smooth the transition from wet, slippery hair, to hair that is more fixed and formable. Then set your styles with cool air to reduce the warmth that curls retain. Retained heat makes the curls pliable and they are likely to "fall" back to their natural bond formation.

- Style and dry in the direction of the cuticle scales, not against them. Keep the dryer's airflow pointing down the hair strand from the scalp to the ends. Drying the hair in the direction of the cuticle scales may help bring out the sheen of hair when its dry.

- Always keep the dryer three to five inches (7.5 cm to 12.7 cm) from the hair and constantly moving back and forth to reduce the potential of both hair and scalp damage from heat.

- Use caution with damaged and bleached hair. The greater the degree of chemical damage, the more susceptible the hair is to breakage, friction and heat damage. Therefore, remove all the water you can from the hair with a towel. Complete drying on the medium setting, style the hair on low, and set the style with cool air. Since this type of hair is easily broken, choose your styling brushes carefully to avoid excessive tension.

Finger Styling

Finger styling is a technique in which the fingers are used to manipulate and style the hair. The hair is lifted or held flat while drying to create the desired finish. The fingers are used to separate and define the texture. **Scrunching, a form of finger styling, involves squeezing the hair to introduce a texture pattern that the hair responds to naturally.** This technique creates the best response on wavy or curly hair. Generally, a diffuser is attached to the blow dryer to soften the air flow while the hair is scrunched with the fingers to create the texture pattern.

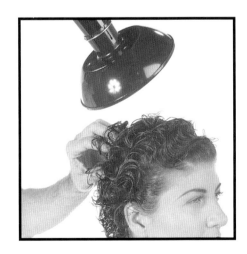

Air Forming with Round Brush

Air forming with a blow dryer in one hand and a round brush in the other hand allows you to dry the hair quickly as you change the form, direction and texture of the hair. The diameter of the round brush you choose will influence the resulting curl pattern. Smaller brushes are used for curlier styles or short hair. Larger brushes are used for smoother results or for longer hair. Some brushes have metal cores, which retain heat and allow you to create stronger curl patterns. Determine the size and firmness of the curl by selecting a brush with the diameter that matches the size of the curl desired and by adjusting the temperature of the blow dryer to set the desired firmness of the curl. For volume, the brush is positioned underneath the hair. For indentation, the brush is positioned on top of the hair. Refer to "Hairstyling Fundamentals" in this chapter for base control information.

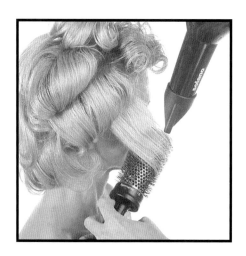

The Hot Brush or Comb

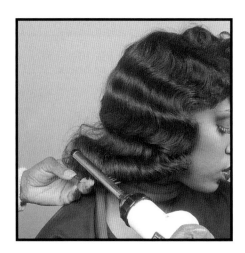

The hot brush, also called a curling brush, and the hot comb are similar to the blow dryer because they create an airflow but they can also curl the hair. Both styling tools have small motors that force air over a heating element and a slotted barrel that holds the brush or metal comb attachment. It is the combination of the airflow that dries the hair and the heat that is retained in the barrel that allows you to introduce the new curl patterns.

These styling tools are used to finish hair that is almost completely dry while simultaneously creating volume, waves or curls anywhere from the scalp to the ends of the hair, which is known as air waving.

Hair Pressing

Hair pressing or "silking" is a form of temporarily straightening overly curly hair. Once the hair is shampooed and conditioned, it is blown dry with tension to begin to reduce the natural curl pattern. A protective oil is applied, and then a hot pressing comb or silking iron (straightening iron) is used on small sections of hair to further straighten the curl. Because the pressing service can require the stylist to heat the hair for a longer period of time than other thermal services, analyzing the type and condition of the hair is particularly important. You need to condition the hair often to protect against breakage, dry scalp, split ends and dull appearance. Avoid pressing chemically damaged hair. Hair pressing results last until the next shampoo.

The diameter of the hair is also very important. Fine hair is especially delicate and must be treated gently. Less heat and pressure should be applied to fine hair than to other types of hair to avoid breakage. Medium hair is the least difficult to press and requires no particular precautions. Coarse, overly curly hair can be quite resistant to hair pressing. It can tolerate more heat and pressure than hair of fine or medium diameter, but be careful! Knowing that coarse hair is more tolerant can lead a stylist to be careless and result in damage to the hair. Remember, burned hair cannot be reconditioned.

The pressing comb is used to apply heat and tension to temporarily straighten overly curly hair. The pressing comb is used on totally dry hair before the service in preparation for the curling iron application, which usually follows. There are two types of pressing combs, regular and electric. Regular pressing combs have a wooden handle since wood does not absorb heat. Regular pressing combs are heated in what is called a "stove heater." Electric pressing combs have either an "on and off" switch or a thermostat with a control switch that allows the stylist to select either high or low heat settings. Test the temperature of the pressing comb by placing it against a paper towel and looking for a change in color. The paper will turn yellow or brown if the comb is too hot. Hair texture will guide you in selecting the right temperature for your client's hair. Remember, fine hair will not require as much heat as coarse hair.

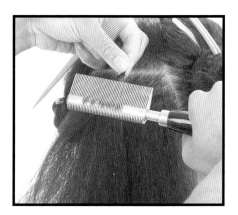

Pressing combs are made of stainless steel or brass.

Smooth effects with a pressing comb are accomplished by the pressing action of the heated spine of the comb against the hair. The number of times you repeat the pressing action on the same subsection depends on the amount of curl you wish to remove. Some stylists prefer to use narrow partings and press once or twice on one side only. Others prefer to take larger sections and press once or twice on both sides of the subsection. Remember to adjust the number of times you press the same section. You'll also need to adjust the pressure and temperature of the iron according to your client's hair condition and texture. A soft press is once with less pressure and heat. A hard or double press is twice with more pressure and heat.

Thermal Irons

There are several ways in which thermal irons may be used to create complete designs and to impart texture patterns on dry hair. Thermal irons include curling irons, which come in a variety of sizes, straightening or flat irons, crimping and undulating irons.

Thermal curling is the process of temporarily adding curl texture to the hair through the use of thermal irons, also called curling irons. Thermal irons were first introduced by Marcel Grateau in 1875 and are now often called "marcel curling irons." These irons are some of the most frequently used styling implements available today. Thermal waving or

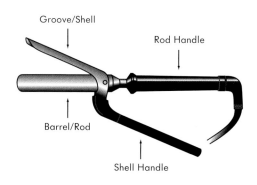

Groove/Shell

Rod Handle

Barrel/Rod

Shell Handle

curling is achieved by applying heat to dry hair from either an electric curling iron or marcel iron heated in a stove to create curls or waves for a finished hairstyle. The curling iron has four parts:

- Rod handle
- Shell handle
- Barrel or rod (the round heating cylinder)
- Groove or shell (the clamp that holds the hair against the barrel)

Electric curling irons have a swivel at the base of the handle that permits the electric cord to turn, without twisting, as the iron is being manipulated. For best performance, curling iron barrels and grooves are made of stainless steel to retain heat. Various barrel sizes and shapes are available, not all of which are intended to create curl patterns. Some barrel shapes straighten the hair while others create a zigzag pattern known as crimping.

The electric curling iron contains a heating element controlled by a thermostat that maintains a constant temperature during use. A good iron should be able to be left on an entire day and still maintain the correct temperature. Remember that testing the temperature of a marcel iron is necessary in order to avoid burning, scorching or damaging the hair. Fine, lightened and damaged hair are able to withstand less heat than healthy hair.

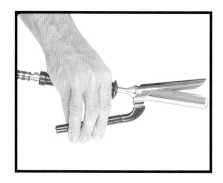

To Properly Hold the Curling Iron

The best method for holding a thermal iron will be determined by your comfort and control. Some stylists prefer to use only the little finger to open the iron, and the other fingers to close the iron (as shown at left). Other stylists find it easier to use the little finger and ring finger to open the iron.

Practice these two methods of holding the thermal iron to determine which is most comfortable for you, while allowing you to maintain the greatest control as you turn the iron to create a curl. As the iron is turned, in downward circular movements, a swivel at the base of the handle will permit the iron to turn without twisting the cord. As you continue to turn the iron, you will need to shift your thumb to aid in the turning motion.

Practice Manipulations with the Curling Iron

Because the thermal iron can be difficult to use and can burn the hair strand if used incorrectly, practice is recommended. Practice with a cold iron in the beginning until you are comfortable with the manipulations.

10

Practice rolling the thermal iron toward you (standing in back of your model, this will be a downward rotation) while opening and closing the clamp at regular intervals.

Practice rolling the thermal iron away from you (standing in back of your model, this will be an upward rotation) while opening and closing the clamp at regular intervals.

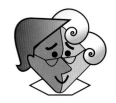

"Take good care of your thermal tools. Dropping them and neglecting to clean them will result in poor performance."

Practice rolling the hair first in one direction and then in another. End each curling rotation by releasing the hair, which is done by opening and closing the clamp in a quick "clicking" movement.

Thermal Iron Considerations

Cleaning marcel irons or pressing combs can be accomplished by running fine-grade steel wool along the barrel of the iron while it is still slightly warm to remove any styling residue. Some stylists like to then place wax paper around the warm iron to put a wax coating on the surface of the barrel, which will allow the comb to glide smoothly through the hair. Clean the iron in the direction that the hair flows across the barrel. That is, move the wool pad around the circumference of the barrel, not vertically (base to tip). This precaution ensures that hair will not flow against the grain and be damaged. This steel wool method should not be used on barrels with Teflon or other coatings. Steel wool can chip and wear off the coating, leading to abrasion during use. Use only a gentle cleaning method on coated irons.

Close a hot iron lightly on a damp towel before curling extremely damaged or bleached hair. This step is not necessary for most hair types, but with damaged hair, you want to cool the iron and assess the heat before it is applied. Some tinted hair, white hair and very fine hair will benefit by testing the iron as well and proceeding with a lower iron temperature. This testing can prevent scorching or dryness.

Choose an iron with even heat distribution. Use appliances that heat up uniformly across the barrel with no cool spots. Uniform heat will avoid uneven curls. Remember that a metal curling iron holder retains heat. If you use a metal holder be sure to test the temperature of the iron before using it on your client's hair. Never test an iron's heat by touching it with your fingers or placing close to your nose to smell if it is hot. You can sufficiently judge the amount of heat it's giving off by bringing your hand very near the barrel, without touching it.

Curling Iron Techniques

Following are examples of different curling iron techniques and various texture patterns that can be achieved by varying the position of the curling iron along the hair strand. Curling irons are usually cylindrical in shape and create the texture pattern that reflects their diameter. Refer to "Hairstyling Fundamentals" in this chapter for volume and indentation base control information.

Base-to-Ends Technique

With the base-to-ends technique, the curling iron is first positioned slightly away from the base. The curling iron is then turned one-half revolution toward the scalp. The curling iron is then turned away from the scalp one-half revolution in the same direction, to make one complete revolution. This technique is repeated until the entire hair strand is gradually fed into the curling iron. A heat-resistant comb is positioned between the curling iron and the scalp to protect the client's scalp from accidental burning. The base-to-ends technique creates volume and support at the base and a consistent curl pattern throughout the strand. For a volume base control, position the barrel of the curling iron underneath the hair strand. For an indentation base control, position the barrel of the curling iron on top of the hair strand.

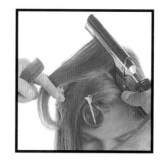
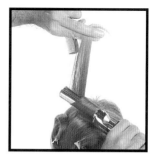
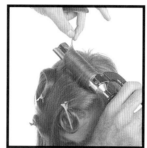
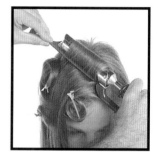

Ends-to-Base Technique

With the ends-to-base technique, the curling iron is positioned at the ends of the hair and then rotated upward, toward the base. For a volume effect, the barrel of the curling iron is positioned underneath the hair strand. For an indentation effect, the barrel of the curling iron is positioned on top of the hair strand. Depending on the hair length, the curl pattern is generally stronger at the ends and weaker toward the base.

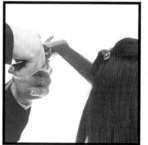
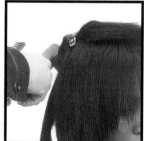

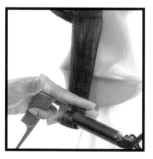
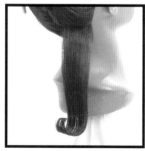

Ends Technique

With the ends technique, the curling iron is positioned to add curl texture at the ends only. This technique can be used to create a curved-under or flipped-up (indentation) effect.

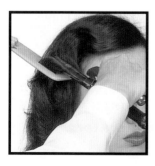

Marcel Technique

The curling iron can be used to create marcel waves or alternating oblongs along the hair strand. The hair strand is placed into the curling iron with barrel of curling iron positioned on top of the strand and the shell of the iron beneath the strand. A comb is used to help direct the hair in alternating directions to form the wave.

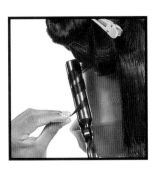
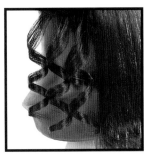

Spiral Technique

The spiral technique can be achieved by positioning the curling iron on the ends of the hair and then turning the curling iron upward in a vertical or diagonal position.

Another way to create the spiral technique is to position the curling iron vertically or diagonally at the base. The curling iron is then turned while gradually feeding the hair strand into the curling iron until the entire strand is fed through and the ends are within the iron.

Special-Effects Thermal Irons

Special-effects thermal irons are available which allow you to create textures other than traditional curvilinear, curled textures. Following are some examples:

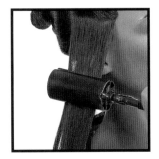

Straightening or Flat Irons

Straightening or flat irons consist of two flat, heated plates. The hair is placed between the two plates near the base and then brought down to the ends in one smooth flowing movement. This technique is referred to as straightening or silking the hair.

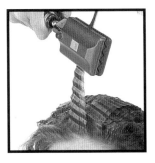

Crimping Irons

Unlike the straightening irons that consist of two flat irons, the crimping irons consist of two irons that have an angular or serrated pattern. The hair is positioned between the two crimped plates, which are then closed upon the hair. The resulting texture is angular, which is often referred to as crimped hair.

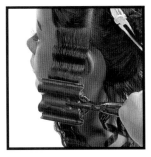

Undulating Irons

Undulating irons consist of two undulating or curved irons that create an "S" pattern. The hair is positioned between the two irons, which are then closed upon the hair. The result produces an undulating wave pattern.

Detangling and combing the hair smoothly prior to applying the thermal iron ensures a consistent texture pattern throughout the hair strand.

Infection Control and Safety

In addition to all of the infection control and safety guidelines that you looked at earlier in this chapter, following are some additional points to consider:

1. Exercise caution when using thermal irons on chemically treated hair. Since this hair is more sensitive, improper usage can cause damage. Wet sets are often recommended.

2. Test the temperature of thermal irons or pressing combs before applying them to the client's hair.

3. Exercise extra caution when working with thermal styling tools near the hairline and especially near the ears to avoid burning the client's skin.

4. Avoid having the teeth of the hot comb or brush come in contact with the client's scalp to avoid burning and/or heat irritation.

5. Remember to disconnect or turn off all appliances and tuck all cords out of reach when leaving your station unattended.

6. Use lower temperatures and shorter contact time on hair that has been chemically altered by perms or color or shows signs of mechanical damage.

7. If you notice brown or black residue on implements, clean metal portions with fine steel wool around the diameter of the barrel. Always use clean combs and brushes for each client.

8. If a burn occurs (on you or your client), flush with cold water and let the skin completely cool. Blot dry and apply a first aid cream to the burn. One percent gentian violet jelly may be applied if the burn is not severe. If blisters appear, see a physician immediately. This is a sign of a severe burn that can scar if left untreated.

9. Avoid pressing hair too often. Frequently pressed hair may suffer progressive hair breakage.

10. Thermal iron procedures are always performed on dry hair.

11. Protect the client's scalp from thermal irons by positioning a hard rubber or nonflammable comb underneath the curling iron.

1 0

Thermal Styling Procedure Overview

The following thermal hairstyles will be demonstrated in this section of the "Hairstyling" chapter. By understanding various thermal hairstyling techniques, such as how to create volume, movement and texture, you will be able to create an array of designs as well as successfully finish other services such as haircutting and hair coloring.

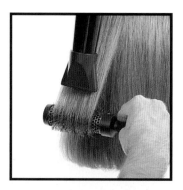
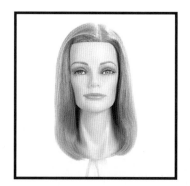

Air Forming Solid Form

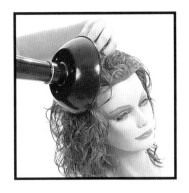 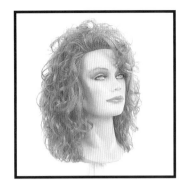

Scrunching Layered Form

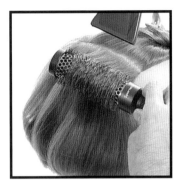 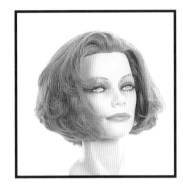

Air Forming Graduated Form: Round Brush

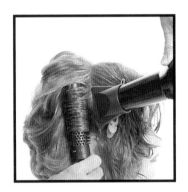 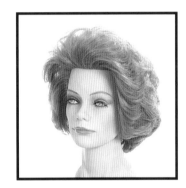

Air Forming Layered Form: Round Brush

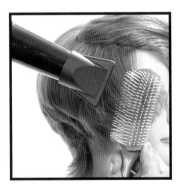 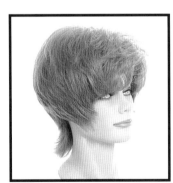

Air Forming Combination Form: 9-Row Brush

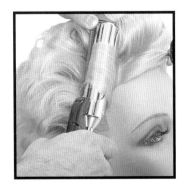 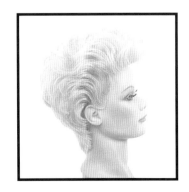

Air Forming Combination Form: Round Brush/Curling Iron

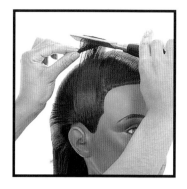
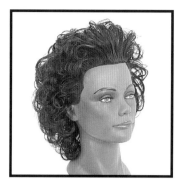

Pressing and Curling

Natural Parts

To strengthen the lasting quality of a style, you may opt to use a natural part. A natural part assumes the direction of the hair's natural growth pattern. You will want to make sure that the natural part is complementary and will enhance the style.

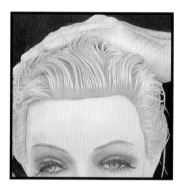
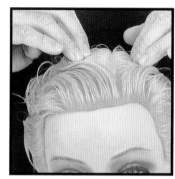
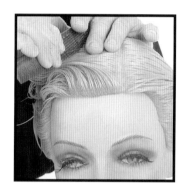

Establishing a Natural Part:

1. Comb and evenly distribute the hair from the hairline. Notice that the hand follows the comb and rests gently on the positioned strands.

2. With even pressure, move your hand forward so that the strands lift naturally at their base. Notice the hair will move in its own growth pattern, and a separation will occur at the natural part line.

3. Continue to hold the bulk of hair in the top and fringe (bang) area as you comb from the part line down through the right side area.

4. Comb and evenly distribute the hair on the left side of the part in the direction of the intended design.

Design Parts

To establish a design part on a client, you must consider the hairline and natural growth pattern. You must also consider that if the part is extended into the crown area, it should be directed toward the center of the natural point of distribution.

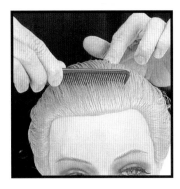
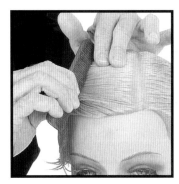
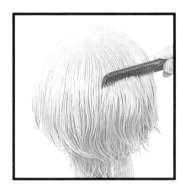

Establishing a Design Part

1. Comb the hair back from the hairline distributing it evenly. Using the large teeth, place the end of the comb at the starting point of the part along the hairline.

2. Place your index finger at the predetermined ending point of the design part. Direct the comb in a straight line toward your index finger.

3. Stop the comb at your index finger and separate the hair at this point.

4. Begin at the ending point of the part line and comb the side hair down as illustrated.

5. Continue combing the top hair away from the part line, working toward the fringe (bang) area.

6. Continue combing and evenly distributing the strands while working around the crown.

Air Forming Solid Form

Air forming is used to finish or highlight the features of a haircut. In this case, you will air form the horizontal solid-form haircut to showcase the smooth unactivated texture and perimeter weight. Consistency of technique is important to achieve optimum results. Partings will reflect or parallel the horizontal form line. The styling products that you choose will be based upon prior assessment of your client's hair and the amount of support and control desired.

A side part can make thin or fine hair look fuller.

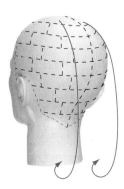

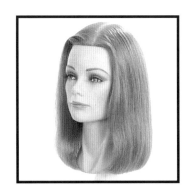

In this exercise, a 9-row styling brush helps attain proper tension to stretch and keep the hair length smooth. A round brush is then used to create a curved-under texture at the ends. Your choice of heat and airflow speed will be influenced by your client's hair type.

Air Forming Solid-Form Preparation

As with any professional service, it is important to have your area, products, implements and equipment in proper order. If the thermal styling service follows a haircutting service, most of your preparation would have taken place prior to the haircut. This exercise assumes that the client is receiving only the thermal styling service. Before you begin air forming the solid form, be sure to satisfy the following points:

- Clean work station with disinfectant
- Arrange implements/supplies including blow dryer, shampoo comb or wide-tooth comb, 9-row and round brushes and appropriate styling products
- Ask the client to remove jewelry and store in a secure place
- Wash and sanitize hands; drape client for a wet service; perform scalp and hair analysis
- Shampoo and condition the hair using products appropriate for client's hair type

Air Forming Solid-Form Procedure

- Remove excess moisture
- Detangle hair
- Apply appropriate styling product and distribute through hair
- Section head
- Take horizontal parting across nape
- Use first few rows of 9-row brush to pick up hair lengths
- Dry base, midstrand and then ends
- Direct airflow on top of brush downward
- Work from center to either side.
- Position brush underneath hair
- Use same technique on subsequent horizontal partings, working up back of head from center to either side
- Use portion of previously air-formed section to blend bases
- Extend horizontal partings to front hairline
- Work to top using same techniques
- Direct the hair back off the face
- Position round brush underneath hair and rotate ends under at least one revolution
- Use same technique throughout design
- Use finishing procedures to style hair as desired

Air Forming Solid Form

1-2. Remove excess moisture from the hair using an absorbent terry cloth towel. Concentrate especially on the ends, which will tend to retain more moisture. **Detangle the hair** using a wide-tooth comb.

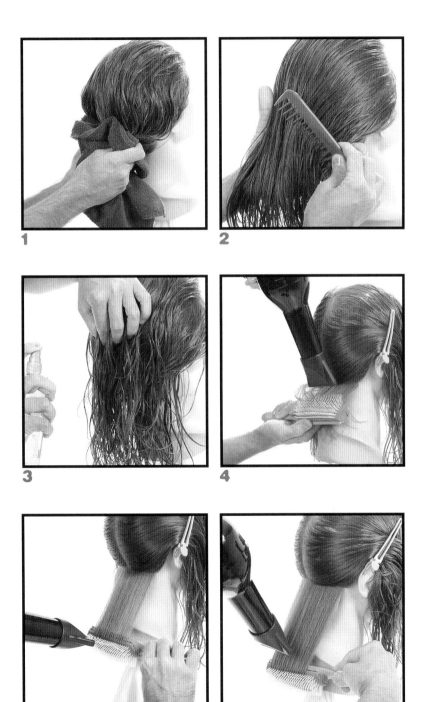

3. **Apply appropriate styling products and distribute through the hair.** In this case a medium-hold spray gel is used.

4. Section the head through the center from the front to the nape. In this case a slightly off-center part is used in the front. **Take a horizontal parting across the nape and use the first few rows of the 9-row brush to pick up the hair lengths.** The size of the parting is determined by the density of the hair. **Dry the base, midstrand and then the ends** using a low projection angle. **Direct the airflow on top of the brush downward,** keeping the cuticle layers smooth and compact for a shiny finish. **Work from the center to either side.**

5. Position the brush underneath the hair when the hair is approximately 90% dry, to create volume and turn the ends under. Note that the hair ends are curved under. A flipped-up effect would be achieved by positioning the brush on top of the ends and turning the ends upward.

6. Use the same technique on subsequent horizontal partings, working up the back of the head from the center to either side. Use a portion of the previously air formed section to blend the bases.

7-8. **Extend the horizontal partings to the front hairline** when you reach the area above the ears. Remember to alter the position of the brush as the hair becomes almost dry and turn the ends under. Work from the center to either side.

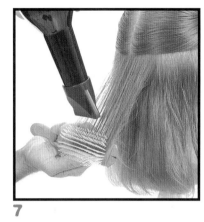

7

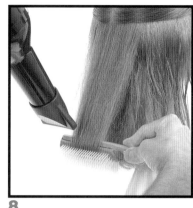

8

9. **Work to the top using the same techniques.**

10. **Direct the hair back off the face** slightly on the lighter side of the part.

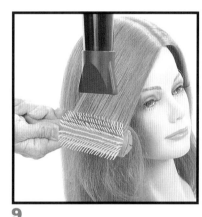

9

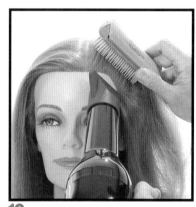

10

11-12. Use a metal-core round brush to impart more defined curved-under texture to the ends of the hair. **Position the round brush underneath the hair and rotate the ends at least one revolution. Use the same technique throughout the design** to create consistent curved-under texture. **Use finishing procedures to style the hair as desired.**

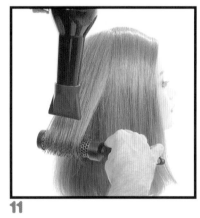

11

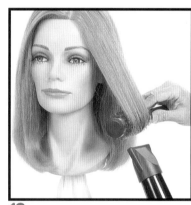

12

Air Forming Solid-Form Completion

- Offer your client a rebook visit
- Recommend retail products for your client
- Disinfect implements and clean work station
- Wash your hands with liquid antibacterial soap

Scrunching Layered Form

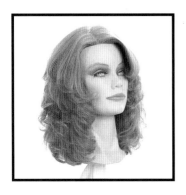

Not all thermal styling and air forming techniques require the use of brushes, partings and base controls. Beautiful finishes can be achieved on naturally wavy, curly or permed hair using the scrunching technique. The scrunching technique uses a nozzle attachment on the blow dryer, called a diffuser, which creates a softer, spread-out (diffused) airflow. The diffuser allows you to dry the hair while maintaining the curl formation. Manipulating the hair as little as possible while air forming will result in a stronger curl formation and reduce the possibility of frizziness.

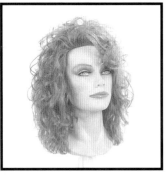

Your choice of styling products will be based on your client's hair type and the results that you wish to achieve. For this design, mousse was used for curl definition without excess weight. Speed and heat settings on the blow dryer can be adjusted according to the hair type. The finished design shows natural-looking, defined curl texture. More expansion in the form is achieved than natural air drying would have accomplished.

Scrunching Layered-Form Preparation

As with any professional service, it is important to have your area, products, implements and equipment in proper order. If the thermal styling service follows a haircutting service, note that most, if not all, of your preparation would have taken place prior to the haircut. This exercise assumes that the client is receiving only the thermal styling service. Before you begin the scrunching, layered-form procedure, be sure to satisfy the following points:

- Clean work station with disinfectant
- Arrange implements/supplies including blow dryer, diffuser, styling combs and appropriate styling products
- Ask the client to remove jewelry and store in a secure place
- Wash and sanitize hands; drape client for a wet service; perform scalp and hair analysis
- Shampoo and condition the hair using products appropriate for client's hair type
- Detangle and remove excess moisture from the hair

Scrunching: Layered-Form Procedure

- Distribute styling product through hair
- Attach diffuser
- Tilt head back
- Position diffuser beneath exterior strands
- Lift dryer up into lengths
- Lift hair at scalp with your fingers

- Dry ends, midstrand and then base
- Work toward interior and complete back using same techniques
- Tilt head to either side and use same techniques
- Work toward interior and complete using same techniques

Scrunching Layered Form

1-2. **Distribute styling product through the hair** lengths. In this case mousse is used. Dispense the product into your hand and gently rub your palms together. Then apply the product through the hair. You may wish to use a wide-tooth comb for more thorough distribution.

3. **Attach the diffuser** firmly to the nozzle of the blow dryer.

4. Tilt the head back to allow the hair to hang freely. Use a medium/high heat setting with a moderate airflow speed. **Position the diffuser beneath the exterior strands and lift the dryer up into the lengths. Lift the hair at the scalp with your fingers,** but do not manipulate the hair excessively. **Dry ends, midstrand and then base.** Proceed somewhat slowly, from one area to the next. **Work toward the interior and complete the back using the same techniques.**

5. **Tilt the head toward either side and use the same techniques** to dry the hair. Remember that increasing the heat, airflow speed and/or manipulating the hair may result in a less-defined curl pattern and frizziness.

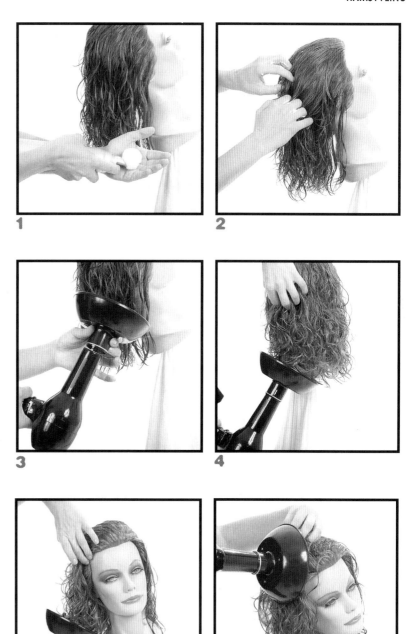

1

2

3

4

5

6

10

6. Note that the lengths should be lifted gently. **Work toward the interior and complete using the same techniques.**

Scrunching Layered-Form Completion

- Offer your client a rebook visit
- Recommend appropriate retail products to your client
- Disinfect implements and clean work station
- Wash hands with liquid antibacterial soap

Air Forming Graduated Form: Round Brush

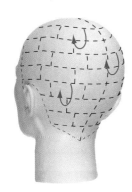

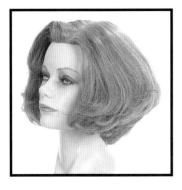

Air forming techniques performed with round brushes are used to highlight the combination of texture and natural expansion of the graduated form. Your choice of styling products will depend on your client's hair type, your own personal design preferences and your familiarity with the various products that are available. In this exercise a medium-hold styling lotion was used. The heat and airflow speed settings of the blow dryer should be adapted to the type of hair with which you are working.

Two different diameter metal-core round brushes are used to create volume and expansion. Initial moisture is first removed with a vent brush, which allows maximum air flow. A smaller diameter round brush is used in the nape and a larger diameter round brush is used to air form the rest of the design. A rake or wide-tooth comb is used to create texture definition, after the hair is completely dry. To accentuate the perimeter line of the haircut, horizontal partings are used in the nape and diagonal-forward partings are used through the upper back, top and sides. Off-base and half-off base control is used to allow less volume and base strength.

Air Forming Graduated Form: Round-Brush Preparation

As with all professional services, it is essential to have your area, products, implements and equipment in proper order. If the thermal styling service follows a haircutting service, note that most, if not all, of your preparation would have taken place prior to the haircut. This example assumes that the client is receiving only thermal styling. Before air forming the graduated form, be sure to satisfy the following points:

- Clean work station with disinfectant
- Arrange implements/supplies including blow dryer, vent brushes, various diameter metal-core round brushes, rake or wide-tooth comb and appropriate styling products
- Ask the client to remove jewelry and store in a secure place
- Wash and sanitize hands; drape client for a wet service; perform scalp and hair analysis
- Shampoo and condition the hair using products appropriate for the client's hair type.
- Towel dry and detangle the hair

Air Forming Graduated Form: Round-Brush Procedure

- Apply medium-hold styling lotion
- Use vent brush and airform hair to remove excess moisture
- Section hair for control
- Release horizontal parting across nape
- Begin with smaller diameter round brush
- Position brush underneath hair and rotate brush from ends to base
- Direct airflow above and below brush

- Work from center to either side
- Use portion of previously air-formed section and a bricklay pattern to blend bases as you work up through nape
- Work from center to either side to complete nape lengths
- Switch to larger diameter round brush on longer lengths
- Extend slightly diagonal forward partings to front hairline
- Continue to use volume base control with round brush
- Stagger bases as you work from center to front hairline on either side
- Position brush parallel to parting
- Continue to use same techniques as you work to top of head
- Complete volume base control with round brush
- Use finishing procedures to style as desired

Air Forming Graduated Form: Round Brush

1. **Apply a medium-hold styling lotion** throughout the hair. Distribute the hair straight back. **Use a vent brush and air form the hair to remove excess moisture.** Work from the front hairline to the back using diagonal back partings. Set the blow dryer on medium heat and high-speed airflow. Work quickly throughout the hair.

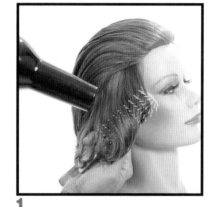

1

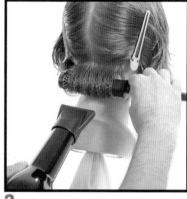

2

2. **Section the hair for control** from the front hairline to the nape. In this case, the front will be slightly off-center. **Release a horizontal parting across the nape and begin with the smaller diameter round brush. Position the brush underneath the hair and rotate the brush from the ends to the base** to create volume. **Direct the airflow above and below the brush** to ensure good curl formation. Use an off-base volume control with a round brush and **work from the center to either side.**

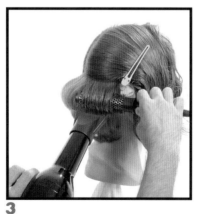

3

3. **Use a portion of the previously air-formed section and a bricklay pattern to blend the bases as you work up through the nape.** Use half-off base volume control with a round brush. **Work from the center to either side to complete the nape lengths.**

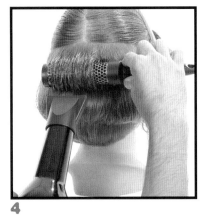

4

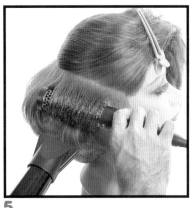

5

4. Switch to a larger diameter round brush on the longer lengths. When you reach the area above the ear, **extend slightly diagonal forward partings to the front hairline. Continue to use volume base control with a round brush.** Note that the brush is positioned horizontally in the center back to blend between the two diagonal forward lines.

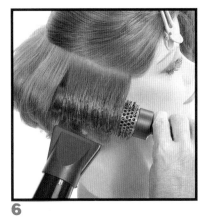

6

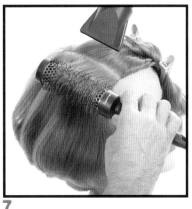

7

5-6. Stagger the bases as you work from the center to the front hairline on either side. Position the brush parallel to the parting and direct the airflow from the top and the bottom of the brush and continue positioning the brush half-off base.

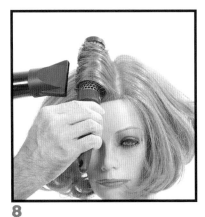

8

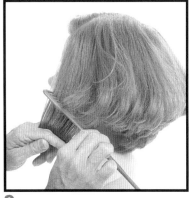

9

7-8. Continue to use the same techniques as you work to the top of the head. Note that the brush is not placed on its base at any point in the air-forming procedure. Excessive volume could distort the shape of the graduated form and lessen the degree of textural contrast. **Complete volume base control with a round brush.**

9-10. Use finishing procedures to style as desired. You may wish to use a wide-tooth comb to backcomb slightly for expansion, especially in the exterior.

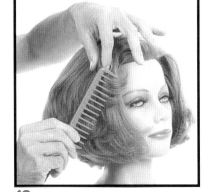

10

Air Forming Graduated Form: Round-Brush Completion

- Offer your client a rebook visit
- Recommend retail products to your client
- Disinfect implements and clean work station
- Wash your hands with liquid antibacterial soap

Air Forming Layered Form: Round Brush

In this style, the hair is directed back off the face without a part. A progression of base controls creates a progression of volume and a medium-diameter, round brush is used to achieve the repetition of curl texture. Horizontal, diagonal forward and vertical partings are used and bases are staggered within each parting for blending.

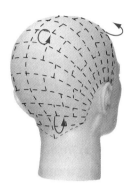 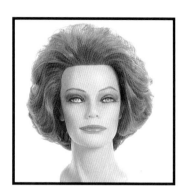

The styling products you choose will depend on your client's hair texture and the amount of support you need to successfully air form this design. Airflow speed and heat settings will be determined by the client's hair type.

Air Forming Layered Form: Round-Brush Preparation

As always, it is necessary to have your area, products, implements and equipment in proper order. This exercise assumes that the client has come in only for the thermal styling. If a haircutting service had preceded the thermal styling, your preparation would have been completed prior to the haircut.

- Clean work station with disinfectant
- Arrange implements/supplies including blow dryer, round brushes, wide-tooth comb and appropriate styling products
- Ask the client to remove jewelry and store in a secure place
- Wash and sanitize hands; drape client for a wet service; perform scalp and hair analysis
- Shampoo and condition the hair using product appropriate for client's hair type
- Towel dry and detangle hair

Air Forming Layered Form: Round-Brush Procedure

- Apply styling product
- Use vent brush and remove moisture from hair
- Section head for control
- Release horizontal parting across nape
- Position brush underneath hair and rotate brush upward
- Dry base, midstrand and ends
- Work from center to either side using volume base control

- Use diagonal forward partings as you work up back of head
- Use portion of previously air-formed section and stagger bases
- Use vertical partings as you work toward crown
- Overdirect the fringe for exaggerated volume
- Use finishing procedures and style as desired

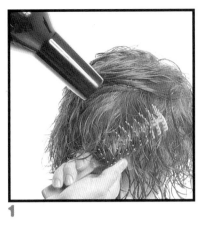

1

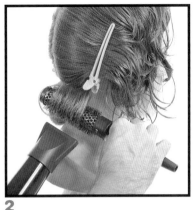

2

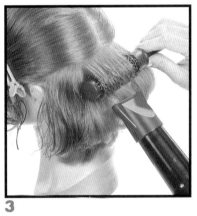

3

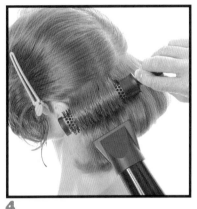

4

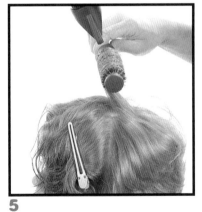

5

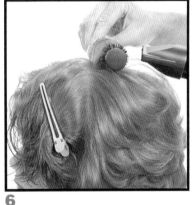

6

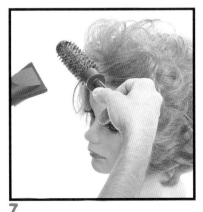

7

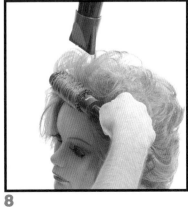

8

Air Forming Layered Form: Round Brush

1. **Apply a styling product** such as mousse. **Use a vent brush and remove the majority of the moisture from the hair.** Set the blow dry on medium heat and airflow. Work quickly throughout the hair.

2. **Section the head for control** down the center from the front hairline to the nape. Then **release a horizontal parting across the nape. Position the brush underneath the hair and rotate the brush upward. Dry the base, midstrand and ends.** Position the brush half-off base. **Work from the center to either side, using volume base control.**

3-4. **Use diagonal forward partings as you work up the back of the head. Use a portion of the previously air-formed section and stagger the bases** to avoid splits. Work from the center to either side.

5-6. **Use vertical partings as you work toward the crown and continue** to use volume base control with a round brush. Use on-base control at the upper crown for maximum volume. Direct the airflow from above and below the brush to ensure strong curl formation.

7-8. Stand in front of the client and **overdirect the fringe for exaggerated volume** and dimension in the design. Direct the airflow from the front and back of the brush.

9–10. Backcomb the hair for support. **Use finishing procedures and style as desired.**

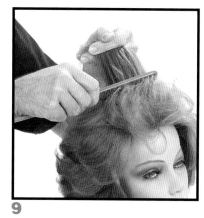

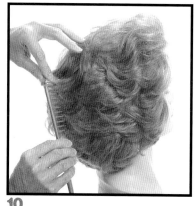

9

10

Air Forming Layered Form: Round-Brush Completion

- Offer your client a rebook visit
- Recommend retail products to your client
- Disinfect implements and clean work station
- Wash your hands with liquid antibacterial soap

Air Forming Combination Form: 9-Row Brush

Combination forms with shorter interior lengths can be styled in any number of ways. Depending upon the client's wishes, the hair can be styled with or without a parting. The hair may also be styled away from the face or toward the face.

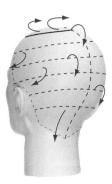

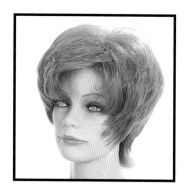

In this exercise, the nape lengths are air formed for closeness while the hair at the front hairline is air formed toward the face from an off-center parting. A 9-row brush is used to create volume, while a round brush is used to achieve additional curved end volume texture throughout.

Air Forming Combination Form: 9-Row Brush Preparation

As with any professional service, it is important to have your area, products, implements and equipment in proper order. Before performing a thermal styling service, be sure to satisfy the following points:

- Clean work station with disinfectant
- Arrange implements/supplies including 9-row brush, round brush, large-tooth comb, sectioning clips, styling and finishing products

- Ask the client to remove jewelry and store in a secure place
- Wash and sanitize hands; drape client for a wet service; perform scalp and hair analysis
- Shampoo and condition the hair with the appropriate products for client's hair type
- Towel dry the hair to remove excess moisture

Air Forming Combination Form: 9-Row Brush Procedure

- Find natural part
- Section back in half
- Position 9-row brush on top of nape lengths and air form
- Above nape, begin at center
- Position brush underneath hair
- Take slight diagonal-forward partings and work from center to behind ear
- Use portion of previous partings and continue to work toward crown
- At sides, use same techniques from horizontal partings
- At front hairline, position brush underneath hair and direct lengths toward face
- Continue to work upward using same techniques
- Lift hair along parting with first few rows of brush
- Repeat same procedures on opposite side
- Use round brush throughout interior
- Use finishing procedures to style hair as desired

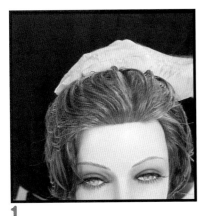

1

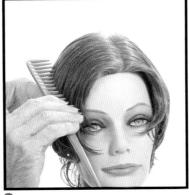

2

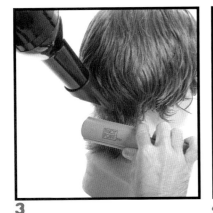

3

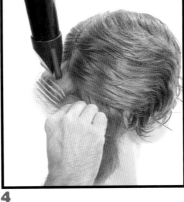

4

Air Forming Combination Form: 9-Row Brush

1-2. Distribute the hair straight back. Push the hair forward to **find the natural part.** Then distribute the hair from the parting.

3. Section the back in half. Position a 9-row brush on top of the nape lengths and air form the lengths to conform to the curve of the head. Direct the air flow to follow the brush.

4. Above the nape, begin at the center and position the brush underneath the hair to create volume end texture. **Take slight diagonal-forward partings and work from the center to behind the ear.**

5. Use a portion of the previous partings and continue to work toward the **crown** using the same techniques.

6. At the sides, use the same techniques from horizontal partings.

7. At the front hairline, position the brush underneath the hair and direct the lengths forward toward the face.

8. Continue to work upward using the same techniques. **Lift the hair along the parting with the first few rows of the brush** to create additional volume.

9. Repeat the same procedures on the opposite side.

10. Use a round brush throughout the **interior** to create additional volume and end texture.

11-12. Lightly backcomb the hair and **use finishing procedures to style the hair as desired.**

Air Forming Combination Form: 9-Row Brush Completion

- Offer your client a rebook visit
- Recommend retail products to your client
- Disinfect implements and clean work station
- Wash hands with liquid antibacterial soap

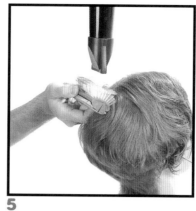
5

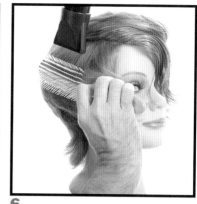
6

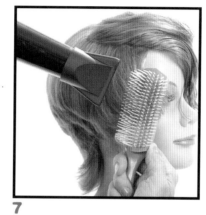
7

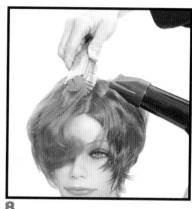
8

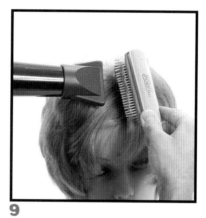
9

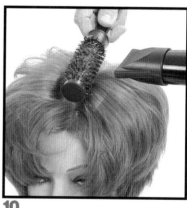
10

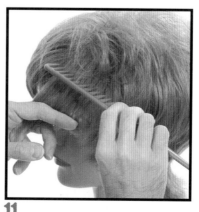
11

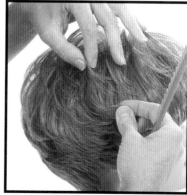
12

1
0

Air Forming Combination Form: Round Brush/Curling Iron

Combination forms with shorter interior lengths are ideal for creating styles that move away or toward the face with or without a part. In this exercise a 9-row brush is used first to create curved end texture along with movement and direction back away from the face. Volume round-brush techniques are then used to create curved end texture and to prepare for the curling-iron techniques. A progression of base controls from diminishing volume at the nape, maximum volume at the crown and overdirected volume at the front hairline is used.

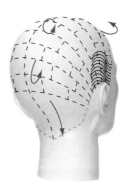
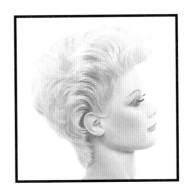

Air Forming Combination Form: Round-Brush/Curling-Iron Preparation

As with any professional service, it is important to have your area, products, implements and equipment in proper order. Before performing a thermal styling service, be sure to satisfy the following points:

- Clean work station with disinfectant
- Arrange implements/supplies including blow dryer, 9-row brush, round brush, curling iron, large-tooth comb, sectioning clips, styling and finishing products
- Ask the client to remove jewelry and store in a secure place
- Wash and sanitize hands; drape client for a wet service; perform scalp and hair analysis
- Shampoo and condition the hair with the appropriate products for the client's hair type
- Towel dry and detangle the hair

Air Forming Combination Form: Round-Brush/Curling-Iron Procedure

- Section hair
- Use 9-row brush to air form nape lengths
- Above nape, work from center to either side from horizontal partings
- Lift hair at scalp to create volume, then position brush underneath the hair to create curved end texture
- Work upward using same techniques from diagonal forward and vertical partings
- Direct hair away from face
- Work toward front using same techniques from vertical partings
- At front sides, create curvature movement away from face

- Complete front sides
- Create volume curved end texture in back using a round brush
- Work toward crown using progression of volume base controls
- Create maximum volume at crown and top
- Overdirect hair at fringe area
- Begin at back for curling-iron techniques
- On shorter lengths, create curved end texture
- Create progression of volume curling-iron base controls as you work upward
- Use portion of previous curl as you work from horizontal partings at center to diagonal partings at sides
- Progress to maximum-volume base control at crown
- Continue to use maximum-volume base control as you work from center top to sides
- Use overdirected-base control at fringe area
- Use finishing procedures and style hair as desired

Air Forming Combination Form: Round-Brush/Curling-Iron

1-2. Section the hair from the center front hairline to the occipital for control. **Use a 9-row brush to air form the nape lengths** to conform to the curve of the head. **Above the nape, work from the center to either side from horizontal partings** to create curved end texture. **Lift the hair at the scalp to create volume, then position the brush underneath the hair to create curved end texture. Work upward using the same techniques from diagonal forward and vertical partings. Direct the hair away from the face. Work toward the front using the same techniques from vertical partings.**

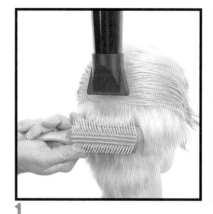
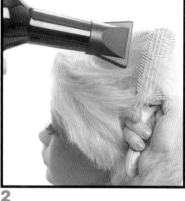
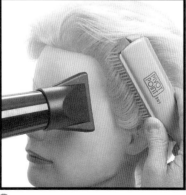
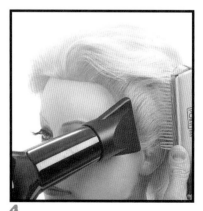

3-4. At the front sides, create a curvature movement that moves away from the face. To create an oblong, position the teeth of the brush at the front hairline and create parallel curved lines. Direct the airflow into the curved lines. Create another set of parallel curved lines behind the first oblong in the opposite direction. **Complete the front sides.**

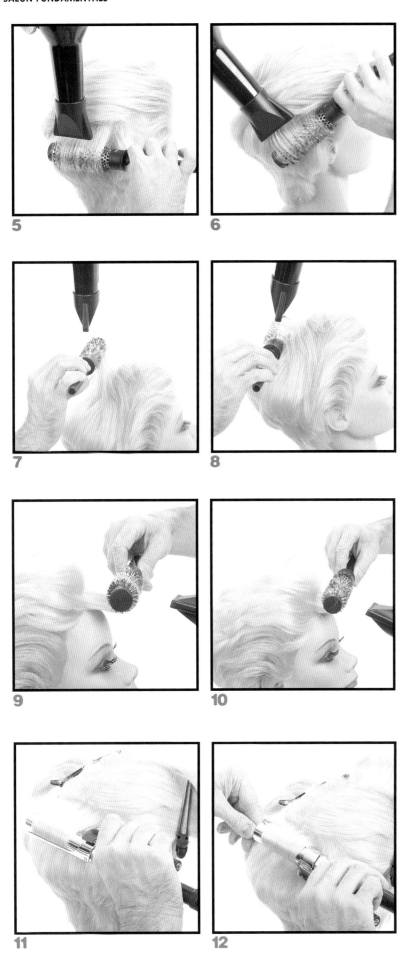

5

6

7

8

9

10

11

12

5-6. Create volume curved end texture in the back using a round brush. Begin at crest area and use half-off base control from horizontal and diagonal partings.

7-8. Work toward the crown using a progression of volume base controls. Create maximum volume at the crown and top.

9-10. Overdirect the hair at the fringe area for exaggerated direction and volume.

11-12. Begin at the back for the curling-iron techniques. On the shorter lengths, create curved end texture. Then create a progression of volume curling-iron base controls as you work upward. Begin with diminished volume and progress to maximum volume. Position the comb underneath the curling iron to protect the scalp. Use only a hard rubber or nonflammable comb. Avoid having the ends of the hair protrude over the iron, which will cause hair to bend (referred to as fishhook ends).

Remember, double-processed hair is more fragile and additional care is required. Use thermal-protectant products and avoid high temperatures from the blow dryer and iron.

13-14. Use a portion of the previous curl as you work from horizontal partings at the center to diagonal partings at the sides to blend the curls and avoid splits.

15-16. Progress to maximum-volume base control at the crown.

17-18. Continue to use maximum-volume base control as you work from the center top to the sides.

19-20. Use overdirected-base control at the fringe area for exaggerated volume and direction. Position the curls in a bricklay pattern to avoid splits in the finished design.

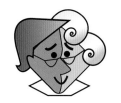

"Using a curling iron after round-brush techniques reinforces the curl pattern."

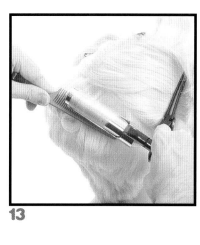

13

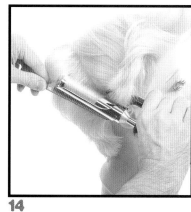

14

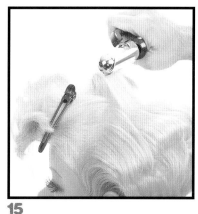

15

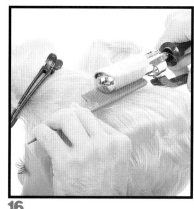

16

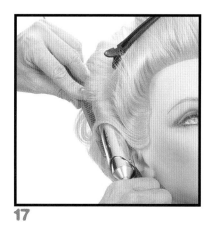

17

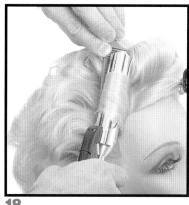

18

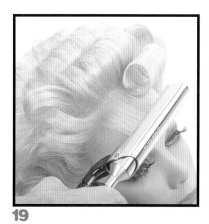

19

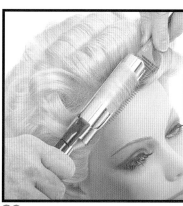

20

1 0

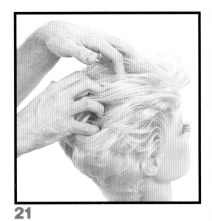

21

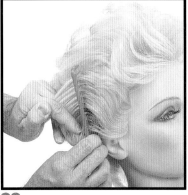

22

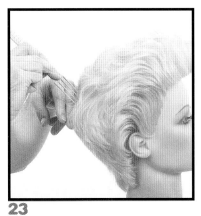

23

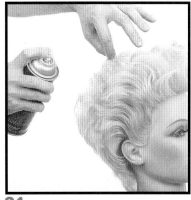

24

21-24. Use finishing procedures and style the hair as desired.

Air Forming Combination Form: Round-Brush/Curling-Iron Completion

- Offer your client a rebook visit
- Recommend retail products to your client
- Disinfect implements and clean work station
- Wash hands with liquid antibacterial soap

Pressing and Curling

Pressing and curling is a natural way to straighten overly curly hair for clients who want to avoid chemicals as well as for children. Once the hair has been pressed straight, it can be curled with marcel irons in any design desired. It is important to plan your style before you begin pressing. Determine if a center or side part is included or if the hair will be worn back off the face. You will want to press the hair to support the final direction it will be worn, especially around the face.

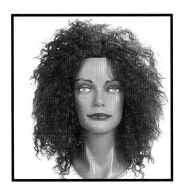

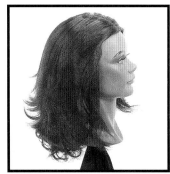

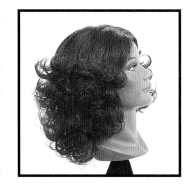

Pressing and Curling Preparation

As with any professional service, it is important to have your area, products, implements and equipment in proper order. Before performing a press-and-curl service, be sure to satisfy the following points:

- Clean work station with disinfectant
- Arrange implements/supplies including blow dryer, 9-row brush, pressing comb, marcel irons, conventional thermal iron stove, large-tooth comb, molding comb, sectioning clips, pressing oil, styling and finishing products
- Ask client to remove jewelry and store in a secure place
- Wash and sanitize hands; drape client for a wet service; perform scalp and hair analysis
- Shampoo and condition the hair with the appropriate products for your client
- Towel dry and detangle the hair

Pressing and Curling Procedure

- Section hair for air forming
- Air form to reduce natural curl pattern
- Section hair for thermal pressing
- Apply pressing oil
- Test temperature of pressing comb
- Insert teeth of pressing comb underneath parting
- Turn comb and press hair with spine as you work from base to ends

- Feed hair slowly through comb as you work down toward the ends
- Complete back using horizontal partings
- Press the front using diagonal partings
- Press hairline last
- Heat marcel irons
- Test the temperature of the irons
- Curl hair as desired
- Complete the combout style

1 0

Pressing and Curling

1-2. Section the hair for air forming. Use a four or five-section pattern depending on your desired style. **Air form the hair to reduce the natural curl pattern.** Use large sub-divisions and apply tension to stretch the hair as you dry it. Work from the bottom to the top of each section.

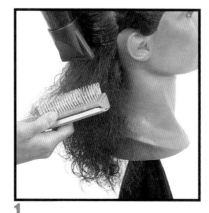

1

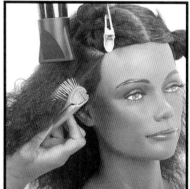

2

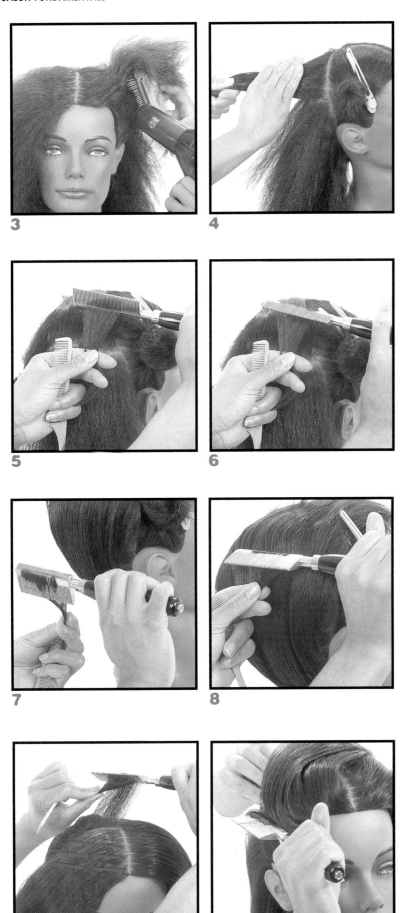

3

4

5

6

7

8

9

10

3. Air form the front sections and blend to the back. Air form the front hairline away from the face. Complete air forming.

4. **Section the hair to prepare for the thermal pressing techniques.** Subdivide the hair from the center front hairline to the nape and from ear to ear. **Apply pressing oil** to the first section.

5-6. **Test the temperature of the pressing comb.** Begin at the top of one of the back sections. Use a tail comb and take a 1/4" (.75 cm) horizontal parting. **Insert the teeth of the pressing comb underneath the parting** near the base. Control the ends of the hair with your opposite hand. **Turn the comb and press the hair with the spine of the comb as you work from the base to** the ends. **Feed the hair slowly through the comb as you work down toward the ends.** Repeat this technique twice for each new subsection. Increase the amount of pressure applied on coarse or extremely curly hair.

7-8. Work toward the bottom of the section, pressing the hair upward, away from you. **Complete the back using horizontal partings.**

9-10. **Press the front using diagonal partings.** Begin at the top of the section. Press away from you. Repeat the same procedures to complete the side sections. Remember that the back or spine of the comb does the majority of the pressing.

11-12. **Press the hairline last.** Once the hair is completely pressed you may perform a haircut. if desired. It is easier to control the lengths once they're straight. Curling the hair with marcel irons is optional.

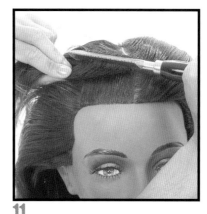
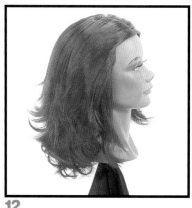

11
12

13-14. **Heat the marcel irons** you wish to use. Section the hair according to the desired style. The same four sections used for air forming are repeated here to create the indentation curls featured in this style. **Test the temperature of the iron. Curl the hair**, choosing the setting pattern that will achieve the results desired. Silk down the lengths of the hair and turn the ends upward slightly. Complete the back using horizontal partings.

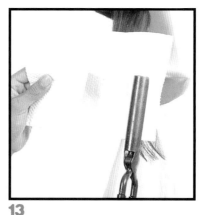
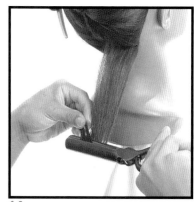

13
14

15-16. Repeat the indentation pattern on the sides. working upward to the center part. **Complete the combout.**

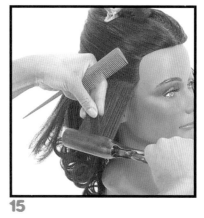
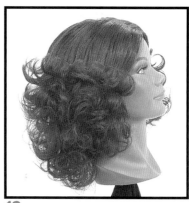

15
16

Pressing and Curling Completion

- Offer your client a rebook visit
- Recommend retail products to your client
- Disinfect implements and clean work space
- Wash hands with liquid antibacterial soap

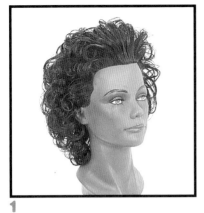

1

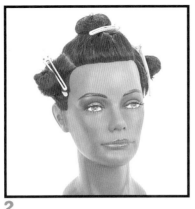

2

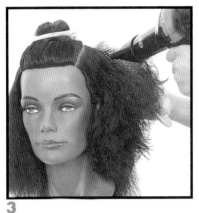

3

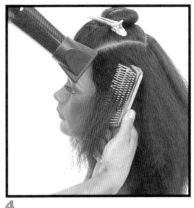

4

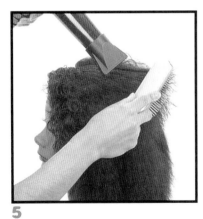

5

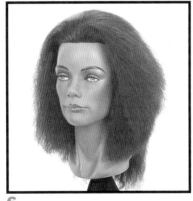

6

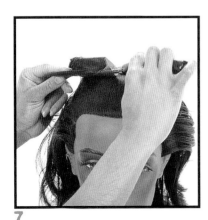

7

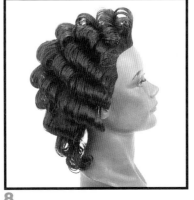

8

Press and Curl Variation: No Part

1-2. For styles that move back off the face or when a part is not desired, a five-section air-forming and pressing pattern offers maximum control.

3-4. Divide the back with a center part and separate the top from the sides. Air forming is completed in the back first, then the sides and, finally, the top.

5-6. Direct top lengths back off the face and complete the air forming. Make sure the hair is completely dry before pressing to avoid burning the scalp. If a haircut is included in the service, it would be performed now.

7-8. Pressing is done the same way as the previous exercise, except in the top area. Here, press the top lengths backward, beginning in the back of the section and working toward the front hairline. **Marcel curling in a bricklay pattern** completes the set.

WET STYLING

Wet styling refers to the area of hairstyling in which the hair is manipulated into the desired shapes and movements while wet then allowed to dry. Wet styling includes molded designs such as fingerwave designs, roller sets and pincurl sets. Once the hair is 'set,' it is allowed to dry completely. Then it is finished using any combination of combs, brushes and/or fingers, in combination with additional liquid tools if desired. Wet setting generally results in the firmest set and the longest-lasting results. In determining the style that will work best and be the most flattering for your client, you will need to consider lifestyle, hair type and the factors discussed in the chapter titled "Design Decisions." Your review of wet hairstyling in this chapter will include fingerwaving, pincurls and roller placements (setting).

Fingerwaves

As an artist, the professional stylist can create beautiful hairstyles using a minimum of tools, relying primarily on his/her skill and dexterity in manipulating the hair for artistic effect. **Fingerwaving, the art of shaping and defining the hair in graceful waves,** is an ageless form of hair design. Once popular for everyday wear, fingerwaves are now most often used in conjunction with other styling techniques.

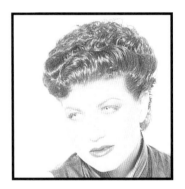

By learning to fingerwave, you're discovering a creative technique for moving and directing hair, using the most basic tools: your own fingers, a comb, waving lotion and hair pins. You're also developing dexterity, coordination and strength in your fingers as you mold and hold the waves. Finally, you're exercising your visual imagination as you design wave patterns to follow the curves of the head.

A complete understanding of the correct fingerwaving procedure is necessary to accurately create a fluid movement or balanced design. The ability to create soft, natural wave movements is a talent that must be developed early in your cosmetology career. Mastery of fingerwaving will give you the foundation you need for all wave patterns. Take the time and exert the effort needed to learn these important procedures.

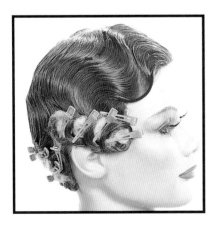

A fingerwave is created by two complete oblong shapings that are joined and connected by a ridge. View the photo to the left. The open end of the oblong is identified by a dashed line and the closed end by a solid line. Notice how the shaping creates a series of parallel curved lines. Also, notice the **hollow (recess) and the ridge (high ledge) areas of each wave-movement. Pinching or pushing the ridge will create overdirection of the wave. Finger waves with low ridges are known as shadow waves.**

10

Pincurls

Pincurls, also known as sculpture curls, are one of many ways you are able to temporarily change the direction and texture of the hair. Generally pincurls are used on straight, permed, or naturally curly hair that has been properly tapered. Pincurls are not recommended to be used on overly curly hair. Used primarily to create long-lasting effects or specialized closeness, pincurls allow a wide range of movement. Forming pincurls relies on your dexterity and smooth handling of the hair to create clean, smoothly wound curls, without the use of a tool such as a roller, to control the consistency of the curl shape. If the pincurls are not smooth, the resulting curl or wave will not be smooth.

Components of a Pincurl

A section of hair that forms a pincurl is commonly described in three parts, the base, the stem (arc) and the circle.

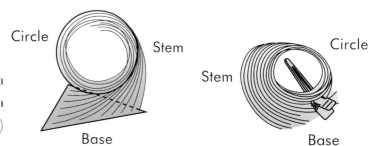

The base of the pincurl is the area of the strand at the scalp between partings within a shape. Pincurl bases may be straight or curved.

The stem (arc) is the beginning portion of the strand that demonstrates the direction of the curl (between base and first turn). The stem determines the amount of movement a pincurl will have.

The circle is the remaining end of the strand that forms the curl. The size of the circle determines the width and strength of the wave. A closed circle will produce a much smaller and stronger wave, for a fluffy effect. An open circle will produce a wider wave pattern with uniform curls.

Types of Pincurls

Consultating with your client will help you determine where she wants or needs lift (volume) and where a closer effect is desired. The three common types of pincurls are flat (sculpture curls), volume (stand-up curls) and indentation.

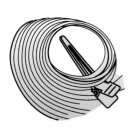
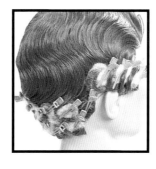

Flat Pincurls

With flat pincurls the base, stem (arc) and circle are flat. Flat pincurls are used for closeness. Since the hair does not travel any distance from the base before the arc begins, the result is a no-stem curl.

With volume pincurls the base and stem (arc) are lifted away from the head and the circle turns under. Volume pincurls are used to create fullness and height. They can be positioned anywhere on the head. Volume pincurls are also referred to as stand-up or cascade pincurls. Barrel curls are large stand-up pincurls, achieving a similar effect to hair wound around a roller, but resulting in weaker (less) volume.

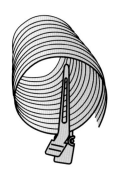
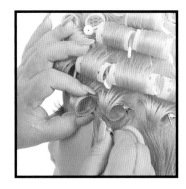
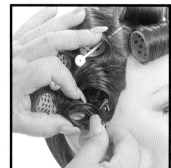

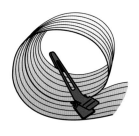
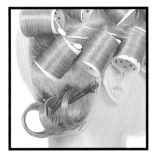

With indentation pincurls the base is flat and the stem (arc) and circle are lifted. Indentation pincurls are used to create hollow space and flare. Generally, indentation pincurls follow volume pincurls in a hairstyle.

In some instances, you will need to create a blend or transition from areas of volume to areas of closeness. Transitional or semi-stand-up pincurls will achieve this blend. These pincurls are not quite stand-up curls and not quite flat curls.

Pincurl Base Shapes

Various shaped bases are used when working with pincurls. The primary reason for this variation of base shapes is to avoid splits in the finished hairstyle. Generally, straight-shaped bases are used within straight shapes and curved-shaped bases are used within curved shapes. Pincurl base shapes that are used most often are triangle, square, rectangle and crescent.

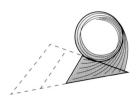

Triangle: Used within straight shapes, and along the hairline; alternating triangles helps to avoid splits

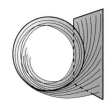

Square/Rectangle: Usually used within an overall square shape.

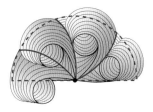

Crescent: Also known as arc, curved, half-moon or C-shaped base; used within curvature shapes such as circles and oblongs. Curvature or carved pincurls are curls that are carved from a curved shaping.

Keeping bases consistent within a shape will allow you to work with equal amounts of hair in each pincurl and therefore have more consistent results in your finished curls and waves.

Base Control - Pincurls

The sizes of pincurl bases are usually related to the diameter of the circle which, in turn, determines the resulting wave or curl. Pincurl base control refers to the size of the base in relation to the size of the circle or curl and the position of the curl relative to the base. The size of the base and the base control used will affect the length of the stem of each pincurl. The length of the stem will determine the movement of the curl. The base controls that are most often used are on base (no stem), half-off base (half-stem), off base (full stem), underdirected and overdirected.

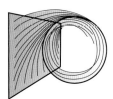

On Base (no stem)

A correct on-base control requires that the entire circle of the curl be positioned on the base. This base control is used to produce a lift or strong curl effect or, when used in a series, to create a strong wave line.

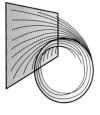
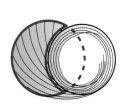

Half-Off Base (half-stem)

Notice that in a correct half-off base control, half of the circle is positioned below the base and pick-up line. This base control is used when an equal degree of predetermined direction and volume is required.

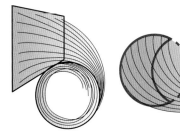

Off Base (full-stem)

With off-base control, the stem and circle are positioned below the base and pick-up line. This base control is used when design closeness and mobility is required, usually in the nape area or along the hairline.

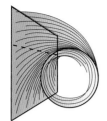

With **underdirected** base control the circle sits on the lower portion of the base. This base control is used to create reduced volume.

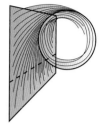

With **overdirected** base control, the circle sits in the upper portion of the base. This base control is used to create exaggerated direction.

Flat, Volume and Indentation Pincurls

Flat, volume and indentation pincurls are set within an alternating oblong pattern to create closeness, fullness and dimension. Flat pincurls are used to create closeness. The base, stem (arc) and circle are flat. Volume pincurls are used to create fullness. The base and stem are lifted and the circle turns under. Indentation pincurls are used to create a hollow space and flare. The base is flat while the stem and circle are lifted.

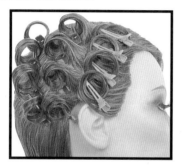
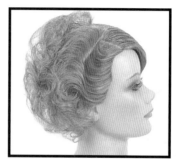

Flat Pincurls

To create a flat pincurl, a clockwise oblong is first molded at the front hairline. Flat pincurls begin at the concave end of the shape. A tail comb is used to part the hair from the center of the shape in the second direction or toward the concave end. The hair is then smoothed to create a ribbon like effect. The base remains flat while the stem is curved and the circle is formed. The flat pincurl is secured in the second direction. This technique is repeated until the remaining shape is completed.

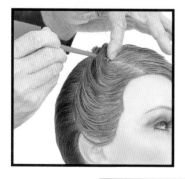
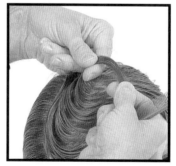
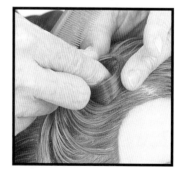
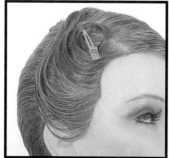
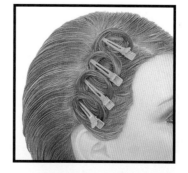

Volume Pincurls

To create a volume pincurl, a counterclockwise oblong is molded first. Volume pincurls begin at the convex end of the shape. A tail comb is used to part the hair toward the first direction or convex end. The comb is used to create lift at the base and to reinforce the stem. The circle is then formed. The volume pincurl is secured inside the circle in the first direction or convex end of the shape. This technique is repeated until the remaining shape is completed.

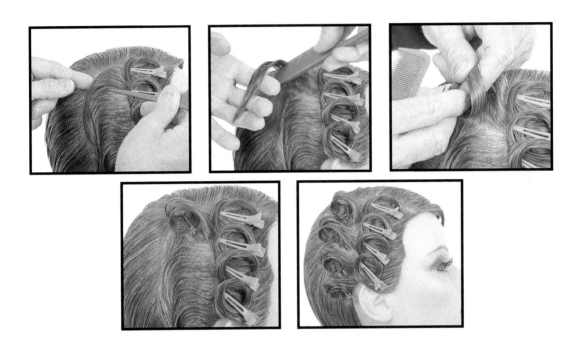

Indentation Pincurls

To create an indentation pincurl, a clockwise oblong is molded first. Indentation pincurls begin at the concave end of the shape. A tail comb is used to part the hair from the center of the shape in the second direction. The index finger is used to keep the base flat while curving the stem with the comb. The circle is the then formed up and away from the base. The indentation pincurl is secured through the circle in the second direction. This technique is repeated until the entire shape is completed.

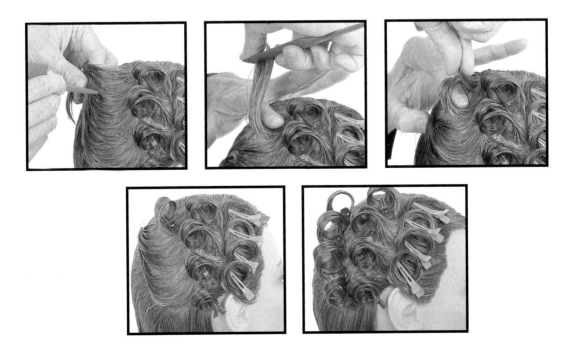

Skip Waves

A wave pattern that combines fingerwaves and flat pincurls is called a skip wave. The first oblong remains molded (skipped) and the next oblong is set in flat pincurls. Skip waves achieve wide, deep-flowing waves and are generally positioned on the side of the head, either vertically or horizontally. **One oblong followed by a row of pincurls is called a ridge curl.** An alternation consisting of at least two oblongs and two rows of pincurls creates a skip wave and produces a strong wave pattern.

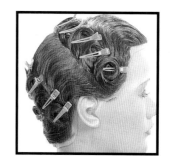 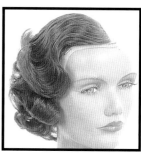

Skip Waves with Flat Pincurls

Skip waves are composed of alternating oblongs connected by a ridge. One of the oblongs is molded and the other is set with pincurls or rollers. The oblong that is set supports the molded shape and gives more dimension to the design. The pattern is repeated in order to create a series of skip waves. Flat, volume or indentation pincurls can be used to create a variety of undulating patterns. Here, flat pincurls are used to create a wave pattern with alternating oblongs that blend and flow in a curvature movement.

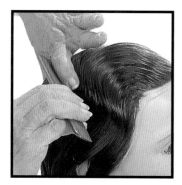 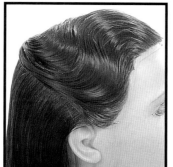

Mold two oblongs with a connecting ridge. The first shape travels in a counterclockwise direction and the second oblong travels clockwise.

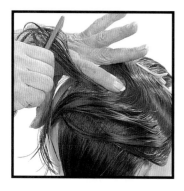 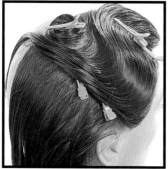

Set flat pincurls in the second oblong. Begin setting at the open or concave end. Do not disturb the shapes or the ridge as you position the pincurls.

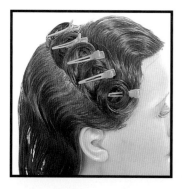 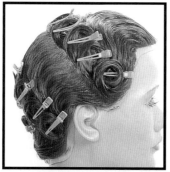

Complete the row of pincurls. Mold two more oblongs. Leave the first oblong undisturbed and set the second in flat pincurls. Dry the hair completely before combing this pattern out.

Rollers

Rollers are used to set the hair and can achieve many of the same effects that are achieved with pincurls. So why would you choose rollers over pincurls? For starters, one roller, depending on its length, sets the same amount of hair as two to four stand-up pincurls. This means that your setting time can be greatly reduced. Secondly, setting with rollers allows you to set the hair with tension, which will result in a firmer, longer-lasting set. Earlier in this chapter, you learned about the components of a roller curl as well as the various base controls that are used when setting the hair on rollers. Now you'll look at some additional points that you will need to know in order to create easy-to-finish roller hairstyles.

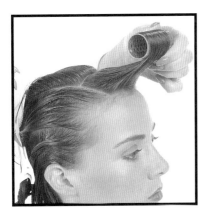
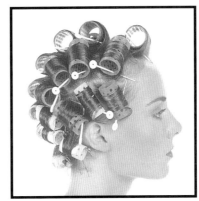
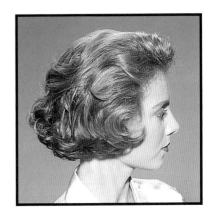

Roller Diameter

The diameter of rollers, just like the diameters of round brushes or curling irons, are chosen according to the desired curl pattern. Smaller rollers usually produce curlier effects, but the exact results will vary according to the length of your client's hair.

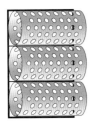

Rollers in Straight Shapes

Cylindrical rollers are usually used within straight shapes such as rectangles and triangles. Within a rectangle, rollers of the same length are used to encompass the shape. Depending on the desired result, the roller diameter you choose can create repetition, alternation or even a progression of curl.

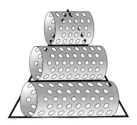

Within a triangle shape, the length of the rollers used will progress from short to long to encompass the shape from the narrow end to the wide end, or a bricklay pattern may be used.

To set a straight shape, the diameter and length of the roller are used to measure the base size. Next, the hair is distributed and projected according to the desired base control. The hair is then wrapped around the roller, which is rolled with even tension to the base and secured.

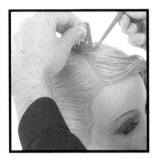 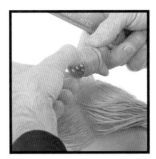 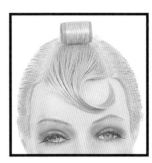 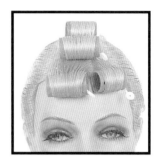

Rollers in Curvature shapes

The most efficient way to set rollers within a curvature shape is to use cone-shaped or conical rollers. These rollers, sometimes called tapered rollers, are narrower at one end and wider at the other. Because of the way conical rollers fit into a curvature shape, they allow you to create a stronger curvature movement. It is essential to know how the application of cone-shaped rollers within a curved shaped differs from setting cylindrical rollers within a straight shape.

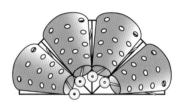

Within circular shapes, such as a half circle, the roller sits one diameter away from the point of origin (point from which the movement radiates). You will use the smaller end of the roller to measure this diameter. The base is, therefore, the length of the roller plus one diameter. The outside of the base is the same width as the larger diameter of the roller. When setting the hair using cone-shaped rollers, angle the smaller end of the roller toward the point of origin, then roll toward the back of the shape.

10

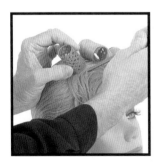 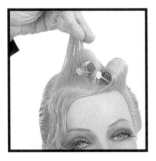 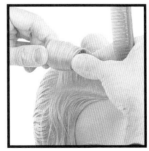 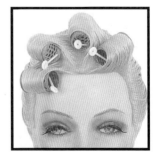

When setting the hair using cone-shaped rollers within an oblong, the rollers sit diagonally within the shape. Measure the base size using the larger end of the cone roller. Create the molded oblong using the roller positioned at a 45° angle.

Wet Styling Procedure Overview

Once you understand the theory behind wet hair styling, you are ready to use your knowledge and apply it to the medium of hair. The following wet hairstyles will be demonstrated in this section of the "Hairstyling" chapter. By understanding wet hairstyling techniques such as how to mold the hair and create straight and curvature volume with pincurls and rollers, as well as finishing techniques, you will be able to create a multitude of designs.

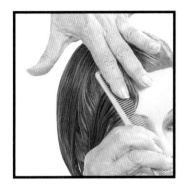 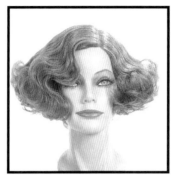

Fingerwaves and Flat Pincurls

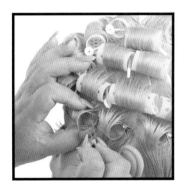 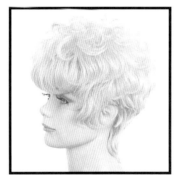

Straight Volume Rollers and Pincurls

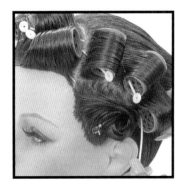 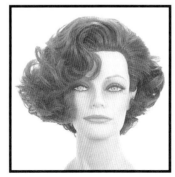

Curvature Volume Rollers and Pincurls

Fingerwaves and Flat Pincurls

Molded fingerwaves or alternating oblongs are timeless and classic. They can be performed throughout the entire head, a portion of the head or combined with pincurls and rollers. The proportions of each texture can vary according to the amount of expansion desired.

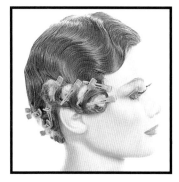 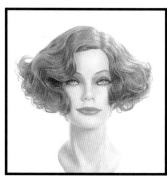

In this exercise, molded horizontal fingerwaves from a side part in the interior are combined with flat pincurls along the perimeter hairline. The finished style shows a flowing wave pattern combined with curl texture that is achieved from the flat pincurls. Prior to beginning the fingerwave design, you should have a mental vision of the proportion of fingerwaves to pincurls. Visualizing the proportions will help you decide where to end the fingerwaves and where to begin the pincurls.

Fingerwaves and Flat-Pincurls Preparation

As with any professional service, it is important to have your area, products, implements and equipment in proper order. Before performing a fingerwave and pincurl exercise, be sure to satisfy the following points:

- Clean work station with disinfectant
- Arrange implements/supplies including molding comb, tail comb, large-tooth comb, single-prong clips, wool crepe, light styling gel and finishing products
- Ask the client to remove jewelry and store in a secure place
- Wash and sanitize hands; drape client for a wet service; perform scalp and hair analysis
- Shampoo and condition the hair using products appropriate for client's hair type
- Towel dry and detangle the hair

Fingerwaving and Flat-Pincurls Procedure

- Apply styling product
- Determine where to begin first oblong
- Mold first direction (toward closed end) of oblong
- Position index finger in center of shape and mold second direction (toward open end)
- Create the ridge, starting at the concave end
- Complete ridge of first oblong
- Continue fingerwaving
- Complete fingerwaves
- Set flat pincurls beginning at concave end of last oblong
- Complete flat pincurls
- Use finishing procedures to style as desired

10

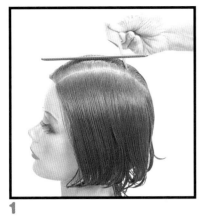

1

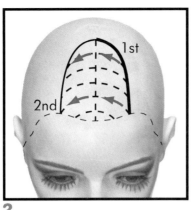

2

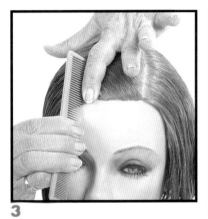

3

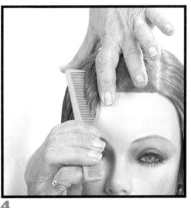

4

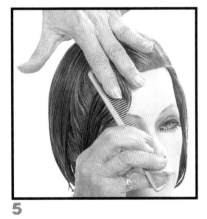

5

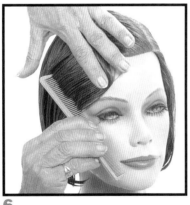

6

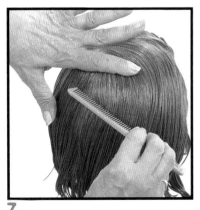

7

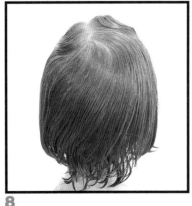

8

Fingerwaves and Flat Pincurls

1. **Apply styling product. Determine where to begin to form the first oblong** by laying a comb on the top of the head at the highest point. Position the comb from the front hairline to the crown. Wherever the comb separates from the head near the crown is where you should begin.

2. **Mold the first direction (toward closed end) of the oblong** toward the crown. **Position your index finger in the center of the shape and mold the second direction (toward open end)** toward the face. The molding of the first and second direction is now complete.

3-4. **Start creating the ridge at the concave end.** Position the teeth of the comb along your index finger and slide the comb approximately one inch (2.5 cm) toward the concave end to begin forming the ridge.

5-6. Flatten the comb and switch fingers. Position the ridge between your index and middle fingers. Turn the comb and distribute the hair in the opposite direction. Note that the first direction of the next oblong is automatically established. **Complete ridge of first oblong.**

7-8. At the crown area pivot carefully to avoid overdirecting the hair. **Continue fingerwaving** as you work around the curve of the head to the other side.

9-10. Begin the ridge of the next oblong at the concave end. Work from the front hairline around the head to the other side.

11. Strive for equally spaced waves. **Complete the fingerwaves.**

12. Begin to **set flat pincurls begin- nign at the concave end of the last oblong.** Be careful not to disturb the ridge.

13-14. **Complete the flat pincurls.** Once the hair has dried, **use finishing procedures to style as desired.**

Fingerwaves and Flat- Pincurls Completion

- Offer your client a rebook visit
- Recommend retail products to your client
- Disinfect implements and clean work space
- Wash hands with liquid antibacterial soap

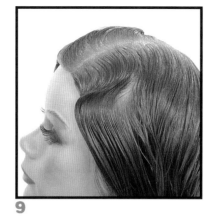

9

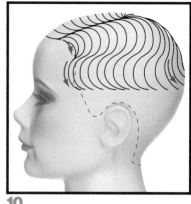

10

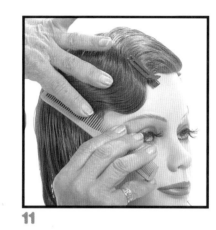

11

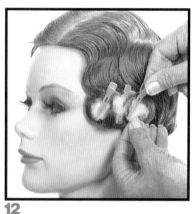

12

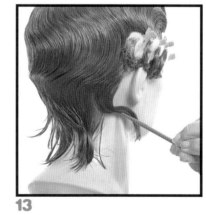

13

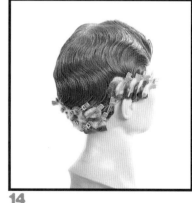

14

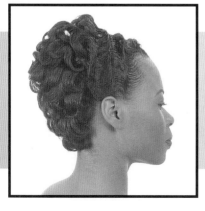

Fingerwave patterns are limitless. They can be designed diagonally, vertically or horizontally. Some patterns include a part, while others move directly off the face. The size of the wave pattern can also vary.

Straight Volume Rollers and Pincurls

Straight shapes such as the triangle are commonly used to create directional movement that moves toward or away from the face. Any base control can be used depending upon the desired results. In this exercise, a bricklay pattern radiating from the crown is set within triangular shapes. Rollers are used to create straight volume, while **semi-stand-up pincurls are used to create a transitional blend** to the molded exterior.

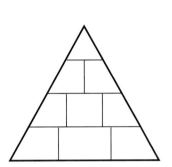 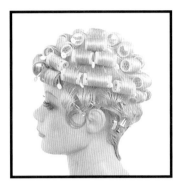 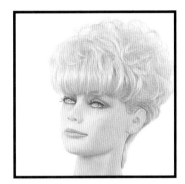

Straight-Volume-Rollers and Pincurls Preparation

As with any professional service, it is important to have your area, products, implements and equipment in proper order. Before performing a roller service, be sure to satisfy the following points:

- Clean work station with disinfectant
- Arrange implements/supplies including various length rollers, picks, clips, tail comb, large-tooth comb, cushion brush, setting lotion and finishing products
- Ask the client to remove jewelry and store in a secure place
- Wash and sanitize hands; drape client for a wet service; perform scalp and hair analysis
- Shampoo and condition the hair using products appropriate for the client's hair type
- Towel dry and detangle the hair

Straight-Volume-Rollers and Pincurls Procedure

- Apply setting lotion
- Mold and section four interior triangular shapes radiating from center crown
- Begin at crown
- Set triangle using straight volume base control within bricklay pattern
- Set remaining triangles using same procedures
- Set a row of straight volume pincurls
- Set a row of semi-stand-up pincurls
- Mold remaining nape lengths in curvature movement
- Position client underneath dryer
- Remove rollers and use finishing procedures to style hair

Straight Volume Rollers and Pincurls

1-2. **Apply setting lotion** to the hair. **Mold and section four interior triangular shapes radiating from the center crown.** Note that there are front, back and side triangles. The outside corners of the eyes are used as a reference to scale the front triangle. Mold the remaining lengths to conform to the curve of the head.

3-4. **Begin at the crown. Set the triangle using straight volume base control within a bricklay pattern.** Part and apply one-diameter, half-off base controls from horizontal partings. Work toward the front hairline.

5. Use a smaller diameter roller and set the last row at the fringe off base.

6. **Set the remaining triangles using the same procedures.** Use a one-diameter, half-off base control from horizontal partings within a bricklay pattern.

7-8. Underneath the back and side triangles, **set a row of straight volume pincurls** half-off base. Mold the remaining nape lengths and determine if additional pincurls are needed.

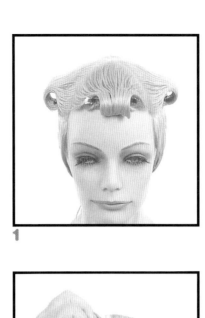

1

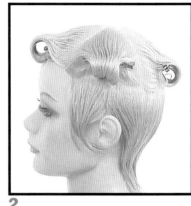

2

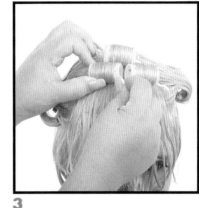

3

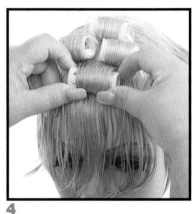

4

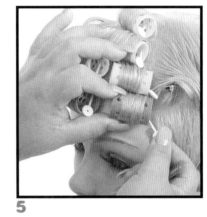

5

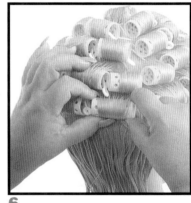

6

10

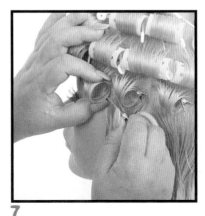

7

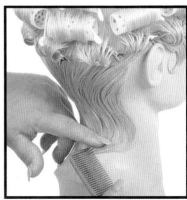

8

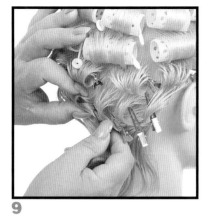

9

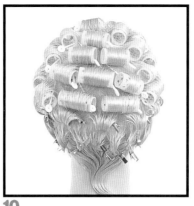

10

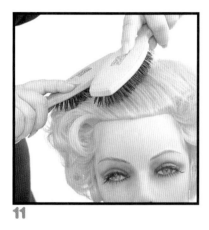

11

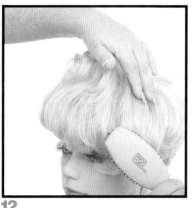

12

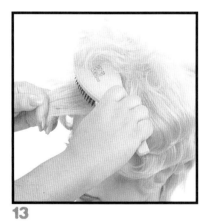

13

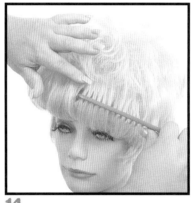

14

9-10. **Set a row of semi-stand up pincurls** for a transitional blend. Then, **mold the remaining nape lengths in a curvature movement.** **Position the client underneath the dryer** to dry the hair. Set the temperature of the dryer so that it is comfortable for the client. Allow the hair to cool once it has dried.

11-14. **Remove the rollers and use finishing procedures to style the hair** as desired.

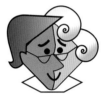

"Some stylists look down their noses at the weekly roller-set as a client. Remember – clients who wish to have roller sets come to you far more frequently than haircut clients or perm clients. These can become your 'bread and butter' clients. Yearly, fifty appointments at ten dollars each brings more money into the salon than three foil highlights at one hundred dollars each!"

Backbrushing Tips

Backbrushing is done on the surface of the hair. Push down toward the base and then remove the brush carefully. Use the bristles of the brush to pick up the next section. Connect the bases.

Other terms for backbrushing are teasing, ratting, matting, French lacing and ruffing.

Straight Volume Rollers and Pincurls Completion

- Offer your client a rebook visit
- Recommend retail products to your client
- Disinfect implements and clean work space
- Wash hands with liquid antibacterial soap

Curvature Volume Rollers and Pincurls

Curvature shapes are generally used along the front hairline to create movement and directions that move away then toward the face. When working with longer fringe lengths, the half circle is a great choice for directing the hair away from the forehead and then toward the forehead.

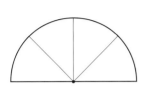 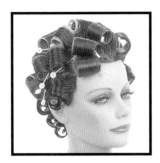 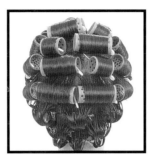 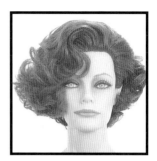

In this exercise a half-circle is set at the front hairline using curvature volume rollers. Expanded circles are set at the sides. The inner circle is set with curvature pincurls and the outer circle is set with curvature volume rollers. The back is set in a bricklay pattern with straight rollers and pincurls.

Curvature-Volume-Rollers and Pincurls Preparation

As with any professional service, it is important to have your area, products, implements and equipment in proper order. Before performing a wet styling roller service, be sure to satisfy the following points:

- Clean work station with disinfectant
- Arrange implements/supplies including straight and conical rollers of various lengths, picks, clips, tail comb, large-tooth comb, cushion brush, setting lotion and finishing products
- Ask the client to remove jewelry and store in a secure place
- Wash and sanitize hands; drape client for a wet service; perform scalp and hair analysis
- Shampoo and condition the hair using products appropriate for client's hair type
- Towel dry and detangle the hair

Curvature-Volume-Rollers and Pincurls Procedure

- Mold and scale half circle at front hairline
- Mold and scale expanded circle at sides
- Mold and scale straight shape between circle shapes
- Mold remaining lengths to conform to curve of head
- Set half circle using curvature volume base control
- At sides, set expanded circle using curvature volume base control
- In back, set straight shape using straight volume base control within bricklay pattern
- Set remaining lengths using straight volume pincurl control
- Position client underneath dryer
- Remove rollers and use finishing procedures to style hair

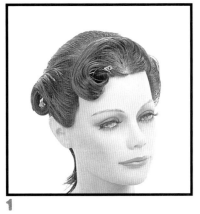

1

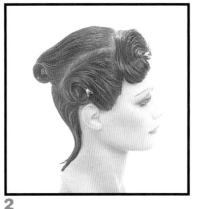

2

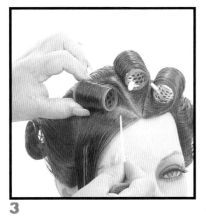

3

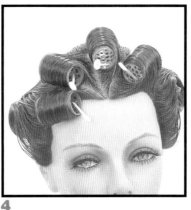

4

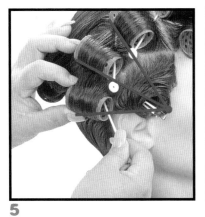

5

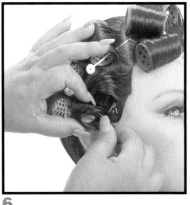

6

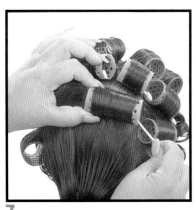

7

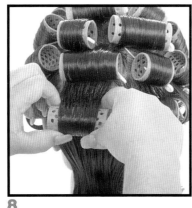

8

Curvature Volume Rollers and Pincurls

1-2. Mold and scale a half circle at the front hairline. Mold and scale an expanded circle at the sides. Mold and scale a straight shape between the circle shapes. Mold remaining lengths to conform to the curve of the head.

3-4. Set the half circle using curvature volume base control. Set the first two rollers one-diameter, on base. Set the next two rollers one-diameter, half-off base.

5-6. At the sides, set the expanded circle using curvature-volume base control. Set the outer circle using one-diameter, half-off base control. Set the inner circle using a half-off and off-base pincurl control.

7-8. In the back, set the straight shape using straight volume base control within a bricklay pattern. Base controls progress from maximum to diminishing volume. Set the first row one-diameter, on-base. Set the remaining rows one-diameter, half-off base. Note that rollers of different lengths are used.

9-10. Set the remaining lengths using straight volume pincurl control. Set the first two rows half-off base, then set the last row with off-base control. **Position the client underneath the dryer** to dry the hair. Set the temperature of the dryer so that it is comfortable for the client. Allow the hair to cool once it has dried.

11-14. Remove the rollers and use finishing procedures to style the hair as desired.

Backcombing Tips

Backcombing is usually performed underneath the surface of the hair. Use the fine teeth of the comb and direct the comb to the base to create a cushion. The cushion expands the form and connects the shapes.

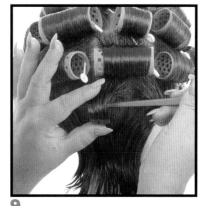
9

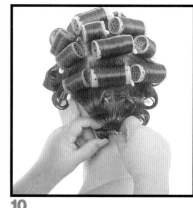
10

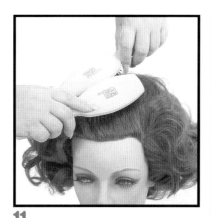
11

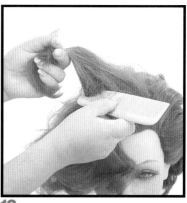
12

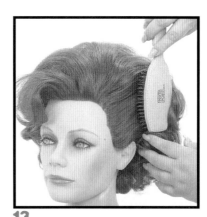
13

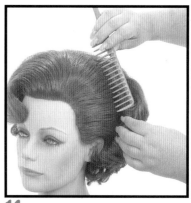
14

1 0

Curvature-Volume-Rollers and Pincurls Completion

- Offer your client a rebook visit
- Recommend retail products to your client
- Disinfect implements and clean work space
- Wash hands with liquid antibacterial soap

LONG-HAIR STYLING

Since ancient times long-hair styles have been a creative art form, often depicting romance, elegance and femininity. Unlike cut, color and perm services, which offer long-lasting effects, long-hair styling offers a temporary change. Styles for long hair can run the gamut from simple braids to intricate, avant-garde designs. The creative possibilities are endless, just let your imagination run wild and have fun creating.

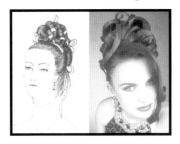 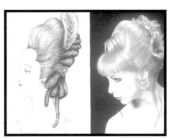 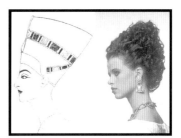

Long-Hair Fundamentals

Since long-hair styling is a service that is performed for special occasions, here are some additional points to keep in mind during your consultation to ensure that successful design decisions will be made:

- Facial features
- Body structure
- Hair length, density and type

- Occasion (formal or informal)
- Wardrobe
- Personal sense of style

Your client's facial features will help you determine whether or not detailing around the face should be a component of the style. Soft facial features may become overpowered with too much detailing. A long-hair style that is pulled away from the face may be more flattering to softer facial features, while bolder facial features can carry off more detail around the face.

Your client's body structure will also play an important role when making your decisions. As you may recall from the "Design Decisions" chapter, there are several different body shapes. When consulting with your client, consider that clients who are short and sturdy need height and volume while just the opposite is true for tall and lanky clients.

The length, density and type of hair (straight, wavy or curly) will also affect your decisions. Clients with short, straight hair who want an upswept design will present more limitations than those with appropriate longer lengths. For short-haired clients, hairpieces are an option. You will learn about hairpieces in the next chapter, "Wigs and Hair Additions."

As mentioned, long-hair styling is generally performed for special occasions, such as weddings, formal dinners, dances and proms. Therefore, special consideration must be given to the occasion and what the client will be wearing. Will she be wearing a long, sleek evening gown or a beaded, lace wedding dress? You may complement the fabric in different ways. For example, if your client has chosen a sleek sophisticated gown, you may chose a smooth, controlled hairstyle. If, on the other hand, she chooses a dress with a romantic feeling, you may choose a softer hairstyle with textural qualities.

Once you offer all of your suggestions, your client's personal sense of style will greatly influence your decisions. In long-hair styling, there is always more than just one choice – the options are endless. Refer to the "Client Consultation" portion of this chapter and to the "Design Decisions" chapter for additional guidelines.

Form

In long-hair styling, it is not the length arrangement but the placement of volume within the style that creates the overall form. Volume may be positioned in a specific area or throughout the style. When volume is positioned in a specific area, such as the crown or nape, it automatically draws the eye to that area. The opposite is true if volume is positioned equally throughout the style. The position of volume within a long-hair style becomes the focal point.

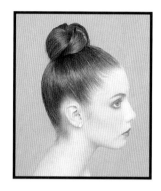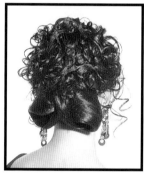

One way to achieve volume is to gather all or some of the hair into a ponytail first. The hair is then formed into shapes to achieve the desired hair style. Another way to achieve volume is to wrap or roll the hair inside itself.

Long-Hair Styling Procedures

Once you understand the theory behind long-hair styling, you are ready to use your knowledge and apply it the medium of hair. Fortunately, long-hair styling is a temporary service, so be creative and have fun practicing on your mannequins and you friends. The more you practice, the more efficient you will become and the more fun you will have.

Three classic long-hair styles are featured next. The three-strand overbraid, the three-strand underbraid and the French twist.

Three-Strand Overbraid

Twine, plait, pleat, weave, intertwine and interlock are just some of the terms associated with the age-old art of braiding. Whether piled high on the head, pinned close in the nape or free-falling past the shoulder, braids offer an artisic, individualistic design opportunity. **The two most common braiding methods are three-strand overbraid, also know as the french or invisible braid, and the three-strand underbraid, also known as the visible braid. The difference between the two techniques is whether a strand of hair is crossed over or under a center strand.**

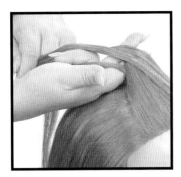
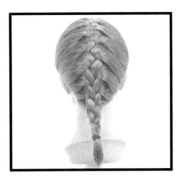
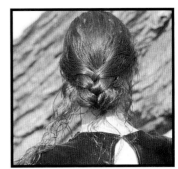

The three-strand overbraid has an inverted appearance. Because of its inverted appearance, the three-strand overbraid is also referred to as an invisible braid. This technique can be used to create one three-strand braid that conforms to the curve of the head or for multiple braids that can either be worn straight or elaborately formed into shapes. In this exercise, the braid is positioned vertically down the center of the head. Three strands are alternately crossed over one another to create an inverted appearance.

Three-Strand Overbraid Preparation

As with any professional service, it is important to have your area, products, implements and equipment in proper order. Before performing a long-hair styling service, be sure to satisfy the following points:

- Clean work station with disinfectant
- Arrange implements/supplies including tail comb, brush, elastic band and finishing products
- Ask the client to remove jewelry and store in a secure place
- Wash and sanitize hands; drape client for a wet service; perform scalp and hair analysis
- Shampoo and condition the hair using products appropriate for client's hair type
- Towel dry and detangle the hair
- Air form the hair
- Re-drape client for a dry service

Three-Strand-Overbraid Procedure

- Distribute hair straight back
- Take crescent-shaped section at fringe area
- Subdivide hair into three equal strands
- Cross right strand over center strand, then cross left strand over center strand
- Cross right strand over center strand again
- Take diagonal parting on right side and join with center strand
- Switch hands and repeat same procedures on other side
- Pick up consistent-size partings and work side to side using same procedures
- Toward nape, conform hands to curve of head
- Continue three-strand overbraid technique toward ends
- Secure ends with coated elastic band

Three-Strand Overbraid

1-2. Distribute the hair straight back. Take a crescent-shaped section at the fringe area. Subdivide the hair into three equal strands. Cross the **right (outside) strand over the center strand, then cross the left (outside) strand over the center.** You have now completed the three-strand sequence. Note that a palm-up hand position is used. Also keep in mind that it does not matter if you cross the right or the left strand over the center first, just as long as you maintain consistency throughout

3-4. Cross the right strand over the center again. Take a diagonal parting on the right side and join it with the center strand. Switch hands and repeat the same procedures on the other side.

5-6. Pick up consistent-size partings and work from side to side using the same procedures. To maintain control and tension on the hair, try to always hold the three strands in one hand.

7-8. As you work **toward the nape, conform your hands to the curve of the head** to create a contoured effect. **Continue to use the three-strand overbraid technique as you work toward the ends. Secure the ends with a coated elastic band.**

Three-Strand-Overbraid Completion

- Offer your client a rebook visit
- Recommend retail products to your client
- Disinfect implements and clean work station
- Wash hands with liquid antibacterial soap

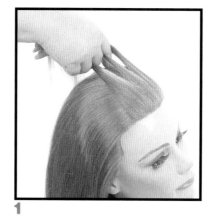
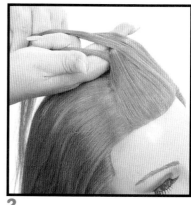
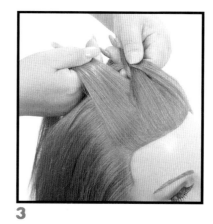
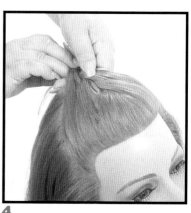
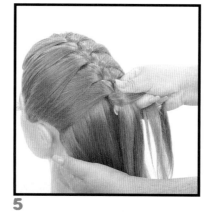
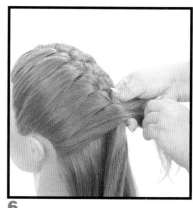
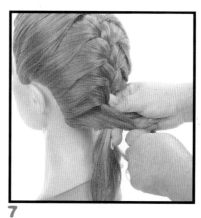
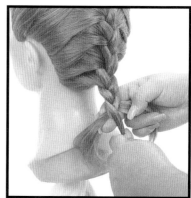

10

Three-Strand Underbraid

Unlike the three-strand overbraid, where the outside strands are crossed over the center strand, for the three-strand underbraid, the outside strands are crossed under the center strand. **Crossing the strands under the center strand creates a projected or visible braid pattern. When performed on the scalp, the three-strand underbraid is also known as cornrowing.** Cornrowing can be a combination of on-the-scalp and off-the-scalp braiding. Three-strand underbraids may be positioned in any number of ways. In this exercise, the three-strand underbraid is positioned vertically down the center of the head.

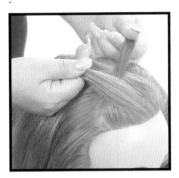 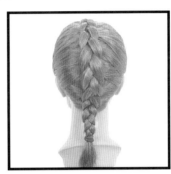 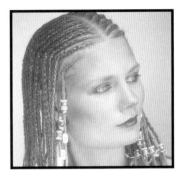

Three-Strand-Underbraid Preparation

As with any professional service, it is important to have your area, products, implements and equipment in proper order. Before performing a long-hair styling service, be sure to satisfy the following points:

- Clean work station with disinfectant
- Arrange implements/supplies including tail comb, brush, elastic band and finishing products
- Ask the client to remove jewelry and store in a secure place
- Wash and sanitize hands; drape client for a wet service; perform scalp and hair analysis
- Shampoo and condition the hair using products appropriate for client's hair type
- Towel dry and detangle the hair
- Air form the hair
- Re-drape client for a dry service

Three-Strand-Underbraid Procedure

- Distribute hair straight back
- Take crescent-shaped section at fringe area
- Subdivide hair into three equal strands
- Cross right strand under center strand, then cross left strand under center strand
- Cross right strand under center strand again
- Take diagonal parting on right side and join with center strand
- Switch hands and repeat same procedures on other side
- Pick up consistent-size partings and work side to side using same procedures
- As you work toward nape, conform hands to curve of head
- Continue three-strand underbraid technique toward the ends
- Secure ends with coated elastic band

Three-Strand Underbraid

1-2. **Distribute the hair straight back.** Take a crescent-shaped section at the fringe area. Subdivide the hair into three equal strands. **Cross the right strand under the center strand.**

3-4. Then **cross the left strand under the center.** You have now completed the three-strand sequence. Note that it does not matter if you cross the right or the left strand under the center first, just as long as you maintain consistency throughout. **Cross the right strand under the center again. Take a diagonal parting on the right side and join it with the center strand. Switch hands and repeat the same procedure on the other side.** Note that a palm-down hand position is used.

5-6. **Pick up consistent-size partings and work from side to side using the same procedures.** To maintain control and tension on the hair, try to always hold the three strands in one hand.

7-8. **As you work toward the nape, conform your hands to the curve of the head** to create a contoured effect. Continue to use the three-strand-underbraid technique as you work toward the ends. Secure the ends with a coated elastic band.

Three-Strand-Underbraid Completion

- Offer your client a rebook visit
- Recommend retail products to your client
- Disinfect implements and clean work station
- Wash hands with liquid antibacterial soap

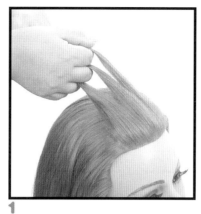

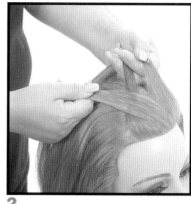

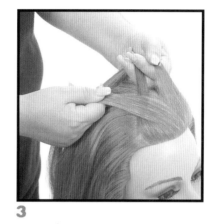

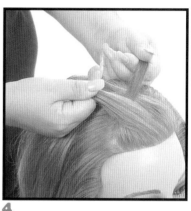

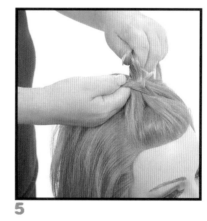

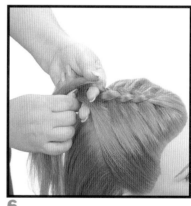

10

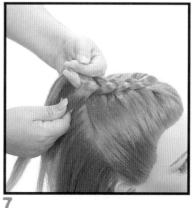

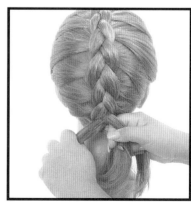

French Twist

The French twist, also known as the vertical roll, is an elegant look that can be adapted in a variety of ways. Worn for special occasions, this design is a popular classic and is requested by women of all ages. When creating a French twist, all the hair can be incorporated into the roll for an elongated smooth finish, or the roll can be positioned up to the crown area and finished with curls for a combination of textures. In this exercise, all the lengths are incorporated in the French twist.

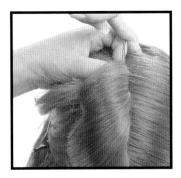 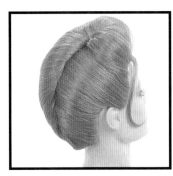 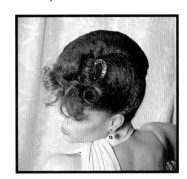

French-Twist Preparation

As with any professional service, it is important to have your area, products, implements and equipment in proper order. Before performing a long-hair styling service, be sure to satisfy the following points:

- Clean work station with disinfectant
- Arrange implements/supplies including tail comb, brush, hair pins, sectioning clips and finishing products
- Ask the client to remove jewelry and store in a secure place
- Wash and sanitize hands; drape client for a wet service; perform scalp and hair analysis
- Shampoo and condition the hair using products appropriate for client's hair type
- Towel dry and detangle the hair
- Air form the hair
- Re-drape client for a dry service

French-Twist Procedure

- Distribute hair to one side
- Secure hair with line of interlocked bobby pins, slightly off center
- Take diagonal parting at nape
- Fold section over bobby pins
- Secure inside of roll near the edge of fold
- Wrap any remaining lengths around finger and secure inside roll
- Continue to take diagonal partings and fold each section slightly over previous section
- Work to front
- Roll remaining lengths away from face
- Finish hair as desired

French Twist

1-2. **Distribute the hair to one side. Secure the hair with a line of interlocked bobby pins, slightly off center,** to prepare for the position of the roll. Interlocking the bobby pins will prevent the bobby pins from slipping and create extra support.

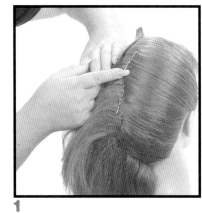
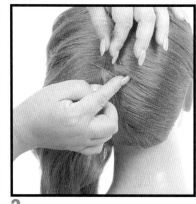

3-4. **Take a diagonal parting at the nape. Fold the section over the bobby pins. Secure the inside of the roll near the edge of the fold. Wrap any remaining lengths around your finger and secure them inside the roll** to act as a filler for the next section. Note, depending on the type of texture and density of the hair with which you are working, as well as the desired results, you may wish to backcomb each section for support and additional volume.

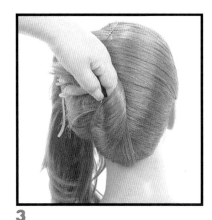
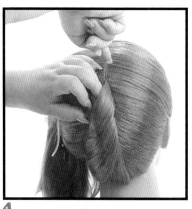

5-6. **Continue to take diagonal partings and fold each section slightly over the previous section** to avoid splits. Secure the inside of the twist each time you fold the hair. Note how the size of the roll begins to increase.

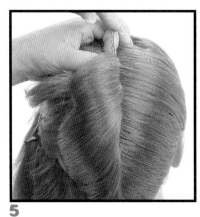
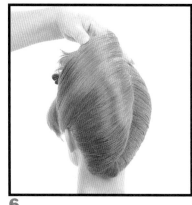

7-8. **Work to the front. Roll the remaining lengths away from the face** and finish the hair as desired.

French-Twist Completion

- Offer your client a rebook visit
- Recommend retail products to your client
- Disinfect implements and clean work station
- Wash hands with liquid antibacterial soap

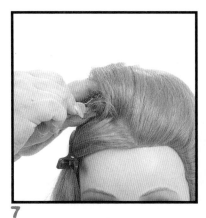
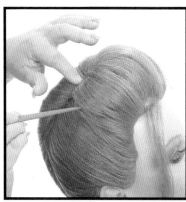

You have explored many new ideas and possibilities in this chapter. As you come to the end of any chapter, it is helpful to hold a mental image of what you have learned. In this chapter, you began with general hairstyling theory before looking more in depth at thermal styling, wet styling and long-hair styling.

As the chapter opened, you heard from Professor Pivot that hairstyling is the heart of your craft. Perhaps you now have a personal sense of how true his statement is and how open-ended the work of any artist is, always joining new vision with steadily improving technique. The many procedures in each practical exercise presented a foundation upon which you can build throughout your career. No one knows yet what hairstyles will be most popular 10 years from now. What you do know, however, is that with what you have learned in this chapter, you can face that future with confidence and skill.

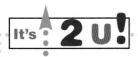

Build Your Critical Thinking Skills

In this chapter you have prepared yourself to meet the following Industry Standards for entry-level cosmetologists:

- Consult with clients to determine their needs and preferences as it relates to cosmetology services
- Provide styling and finishing techniques to complete a hairstyle to the satisfaction of the client
- Use safely a variety of salon products while providing client services

It's Up to You to know what to do. Using your training to this point, review the following case scenarios and think through how you would handle the challenge.

1. Your client usually receives a thermal style after her haircut, but today she has asked you if you could do something to help the style last longer, since she is leaving on vacation. Her hair is very fine with subtle highlights, approximately five inches in length in the crown and decreases to approximately two inches in the perimeter. In order to help this client meet her goal of a longer-lasting style, what would you do?

2. A client that normally has her hair styled by another stylist in the salon is visiting you today because her stylist is ill. This client has very fine, thin hair that has been relaxed and colored with a permanent tint. She has an appointment for a very special photograph, followed by three days of very busy business meetings. In other words, she really wants to look extra nice and have the style last as long as possible. What would you do?

3. This is the very first time you have styled the client's hair that is in your chair right now. She has brought a photo from a magazine with her and after viewing the photo and doing a preliminary analysis of the client's hair type and facial shape, you have determined that the style shown in the photo is not at all appropriate for this client. You want to make sure that you do not insult or offend the client, but at the same time feel that a style with much less volume on top and attention to detail on the sides and nape area would be more appropriate. What would you do?

Chapter 11
WIGS AND HAIR ADDITIONS

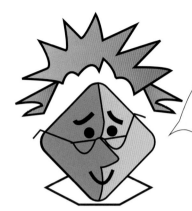

After studying this chapter you will be able to . . .

1. Explain why clients wear wigs and hairpieces and list the professional wig services performed in the salon.

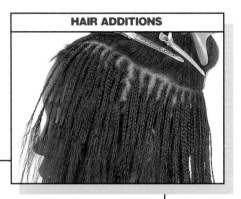

HAIR ADDITIONS

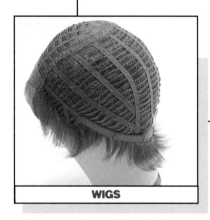

WIGS

2. Define hair additions and describe five methods of attachment.

11

Change is in the air! Can't you just feel it? What better way to experiment with a possible image change than with a wig, a hairpiece or hair additions? This book of Salon Fundamentals would be lacking if we didn't include a chapter on wigs and hair additions. Even though this service is a small part of salon life and business, it is a very important one. You will be able to help people experiencing temporary or permanent hair loss as well as those wanting an exciting or daring change in their looks.

After gaining knowledge and skill with wigs and hair additions, you will be prepared to meet the needs of clients who desire a variety of hairstyle changes but also of those in need of looking and feeling better following any kind of hair loss.

Many people who consult with you concerning wigs or hair additions will be experiencing stress of some kind. Perhaps they are fighting or emerging from a serious illness. What a VALUE you have to offer them through your creative suggestions about ways to deal with hair loss.

Helping clients by offering a variety of wig styles and hair additions will assist them in looking and feeling better.

Nothing hard about this BIG IDEA, is there? So often our outlook improves with a change in our looks. We may not even understand why. We just know we feel better as we look better.

WIGS AND HAIRPIECES
History
Composition, Colors and Construction
Wig and Hairpiece Essentials
Infection Control and Safety
Client Consultation
Wig Services
Hairpieces

HAIR ADDITIONS
Hair Addition Methods

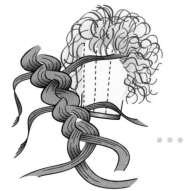

WIGS AND HAIRPIECES

Maybe you have always wanted to work with community theater or help cancer patients who have experienced hair loss following medical treatments. Maybe premature hair loss runs in your family. Whatever the reason for your interest, now is the time to start thinking about all the ways you will be able to use information about wigs and hair additions. The first section of this chapter deals with wigs and hairpieces. **Wigs are designed to cover the entire head and are worn for specific purposes. Hairpieces are designed to cover specific areas of the head and are also designed for definite purposes.**

History

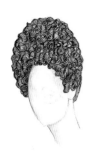

Wigs have been worn, by women and men, for both aesthetic and practical reasons for as long as history has been recorded. It is believed that ancient Egyptians began to wear wigs to protect their heads from the heat of the sun. Originally worn by the upper classes, wigs were eventually worn by all levels of Egyptian society, other than priests and laborers.

Other ancient cultures, such as those of the Romans and the Greeks, also wore wigs to varying degrees, depending on the fashions and customs of the moment. In Imperial Rome, the 'orbis' hairstyle required that a woman brush her hair forward and create a mass of tight curls at the front. Usually built up on a wire frame (a very early hairpiece), these curls were quite often not the wearer's own hair.

Several centuries later, during the Elizabethan era, the aristocracy sported curled wigs generously studded with precious gems.

Historically, wigs and hairpieces have risen and fallen in popularity according to trends, fashions and even politics. During various periods, those that created and tended to the making of wigs for the aristocracy have been both reviled and revered. In ancient times, slaves were often responsible for the care and styling of their master's wigs and hairpieces. While they may have possessed talents and skills, they were still treated as slaves. Later, particularly in the French courts, hairdressers had a more elevated status. Their creations were instrumental in establishing fashion trends and indicating a lady's or gentleman's social status.

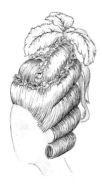

The extraordinary height and complexity of wig designs were, in many ways, indications of the extremes that led to the French Revolution. Yet the prevailing trends (regardless of the extravagant expense and effort) were still followed by those who wished to maintain their status as fashion-conscious members of the aristocracy.

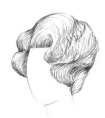

During the 1950s and 1960s, wigs and hairpieces rose tremendously in popularity. The development of synthetic fibers, known as modacrylics, made mass production and lower prices a possibility. Wigs and hairpieces were worn as fashion accessories, especially for evening, with no social stigma.

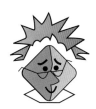

"During the 1950s and 1960s, many women even had 'wardrobes' of false hair, to suit every occasion, outfit or mood."

The majority of clients that schedule salon visits for wigs services do so because they are experiencing hereditary hair loss or hair loss due to illness. For other clients, wigs can offer a quick color or length change

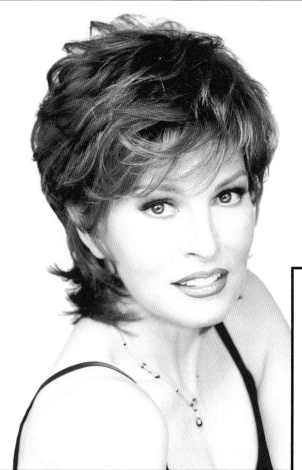

Wigs have also been worn by actors and actresses, to great effect, throughout the ages. Theatrical wigmaking, especially of period styles, for theater and opera stages, is an art form in itself. Many of these actresses and celebrities have come to know the benefits of wearing wigs in their personal lives as well. The advances in technology and design have made it so much easier for them (and your clients) to take advantage of the wide range of wigs available.

Photos: Courtesy of Celebrity Signatures International

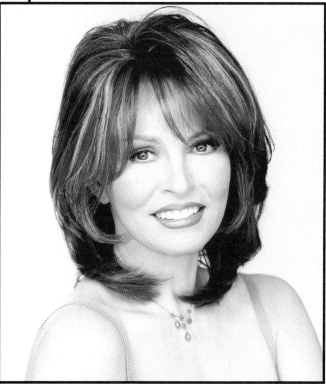

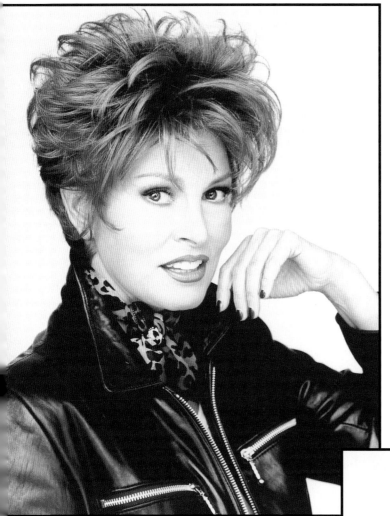

The beautiful actress, Raquel Welch, is so appreciative of the benefits of wigs that she has endorsed a line of them! The examples that we see here were personally chosen by Ms. Welch for inclusion in her signature collection. Note the natural effects of the color designs and the softness and fluidity of the haircuts. Whether your client just wants to change her look, like Ms. Welch, or she needs to wear a wig for prescriptive purposes, wigs that look this real make it so much easier for you to offer this service confidently to your clientele.

Now that you've seen how wigs have been used throughout history and how natural they can look today, you are ready to learn about the composition and construction of wigs.

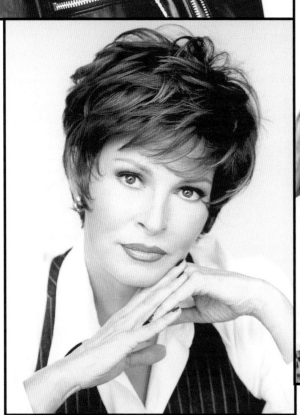

11

Composition, Colors and Construction

Before performing wig services for your clients, it is important to have a good understanding of the composition, colors and construction of wigs.

Wig Composition

Hairpieces can be made of human hair, animal hair, synthetic fibers or a blend of each. Asian, Indian or European hair is generally used to make human hair wigs, European being the most costly. Generally, hair from India is wavy while hair from Asia is straight. The hair is specially treated to protect against possible damage from styling services. Since the appearance and texture of human hairpieces is the most natural, they are preferred by those wanting a wig to look like their own hair. Since the supply of human hair for the manufacturing of wigs is more limited, these wigs are the most expensive.

Modacrylic (synthetic) wig fibers are formulated from petroleum products and are produced as very long threads (monofilaments), which are then rolled onto spools. These fibers make it very cost effective and efficient to produce wigs. Shades are almost unlimited, so human hair colors can be closely duplicated. While modacrylic fibers may not always resemble human hair, modern technology has produced very realistic results.

If you're not certain whether a hairpiece is made of human hair or modacrylic fiber, pull out several strands and hold them over a match flame. **A human hair strand will burn slowly and produce an odor. A synthetic fiber will either "ball up" on the end (melt) and extinguish itself or burn very rapidly and produce no odor.**

Animal hair wigs and hairpieces, most often made of yak, angora, horse or sheep hair, have even less resemblance to human hair than modacrylic fibers. Animal hair is most often used to produce fantasy hairpieces, theatrical wigs or wigs meant to be worn by display mannequins.

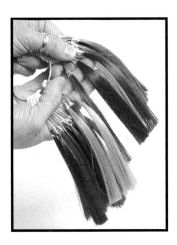

Wig Colors

All the colors used for wigs and hairpieces are standardized according to the seventy colors on the J and L ring (the standard hair color ring used by wig and hairpiece manufacturers). The ring contains numbered samples from black to palest blond. This ring allows wig manufacturers to select from a variety of colors and to create special effects such as highlighted hair.

Wig Construction

Wig construction falls into two general categories, cap wigs and capless wigs. Cap wigs consist of an elasticized mesh-fiber base to which the hair fiber is attached. Cap wigs are available in several sizes and are produced most often as handmade wigs.

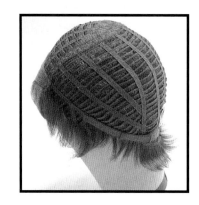

In recent years, capless wigs have become the most prevalent and popular form of wigs. Capless wigs consist of rows of hair wefts sewn to strips of elastic. Because of their construction, many capless wigs weigh only a few ounces and are, therefore, very light, cool and comfortable.

Hair and/or synthetic fibers may be attached to the wig cap or base in one of three methods. They may be hand tied, machine made, or semi-hand tied. A hand-tied (hand-knotted) wig or hairpiece is produced by actually hand tying strands of hair into a fine meshwork or foundation. Patterns are used to simulate natural growth patterns that closely resemble human hair growth and create a natural look. The hair is attached at close intervals and generally duplicates the density of a fairly thick head of human hair. Since this process is labor intensive and time consuming, these wigs tend to be the most expensive.

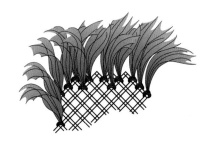

Wigs known as 'machine made' consist of hair fiber sewn into long strips called wefts, which are then sewn to the cap of the wig in a circular or crisscross pattern. Machine-made wigs can be very difficult to style since the direction of the hair is determined by the position in which the weft is sewn to the cap.

Combinations of hand-tied and machine-made wigs and hairpieces are called semi-hand tied. The best toupees (a wig or patch of false hair worn to replace a bald area) are semi-hand tied to create sturdy, natural-looking, reasonably priced hair replacements.

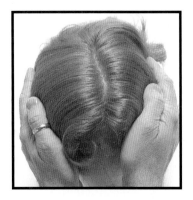

When helping your client select a wig, the wig's construction is significant in determining the best value in the client's price range. Capless wigs or caps that allow the scalp to 'breathe' prevent excessive perspiration that may cause odors. These wigs need to be cleaned less frequently. Another factor of importance is that many wigs have flesh-colored sections designed to look like human skin. These sections give a realistic look when the hair is parted or moves. Most clients, of course, desire as natural a look as possible.

Wig and Hairpiece Essentials

To perform a professional service for a client with a wig, you need a selection of products, implements and equipment. Refer to Material Safety Data Sheets (MSDS) for all products used in the salon.

Wig and Hairpiece Products

PRODUCT	FUNCTION
Nonflammable Liquid Shampoo	Cleans human hair wigs and hairpieces
Conditioner	Keeps the wig in good condition
Mild Shampoo	Cleans synthetic wigs and hairpieces
Synthetic Wig Shampoo	Cleans synthetic wigs and hairpieces
Synthetic Wig Conditioner	Keeps synthetic wigs and hairpieces in optimum condition
Holding Spray	Holds finished wig styles in place

Wig and Hairpiece Implements/Supplies

IMPLEMENTS/SUPPLIES	FUNCTION
Comb	Detangles and styles wigs and hairpieces
Brush	Styles wigs and hairpieces
Shear	Cuts and customizes wigs and hairpieces
Thinning Shear	Tapers and blends; removes bulk and excess fiber
Razor	Tapers and blends; removes bulk and excess fiber
Rollers	Allow temporary curl placement for human hair wigs
Pincurl Clips	Allow temporary curl placement for human hair wigs
Wig Cap	Holds client's hair in place and helps wig to stay in place
Bobby Pins	Secure client's hair under wig; sometimes used to hold wig in place
Hairpins	Secure hair, especially for chignons and other 'updo' effects
Needle and Thread	Create darts and tucks in wigs; secure wefts in track-and-sew technique; used to sew wefts for fantasy hairpieces
Wig Pins	Hold wigs and hairpieces in place on canvas block during styling, cleaning and maintenance services
Styrofoam Heads	Store and display wigs
Chin Strap	Holds wig in place on client's head during services
J and L (JL) Color Ring	Allows client and stylist to choose wig or hairpiece color

IMPLEMENT/SUPPLIES	FUNCTION
Measuring Tape	Measures client's head to determine correct wig size
Plastic Bag	Covers and protects canvas blocks
Porcelain or Glass Bowl	Holds cleaning solution and wigs or hairpieces during cleaning and sizing service
Cloth Cape	Protects client during styling and fitting services

Wig and Hairpiece Equipment

EQUIPMENT	FUNCTION
Canvas Blocks (various sizes)	Hold wig while services are being performed
Wig Dryer	Dries wigs that have been wet set (on canvas blocks)
Hydraulic Chair	Allows client to sit at proper height for stylist to perform services

Infection Control and Safety

The majority of wig services are performed while the wig is on a wig block, so safety concerns are somewhat minimized. However, it is essential to keep your client's safety in mind at all times.

- Disinfect all tools and implements properly.

- Explain to your client points of maintenance and hygiene specific to each service.

- Ensure that a wig or hairpiece has sufficient air flow if it will be worn for long periods of time.

- Work with products, such as liquid dry shampoos, in a well ventilated area.

- Observe carefully, when performing a hair addition service, the direction in which the client's hair grows naturally. Avoid going against the natural growth pattern, since doing so could cause discomfort to the client and damage to the hair.

- Teach your clients how to maintain and care for any hair addition service. Although your artistry may make the additions look like their own hair, they cannot treat the additions in the exact same way!

Client Consultation

There are several things to keep in mind when doing a consultation with a client for a wig, toupee or hair addition service. Regardless of the reason(s) that the client desires the service, discretion is of great importance. Whether hair loss is hereditary, caused by illness or medication, many clients will be very self-conscious about their need to seek your services. First and foremost, you must make sure the client feels comfortable and safe in the environment of the salon. Second, the client must feel trust in you as his/her stylist.

11

Since you will often be dealing with the adverse conditions that cause hair loss, you need to be especially sympathetic and emotionally supportive.

For example, when client's are going through chemotherapy, you might think the physical challenges would be their only concern. However, loss of hair during such treatments can be emotionally devastating as well. Many clients will seek your services in anticipation of hair loss, prior to beginning treatments. Unlike clients who simply want to change their appearance, these clients usually want to duplicate, as closely as possible, their own hair prior to hair loss.

Carefully observe and record details about hair length, texture and colors during your consultation. Discuss with your client certain styling options that may make it easier to attain realistic-looking results. In the case of illness or hereditary hair loss, most clients are not looking forward to the prospect of wearing a wig. It is your job to help them realize how very helpful and positive the experience can and should be. Much of the client's comfort level with the service and the wig itself will be determined during the consultation, so make the most of this opportunity. Serve your client with dignity, respect and a positive, supportive attitude.

Wig Services

Hand-tied wigs may be custom-made or purchased "ready to wear." When selecting and/or designing a wig for a client, remember that your client's comfort is as important as the way the wig looks. Therefore, it is important that you can offer special wig services that will help ensure your client's satisfaction. These services may include wig measurement and fitting, instructions on how to put on a wig, as well as blocking, cleaning, cutting, coloring and styling wigs.

Wig Measurement and Fitting

In order that your client's wig fits comfortably, it is important that you understand how to properly measure and fit the wig to your client's particular head size and shape. Although wig manufacturers may require additional, specific measurements for their products, following these basic measurement guidelines will allow you to properly fit the majority of wigs for your clients.

Wig Measurement and Fitting Guidelines

* Brush the client's hair as smoothly as possible. If the hair is long, pin it flat.

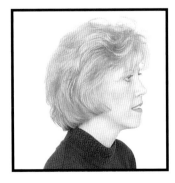 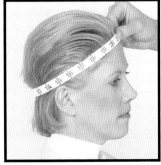

* Measure the circumference of the head, beginning at the hairline in the middle of the forehead and circling the entire head, running the tape just above the ears, around the back and returning to the starting point. Be sure the client's ears are not caught under the tape measure. The average hairline circumference is twenty two inches.

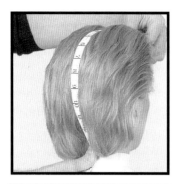

- Measure the distance of the hairline from the center of the forehead over the crown to the nape hairline. For the most comfortable fit possible, bend the client's head back to find the spot at the base of the skull where the wig will rest.

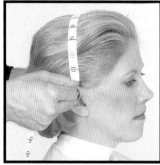

- Measure the distance from temple to temple (just above the ear) over the crown of the head.

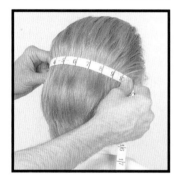

- Measure the distance from ear to ear (just above the ear) over the occipital bone. Some manufacturers may request that you measure the distance from ear to ear, along the nape hairline, and also the width of the nape area.

Putting on a Wig

Along with selecting and/or creating the perfect wig for your client, it is important to teach your client the easiest way to put on a wig. This will help the client feel more comfortable wearing the wig and eliminate frustrations.

Putting on a Wig Guidelines

- Brush your client's hair back from the face and up from the back hairline. Pin to secure. Long hair can be swept up or secured in large, flat pincurls.

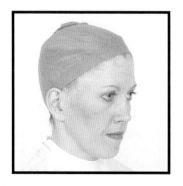

- Cover the client's hair with a fine net or wig cap made specifically for the purpose of controlling the client's hair and making the wig stay more securely in place.

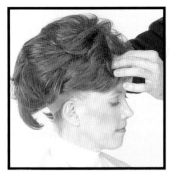
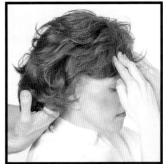

- Place the front hairline of the wig over and slightly lower than the client's front hairline. Hold the front of the wig in place and position the wig over the rest of the head to the nape. You may also ask the client to hold the front of the wig in place as you position the wig over the sides, back and nape. Adjust the wig as needed for security and comfort.

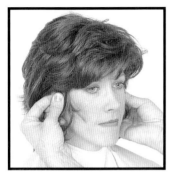
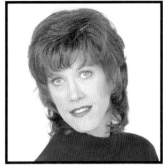

- Adjust and form the wig perimeter to better fit the client's head shape and hairline. Many wigs contain wire at the sideburn area for this very purpose.

Wig Blocking

When performing wig services, such as styling or cleaning, it is important that the size and shape of the wig are not compromised. Proper sizing procedures, called blocking, will help maintain the wig's original size. Canvas-covered wig forms, called wig blocks, are manufactured for use during these services. The blocks are available in six sizes: 20", 20.5", 21", 21.5", 22", 22.5" (50, 51.25, 52.5, 53.75, 55 and 56.25 cm). One of these sizes should closely match the circumference measurement of the client's head. If the wig needs to be stretched, it is placed on a block larger than the client's head, if shrunk, on a smaller block. The block is placed on a swivel clamp for control.

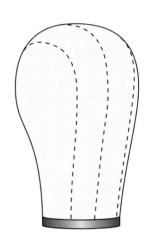

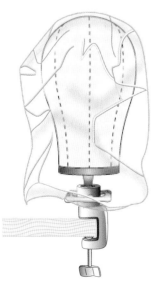

Wig Blocking Guidelines

- Select the correct size canvas block. You may need slightly larger or smaller blocks than the wig for stretching or shrinking.

- Cover the block with clear plastic and then secure the plastic tightly with wig pins to protect the canvas during the service.

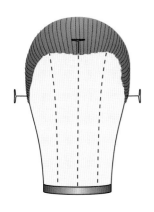
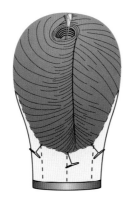

- Place the wig on the block and secure it with wig pins at the following places:
  - Center front
  - Both temples
  - Center of the nape
  - Corners of the nape

Customizing or Fitting a Wig

Custom-ordered wigs can be quite expensive and, therefore, cost-prohibitive for many clients. Fortunately, the majority of clients will be able to use a ready-to-wear wig, one that will not require any alterations from a stylist. However, if alterations are necessary, you will want to be able to offer this service to your clients.

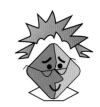

"I wonder if I could find a ready-to-wear wig to fit my particular head size and shape."

Many wigs have elastic bands through the nape or crown that allow for easy adjustments. Almost all have adjustable elastic bands at the bottom back or at either side of the nape. Some are secured with small hooks and many are adjusted with small strips of Velcro™. Many stylists will use a small safety pin for added security. The elastic may be sewn in place with top-stitching that allows the stitches to be removed, since occasional readjustments may be needed. Also the elastic band itself may need to be replaced occasionally.

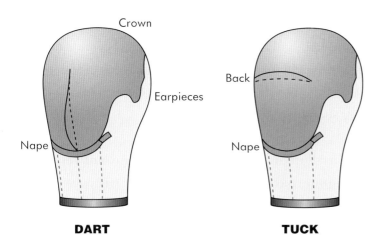

DART   TUCK

Darts are alterations made vertically to remove width in the nape area (from ear to ear). Tucks are alterations made horizontally to shorten a wig from the front to the nape. Both darts and tucks are made by turning a wig inside out and sewing a fold, like a seam, inside the cap. Horizontal alterations are usually made with the tuck near the crown to avoid excess bulk close to the perimeter.

These simple adjustment techniques will help ensure your clients' satisfaction with their wig purchases, as well as their confidence in your abilities as a professional cosmetologist.

Stretching or Shrinking Cap Wigs

In some instances you will be able to adjust the size of a wig without making tucks or darts, by either stretching or shrinking the wig. You might need to stretch a wig if it is just a little too tight or if it has somehow shrunk a bit.

1 1

Stretching Cap Wig Guidelines

- Turn the wig inside out and thoroughly moisten the cap of the wig by spraying with hot water.

- Turn the wig right side out and carefully stretch it over a wig block one size larger than the circumference of the wig itself.

- Secure the wig to the block along the hairline using wig pins.

- Style the hair if desired and allow the wig to dry.

Shrinking Cap Wig Guidelines

- Select a block one size smaller than the wig's circumference.

- Turn the wig inside out and moisten the cap with hot water.

- Turn the wig right side out and place it on the smaller block.

- Dry the wig under a warm dryer (only if the wig is human hair; heat can distort curl patterns of synthetic fibers).

- Adjust the wig, if it is still too big, by sewing darts and tucks into the over-stretched areas.

Cleaning and Conditioning

Many wig and hairpiece manufacturers will give you guidelines as to the proper care of their product. Some manufacturers also have specific products available that you can offer your clients. Regardless of the specific brand of products, the following information will serve you well as you work with your clients' wigs and hairpieces.

Human hair wigs and synthetic wigs will require slightly different methods of cleaning and conditioning. **Human hair wigs or hairpieces should be cleaned every two to four weeks, depending on how frequently the piece is worn.** Conditioning should follow each cleaning, since some wig-cleansing products, like liquid dry-cleaning shampoos, can be very drying.

Because modacrylic fibers aren't as porous as human hair, synthetic wigs do not require cleaning as frequently as their human-hair counterparts. Cleansing a synthetic wig once every 6 to 12 weeks should be sufficient in most cases. Synthetic wigs do not require conditioning as human hair wigs do. However, many manufacturers recommend synthetic conditioning sprays that will keep the fibers in optimum condition.

Human Hair Wigs: Cleaning and Conditioning Guidelines

Since hand-tied wigs generally have a delicate construction and are more expensive, extra care should be taken in their cleaning.

- Clean the perimeter of the wig and the inside foundation with a toothbrush or cotton ball, using liquid cleaner. The remainder of the cleaning is done with the wig on the block.

- Prepare the canvas block by covering it with a plastic bag and securing the bag with wig pins.

- Block the wig and secure it to the form with wig pins. Mark the block with additional wig pins along the hairline to assist you in proper blocking after you've cleaned the wig. Brush or comb the wig to remove tangles and to loosen dirt and styling product residue.

- Place three to five ounces of nonflammable liquid dry shampoo or cleanser in a large porcelain or glass bowl.

- Remove the wig from the block and turn it inside out. Soak the wig for three to five minutes while very gently rubbing the hairline to remove debris and stains. Swirl the hair gently in the product for about one minute and remove the wig from the liquid.

- Blot the inside of the cap of the wig thoroughly to remove excess moisture. Turn the wig right side out and blot the hair gently.

- Stretch the wig gently over the block. Use the hairline markings you made on the plastic to guide your placement of the wig. Secure with wig pins.

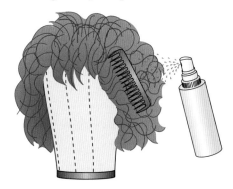

- With the wig on the block, use a wide-tooth comb to distribute conditioner through the hair. Be sure to follow manufacturer's directions.

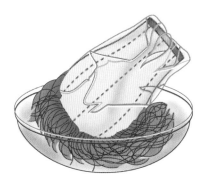

Another option:
Hand-tied wigs may also be soaked right on the wig block, after gently cleaning the hairline with cleaner and a small brush.

Synthetic Hair Wigs: Cleaning Guidelines

- Cover the canvas block with plastic and secure with wig pins.

- Block the wig and secure it to the form with wig pins. Mark the block along the hairline to assist you in proper blocking after you've cleaned the wig. Brush the hair to remove tangles and loosen dirt and wig spray residue. Remove the wig from the block.

- Shampoo the wig by turning it inside out and soaking it in a mild shampoo solution. Work the debris from the hairline and inside with a toothbrush.

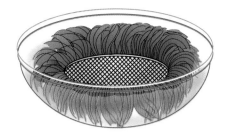

- Turn the wig right side out and swish hair in the solution. Allow the wig to soak for 5 to 10 minutes and then rinse thoroughly with lukewarm water.

- If necessary, repeat cleansing and soak longer.

- Rinse and blot the excess moisture with a towel.
- Place on the block to dry, following the blocking guidelines you indicated on the plastic-covered canvas head form.

Coloring Services

Although most wig manufacturers can custom color their wigs and hairpieces in almost any shade you can imagine, it is an extra benefit to your clients if you can offer this service to them in cases where a desired color doesn't exist for their particular choice. Color should not be applied to synthetic wigs and hairpieces, since the non-porous fiber will not allow the hair shaft to be coated or penetrated.

Human-hair wigs and hairpieces can be effectively colored with temporary rinses that last from shampoo to shampoo, semi-permanent colors, fillers or low-level (darker) oxidative colors. The hair used to create human hairpieces and wigs has already been chemically treated and has most likely been decolorized and bleached. Therefore, it is advisable to avoid oxidative colors and lighteners since it may be hard to predict the results. Refer to the "Hair Coloring" chapter for more information on these types of colors. Before coloring a wig or hairpiece, be sure to perform a strand test. Also keep color off the wig cap as much as possible, since color may eventually dissolve the fabric.

Human-Hair Wigs: Coloring Guidelines

- Clean the wig following the "Cleaning and Conditioning Guidelines."

- Apply the appropriate color on the wig hair according to product directions, distributing evenly through the hair with a wide-tooth comb. Allow the color to process and remain on the hair according to manufacturer's instructions.

- Remove the color and condition hair according to the manufacturer's directions.

- Apply desired styling products and set the hair with rollers, or comb it in the desired direction and allow the wig to dry.

Cutting and Shaping

The majority of wigs are available 'pre-cut.' The hair or fiber is attached to the cap so that the resulting length arrangement creates a finished hair sculpture. Keep in mind, though, that human hair wigs are more likely to require a full shaping than their synthetic counterparts.

Most wigs are produced with about twice as much hair as on a typical human head. Therefore, it is often necessary to taper or thin a wig in order to decrease bulk and create a more natural-looking appearance. You may use a razor or thinning shears to thin a human hair wig. It is not recommended to use a razor on synthetic wigs, since they tend to frizz easily. Be sure to cut synthetic fiber when it is dry to avoid additional frizzing

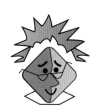

"Unlike a human head of hair, the hair on a wig does not grow back! So, you'll want to plan your cutting procedure carefully before actually removing any hair."

The majority of thinning should be done near the base to remove bulk, especially near the front hairline and behind the ears. Be especially careful to avoid cutting into the cap or the wefting. On a hand-tied wig, be sure that the knotting remains secure and that you have not cut any of the knots.

You may need to do some customizing on a pre-cut wig so that it perfectly suits your client's features. The fringe and front hairline areas are very common areas that require customizing. Thinning or tapering may also be performed closer to the hair ends as needed.

If a full cut is required, it is best to establish the length and basic lines while the client is wearing the wig so you can relate to your client's facial features. Moving the wig to a block after the basic lines have been established will simplify the remaining blending and shaping efforts by allowing you more movement and control. Remember, make sure the wig is properly positioned and secured to the block.

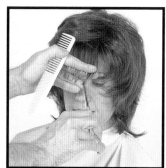
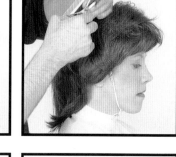
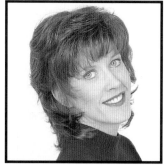
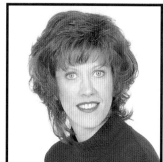

1 1

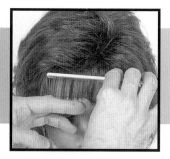

Helpful Tip: Backcombing the hair very close to the front hairline of the wig can help you soften the hairline and create a more natural-looking result.

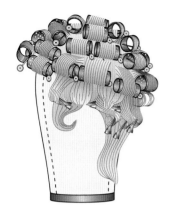
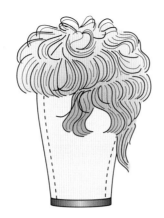

Setting and Styling

Human hair wigs can be either wet set or set when dry. Setting a human hair wig is very much like setting the hair growing on a human head, except that particular attention must be paid to creating closer shapes at the nape and making sure styles cover the hairline. Note that pincurls can be used where closeness is required and that wig pins can be used on the block instead of picks to hold rollers or pincurls in place.

Synthetic wigs are pre-styled with predetermined curl patterns. This curl pattern is not intended to be altered by the client or the stylist. The predetermined curl patterns in synthetic wigs require only minimal styling after cleaning.

Wigs provide a wide range of solutions and fashion statements for you and your clients. Understanding how to provide customized services for your clients allows you another method of retaining a satisfied, loyal clientele.

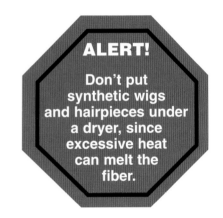

ALERT!

Don't put synthetic wigs and hairpieces under a dryer, since excessive heat can melt the fiber.

Hairpieces

Hairpieces are worn for coverage in specific areas or simply to create particular effects. They consist of a man-made base with attached hair fiber. Hairpieces are most often worn with your client's own hair to create a fashion statement or a special-occasion look. Synthetic hairpiece manufacturers usually produce their own color samples based on the modacrylic fiber they use. A full range of colors and special effects is available.

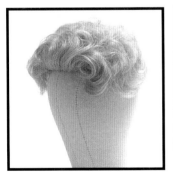
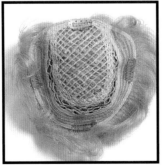

- **A wiglet consists of hair fiber usually six inches or less in length attached to a round-shaped, flat base. A wiglet is a hair piece ususally worn to create fullness or height at the top or crown area of the head. Wiglets are designed to be blended into the wearer's own hair. Most wiglets have clips attached in order to secure them to the client's own hair.**

- **A cascade consists of long hair fiber attached to an oblong-shaped dome base. A cascade is a hairpiece worn to create bulk or special effects.**

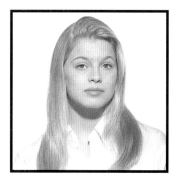 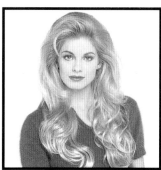

- **A fall is a hairpiece with a base that covers the crown, occipital and nape areas.** Falls are available in various lengths, usually between twelve and twenty-four inches, and create the look of a full, thick head of hair. Variations of the fall include demi-falls, demi-wigs and three-quarter wigs. The front of your client's hair is incorporated into the styling of these pieces.

- **A switch is a long weft of one to three swatches of hair, mounted on a loop base, worn primarily as a braid or ponytail.** Switches may be worn hanging or incorporated into an updo and are used particularly for evening styles.

- **A chignon is a fairly long, bulky segment of looped hair, usually sewn to a wire base or tied into a strong cord.** Chignons are usually pre-formed into a specific shape and are most often worn at the crown of the head or at the nape.

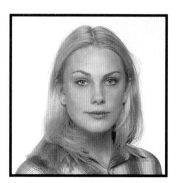 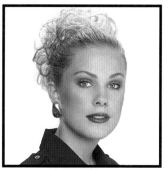

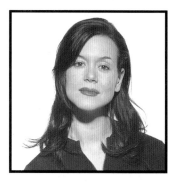 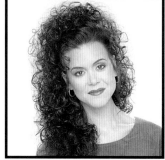

- **A curl segment consists of individual pieces of curly hair that vary in bulk depending on the desired effect.** Colors can be natural or dramatic fantasy colors since curl segments are most often worn to create specific fashion statements.

- **A braid is a switch that has three swatches of hair braided together, often with a thin wire running through it.** The wire helps hold the braid in the shape that you have designed.

- **A toupee is a hairpiece worn by men to cover bald or thinning hair spots, particularly on top of the head.** Some men, however, may require a full wig. Toupees are usually attached with an adhesive.

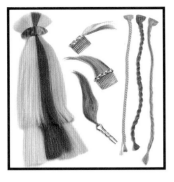
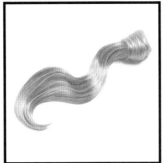

- Many manufacturers offer a variety of hairpieces that do not fall into the more traditional categories. These include small clip-on pieces, ponytail wraps, artificial ponytails, and many other designs worn for fun and fashion!

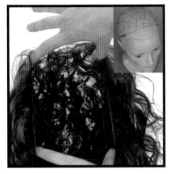
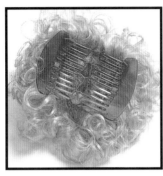

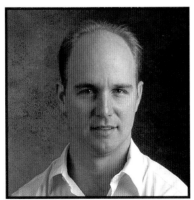
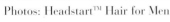
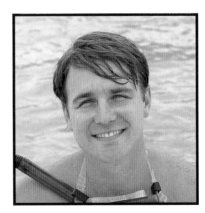

- An integration hairpiece has many openings in the base that allow the client's hair to be pulled through for blending purposes. Primarily used to add length and volume to a hairstyle, the integration hairpiece is lightweight and adaptable to many hairstyles.

  Many fashion hairpieces are designed so that attachment is as simple as possible. A variety of clips, combs or interlocking combs is used to allow for quick and easy changes.

- Other hairpieces can include elaborate hair ornaments like those used in the HairWorld Championships or International Hairstyling Competitions. These hairpieces are often custom-made by the contestants and incorporated into the overall design according to the rules of the competition.

Toupees

Toupees are hairpieces designed specifically to cover balding areas, especially for men. Many men will wish to be as discreet as possible about attaining this particular service from you, so again you must exercise discretion and propriety during your consultation and follow-up services.

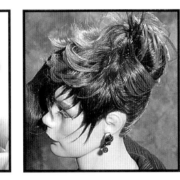
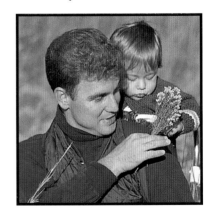

Photos: Headstart™ Hair for Men

Guidelines for Measuring Toupees

Most toupee manufacturers require that the stylist submit an impression of the client's head. This impression is used to customize the toupee to the specific size and shape of the client's head and his particular needs. When creating a plastic head form, accuracy is obviously very important.

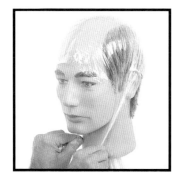

- Place a length of clear plastic wrap over your client's head, from ear to ear. Twist the ends until the plastic molds tightly to the head.

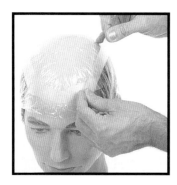

- Create an 'outline' of the intended shape of the toupee by placing tape over the plastic parallel to and slightly beyond the area of hair loss.

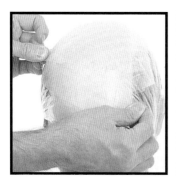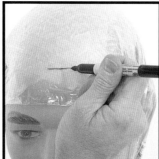

- Create a cap for the toupee by criss-crossing strips of plastic tape within the outlined area. Position each strip, one at a time, and mold to the head. Create a complete cap with tape. Once the 'impression' is complete, use a felt tip pen to indicate the exact size and shape of the toupee.

1 1

To establish a front hairline:

- Have the client raise his brows to wrinkle his forehead. Approximately 1/2" (1.25 cm) above the top wrinkle indicates a generally ideal position for the center hairline. An alternative is to measure four finger widths above the brow line. Generally, this will give you an appropriate and acceptable front hairline position. An extremely low hairline position is one of the 'giveaways' of a poorly fitted toupee.

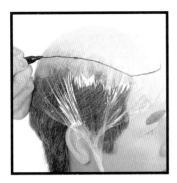

- Extend the line to cover the bald area. It is advisable to extend the pattern 1/2 inch (1.75 cm) over the hairline. If the client's hairline continues to recede, he will still be able to wear the toupee.

- Identify the crown/cowlick area by clearly marking this area on your form.

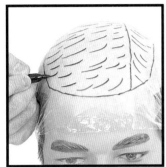

- Carefully draw a part, if it is desired, and indicate the hair growth direction to be positioned on either side.

- Remove taped form carefully and trim excess. Tape underside if necessary.

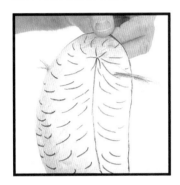

- Clip hair samples from behind the ear and nape to guide the manufacturer in blending the right color for the client.

NOTE: Some manufacturers require a plaster form of the client's head. This form is sent to the manufacturer who creates a latex cap and attaches hair to the cap. A latex cap creates the best fit but may not allow perspiration to escape.

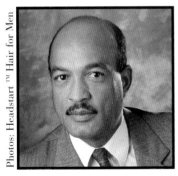
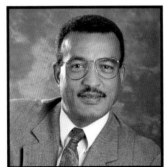
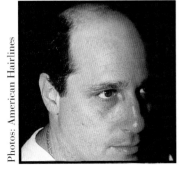
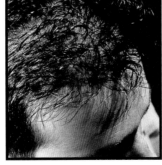

Photos: Headstart ™ Hair for Men

Photos: American Hairlines

Clients who wear toupees are in need of your continued expertise, even after the toupee has been created. Careful sculpting and blending with the client's own hair is an absolute necessity to ensure that the finished design looks as natural as possible. Advise your client to maintain the natural hair with regular haircut appointments. If the natural hair becomes too long, it will not blend with the perimeter lengths of the toupee. It is also necessary to advise the client that his natural hair may alter in color, possibly through graying. Color change may create a situation in which the toupee and the client's hair no longer match or blend. At that time it may become necessary for your client to invest in a new toupee.

HAIR ADDITIONS

Unlike wigs and hair pieces, hair additions consist of loose hair fiber intended for attachment to the base of the client's own hair. Hair additions offer a whole new spectrum of designing options for you and your clients. You can add length, density, texture and/or color, all over, or in just the right places to accent your design. Match the color and texture of your client's hair for the most natural-looking results, or create stunning new effects by introducing contrasting elements in the hair additions.

Hair Addition Methods

On these pages, you will find highlights of several of the most popular and commonly used methods of creating hair additions. Keep an eye on industry publications to learn about new methods that are being developed on an ongoing basis.

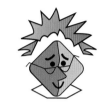

"For more information and step-by-step technicals on the techniques highlighted here, look at Pivot Point's *Hair Additions* course book."

Off-the-Scalp Braiding, Loose Hair/Fiber

Off-the-scalp braiding uses a standard three-strand braiding technique to attach loose fiber or hair. It is achieved by incorporating the hair or fiber, along with the natural hair, as it is braided. The additional hair can be added to one side or both sides of the braid.

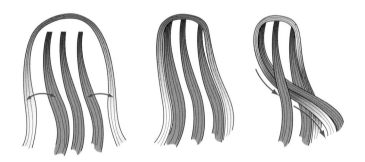

The size of the base is determined by the desired thickness of the braid. Divide the base into three sections. Then select the length and density of the hair to be added. Position the addition as shown, joining it with the outside strands. An underbraid technique is used in this example. Grasp the center strand with the thumb and index fingers of your left hand. Then turn your right hand in order to cross the outside right strand (with the additional hair) under. This now becomes the center strand. Next, turn your left hand to cross the left strand (with additional hair) under. This now becomes the center strand. Continue this alternating pattern to the ends.

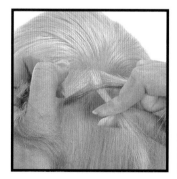
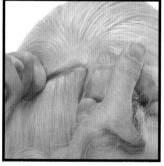

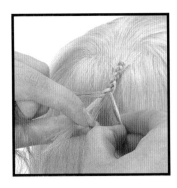
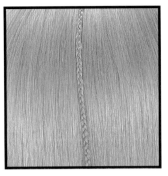

As you work, you may equalize the density of the strands by 'borrowing' a small amount of hair from the added strands and joining this hair with the strand that did not get additional hair.

This model's hair additions combine on-the-scalp and off-the-scalp braiding with loose fiber. Note the consistency of the base sizes and the tension used to create these additions. Notice that the ends are not braided, since they will be incorporated into the finished, sculpted design.

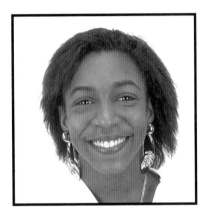
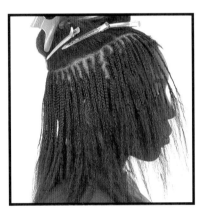
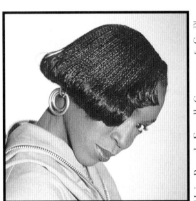

Hair: Pamela Ferrell, Cornrows & Co.™

On-The-Scalp Braiding, Loose Hair/Fiber

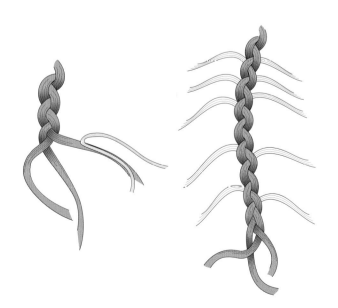

With this technique (known as interlocking), a three-strand, on-the-scalp braid is used as a base to which fiber or hair is added. You can add loose fiber to every left and right strand for maximum density or you can space the additions along the braid to create a progression of density.

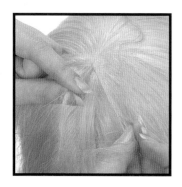

Begin by parting off a strip of hair to be braided. This strip is called a track. At the top of the track, part off a small square and section it into three strands. Begin a three-strand underbraid, crossing the right strand under the center and then the left strand under the center.

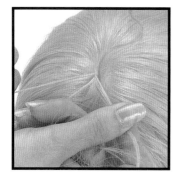

Join a strand of hair or fiber to the right strand, with the end of the fiber at the ends of the outside strand. Then cross these combined strands to the center.

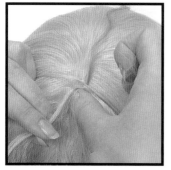
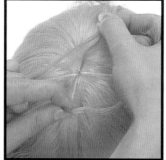

Use your thumb and index finger to pick up hair from the track, and add it to the center strand.

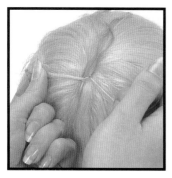
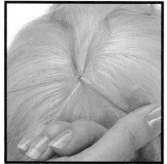

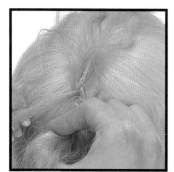
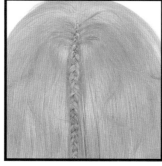

Then add a new strand of fiber to the left strand and cross the combined strands to the center to lock the new strands at the base. Continue using the same technique, picking up hair at the scalp, as you work through the track. You may alter the pattern by adding more or less fiber. You can also alter the number of crosses between the added fiber, depending on the desired results. Remember: the amount of fiber you add along the braided track will determine the density in any given area.

11

This model is wearing a beautiful example of on-the-scalp braids with loose fibers. Note that the hair additions create a fashionable texture statement as length is added.

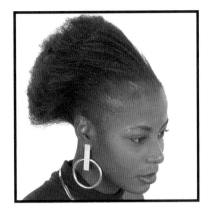 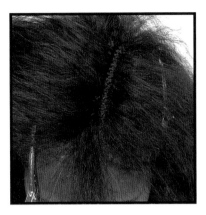 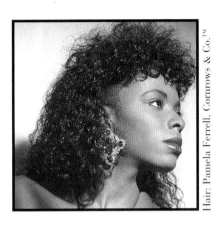

Hair: Pamela Ferrell, Cornrows & Co.™

Track and Sew

With this method, a three-strand on-the-scalp braid is used as a support structure to which a hair weft (a strip of human or artificial hair) is then sewn.

Tracking

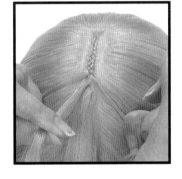

The tracks used in this technique are similar to the tracks described in on-the-scalp braiding. The difference is that these tracks will be used to support hair wefts as opposed to having loose fiber added to them. Tracks can follow the curves of the head or relate to the desired form line. They may be positioned horizontally, vertically or diagonally as well as along convex or concave curved lines. Clean precise tracks depend on clean precise parting lines. Once you have parted the track, secure the remaining hair on either side out of the way.

Plan your track so that the ends of the braids can be camouflaged by the sewn-on wefts. Generally, position the tracks one inch (2.5 cm) behind the hairline so they are not visible.

On finer or straighter hair, crimped fiber may be added to the braided track for additional stability.

Sewing Methods

Straight and/or curved needles with blunted ends are used to sew weft to the braided tracks. These blunted ends help avoid discomfort or injury to you or your client. Generally, a cotton/polyester blend thread is used to sew the wefts to the tracks.

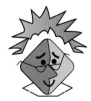

"Make sure your needles, whether straight or curved, have blunt ends. This avoids damaging the hair and injuring your client...or yourself!"

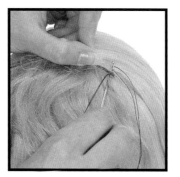

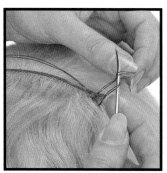

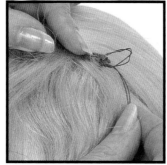

LOCK STITCH

Thread the needle, making sure the thread is long enough to be doubled across the length of the weft/track. Sew through the weft first and then bring the needle through the track. Pull the thread through, forming a small loop. Bring the needle through the loop and wrap the thread around the needle. Pull the loop tight to form a 'lock stitch' that will keep the end of the weft more secure.

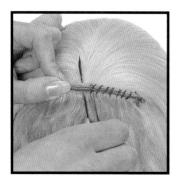

OVERCAST STITCH

An 'overcast' stitch is used to secure the weft to the track. For this stitch, the needle and thread are passed under the track and the weft and then brought back over. Move slightly to one side to complete the next stitch. This is the simplest and quickest stitch used to secure the weft to the track. A lock stitch is used at either end of the track for added security.

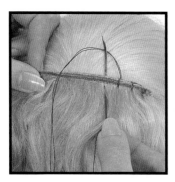

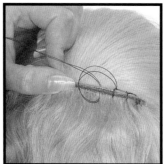

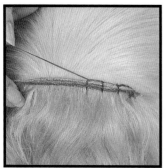

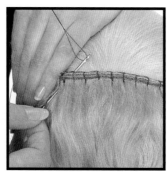

LOCK STITCH THROUGHOUT

You may also use a lock stitch across the length of the entire weft/track. Spacing the stitches equally will help to distribute the weight of the weft more evenly.

11

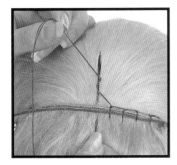

DOUBLE-LOCK STITCH

A double-lock stitch can be used to secure a weft at either end or across the length of the weft/track. This stitch is similar to the lock stitch except that the thread is wound around the needle as shown to create a 'double lock.'

For this model, the track-and-sew technique is used to attach synthetic hair that matches her color and curl texture. Three curved tracks are braided and an overcast stitch is used to secure the wefts to the tracks.

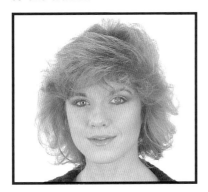 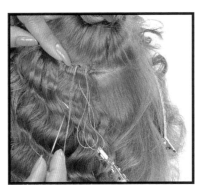 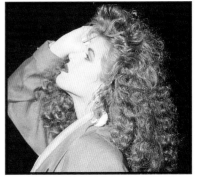

Hair: Pamela Ferrell, Cornrows & Co.™

Make sure that the partings are clean and neat. Keep the hair outside of the track isolated with clips to ensure accuracy. Note that the loose ends of the braids have been crossed over and sewn as the weft is being sewn on.

Bonding - Wefts

Bonding is the attachment of additional hair fiber to a client's own hair with a special adhesive. The adhesive is applied along partings of the client's hair and to the sewn edge of the weft being added. Since some clients may have an allergic reaction to ingredients in the adhesive, it is necessary to perform a patch test prior to the application of bonded hair additions. It is also necessary to advise your clients of the duration and longevity of this type of hair-addition service, which may vary according to factors such as frequency of shampooing, oiliness of the scalp and of products used. Note that oil will break down the adhesive.

After creating the part, measure the length of the weft and cut it accordingly. Note that both the client's hair and the weft must be completely dry prior to performing the service.

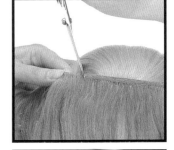

Apply the liquid adhesive to the hair along the parting. Make sure the adhesive is applied consistently to ensure proper bonding.

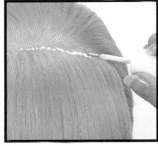

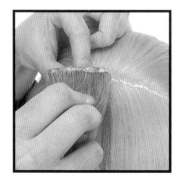
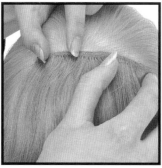

Apply the adhesive along the sewn edge of the weft, then place the weft along the part and apply gentle pressure. Make sure that contact is made along the entire length of the weft.

For this model, bonded additions are performed in the back and layered to blend with the rest of the design in order to add length to her fine hair, while maintaining her professional image.

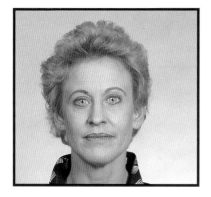
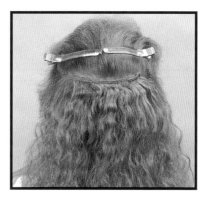
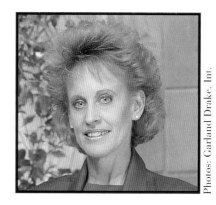

Photos: Garland Drake, Int.

Bonding - Strand by Strand (Fusion Method)

This technique utilizes a bonding agent that is activated by a heating element to affix loose hair fiber to small sections of the client's own hair. Since the hair is attached in such small increments, the results can be very natural-looking and undetectable.

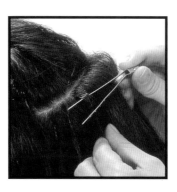

Small rectangular sections are taken within rows and isolated with a plastic disc. The additions are placed behind the sections of hair. The heating element (in this case 'tongs') is applied until the bonding agent has softened. Then the fingers are used to roll the bonded area until the natural and added hair have bonded. It is essential that natural growth patterns are carefully observed and noted prior to the service. Going against these patterns can result in discomfort to your client and possible damage to the hair and scalp.

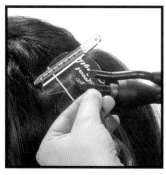
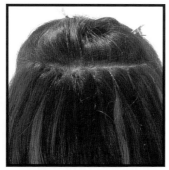

11

The placement of color within the pattern of additions is also important to consider so that the additions blend with the client's natural or artificial colors attractively. This model gets it all–additional length, texture and color! Strand-by-strand bonded additions are terrific for achieving high fashion looks but are also used for 'prescriptive' purposes to improve self-esteem.

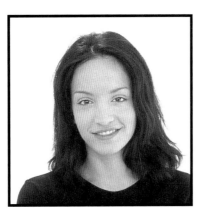 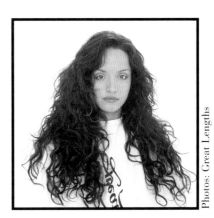

Photos: Great Lengths

This model will not be alone in 'getting it all' once you add wig services to your resume. With most people, hair loss for any reason carries strong consequences, emotional as well as physical. Imagine their relief if you as their stylist know not only the background and history of wigs and hairpieces but also how to fit, clean, style and maintain the wig, hairpiece or hair addition you have helped them select.

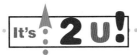

Build Your Critical Thinking Skills

In this chapter you have prepared yourself to meet the following Industry Standards for entry-level cosmetologists:
- Consult with clients to determine their needs and preferences
- Provide non-surgical hair additions
- Market professional salon products

It's Up to You to know what to do. Using your training to this point, review the following case scenario and think through how you would handle the challenge.

One of your clients has just stopped by the salon with a wig that she received from her elderly aunt. Her aunt has kept the wig in a very nice wig case over the years but cannot remember if the wig is made of human or synthetic hair. Your client wants you to look at the wig and determine if you could color the wig to match her hair color, since her aunt's hair is a few shades lighter than hers. What would you do?

Chapter 12
CHEMICAL TEXTURIZING

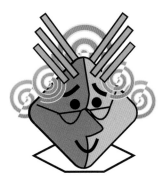

After studying this chapter you will be able to . . .

1. **Explain and demonstrate the fundamental theory and procedures of perming**

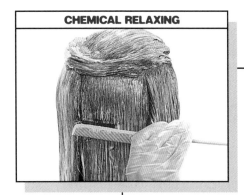

PERMING

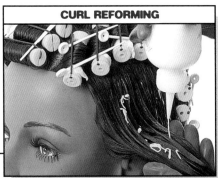

CURL REFORMING

3. **Explain and demonstrate the fundamental theory and procedures of curl reforming**

CHEMICAL RELAXING

2. **Explain and demonstrate the fundamental theory and procedures of chemical relaxing**

1 2

Did you think you had seen the last of chemistry once you finished Chapter 5? Guess again! Now you come to the chapter where chemistry really becomes fun and exciting because you take it into your own hands. In this chapter, your knowledge of chemistry translates into your ability to successfully perm or relax a client's hair.

Your study and practice of chemical texturizing gives you the ability to chemically alter the texture of hair, greatly expanding the services you are able to offer your clients and the number of clients seeking your services.

Because of the wonders of chemical texturizing, no head of hair has to stay in its original condition. People can successfully answer for themselves with your help the intriguing question: How would I look if...? If my straight hair could be wavy or curly... If my thin hair could look full... If my thick hair could become more manageable... What a VALUE for the client! What a VALUE for you!

Perming, Chemical Relaxing and Curl Reforming provide major chemical changes for the hair that, in turn, offer a client new options for cuts and styles.

This chapter's three very clear-cut sections - Perming, Chemical Relaxing and Curl Reforming - make its BIG IDEA easy to grasp. You need to learn a way to add texture, body and curl, to remove it or to tone it down a bit. That you'll do by executing the PLAN I have laid out for you.

PERMING

History of Perming
Perm Theory
Perming Essentials
Infection Control and Safety
Client Consultation
Perm Wrap Overview
Rectangle Perm Wrap
Bricklay Perm Wrap
Spiral Bricklay Perm Wrap
Oblong and Spiral Bricklay
    Perm Wrap
Perm Problems and
    Solutions

RELAXING

Chemical Relaxing Theory
Chemical Relaxing Essentials
Infection Control and Safety
Client Consultation
Product and Application
    Overview
Virgin Sodium Hydroxide
    Relaxer
Virgin Thio Relaxer
Relaxer Retouch

CURL REFORMING

Curl Reforming Theory
Curl Reforming Essentials
Infection Control and Safety
Client Consultation
Curl Reforming Service:
    Contour Wrap

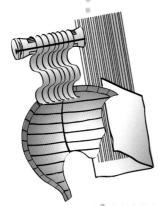

"Chemical Texturizing" may seem like a strange title for a chapter in a cosmetology textbook until you realize what it involves. You all know people with straight hair who wish it were curly and those with curly hair who dream about having it straight. What exactly do these people want? They want their hair chemically texturized! **Chemical texturizing (reforming) is simply the process of using physical and chemical actions to permanently change the texture of hair.**

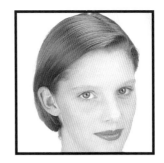
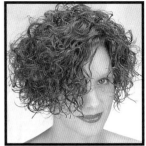
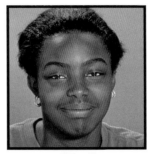
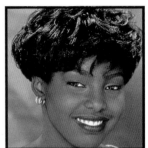
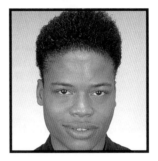
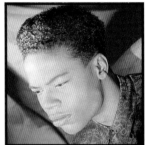

There are three major classifications of chemical texturizing – perming, hair relaxing and curl reforming. With this information you will be able to make straight hair curly (perming) and curly hair straight (relaxing) as well as to change the types of curls and configurations in the hair (curl reforming). In this chapter you will learn how perming, hair relaxing and curl reforming have become some of the most important and popular salon services. You will also look at the different types of hair, the kinds of products to be used and the procedures that yield professional results.

PERMING

Perming is a highly valued service in the salon. Not only does it create changes in the client's appearance, it is also a significant revenue generator. Today's clients request perms to add volume, texture and movement to their hair. Fortunately, manufacturers have created perm formulas that remove the chemical guesswork and allow you, as a stylist, to concentrate on the creative side of the service, such as determining how much curl is introduced and what direction it moves. Perming is a chemical service that you can successfully use throughout your entire salon career.

History of Perming

Perming (or permanent waving) the hair has a fascinating history and a solid future in the salon industry. As people seek ways to improve their appearance, they will continue to request professional services to add fullness, waves or curls to their hair.

The desire for curly or wavy hair dates back to ancient cultures. The ancient Egyptians wrapped hair around wooden sticks, applied mud from hot springs and then baked it in the sun. When the mud was dry, it was removed. Sometimes the results lasted a few weeks, possibly because of sulfur derivatives in the mud.

1
2

Three to four hundred years ago, wigmakers achieved permanent curl in hairpieces by wrapping hair on rods and then boiling them in solutions of hot alkalis. It was believed that the caustic qualities of the chemicals caused the curls to be permanent. Obviously, this process was not safe to use on people.

The ability to create curls and waves with long-lasting results, which today is called perming or permanent waving, didn't become a reality until the 20th century. **In 1905, Charles Nessler made the first real breakthrough with his heat permanent waving machine.** The machine heated the rollers, around which the hair was tightly wrapped in a spiral fashion. **This spiral method involved wrapping the hair from scalp to ends,** which was only suitable for clients with long hair. These first permanents consisted of a solution of strong alkalis not unlike the sodium hydroxide used today for hair relaxing. Once applied, the solution was heated to about 212°+ F (100°+ C) with the aid of electrical heaters.

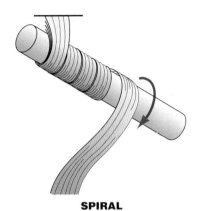

SPIRAL

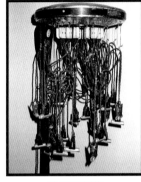

ELECTRIC PERMANENT WAVING MACHINE

After World War I, women began cutting their hair much shorter, so the spiral method did not work well with these new lengths. Consequently, in 1926, **the croquignole method of wrapping hair from the ends to the scalp** became practical and popular. **This croquignole method led the way to the use of clamps that were preheated on a separate electric unit and then placed over the hair. This preheated clamp process was called the pre-heat or machineless method.** Again strong alkali chemicals were used with the heat to produce a lasting curl.

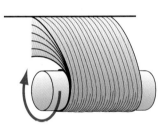

CROQUIGNOLE

In 1931, at the Midwest Beauty Show in Chicago, Ralph I. Evans and Everett G. McDonough introduced another method of perming. Instead of electricity, this heatless technique used bi-sulphides that worked fairly well. The process produced a chemical reaction, which reformed the hair from straight to curly or wavy. Sometimes, the client would have the wave wrapped in the salon, go home and then return in the morning for her finished style, which led to the name the "overnight wave."

All three methods used various combinations of strong alkalis, heat, tightly wrapped hair and long processing times to produce a permanent curl. These often caused scalp burns and severe hair damage.

Cold Waves

Because of the many drawbacks and unwanted side effects of the early perms, there was an increasing need for a safer and more practical perm process. Research for better procedures continued and by 1938 Arnold F. Willatt invented the first cold wave. Its name meant that no machines were used and chemicals created no heat reactions. **With this machineless method, the hair was still wrapped on rods while a waving lotion (thioglycolic acid or its derivatives) processed the hair without heat.** Once the hair was processed, it was rinsed. Then a chemical with an acid pH, called a neutralizer, was applied to reform the hair and take on the shape of the rod. Even so, those first cold waves took six to eight hours to complete at room temperature. Today's highly improved cold waves are called alkaline waves.

Alkaline waves are currently formulated with thioglycolic acid or its derivatives and ammonia, which creates a compound called ammonium thioglycolate. Ammonia is a strong alkaline and, when added to thioglycolic acid, creates a waving lotion with a pH between 8.0 - 9.5 that penetrates the hair much faster without heat. Generally, alkaline waves on today's market process within 15 to 30 minutes. Neutralizers bring down the pH of the hair and rebond the curl pattern to make it permanent.

Heat Waves: Acid and Exothermic

To satisfy a growing need for perms that would leave the hair shiny and healthy, acid waves appeared on the market in the early 1970s. **Acid waves contained a thioglycolic derivative, called glycerol monothioglycolate,** and did not contain ammonia. Many were called "buffered waves" because they were more gentle on the hair and penetrated the hair strand more slowly. To speed up the processing time, **heat was added by placing a plastic cap on the client's head and placing her under a pre-heated dryer. This method of heat is called endothermic.** Heat caused the pH to gradually rise, leaving the hair in a much healthier condition. **Today's acid perms are in the range of 6.9 to 7.2.**

Exothermic perms appeared on the market next. These were self-timing and self-heating. An additive that created heat through a chemical reaction was mixed with the perm solution. Exothermic perms range from acid to alkaline, depending upon the manufacturer.

New Technology

Perm technology and products are continually evolving. More recent perm products on today's market include neutral, low pH alkaline and thio-free perms (which may or may not require heat). As a professional cosmetologist, it is your responsibility to stay current with the latest technology and products and always follow manufacturer's directions.

1 2

Perm Theory

Today's perms involve two major phases. The first phase is the physical action, the wrapping of the hair around the perm tool, using end papers. The second step is the chemical phase, which involves applying the perm solution, rinsing it from the hair, applying the neutralizer and rinsing it from the hair. Both phases of the perm process are of equal importance.

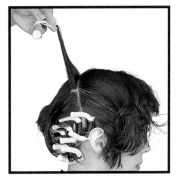
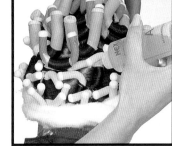
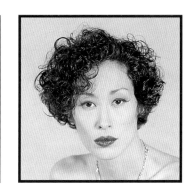

PHYSICAL PHASE **CHEMICAL PHASE** **FINAL RESULT**

Physical Phase

In order to perform the physical phase of a perm service, you will need to become familiar with perm tools (rods), end paper techniques, base sizes, tool positions and wrapping patterns. In perming the goal is to have the hair assume the size and shape of the tool used. Therefore, it is important to wrap the hair smoothly and evenly around the tool, using appropriate tension without stretching the hair. There are two basic methods of wrapping hair around a perm tool: The croquignole, also called the overlap, and the spiral.

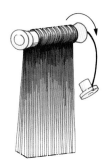

Croquignole

As you'll recall, when performing the croquignole (overlap) method, the hair is wrapped from the ends up to the scalp. With this method the hair overlaps itself with each revolution. To create a complete curl pattern, the strand should overlap around the perm tool at least 2.5 times. This overlap method creates an undulating wave and volume at the base.

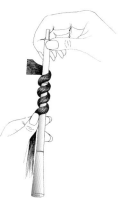

Spiral

There are two types of spiral wrapping methods, base-to-ends and ends-to-base. With the base-to-ends method, you begin at the base and wrap the hair around the tool. The ends are then secured.

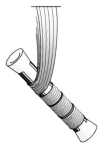

With the ends-to-base spiral method, you begin at the ends and rotate under twice and then position the tool vertically before wrapping the hair around the tool in a corkscrew fashion. Both methods produce a hanging curl with reduced volume at the base.

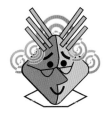

"When wrapped properly, the hair around a perm tool should look like thread around a spool."

Perm Tools

Perm tools come in various lengths, diameters and shapes. The most common is the perm rod. Each size is color-coded for easier selection of the correct diameter. Colors will vary with individual perm tool manufacturers. **Small diameter rods produce small, firm curls and large diameter rods produce large curls, wave formations or body waves.**

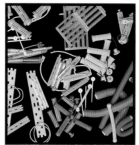
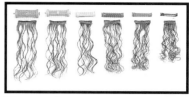

The smaller the rod, the greater the length reduction.

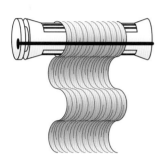

Perm rods are either straight or concave. Straight rods produce curls or waves that are uniform throughout the hair strands. The hair on the ends travels approximately the same distance as the hair in the center, producing a consistent curl throughout the strands.

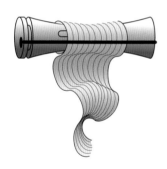

Concave rods produce a smaller, tighter curl in the center. With concave rods, the hair on both ends must travel farther to make one complete turn around the rod than the hair in the center. This difference creates the wider and more spiraling pattern on the ends of the rod.

End Paper Techniques

End papers are used to control the hair ends and keep the hair smoothly wrapped around the perm tool. End papers are available in several sizes and are chosen according to the hair length and the amount of hair being wrapped. Proper end paper techniques will eliminate crimps or "fishhooks" on the ends of the hair.

1 2

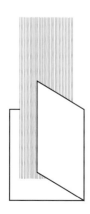

A **bookend technique** uses one end paper folded in half. This technique is used to control sections of hair when a shorter rod length is selected or to wrap sections of very short hair.

- Either pre-fold an end paper and place it over the strand, or position the end paper and fold it over the ends.

- Slide the end paper past the ends of the strand without converging (bunching) the hair. Keep the ends flat and completely covered.

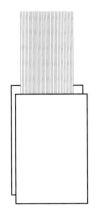

A **double-flat end paper technique** incorporates two end papers, one on the top and one on the bottom. It is the most common end paper technique because it allows you maximum control of tapered ends and avoids bunching the ends. Note that longer end papers are available for this technique.

- Position the first end paper under the strand, past the ends of the hair.
- Position the second end paper on top of the strand, slightly past the first end paper.

A **cushion end paper technique** incorporates several end papers. It begins with a double-flat technique and then additional end papers are positioned on top of the strand as you wrap the tool. This technique is known as cushion wrapping because it provides an extra layer of protection between the revolutions of hair wrapped around the rod. It is recommended for chemically treated or highly porous hair to allow even absorption of the solutions and is used primarily in alkaline waving to keep the hair smooth and provide for expansion when the hair swells.

- Wrap the rod to within 1/4" (.66 cm) of the end of the first two papers. Place a paper on the top of the strand overlapping the first paper.
- Wrap the hair toward the scalp. Continue the cushion technique up the strand as needed.

When using multiple end papers, it is important to rinse and blot the hair thoroughly since the extra papers hold more moisture. Water left in the end papers after rinsing the perm solution will dilute the neutralizer and weaken the curl formation.

Base Size

The area between two partings for an individual perm rod is called a base, panel, blocking or subsection. It is important that the base is not longer than the length of the rod being used. If the base is longer than the rod length, excess hair at both ends of the rod will be dragged toward the center. This extended drag creates an uneven curl pattern that is wider at both ends than it is in the center.

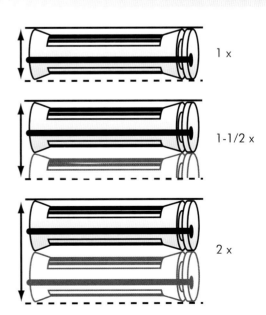

1 x

1-1/2 x

2 x

Generally, the width of the base is determined by the diameter of the rod. A one-base size is equal to the diameter of the rod. A larger base size, 1.5 to 2 times the diameter of the rod, will reduce the strength of the curl, which may be a desired option. Be careful, however, since too much hair on the rod will prevent the solutions from penetrating properly, weakening the curl. Too much hair on the rod can also cause the rod bands to cut into or crease the hair. This creasing produces a crimp or a ridge causing a stress point on the hair, which may eventually cause the hair to break.

Tool Position

Tool position, or base control, is determined by the size of the base and the angle at which the hair is held while wrapping. There are four basic tool positions: On base, half-off base, underdirected and off base.

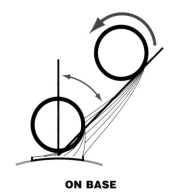

ON BASE

To achieve an **on-base** tool position, a one-diameter base is directed 45° above the center of the base and wrapped so the tool sets between the two partings. **An on-base tool position is used to create more volume.** On-base control is not recommended for alkaline perms, since expansion is limited at the base and tension may cause breakage.

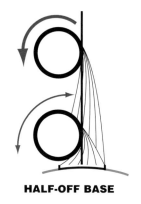

HALF-OFF BASE

The most common base control is a **half-off base,** one-diameter base size. With half-off base control, a one-diameter base is held at a 90° angle from the center of the base. This base control produces the maximum amount of curl from the scalp to the ends with minimum stress on the hair. **With half-off base control, the rod will be positioned half on its base and half off its base, directly on the bottom parting.**

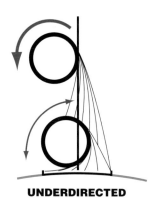

UNDERDIRECTED

With an **underdirected** tool position, the base size is at least 1.5 diameters. The tool is positioned in the lower half of the base to achieve moderate base lift. This base control is used in perimeter areas where closeness is desired.

1
2

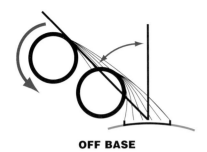

OFF BASE

With an **off-base** tool position, there will be no curl at the scalp. The hair is held at 45° below the center of the base while wrapping so that the tool sets completely off its base. **An off-base tool placement is used only where you want a minimal degree of volume** and a curl pattern concentrated on the midstrand and ends. Any base size can be used for the off-base tool position.

Wrapping Patterns

Proper sectioning and parting patterns are important to successful perming. Sectioning begins with combing the hair in the direction you want it to move and then dividing the head according to the length of the rod or the wrapping pattern you've chosen. The parting pattern within the sections creates the bases, or subsections, for each tool. These partings are sometimes called blockings.

There are many wrapping patterns, also called rod placement patterns. A few of the more common patterns are illustrated below.

The **rectangle, or 9-block pattern,** consists primarily of rectangular shapes throughout the pattern. The basic direction is downward. The rectangle pattern is generally considered to be the most basic perm pattern.

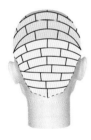

The **bricklay pattern** positions tools in a staggered configuration. This pattern can be compared to the way a bricklayer arranges the bricks in a building, alternating their position row by row. This wrapping pattern can move in any direction and is chosen to avoid splits in a design.

The **spiral bricklay pattern** features horizontal rows that are subdivided in a staggered bricklay pattern. Tools are positioned vertically within the square bases.

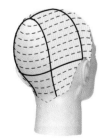

The **double-halo pattern** features a center part with two rows of perm rods that follow the curves of the head.

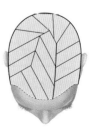

The **oblong pattern** positions rods within oblongs using diagonal partings. Oblongs are elongated shapes that create strong wave patterns.

Custom Wrapping Patterns

Partial perms position new texture only where it is desired. These wraps are excellent for short hair.

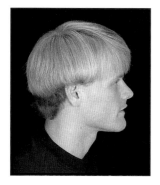 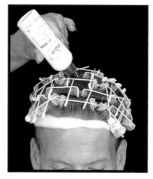 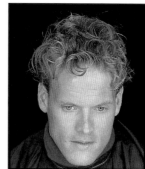

Perimeter perms, also called a drop crown wrap, eliminate texture in the top and crown and focus on the perimeter and ends of the hair.

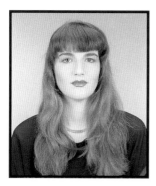 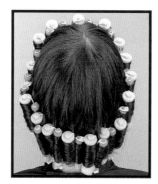 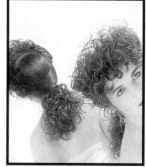

Piggyback perms position two rods along a single strand. This is designed for longer lengths to ensure complete saturation of chemicals. The rods are wrapped in alternate directions to create a continued wave pattern. Both rods can be the same diameter or can be customized. Here, a smaller tool is positioned at the base and a larger one on the ends.

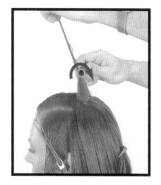 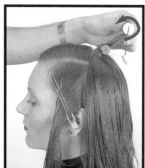 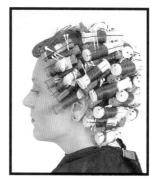 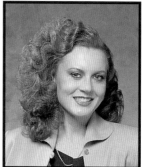

Always read and follow manufacturer's directions before you begin wrapping. A special shampoo or a pre-wrap solution designed to be applied before you wrap the hair may be included in the perm you have selected. Some perms may recommend applying the perm solution to individual sections prior to wrapping.

Ergonomic Tips

- When wrapping the hair, stand directly behind the section to be wrapped, not to one side or the other.

- Be sure the rods, end papers and spray bottle are within easy reach of your free hand. You cannot create a smooth, even wrap if you must shift to reach for supplies.

- Do not bend over, stoop or raise your shoulders uncomfortably while wrapping. Raise or lower the styling chair and tilt the client's head in a position to achieve the proper angle. This adjustment keeps your back erect, distributes weight evenly on your legs and eliminates shoulder cramps.

Chemical Phase

Once the hair has been wrapped on perm tools, the chemical phase begins. The basic steps of the chemical phase include:

- Applying perm solution
- Setting timer/taking test curl
- Rinsing
- Blotting
- Applying neutralizer
- Removing rods
- Rinsing

Perm Solution

To permanently change the hair from a straight to a curly state, strong disulfide bonds found in the cortex of the protein chains of hair must be broken. The disulfide bond is a chemical bond formed between two sulfur (S) atoms found in the amino acid, cystine. The perm solution (waving or reforming lotion) breaks the disulfide or S-S bonds.

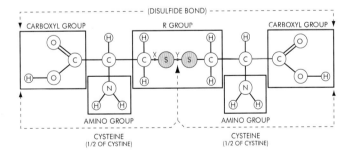
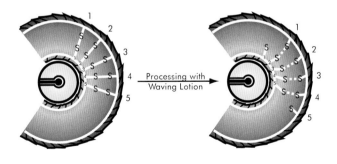

In alkaline (cold) waves, the perm solution chemically breaks (or reduces) the strong disulfide bonds while the hair is wrapped on the perm rods. With acid (heat) waves, heat, tension, and the perm solution break the disulfide bonds. With both types of perm solutions, the processing action softens the protein structure and allows the disulfide bonds to shift, assuming the shape of the rod.

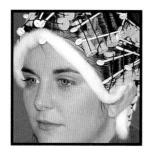

A smooth wrapping pattern will allow for proper saturation of the perm solution. Once the hair is wrapped, a protective cream is applied around the client's hairline and cotton is positioned on top of that. Keep in mind that the cotton should be replaced once it becomes saturated. Leaving it on your client's skin could cause chemical burns.

The perm solution is applied to both the top and bottom of each rod. It is important to work carefully and not to skip any rods because this will produce an inconsistent curl formation.

If the manufacturer requires heat for processing, a plastic bag should be attached around the hairline and the client should be placed under a hooded dryer. Heat is sometimes required for acid perms but generally not for alkaline perms. Resistant hair may require heat and a longer processing time.

Test Curl During Processing

Some perms are self-timing and others require you to take a test curl to determine complete processing. A good test curl occurs when chemical bonds have been broken to allow the strands to assume the shape of the perm tool. When performing a test curl, the tool is unwound one and one-half times, allowing the hair to unfold naturally. A positive test curl shows a definite "S" pattern and tends to subdivide into groupings. The wave dimension of a positive curl matches the diameter of the tool.

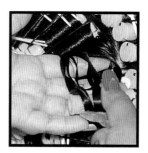 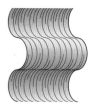

Rinsing

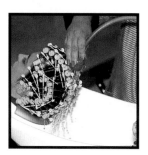

The rinsing step takes place after the waving (or reforming) lotion has broken the disulfide bonds, creating a strong test curl. Rinsing removes excess waving (or reforming) solution from the hair before neutralizing or rebonding. Some perms require you to rinse for a full five minutes. Longer hair may require a longer rinsing time. At this stage, it is important not to disturb the position of the rods because the hair is in a swollen and softened state.

Blotting

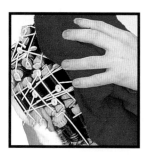

The next step is to towel blot the hair after it is rinsed. Blotting removes excess water before you apply the neutralizing solution. Blotting is a very important step because excess water left in the strands dilutes the neutralizer and results in incomplete rebonding. Insufficient blotting can lead to weak curls that relax prematurely.

1
2

Neutralizing or Rebonding (Oxidation)

Neutralizing (rebonding or oxidation) is the final chemical step in the perm process. It reforms the disulfide bonds while lowering the pH of the hair. **The main ingredient found in most neutralizers is hydrogen peroxide, sodium perborate or sodium bromate. The pH can range from 2.5 to 7,** depending on the type of neutralizer.

The neutralizer serves two functions:

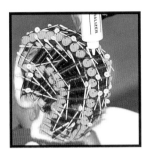

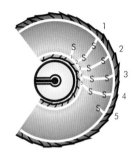

1. **Neutralizer rebonds and restores the disulfide bonds. This change fixes the hair in a new position, which is determined by the size of the rod, making the change 'permanent.'**

2. **Neutralizer reduces the swelling caused by the alkalinity of the perm solution (or reforming lotion) and hardens the bonds in the new shape.**

It is interesting to know that oxygen from the air (air oxidation) can be used to achieve the same results as the neutralizer. However, it is an impractical process because the hair must dry naturally on the rods, without heat, for 24 - 48 hours, depending on the length and texture of the hair.

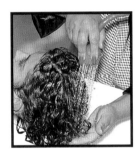

Rinsing

After it is neutralized, the hair will need to be rinsed again to remove all chemicals. Again, it is important to handle the hair carefully since it is still swollen and can be easily damaged. Remove the rods and work the neutralizer through the ends and rinse. An optional method is to leave the rods in position during rinsing and then remove them.

ALERT!

Always read manufacturers' directions to achieve the best results from their perm products.

Categories of Perm Solutions

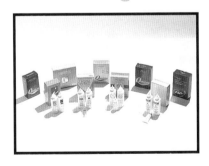

Manufacturers have created a wide variety of perm solutions so that you can select the most appropriate one according to the pre-perm analysis of your client's hair and the strength of the curl desired. There are two general categories of perms used in the salon, alkaline (cold) waves and acid (heat) waves. As their names in parentheses imply, **alkaline waves are processed without heat and acid waves are generally processed with heat.**

Alkaline Waves

Alkaline waves carry a pH of approximately 8.0 to 9.5. The alkalinity softens and swells the hair fibers, making it easier for the chemicals to penetrate the hair structure. These perms are excellent for resistant hair or when strong curl patterns are desired. **Because of the high alkalinity, it is necessary to use caution and skill to prevent damage to the hair structure or chemical burns to the skin.** Alkaline waves are not recommended for highly porous hair. Another kind of perm in this category is the low pH alkaline wave, created for textures and types of hair that do not respond well to other kinds of wave solutions. With a pH of 8, it is less alkaline than the typical cold wave.

Alkaline waves should be wrapped without tension (minimal stretching or straining of the hair) because alkaline reforming lotion causes the hair to swell. This swelling creates the necessary tension on the hair. Wrapping the hair with too much tension prior to applying an alkaline perm solution could result in an uneven penetration of the lotion and lead to breakage. Instead, hair should be held just taut enough to control the hair, creating a smooth, even wrap from ends to scalp.

With alkaline waving, the hair starts to process as soon as the solution is applied. Because of its higher pH, it processes faster than an acid wave, increasing the risk for hair damage. Therefore, it is important to watch the process carefully. Remember that **alkaline waves are applied without heat.**

Keep in mind that it is easier to rinse and/or blot an alkaline solution, since the hair is swollen. It is critical that you never leave neutralizer on longer than indicated by the manufacturer since extra time can lead to hair damage.

Acid Waves

Acid perms are in the pH range of 6.9 to 7.2. Current acid waves are *now* capable of processing without heat. They start out with a higher pH and heat is an option for a firmer curl. Unlike alkaline waves, **acid waves cause only minimal swelling. Therefore, it is essential that the hair be wrapped with firm, even tension.** Without uniform tension throughout the strand, the curls will not process correctly and/or there will be an uneven curl pattern.

Heat and wrapping with even tension boost the penetration of the glycerylmonothioglycolate into the hair strands where it breaks the disulfide bonds. The heat needed for acid waves is often just the body heat that is trapped by placing a plastic bag over the perm wrap. Additional heat is achieved by placing the client under a hooded dryer. Acid waves are slower acting than alkaline waves and are recommended for damaged, highly porous and previously permed hair. Since the lower pH of an acid wave requires longer processing time, there is less chance of damage from overprocessing. However, always monitor the process carefully.

It is essential to completely rinse the perm solution from the hair before neutralizing. Since acid waves cause little swelling, rinsing is harder and takes longer (at least 5 minutes) to remove the solution from the hair. Improper rinsing before neutralizing can trap odor in the hair.

As with alkaline waves, the neutralizer in acid waves restores the disulfide bonds. A real benefit of working with the lower pH in an acid wave means that you avoid exposure to higher alkaline pH solutions and excessive hair swelling, which would need to be counteracted during neutralizing. However, as with alkaline waving, if the neutralizer is left on longer than specified, damage can occur.

1
2

Advantages of Alkaline and Acid Perms

Alkaline Perms

- Strong curl patterns
- Faster processing time
- Better for resistant hair
- No need for heat

Acid Perms

- Soft, natural curl patterns
- More control due to slower processing time
- Better for fragile or tinted hair

The first thio-free perm was introduced in 1992. This perm has a different reducing agent known as cystemine hydrochloride (hi-dro-CLOR-id). There were many benefits to using this type of perm, such as deeper penetration of waving lotion for longer-lasting curl results and more curl pattern consistency; less dilation of the cuticle layer and the ability to reform up to 60% more of the bonds during neutralization. For people who may have an allergic reaction to thioglycolic acid, which is found in both alkaline and acid waves, thio-free perms are an option.

Hair Analysis

In order to help you select the proper perm solution, it is important that you analyze the type and condition of your client's hair. Refer to the "Trichology" chapter for additional information.

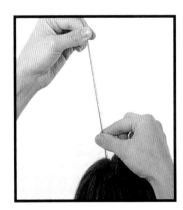

Porosity

Porosity refers to the hair's ability to absorb and/or retain liquids. The more porous the hair, the less resistant it is to absorbing the perm solution. Therefore, a mild acid perm would be desired. If the hair is resistant, it will require a stronger alkaline solution in order to pre-soften the cuticle and allow absorption. Hair with excessive porosity is usually in some stage of chemical or physical damage from highly alkaline shampoos, hair color treatments or excessive thermal styling. Highly porous hair needs to be reconditioned before any perm service with a prewrapping product to equalize porosity. In addition, you will need to select a gentler, slower-acting perm that gives greater control during processing.

Elasticity

Elasticity is the hair's ability to be stretched and return to its original condition. If hair has poor elasticity, it means that it will not return to its original state after it is gently stretched. Therefore, it will react adversely to the perm solution. It is not advisable or safe to perm hair that is weak or shows any signs of breakage.

Texture

Hair texture is essential to consider when selecting the proper perm formula as well as the size of the rod used. Hair texture is generally classified as fine, medium or coarse. Although it is not a rule, most of the time you will see that fine hair and coarse hair are the

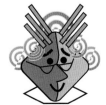

"As a rule, you will find excessive porosity and poor elasticity together."

two hair types that can be most challenging to perm. Manufacturers will often label their perms according to the results you can expect to achieve for fine, medium or coarse hair.

Density

You know from an earlier chapter that hair density refers to the number of hairs per square inch. Remember that **hair density does not always match hair texture.** Hair with a fine texture can be very dense (thick) or not very dense (thin). It also means that hair with a coarse texture can be thick or thin. Density also plays an important role in sectioning and wrapping a perm tool. Smaller base sizes are needed for hair with heavier density.

Manufacturers have labeled their perms according to hair texture, porosity and desired curl:

Texture:	Fine, medium, coarse
Porosity:	Normal, resistant, previously permed, tinted, bleached
Desired Curl:	Firm, true to rod size; soft, body waves

Analyzing your client's hair and choosing the desired curl formation will help you select the appropriate perm product for your client.

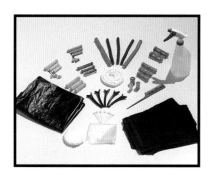

Perming Essentials

To deliver a professional perm service, you need an organized selection of products, implements and equipment. Manufacturers produce a wide range of perm products designed for all types of hair. Refer to Material Safety Data Sheets (MSDS) for all chemical products used in the salon. Perm service equipment includes furnishings and provisions necessary to provide a professional service.

Perming Products

PRODUCTS	FUNCTION
Perm Solution	Reduces disulfide bonds so hair can assume new shape of rod
Neutralizer	Fixes, locks in, restores bonds to make new shape of hair permanent
Protective Skin Cream	Protects client's skin when applied to hairline before using chemicals

Perming Implements/Supplies

IMPLEMENT/SUPPLIES	FUNCTION
Applicator Bottle	Controls and applies perm solution or neutralizer
Perm Rods (Tools)	Determine the size and shape of new curl configuration
Plastic Shampoo Cape	Protects client from chemicals

1
2

IMPLEMENT/SUPPLIES	FUNCTION
Cloth Towels	Absorb and remove water, perm solution and neutralizer through blotting
Perm Bib/ Neutralizing Cape	Catches excess chemicals as they run off the scalp; protects client
Cotton Strips	Protect client's face from chemicals when applied around hairline
Plastic Sectioning Clips	Hold hair in place in controlled sections before and during wrapping procedure
Styling Comb	Controls, distributes and parts hair to be wrapped within a section
Tail Comb	Parts off sections of hair and individual bases when wrapping
End Papers	Control the hair ends when wrapping; equalizes porosity and absorbency during processing, rinsing and neutralizing
Spray Bottle	Holds water used to keep hair damp for more control of hair while wrapping
Protective Gloves or Creams	Shield stylist's hands from chemicals during processing

Perming Equipment

EQUIPMENT	FUNCTION
Infrared Lamps	Provide heat for acid waves during processing, as required by the manufacturer's instructions
Timer	Alerts stylist to check for test curls, processing and neutralizing times as recommended by the manufacturer
Shampoo Bowl	Holds client's head and hair for shampooing prior to service and for rinsing perm solution and neutralizer from hair
Styling Chair	Provides comfortable seat for client; adjustable for best working height

Infection Control and Safety

The following is a list of safety precautions to be followed prior to and during a perm service.

- Practice infection control guidelines. Wash your hands with liquid antibacterial soap.
- Protect yourself. Wear gloves when applying chemical solutions.
- Protect your client's clothing with proper draping.
- Check the scalp for abrasions or diseases. Do not proceed with the perm services if abrasions or diseases are present.
- Avoid perming damaged hair that shows breakage. If the hair is dry, brittle or over-porous, recondition it first. Cut off damaged hair ends and select a mild perm formula.
- Never perm hair that has been treated with a sodium hydroxide or a no-lye relaxer.

Relaxers and perms break different bonds in the hair. Using both products on the same head of hair can result in severe hair damage or breakage.

- Analyze your client's hair to determine the correct perm formula to be used. Identify if the hair has been tinted, bleached, highlighted/frosted or previously permed.
- Perform a test for metallic salts if there is a possibility that such a product is on the hair. See "Testing for Metallic Salts" in this chapter.
- Determine if a client has experienced an allergic reaction to any other previous perm service prior to beginning the current perm service.
- Protect your client's skin by applying a protective cream and cotton around the hairline. Replace after it becomes saturated. Note that solution-saturated cotton could cause chemical burns if left on the skin too long.
- Throw away any opened, unused waving solution or neutralizer. These products can change in strength and effectiveness if they are not used soon after being opened.
- Follow manufacturer's directions. Do not dilute or add anything to the solution or the neutralizer unless indicated by the manufacturer's instructions.
- Keep all products out of the eyes and away from the skin as much as possible. If the products contact these areas, rinse immediately and thoroughly with cool water.
- If a plastic bag is used during processing, do not allow it to rest on the skin. It should be attached over the cotton strip that is positioned around the hairline.

Scalp Analysis

Since perming is a chemical service, it is important to perform certain preliminary steps, including tests and proper draping, in order to ensure client safety. It is equally important to examine the condition of the scalp. When the scalp is healthy, you may proceed with the service if the hair is structurally competent. Look for any abnormalities on the scalp, such as cuts, scratches, sores or abrasions. If you find any of these irregularities, postpone the perm service until the scalp is healthy again. **Never apply chemicals over any abnormal scalp condition.** To do so will create chemical burns and scalp problems.

Draping for Chemical Services

Proper draping procedures for chemical services protect the client's clothing as well as help prevent skin irritations or burns caused by the chemicals you apply. Draping for chemical services is not the same as draping for a shampoo.

- Ask the client to remove her neck jewelry, earrings or eyeglasses, and place them in her purse or pocket for safekeeping.
- Turn client's collar under.
- Place a towel around the client's neck and fasten the shampoo cape over the towel. Be sure the cape covers the back of the chair. Check with the client to be sure that the cape is not too tight, yet fits snugly enough to prevent water or solution from dripping onto clothing.
- Fold the edge of the towel down over the cape and drape a second towel over the shampoo cape. Fasten it securely with a clamp.
- Check before applying chemical solutions and performing rinsing procedures that the cape has not fallen inside the back of the chair.

Test for Metallic Salt

Color products that contain metallic salts (see "Hair Coloring" chapter) form a residue on the hair that interferes with the chemical action of a perm. The results can be uneven curls, distinct discoloration, hair damage or breakage. If you suspect metallic salts are present, perform a 1:20 test prior to performing a perm service. This test is done by mixing 1 ounce (30 ml) of 20 volume (6%) peroxide and 20 drops of 28% ammonia in a glass bowl. Immerse at least 20 strands of hair in this mixture for 30 minutes. At the end of 30 minutes, look for any of these possible results:

- If there are no metallic salts, the hair will lighten slightly. You may proceed with the perm.

- If the hair strands lighten quickly, the hair contains lead. Do not perm.

- After 30 minutes, if there is no reaction, the hair contains silver. Do not perm.

- If the solution begins to boil within a few minutes, giving off an unpleasant odor and if the hair degrades and pulls apart easily, the hair contains copper. Do not perm.

ALERT!

Do not perm until the metallic product has been cut out of the hair. Before giving any future perms, repeat the test for metallic salts.

Preliminary Test Curls

Preliminary test curls help determine how your client's hair will react to a perm. Take the time to test hair that is bleached, overporous, damaged or has been colored with henna.

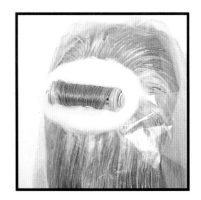

- Shampoo the hair once and gently towel dry it. Use light manipulations.

- Wrap one rod in a concealed area that represents the overall condition of the hair, following perm directions.

- Apply barrier cream to the surrounding area and cover with plastic.

- Wrap a coil of cotton around the rod to protect the surrounding hair from the chemicals.

- Apply waving lotion to the wrapped hair; keep the chemicals away from the unwrapped hair.

- Set a timer and process according to manufacturer's directions.

- Check the hair at least every five minutes by taking a test curl.

To check a test curl, unfasten a rod and carefully unwind the curl 1.5 to 2 turns of the rod diameter. Do not permit the hair to loosen or unwind from the rod completely. Hold the thumbs together on the back of the tool and turn it back toward the head. Do not push the rod toward the head. If a 'C' or 'S' shape (undulation) is not evident, rewrap the rod and allow it to continue processing. Observe the hair carefully and look for overly softened hair. When the undulation is ready, the hair will automatically form a strong, well-defined 'C' or 'S' shape. This is the same procedure used for testing curls during the actual processing time as well. If you achieve a positive test curl, proceed with the rinsing and neutralizing steps. Examine the finished curl. If desired results are achieved, proceed with perm service.

Client Consultation

As with all hair services, consulting with your client prior to the actual service will ensure predictable results and will help you avoid any misunderstandings that may arise. To ensure client comfort, you should perform your consultation in a private area. Use photos and magazines while communicating with your client to allow your client to clearly visualize your design intentions. To help you remember the important steps in the consultation process, remember: Great Artists Always Draw Creatively. As you review the five basic steps for the consultation, remember the importance of active listening, critical thinking and analysis on the overall success of the service.

Greet

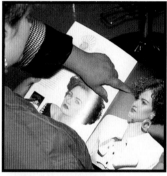

- Meet and greet the client with a firm handshake and pleasant tone of voice.

- Communicate to build rapport and develop a link with the client.

- Help client fill out consultation form.

Ask, Analyze and Assess

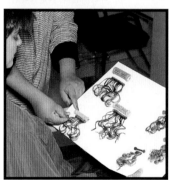

- Ask questions to discover client needs.

- What type of hair style does your client expect? Determine how much curl is needed. Use photos or a stylebook for clear communication.

- Consider your client's lifestyle. Is your client a busy business executive or is there leisure time to spend styling the hair? Will the style be low or high maintenance?

- Check into your client's perming history. Have there been problems with perming in the past? Are there particular details that your client would like to share about her hair?

- Analyze client's, face and body shape, physical features, lifestyle, climate effects, hair and scalp type, condition, prior product usage and results from previous services.

1
2

- Assess the facts and thoroughly think through your recommendations.

- Document on the record card everything that is important to the successful outcome of this service, as well as future services.

- Have your client sign the Release Form, which is required by some malpractice insurance companies. This release form states that the school or salon is not responsible for damages that may occur. Always use extreme care when working with chemical services.

Agree

- Explain your recommended solutions as well as the price for the service(s). Think not of just today's service, but also future services.

- Return to step 2 (Ask, Analyze, Assess) if your client is hesitant with your recommendation.

- Gain feedback and approval from your client.

Deliver

- Ensure client protection by draping the client with a plastic cape and towel.

- Ensure client comfort during the service.

- Stay focused on delivering the service to the best of your ability.

- Teach the client how to perform home hair care.

Complete

- Request satisfaction and feedback from your client.

- Recommend products to maintain the healthy condition of your client's hair.

- Suggest a future appointment time for your client's next visit.

- Offer appreciation to your client for visiting the school or salon.

- Complete the record card with accurate information for future services and file it in a secure area with other record cards.

CLIENT CHEMICAL PERMANENT RELEASE FORM

Name _____ Phone Number _____
Address _____ City, State, Zip _____

I request a permanent and I fully understand that this service is to be given by a student of cosmetology at Your Name Beauty School. I hereby express my willingness for a student to do this work. I furthermore understand that I will assume full responsibility thereof.

Your Name Beauty School

Witness _____ Client Signature _____
Date _____ Date _____

CLIENT CHEMICAL PERMANENT RECORD CARD

Date	Wrap	Rod Size	Products	Process Time	Results
					___ Good
					___ Poor
					___ Too Tight
					___ Too Loose

Description of Hair

Length	Density	Texture	Porosity	Tress-Tester Results	Test Curl Results
•Short	•Light	•Fine	•Average	•Strength ___	•Negative
•Medium	•Medium	•Medium	•Resistant	•Stretch ___	•Positive
•Long	•Heavy	•Coarse	•Extreme Porosity		

Medications _____
Vitamins _____
Comments _____
Home Care _____

Price of Service $ _____

Signature of Student _____ Signature of Instructor _____

Perm Wrap Overview

The basic perm patterns you learned about in the theory portion will be applied to the following perm wraps, which will be outlined in detail in the upcoming procedure portion of this chapter. Keep in mind that these patterns can be used alone or combined to create any number of perm wraps for your clientele. To increase your wrapping speed, practice these patterns over and over. Try to reach the salon speed indicated next to each wrapping pattern. Hair length and density will affect your speed.

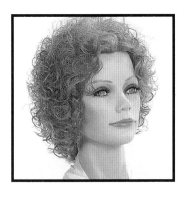 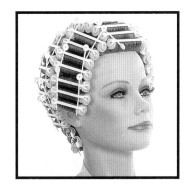

Rectangle Perm Wrap

Salon Speed 30 minutes

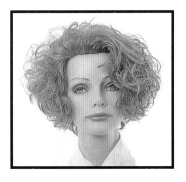 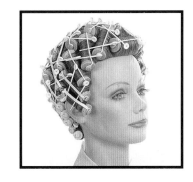

Bricklay Perm Wrap

Salon Speed 40 minutes

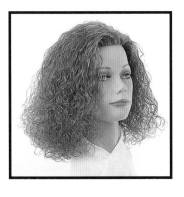 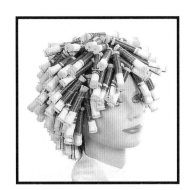

Spiral Bricklay Perm Wrap

Salon Speed 75 minutes

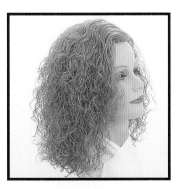 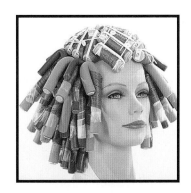

Oblong and Spiral Bricklay Perm Wrap

Salon Speed 60 minutes

1
2

Rectangle Perm Wrap

The rectangle pattern is generally considered the most basic perm pattern and can be performed on any haircut. It consists primarily of rectangular shapes throughout the pattern. The basic direction is downward. A rectangular shape is generally positioned from the front hairline to the nape. The hair in the center front rectangle can be wrapped away from or toward the face. The remaining hair at the sides is subdivided in half. Rectangular-shaped bases are used throughout. When using the rectangle pattern on longer lengths, you may wish to increase the diameter of the rod. In this exercise, the rectangle pattern consists of five sections. A half-off base control is used from horizontal partings.

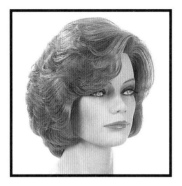
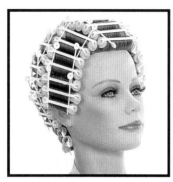
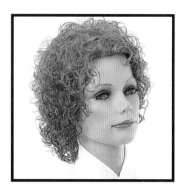

Rectangle Perm Wrap Preparation

As with any professional service, it is important to have your area, products, implements and equipment in proper order. Before performing a rectangle perm wrap, be sure to satisfy the following points:

- Clean work station with disinfectant
- Arrange implements/supplies including perm rods, picks, end papers, sectioning clips, tail comb, plastic cap, gloves, barrier cream, cotton, perm solution and neutralizer
- Wash your hands with liquid antibacterial soap
- Perform analysis of hair and scalp
- Ask the client to remove jewelry and store in a secure place
- Drape your client for a chemical service
- Shampoo hair lightly without scalp manipulations

Rectangle Pattern Perm Wrap Procedure

- Subdivide hair into five sections
- Begin at front hairline of center section
- Use the diameter of the rod to measure the base size
- Take horizontal parting and project hair at 90° from center of base
- Apply end papers and use overlap technique
- Position rod half-off base
- Secure each rod with picks
- Use same techniques and complete center section

- Adjust size of rod to size of section
- Complete back side section at the back
- Complete front side section using same techniques
- Repeat same procedures on opposite side
- Apply barrier cream and cotton around entire hairline
- Apply perm solution to each rod
- Follow manufacturer's directions regarding plastic cap, processing and timing
- Take test curl
- Rinse hair thoroughly
- Towel blot each rod
- Apply neutralizer to each rod
- Set timer according to manufacturer's directions
- Remove rods
- Work remaining neutralizer through ends
- Rinse thoroughly

Option: The neutralizer may be rinsed from the hair while the rods are in place. The rods are removed after rinsing is complete.

Rectangle Perm Wrap

1-3. Subdivide the hair into five sections. Use the length of the rod to measure and scale out a center rectangle section from the front hairline to the nape. Use the length of the rod to measure and scale out the front side section. Section the remaining hair.

4. Begin at the front hairline of the center section. Use the diameter of the rod to measure the base size. Take a horizontal parting and project the hair at 90° from the center of the base. Apply end papers and use the overlap technique. Position the rod half-off base.

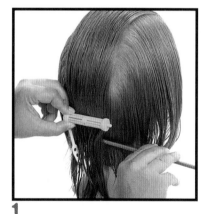

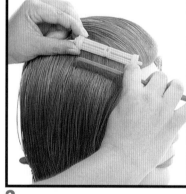

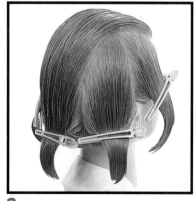

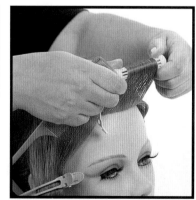

1
2

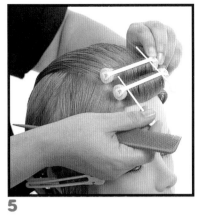

5

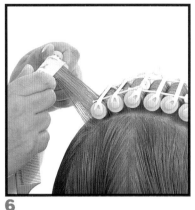

6

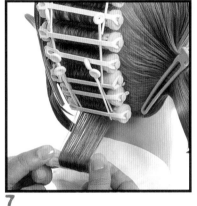

7

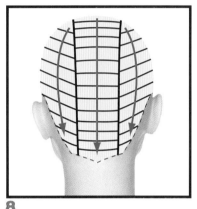

8

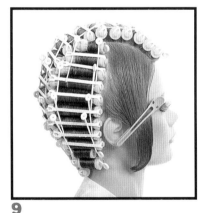

9

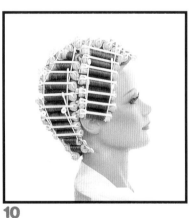

10

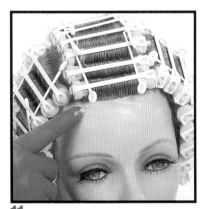

11

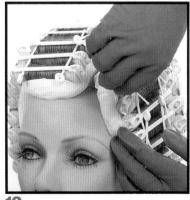

12

5. **Secure each rod with picks** in the direction the hair is wrapped. Picks will lift the elastic band off the hair and avoid the pressure which may lead to hair breakage.

6-7. **Use the same techniques and complete the center section.**

8. Move to the adjacent section in the back and repeat the wrapping technique.

9-10. Adjust the length of the rod to the size of the section at the back. Complete the back side section. Then complete the front side section using the same techniques. Repeat the same procedures on the opposite side.

11-12. Apply barrier cream and cotton around the entire hairline.

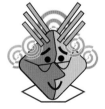

"Don't forget to replace the cotton around your client's hairline after you are through applying the perm solution. Cotton soaked with chemicals can irritate the skin."

13-14. Carefully **apply the perm solution to each rod.** Use a towel as you apply the solution to prevent the product from splashing. **Follow manufacturer's directions regarding a plastic cap, processing and timing.**

15-16. **Take a test curl.** Once you reach the desired curl pattern or "S" formation, **rinse the hair thoroughly.** Then towel blot each rod.

17. Apply the neutralizer to each rod. Set the timer according to manufacturer's directions. Remove rods and distribute remaining neutralizer through ends. Rinse thoroughly.

18. Style as desired.

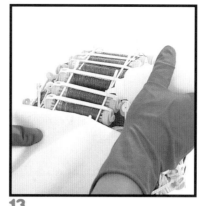

13

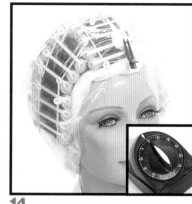

14

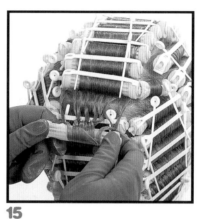

15

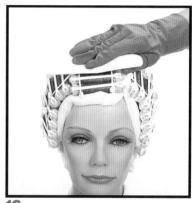

16

Rectangle Perm Wrap Completion

- Offer a rebook visit to your client
- Recommend retail products to your client
- Discard non-reusable materials, disinfect implements and arrange work station in proper order
- Wash your hands with liquid antibacterial soap

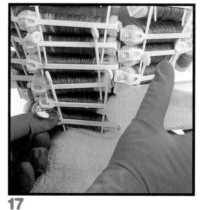

17

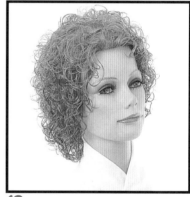

18

Bricklay Perm Wrap

The bricklay pattern can be compared to the way a bricklayer artfully arranges the bricks in a building to create a staggered effect. The bricklay pattern is used to create a consistent curl pattern and to help avoid splits between the bases. An overlap or spiral pattern can be used within a bricklay pattern from rectangular or trapezoid-shaped bases. The wrapping pattern can move toward or away from the face.

1
2

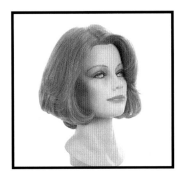 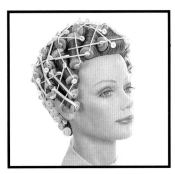 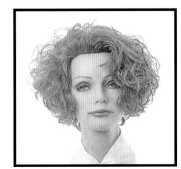

In this procedure, an overlap technique is used within the one-two bricklay pattern. A progression of rods is used to accommodate the lengths and to create a progression of curl patterns. A half-off base control is used throughout from horizontal and diagonal partings. The wrapping direction is back away from the face.

Bricklay Perm Wrap Preparation

As with any professional service, it is important to have your area, products, implements and equipment in proper order. Before performing a bricklay perm wrap, be sure to satisfy the following points:

- Clean work station with disinfectant
- Arrange implements/supplies including different diameter perm rods, picks, end papers, sectioning clips, tail comb, plastic cap, gloves, barrier cream, cotton, perm solution and neutralizer
- Wash your hands with liquid antibacterial soap
- Perform analysis of hair and scalp
- Ask the client to remove jewelry and store in a secure place
- Drape your client for a chemical service
- Shampoo hair lightly without scalp manipulations

Bricklay Perm Wrap Procedure

- Distribute hair straight back
- Begin at center front hairline
- Measure base size with diameter and length of rod
- Wrap first rod away from face using overlap technique
- Position rod half-off base
- Part diagonally to include hairline in next row
- Wrap two rods behind center of first rod using one-two bricklay method
- Begin at the center of the next row

- Secure rods with picks in direction hair was wrapped
- Continue same procedures and one-two bricklay method as you work from the center to either side
- Work toward lower crown and nape using one-two bricklay method along horizontal partings
- Complete back
- Follow manufacturer's directions for processing

Bricklay Pattern Wrap

1. **Distribute the hair straight back. Begin at the center front hairline.** Measure the base size with the diameter and the length of the rod. Apply end papers to the ends. **Wrap the first rod away from the face using the overlap technique and position the rod half-off base.**

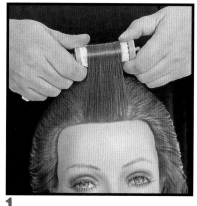
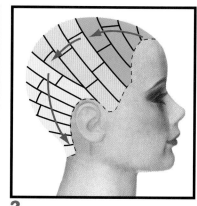

2-3. **Part diagonally to include the hairline in the next row. Wrap the next two rods behind the center of the first rod using the one-two bricklay method.** With the one-two method, wrapping is performed in rows. The first rod is positioned in the center. In the next row, beginning from just off-center, the rods are staggered. In the next row, a rod is positioned in the center again.

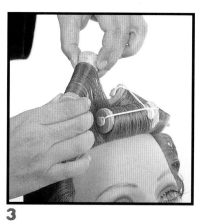
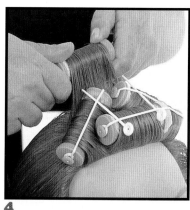

4. Begin at the center of the next row. Secure the rods with picks in the direction the hair has been wrapped.

5-6. **Continue to use the same procedures and the one-two method as you work from the center to either side.** Adjust the diameter of the rod to accommodate the lengths.

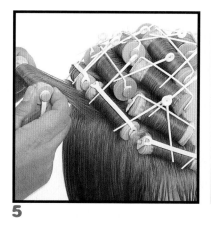
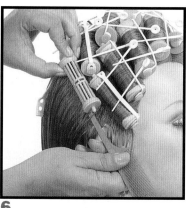

7-8. Continue to **work toward the lower crown and nape using the one-two brick lay method along horizontal partings.**

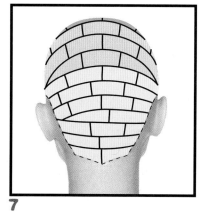
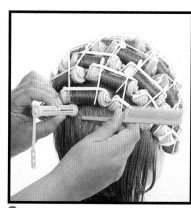

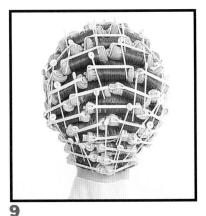

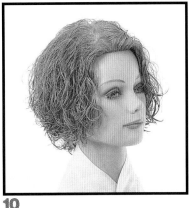

9

10

9. Complete the back. Apply barrier cream and cotton around the hairline. **Follow the manufacturer's directions for processing.**

10. Remove rods and style as desired.

Bricklay Perm Wrap Completion

- Offer a rebook visit to your client
- Recommend retail products to your client
- Discard non-reusable materials, disinfect implements and arrange work station in proper order
- Wash your hands with liquid antibacterial soap

Spiral Bricklay Perm Wrap

Spiral wrapping is used on medium to longer lengths of hair to achieve an elongated curl pattern. Spiral wrapping can be accomplished by wrapping the hair from base to ends or from ends to the base, depending on the tool used. For this exercise cylinder rods are used with an ends-to-base wrapping method. The rods are wrapped within a bricklay pattern.

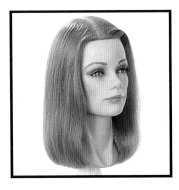
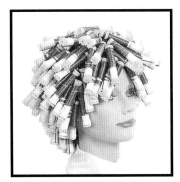
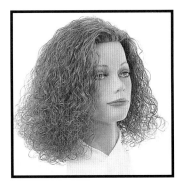

Spiral Bricklay Perm Wrap Preparation

As with any professional service, it is important to have your area, products, implements and equipment in proper order. Before performing a spiral bricklay perm wrap, be sure to satisfy the following points:

- Clean work station with disinfectant
- Arrange implements/supplies including perm rods, end papers, sectioning clips, tail comb, plastic cap, gloves, barrier cream, cotton, perm solution and neutralizer
- Wash your hands with liquid antibacterial soap
- Perform analysis of hair and scalp

- Ask the client to remove jewelry and store in a secure place
- Drape your client for a chemical service
- Shampoo hair lightly without scalp manipulations

Spiral Bricklay Perm Wrap Procedure

- Section hair for control
- Release horizontal parting across nape
- Use rectangular-shaped bases, one-diameter base size and spiral wrap technique
- Work from one side of nape to other
- Wrap first row in same direction
- Wrap next row in opposite direction
- Above the ear, work from one side of head to other
- Alternate the wrapping direction of each row
- Use horseshoe-shaped partings at the top
- Work from one side of front hairline to other
- Use zigzag parting at center top
- Complete spiral wrap
- Follow manufacturer's directions for processing

Spiral Bricklay Perm Wrap

1-2. Section the hair for control. Release a horizontal parting across the nape. Use rectangular-shaped bases, a one-diameter base size and the spiral wrap technique.

3. Apply end papers and **work from one side of the nape to the other. Wrap the first row in the same direction.**

4. Wrap the next row in the opposite direction beginning at the top of the last positioned rod.

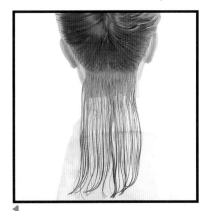

1

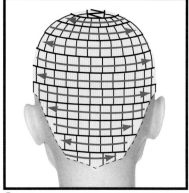

2

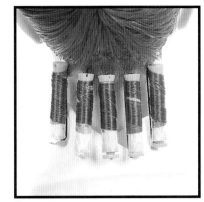

3

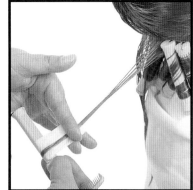

4

1
2

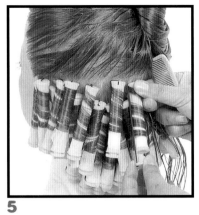

5

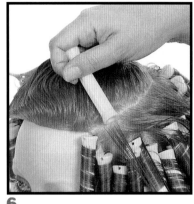

6

5-6. Above the ear, work from one side of the head to the other. Alternate the wrapping direction of each row.

7. Use horseshoe-shaped partings at the top. Work from one side of the front hairline to the other.

8. Use a zigzag parting at the center **top** to avoid a split.

9-10. Complete the spiral wrap. Apply barrier cream and cotton around the hairline. **Follow manufacturer's directions for processing.** Finish as desired.

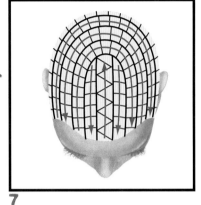

7

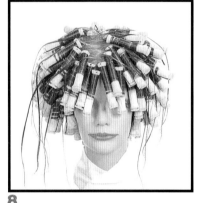

8

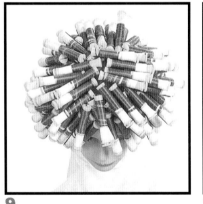

9

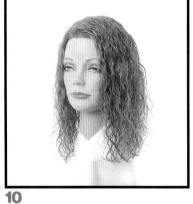

10

Spiral Bricklay Perm Wrap Completion

- Offer a rebook visit to your client
- Recommend retail products to your client
- Discard non-reusable materials, disinfect implements and arrange work station in proper order
- Wash your hands with liquid antibacterial soap

Oblong and Spiral Bricklay Perm Wrap

An oblong consists of a succession of parallel "C" lines and has a convex (closed) end and a concave (open) end. Oblongs can move toward or away from the face. When two oblongs are positioned next to one another in opposite directions, an alternating curvature movement or "S" pattern is created. For this exercise, an oblong pattern is used in the interior. A spiral bricklay pattern using soft rods and an ends-to-base wrapping technique are used in the exterior.

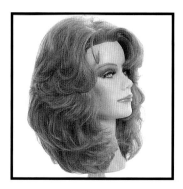 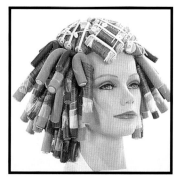 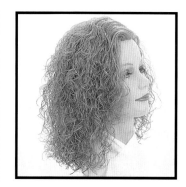

Oblong and Spiral Bricklay Perm Wrap Preparation

As with any professional service, it is important to have your area, products, implements and equipment in proper order. Before performing an oblong and spiral bricklay perm wrap, be sure to satisfy the following points:

- Clean work station with disinfectant
- Arrange implements/supplies including different diameter perm rods, picks, end papers, sectioning clips, tail comb, plastic cap, gloves, barrier cream, cotton, perm solution and neutralizer
- Wash your hands with liquid antibacterial soap
- Perform analysis of hair and scalp
- Ask the client to remove jewelry and store in a secure place
- Drape your client for a chemical service
- Shampoo hair lightly without scalp manipulations

Oblong and Spiral Bricklay Perm Wrap Procedure

- Mold two oblong shapes at top in alternating directions
- Wrap first shape toward face using overlap technique
- Begin at closed end of first shape
- Use one-diameter, half-off base control from diagonal partings
- Secure rods with picks
- Wrap next shape in opposite direction
- Begin at closed end of shape
- Work from one side of hairline toward other
- Continue half-off base control
- Complete top
- Subdivide and section remaining hair for control

1 2

- Release horizontal parting across nape
- Use spiral technique from rectangular-shaped bases
- Work from one side to other
- Release next horizontal parting
- Use a bricklay pattern and wrap hair in opposite direction
- Continue to work from side to side
- Above ear, release horizontal parting from one side of head to other
- Continue to use spiral technique and alternate direction of each row
- Complete spiral wrap
- Follow manufacturer's directions for processing

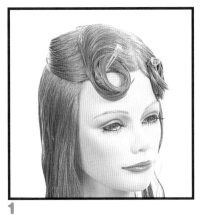

1

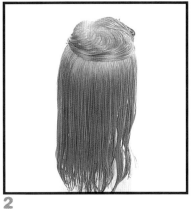

2

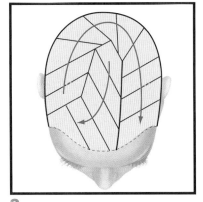

3

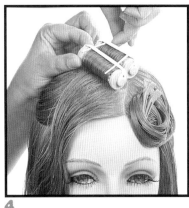

4

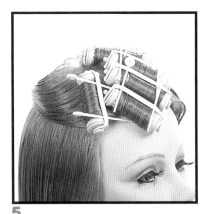

5

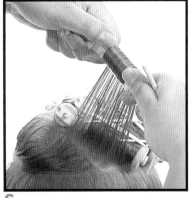

6

Oblong and Spiral Bricklay Wrap

1-2. Mold two oblong shapes at the top in alternating directions.

3-4. Wrap the first shape toward the face using the overlap technique. Begin at the closed end of the first shape. Apply end papers to the ends. Use a one-diameter, half-off base control from diagonal partings. Secure each rod with picks. Adjust the length of the tool as necessary.

5-6. Wrap the next shape in the opposite direction. Begin at closed end of next shape. Work from one side of the hairline toward the other. Continue to use a half-off base control. Use shorter length rods at the crown.

7. Complete the top.

8. Subdivide and section the remaining hair for control. Release a horizontal parting across the nape.

9-10. Use the spiral technique from rectangular-shaped bases. Use a one-diameter base size. Apply end papers and wrap the hair from the ends to the base. Bend the tool in the opposite direction that the hair was wrapped to secure. **Work from one side to the other.**

11-14. Release the next horizontal parting. Begin at the top of the last positioned tool. **Use a bricklay pattern and wrap the hair in the opposite direction.** Work from one side of the parting to the other.

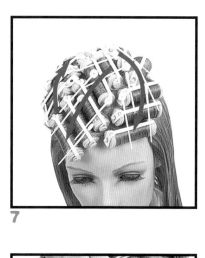

7

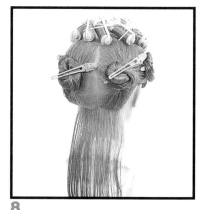

8

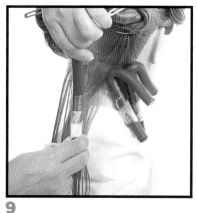

9

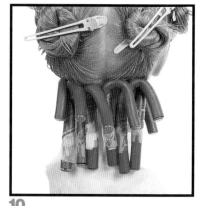

10

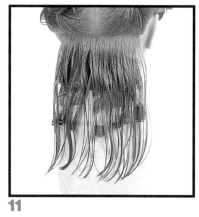

11

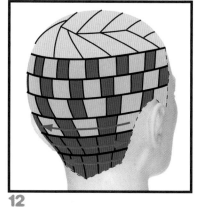

12

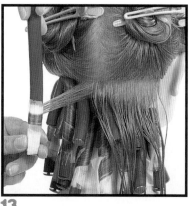

13

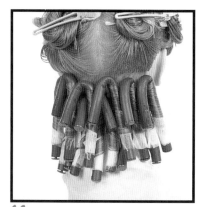

14

1
2

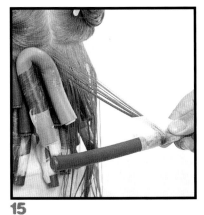
15

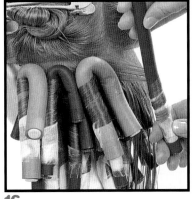
16

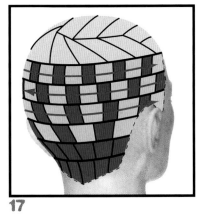
17

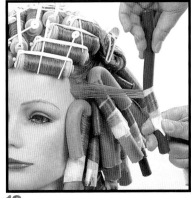
18

15-16. **Continue to work from side to side** using the spiral technique within a bricklay pattern. You may wish to alternate tool diameters to achieve a more natural result.

17-18. Above the ear, release a horizontal parting from one side of the head to the other. Continue to use the spiral technique and alternate the direction of each row.

19. **Complete the spiral wrap.** Apply barrier cream and cotton around the hairline.

20. **Follow manufacturer's directions for processing.** Finish as desired.

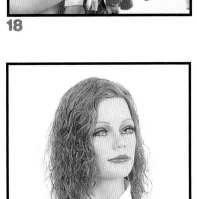
19

20

Oblong and Spiral Bricklay Perm Wrap Completion

• Offer a rebook visit to your client
• Recommend retail products to your client
• Discard non-reusable materials, disinfect implements and arrange work station in proper order
• Wash your hands with liquid antibacterial soap

Perm Problems and Solutions

The following are a few problems that may occur with perms, along with some possible solutions.

Problem: Weak or Limp Curl

Cause: Underprocessing – perm solution not left on long enough

Solution: Follow manufacturer's self-timing recommendations; use a timer for accuracy; take accurate test curls

Cause: Rods too large for desired curl

Solution: Make sure hair completes 2.5 revolutions around the rod, or reduce rod diameter

Cause: Hair wrapped too loosely around rods

Solution: Wrap with smooth, even tension; acid waves generally require more tension than alkaline waves; always read and follow manufacturer's directions

Cause: Incorrect choice of perm product

Solution: Analyze your client's hair and match your findings to the perm performance description listed by the manufacturer

Problem: Uneven Curl

Cause: Inconsistent application of perm solution and/or neutralizer

Solution: Apply chemicals in a systematic method to avoid missing rods

Cause: Incomplete rinsing or blotting

Solution: Be consistent; rinse and blot all rods thoroughly

Cause: Too much hair on the rods or hair not evenly distributed around the rod

Solution: Base sizes equal to the diameter of the tool will give you the most consistent curl pattern; avoid bunching the hair and wrap the hair as smoothly as possible around the rod

Problem: Frizziness

Cause: Overprocessing – perm solution left on too long; may look curly when wet, and frizzy when dry

Solution: Take frequent test curls; use timer to accurately track time

Cause: The hair is stretched or manipulated too much after perm when thermal styling

Solution: Use finishing products designed to define curl patterns; dry with warm heat using little tension on the hair

Problem: Breakage or Dryness

Cause: Hair wound on rods with too much tension

Solution: Avoid excessive stretching; moderate tension is advisable

Cause: Hair too fragile for perming

Solution: Perform thorough pre-perm analysis of the hair to determine if perming is advisable; perform preliminary test curl if in doubt

Cause: Perm band places pressure on the hair during processing

Solution: Lift the band off the hair by placing picks under it

Problem: Skin Irritation

Cause: Cotton or neck towel was allowed to remain on the skin after it was saturated with perm solution

Solution: Replace with fresh cotton or towel as needed; do not allow perm soaked cotton to remain on skin, especially under plastic cap

Problem: Unpleasant Odor After Perming

Cause: Insufficient rinsing of perm solution before neutralizing

Solution: Rinse hair for a full 5 minutes or longer; check for proper rinsing by smelling the hair, you should not smell perm solution; rinse more carefully when using acid or thio-free perms since they take longer to remove from the hair

Problem: Hair Lightens After a Perm Sevice

Cause: Many neutralizers contain hydrogen peroxide which will lighten the hair slightly; lightening effect is more apparent on porous hair

Solution: Apply a temporary color to deposit missing tones; book hair color appointment, if needed, one or more weeks after perm; follow manufacturer's directions for same day perm and color services

Problem: Perm Did Not Last as Long as Expected

Cause: Hair not in proper condition before wave

Solution: Recondition weak hair before perming

Cause: Incomplete neutralization; insufficient blotting after rinsing perm solution, which dilutes the neutralizer

Solution: Remove excess water by blotting the entire head first and then each rod before applying neutralizer

CHEMICAL RELAXING

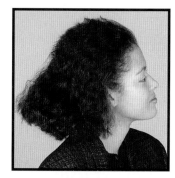

Chemical hair relaxing appeared early in the twentieth century as a means of controlling excessively curly hair. The first chemical relaxers were made of potash (wood ashes), lye, white potatoes and lard. The process was also known as a 'conk.' Mixed together, these ingredients produced a harsh mixture strong enough to chemically straighten overly curly hair. In its pure form, lye is a caustic chemical with a pH 14. It has the ability to eat away or erode the cuticle layer of the hair, making it very limp and straight, as well as easier to manage.

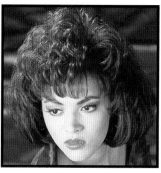

Because the mixture contained domestic household ingredients, it was an unstable formula that produced unpredictable results. The mixture was usually so strong that it caused hair loss and severe scalp burns. Yet, in spite of these risks, people were willing to accept the consequences in order to achieve the desired results.

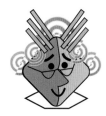

"Did you know that Madam C. J. Walker was the first black female millionaire in the United States?"

With time, entertainers, athletes and other celebrities made the straightened look popular for both men and women. People saw clearly that chemical relaxing did more than simply control overly curly hair. It offered a variety of hairstyles as well.

In the early 1900s a temporary method of hair relaxing, called hair pressing, was conceived by Sarah Breedlove (1867-1919), who was better known as Madam C. J. Walker. After the hair was washed and dried, petroleum jelly was applied. Then a metal comb, heated over a small gas burner, was pressed against and pulled through the hair using tension, temporarily straightening it. Refer to the "Hairstyling" chapter for more information on this straightening (pressing) method.

By the late 1950s, several commercially produced chemical relaxers were available. Even though they remained highly caustic with the potential to cause damage to hair and scalp, the new formulas were more consistent, making the results more predictable.

Chemical Relaxing Theory

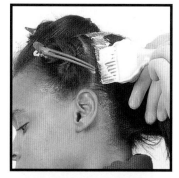

CHEMICAL PHASE

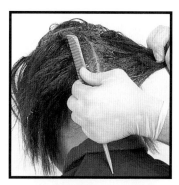

SMOOTHING PHASE

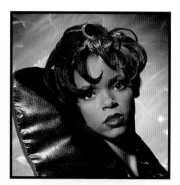

FINAL RESULT

Chemical relaxing involves two major phases: the chemical phase, which begins when the straightening product is applied to the hair, and the physical phase, which is smoothing the hair, rinsing the product from the hair and applying the neutralizer or neutralizing shampoo (also known as fixative or stabilizer). As you learned in the "Perming" section of this chapter, the neutralizer causes oxidation, which restores the broken disulfide bonds. Keep in mind that the chemical and physical phases of relaxing are of equal importance.

Types of Relaxers

Although there are many types of relaxers used in the professional salon, there are two primary results, the first of which completely straightens the hair and the second of which reduces the curl pattern. The most common ingredient found in products that completely straighten the hair is sodium hydroxide. The most common ingredient found in products that reduce the curl pattern is ammonium thioglycolate (thio).

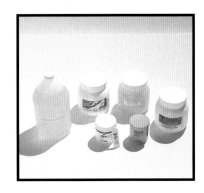

Sodium Hydroxide

Sodium relaxers prior to the 1960s were called base relaxers. These relaxers required that a protective cream (base) be applied to the scalp prior to the relaxer service. Following the 1960s no-base chemical relaxers were developed. They have a high oil content (the base) and conditioning agents that help protect the hair and scalp from irritation. No-base chemical relaxers are generally the choice of salon professionals because they are gentler to the hair and scalp. Keep in mind, however, that they still contain a caustic chemical, so skill and thorough product knowledge are required. Appropriate use of base cream may still be needed for clients with sensitive scalps. Sodium hydroxide relaxers are also known as lye relaxers and have a ph of 10.5 - 14. Always follow manufacturer's directions.

Ammonium Thioglycolate

Ammonium thioglycolate relaxers, also called thio relaxers, is a chemical reducing agent that causes the hair to soften and swell. Hydrogen and disulfide bonds in the hair are affected during this process. With the thioglycolate relaxer, the disulfide bonds break between the two sulfur atoms in the cystine amino acids. As you learned in "Perming," the neutralizing process causes the split cystine amino acids to rejoin.

Other Relaxers

No-lye relaxers contain a derivative of sodium hydroxide. No-lye relaxers contain calcium, potassium, guanidine, lithium hydroxide, or bisulfate as the active ingredient. The name, no-lye, derives from the fact that sodium hydroxide is not the active ingredient. No-lye chemical relaxers are usually recommended for less resistant hair and require frequent conditioning follow-up treatments. It is important to have an understanding of each of these relaxers so that you can choose the best product for your clients.

These relaxer formulas consist of three principle ingredients: an alkaline agent (sodium, potassium, lithium or guanidine hydroxide), oil (surfactants or surface-acting agents that protect the hair and scalp) and water, the active alkaline component. These components control the chemical relaxer's effectiveness and efficiency. It is important to remember that the formulation of the chemical relaxer requires quick application, processing and removal to prevent damage. Correctly applied, relaxers provide maximum straightening action as well as optimum conditioning effects with minimal or no scalp irritation or hair loss. As a result, the hair is soft, shiny and in good condition.

Relaxer Strengths

During hair analysis, each client's hair should be properly assessed. The texture, porosity, elasticity, density, type and overall condition of the hair will determine the processing time and the proper relaxer strength to use. Refer to "Infection Control and Safety" in this chapter for more information on how to assess the hair for a chemical relaxer service.

Relaxer strengths for ammonium thioglycolate are usually categorized as mild (delicate), regular (normal), and super (resistant).

- Mild is used on healthy, color-treated hair, fine-textured or porous hair.
- Regular is used on curly to medium-textured hair.
- Super is used on overly curly, coarse-textured or resistant hair.

Semi-permanent hair color can be applied over hair that has been relaxed with sodium hydroxide. Hair color mixed with 20 volume (6%) developer or less can be applied to hair that has average porosity, is in good condition and has been straightened with a mild relaxer. Note that haircoloring services requiring hydrogen peroxide are not generally performed on the same day of the relaxer service. Follow manufacturer's directions for specific guidelines.

ALERT!

Do not apply sodium hydroxide relaxer to extremely porous hair that has been colored with permanent hair color or lightened hair (decolorized, bleached). Also, do not apply sodium hydroxide to hair that has been permed with ammonium thioglycolate or to hair that is going to be permed with ammonium thioglycolate. Multiple services performed over the hair reduces the number of bonds in the hair, which can cause severe breakage.

1
2

Hair Analysis

Consider giving several preliminary tests before a chemical service to determine the hair's porosity, elasticity, density, texture and type. The information gained from these tests is necessary to help ensure successful results. As you perform these tests, carefully analyze the condition of the hair and scalp. If the hair shows signs of breakage, postpone the service until the condition of the hair and/or scalp improves. Refer to the "Trichology" chapter for additional information on hair analysis testing.

Porosity

Porosity refers to the ability of the hair to absorb liquids or chemicals. It's also one of the determining factors in selecting the appropriate chemical relaxer strength and processing time. The more porous the hair, the faster the hair will accept the product. With porous hair, choose a product that has a lower alkaline content. When the hair is more resistant, you will need to use a product with a higher alkaline content. The porosity test is also known as the finger test.

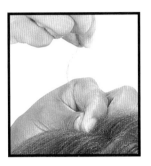

Elasticity

Elasticity describes the hair's ability to stretch and return without breaking, much like the action of a rubber band. Elasticity can range from very good to very poor. If the hair flexes back and forth as it is gently pulled, it shows good elasticity. Hair with good elasticity can usually tolerate stronger chemicals, while hair with weaker elasticity requires milder chemicals. Note that if the hair lacks elasticity, chemicals should not be used. **The elasticity test is also known as the pull test.**

Texture

Texture relates to the actual size or diameter of an individual hair strand. When analyzing the hair for a chemical relaxing service, texture can be categorized as fine, medium and coarse. It is common for one head of hair to have several different textures, such as very fine hair in the nape area and coarse hair in the crown. Therefore, it is important to test in several areas of the head with the proper strength of relaxer on the appropriate hair texture.

Density

Density refers to the number of hair strands per square inch, which can be classified as either light, medium or heavy (sometimes thin, medium, thick). Knowing the density helps you determine what size partings to use during the relaxer application. Partings can range from 1/4" to 1/2" (.75 to 1.25 cm). For example, thick hair will require more partings than thin hair.

Identifying and Changing Existing Curl Patterns

Natural curl patterns can be identified by their visual characteristics. The four major texture patterns that can be determined by the shape of the hair follicle are:

- Straight–Round Follicle
- Wavy–Oval Follicle
- Curly–Elliptical Follicle
- Overly Curly–Elliptical Follicle

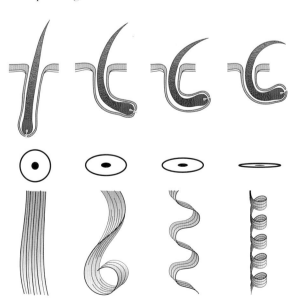

Each one of these types of texture patterns can be found in every ethnic race. It is also common for one head of hair to have several different texture patterns. Straight hair is also referred to as round-cell hair because of its round shape, and overly curly hair is also referred to as flat-cell hair because of its almost flat-like shape.

Generally, sodium hydroxide relaxers are used on curly, overly curly and resistant hair, while thio relaxers are used on wavy, curly or non-resistant hair.

Creating a reduced curl pattern consists of a chemical phase (applying the proper relaxer strength according to the hair type) and the physical phase (smoothing), while taking into consideration the existing curl pattern.

Stages of Reduction

The following chart can be used as a guide when relaxing overly curly hair to achieve the new reduced curl pattern. Keep in mind that relaxing doesn't mean that you must remove 100% of the natural curl pattern, which could result in totally limp hair and even breakage.

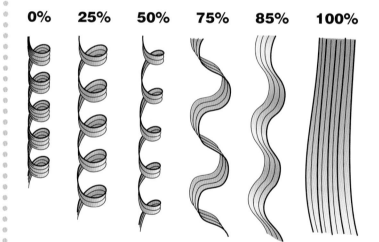

0% 25% 50% 75% 85% 100%

Overly Curly Texture Pattern
- 0%

Texturizing
- 25%–Minimum Relaxing
- 50%–Curl Diffusion (also known as chemical blow out)
- 75%–S-Curl Pattern

Optimum Relaxing
- 85%

Over Processed
- 100%

The following are steps that you can use to create the new curl pattern.

1. Determine the Existing Curl Pattern
   Wavy, Curly, Overly Curly

2. Determine the Desired Curl Pattern
   Wavy, Curly

3. Choose the Formula
   Thio or Sodium (Mild, Regular, Super)

4. Determine processing time and amount of smoothing

12

Chemical Phase

As mentioned earlier, the chemical phase of the relaxer service takes place when the chemical relaxer product is applied to the hair. There are three methods for applying the relaxer: the brush, comb or fingers. The relaxer product is applied to one or both sides of the strand.

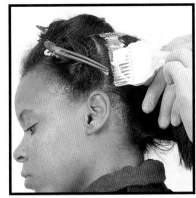

APPLYING

However, **before applying the chemical relaxer product on the client's hair and scalp, it is important to protect the skin around the hairline and ears with a protective base cream (basing).** Sometimes it is applied to the entire scalp if the client has a history of scalp sensitivity. Petroleum is the main ingredient in base creams. Body heat liquefies the base, providing a light, oily film that helps protect the scalp from irritation during chemical processing.

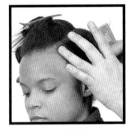

BASING

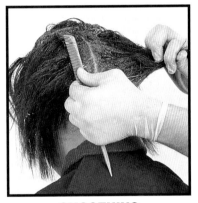

SMOOTHING

Physical Phase

The success or failure of a chemical relaxer service is strongly influenced by the physical phase of the service. The action of spreading the chemical relaxer through the hair with the back of a comb or your fingers as it processes is called smoothing. Smoothing redistributes the relaxer on the hair strand and helps relax and reform the bonds to a new straighter position.

Relaxation Test

The relaxation test, also known as the comb test, allows you to determine if additional smoothing is required. The relaxation test is performed with the back of the comb. The first step is to smooth excess product from the scalp area. The second step is to press the back of the comb against the scalp area to determine the degree of relaxation. If a minimal amount of indentation occurs, and the curl pattern reverts or "beads," additional smoothing may be required depending upon the desired results. If a strong amount of indentation occurs, the hair has thoroughly reached optimum relaxation. You are now ready to thoroughly rinse and blot the hair.

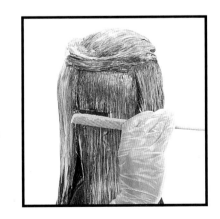

Relaxer Application Methods

There are four basic methods of application, virgin relaxer, relaxer retouch, partial relaxer and curl diffusion.

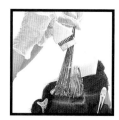

A **virgin relaxer** is applied to untreated or 'virgin' hair. The chemical relaxer is applied to the most resistant area (usually the crown or lower) and 1/4" (.75 cm) to 1/2" (1.25 cm) away from the scalp area and up to the porous ends. Next, the product is applied to the scalp area, if necessary. Chemical relaxers have a tendency to spread toward the scalp due to body heat, so further application may not be needed. The hair is then smoothed with light, even strokes from the scalp to the ends.

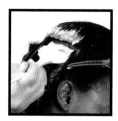

A **relaxer retouch** uses the same procedures as a virgin application, except that the product is applied only to the new growth area at the scalp. Each major section may be outlined to assist in parting and product control. Avoid allowing the relaxer to come in contact with the previously treated hair. Contact with treated hair, known as overlapping, may result in breakage.

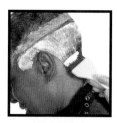

A **partial relaxer** is a virgin relaxer applied only to selected areas of the head. The partial relaxer technique is used mainly when the nape area and sides are closely tapered or when the perimeter hairline is frizzy. When used on tapered areas, it is applied every 2-3 weeks.

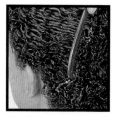

Curl diffusion, also known as chemical blow-out, is a technique used to loosen or relax overly curly hair patterns by approximately 50% of their natural shape. With this technique the chemical relaxer is applied and gently combed through the lengths for even distribution and coverage. As the hair is combed in its growth direction, you will need to carefully watch for the desired texture pattern. When the hair attains the desired texture pattern, the product will need to be rinsed out before you apply a neutralizing shampoo. You will then need to comb the hair in the final style direction and allow it to air dry.

Rinsing and Blotting

Because of the high alkalinity of relaxers, the hair must be rinsed for a long period of time to stop the chemical action and completely rid the hair of any chemical residues. It is important to check closely in the nape area and behind the ears, which are areas more difficult to rinse. Any chemicals left in the hair will remain active and could cause serious skin and/or hair damage.

The blotting process is also very important. Unlike perming when you blot the hair wrapped around the rods, the hair is now free and easier to blot. The blotting process allows you the opportunity to check carefully throughout the entire scalp area to detect any chemicals that have not been rinsed.

1
2

Neutralizing

When you are certain the hair is free of chemicals, proceed with the neutralizing shampoo procedure. **It is important to use an acid-balanced neutralizing shampoo or stabilizer to re-harden (lock) the hair into its new, straight shape.** Neutralizing shampoos or stabilizers contain an oxidizing agent, often sodium bromate or hydrogen peroxide. Always be guided by the manufacturer's instructions about how many times you must shampoo the hair and how long the product is to be left on the hair.

Timing Guide

When the chemical relaxer is applied to the hair, it softens and swells the hair, allowing penetration through the cuticle into the cortical layer where the sulfur and hydrogen bonds are altered. These bonds contribute to the hair's elasticity, strength and resilience, while helping retain its curly state. How fast or how slow the chemical relaxer penetrates depends on the hair's texture and porosity. Coarse-texture hair generally has more cuticle and more cortex than fine hair, which slows product absorption. Slower absorption increases the processing time, especially if the hair is non-porous or highly resistant.

By contrast, fine-texture hair has more cuticle and less cortex. Initially, the relaxer product may take longer to penetrate to the cortex, yet the product can quickly damage the inner layer of hair. This type of hair requires a sound knowledge of its structure and the effects of chemicals on it. The following charts overview the different relaxer strengths and the timing for application.

For Thio Relaxers (includes application and smoothing)

STRENGTH	CONDITION OF HAIR	TIMING
Mild	Fine Texture Hair	Up to 15 Minutes
Regular	Curly - Medium Texture Hair	Up to 20 Minutes
Super	Overly Curly - Coarse Texture Hair	Up to 25 Minutes

For Hydroxide Relaxers (includes application and smoothing)

STRENGTH	CONDITION OF HAIR	TIMING
Mild	Color Treated - Fine Texture Hair	Up to 10 - 15 Minutes
Regular	Curly - Medium Texture	Up to 15 Minutes
Super	Curly - Coarse Texture Hair	Up to 20 Minutes

Chemical Relaxing Essentials

To deliver a professional chemical relaxing service, you need an organized selection of products, implements and equipment. Refer to Material Safety Data Sheets (MSDS) for all products used in the salon. Perm service equipment includes furnishings and provisions necessary to provide a professional service.

Chemical Relaxer Products

PRODUCTS	FUNCTION
Protective Base Cream (if using lye, base chemical relaxer)	Protects scalp and hairline from caustic chemicals
Protective Cream	Protects hairline and top of ears from caustic chemicals
Chemical Relaxer Product	Straightens overly curly hair
Neutralizer or Neutralizing Shampoo	Rehardens and fixes hair in its new, straight shape
Moisturizing Conditioner/Sealer	Restores moisture balance
Styling Lotion	Provides extra control and lasting quality of hairstyle
Hairspray or Styling Product	Provides extra flexibility and holding qualities of design

Chemical Relaxer Implements/Supplies

IMPLEMENT/SUPPLIES	FUNCTION
Protective Shampoo Cape	Protects client from chemicals; large, loose protective covering fastened at the neck area
Cloth Towels	Absorb and remove water, relaxer product and neutralizer through blotting
Protective Gloves	Shield stylist's hands from chemicals during processing
Spatula	Removes relaxer and/or other products from containers for application, keeping supply of original product uncontaminated
Sectioning Clips	Hold hair in place in controlled sections for easier application of relaxer products

1
2

IMPLEMENT/SUPPLIES	FUNCTION
Applicator Brush	Applies relaxer to hair with less product waste, greater control and time savings
Tail Comb (non-metal)	Parts out sections of hair used for smoothing during processing.
Shampoo Comb	Distributes neutralizer through the hair, eliminating tangles and minimizing damage to swollen hair by using smooth, wide teeth of the comb
Bowl	Used to hold relaxer for application
Styling Implements	Provide manageability during styling

Chemical Relaxer Equipment

EQUIPMENT	FUNCTION
Heat equipment: plastic cap, infrared lamps, hooded dryer	Provide and capture heat for conditioning services following relaxer service; help restore hair's structural integrity
Timer	Alerts stylist to check for maximum amount of time allowed for relaxer to be on hair and scalp; also for keeping check on neutralizing times as recommended by the manufacturer
Shampoo Bowl	Allows client's hair to be rinsed and shampooed; needed for rinsing relaxer chemicals and neutralizer from hair
Styling Chair	Provides adjustability for stylist's working needs and comfortable seating for client

Infection Control and Safety

It is important to practice infection control and safety procedures in order to prevent the spread of any harmful bacteria. Always use sanitized combs, brushes and cutting implements for every client, every time.

Special Safety Considerations
1. If a client experiences burning during a sodium hydroxide relaxer service, rinse the hair with warm water, apply neutralizing shampoo and proceed with remaining service.
2. Avoid brushing the hair before any chemical service.

3. Perform several test strands to avoid overprocessing.

4. Avoid pulling the hair, which can cause irritation and make the scalp sensitive.

5. Wear protective gloves during chemical services.

6. Never exceed timing guidelines.

7. Use caution while applying the chemical relaxer and prevent it from contacting the skin. If it accidentally gets on the skin, wash the area immediately with warm water and neutralizing shampoo.

8. If the chemical relaxer gets into the eyes, flush them thoroughly with lukewarm water and consult a physician immediately.

9. Never attempt to relax hair that has been bleached.

10. Never use sodium hydroxide to relax hair that has been treated with a thio product or vice versa. The results could be severe breakage and/or irreversible damage.

11. Apply relaxer evenly without missing any areas. If the relaxer is not evenly applied or if areas are missed, there will be an uneven pattern of straight or curly hair or ridges that could be hard to control.

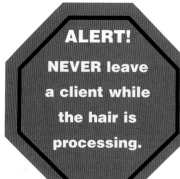

ALERT!
NEVER leave a client while the hair is processing.

12. Advise client not to shampoo before 48 hours of the chemical service. The natural oils can help protect the scalp.

13. Avoid performing any chemical services when any cuts, open sores or abrasions are present on the scalp.

Draping for a Chemical Service

Refer to the "Perming" portion of this chapter for details on this draping procedure.

Testing for Metallic Salts

Applying a relaxer over hair with metallic salts will cause severe damage if not a total destruction of the hair fiber. Therefore, it is critical to test the hair for metallic salts if you suspect they are present. Refer to "Test for Metallic Salts" in the "Perming" portion of this chapter.

Preliminary Strand Testing

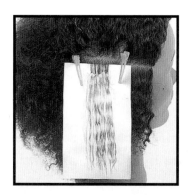

Strand testing evaluates the overall condition of the hair to determine if it can withstand the chemical service. To strand test, part off a small section of hair in the most resistant area of the head. Apply the chemical relaxer to the test strand. Follow the manufacturer's timing guide and check the test area frequently. Process (smooth) the hair to straighten it. Rinse, then use a neutralizing shampoo and towel dry the test area thoroughly. If the test strands did not relax enough, test in another area using a stronger relaxer strength.

Client Consultation

Before applying any chemicals to the hair, conduct a thorough consultation with the client. You'll want to remember that a consultation is a two-way conversation between you and the client. Success comes from listening carefully and recording all the important information on the record card. As you may recall, some important considerations for a relaxing service include determining the new curl texture pattern that your client desires. Asking the client how much of the existing curl pattern he/she would like reduced and gathering your client's chemical relaxing history, such as any problems he/she may have had in the past, will enable you to make the proper decisions during the consultation phase.

The five steps of the consultation are:

Greet

Ask, analyze and assess

- Have the client sign the Release Form before the service begins. A standard Release Form, required by some malpractice insurance companies, states that the school or salon is not responsible for damages that may occur.

Agree

Deliver

Complete

- Complete the client record card with accurate information for future services and file it in a secure area with other record cards.

Review the "Perming" portion of this chapter and the "Design Decisions" chapter for more information on Client Consultation.

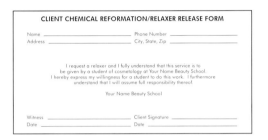

Product and Application Overview

In this portion of the chapter you will overview the relaxer products and application techniques you will perform in the exercises that follow. These products and application techniques will help prepare you for the chemical relaxer services you'll encounter in the salon.

The following chart summarizes and categorizes the different types of relaxers along with their advantages and disadvantages. This chart can be used as a guide when choosing the proper relaxer for any type of hair. The strength of the relaxer must also be considered.

Note: prior to thio application, the hair should be pre-shampooed and base applied only to the hairline and ears. Whereas, for sodium hydroxide application, the hair should not be pre-shampooed and base should be applied to the entire hairline, scalp and ears.

TYPE AND DESCRIPTION (listed by main ingredient)	ADVANTAGE	DISADVANTAGE
Sodium Hydroxide Category: Lye, Base pH: 10.5 - 14	Faster processing time; better for resistant hair and/or coarse hair	Irritates the scalp; may cause severe damage; strict time constraints; requires base application
Sodium Hydroxide Category: Lye, No Base pH: 10.5 - 14	Faster processing time; better for resistant hair and/or coarse hair	Irritates the scalp; may cause severe damage; strict time constraints
Calcium or Potassium Hydroxide Category: No Lye	Better for less-resistant hair; less irritating to scalp	May be more drying; slower processing time; requires frequent conditioning treatments
Guanidine Hydroxide Category: No Lye, Mix (contain calcium hydroxide and guanidine carbonate)	Better for less-resistant hair; less irritating to scalp	Processes slowly; not recommended for overly curly hair
Lithium Hydroxide Category: No Lye, No Mix	Better for less-resistant hair; less irritating to scalp	Processes slowly; not recommended for overly curly hair
Ammonium Bisulfate Category: No Lye, No Mix	Better for less resistant hair	Requires the addition of heat; not recommended for overly curly hair
Ammonium Thioglycolate	Better for less resistant hair; more control due to processing time; better for fragile, fine or tinted hair	Not recommended for overly curly hair

ALERT!

Never apply a thio relaxer over hair that has been relaxed with a sodium hydroxide relaxer or vice versa, since these two chemicals are not compatible. Severe damage and breakage can occur.

1
2

Relaxing Application Techniques

A chemical relaxer should be considered part of a total design. The final design that you choose should complement the shape of the haircut as well as your client's wishes. Here we've overviewed the application techniques you will learn in this portion of the chapter.

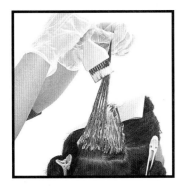
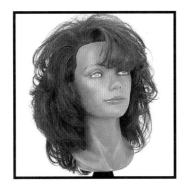

Virgin Application
MIDSTRAND, BASE THEN ENDS

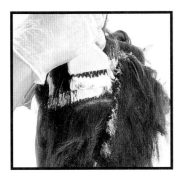
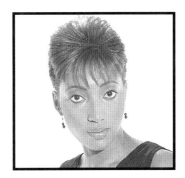

Retouch Application
BASE ONLY

Virgin Sodium Hydroxide Relaxer

Sodium hydroxide relaxers can be used on any type of hair but are especially designed for overly curly hair. A sodium hydroxide relaxer is a progressive product, which means that once you apply the product, the hair cannot return to its original state nor can you perform a curl reformation service afterward. Therefore, a sodium hydroxide relaxer is used to permanently straighten the hair.

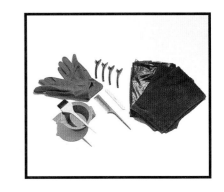

For a virgin application of a sodium hydroxide relaxer, the product is applied to the most resistant area and 1/4" (.75 cm) to 1/2" (1.25 cm) away from the scalp up to the porous ends. To ensure a thorough application, partings should be approximately 1/4" (.75 cm) and product should be applied to both sides of the strand. The heat from the scalp will allow the product to spread upward toward the scalp. However, if you need to apply product closer to the scalp, do so only after you have applied it to the midstrand throughout the head first. Never apply product directly on the scalp. The relaxer product is applied to the perimeter hairline last since the hairline is sensitive to breakage and is usually finer in texture.

The above application procedure is a guideline. However, other application techniques are also acceptable. For example:

- You may begin the application at the ridge of the first curl.
- To equalize processing time on long hair, you may begin application farther away from the scalp to avoid overprocessing the hair.

Your instructor may have additional guidelines that are equally acceptable for you to follow.

Virgin Sodium Hydroxide Relaxer Guidelines

- Perform strand test.

- Disinfect work station; arrange implements and supplies including sectioning clips, non-metal tail comb, gloves, base, sodium hydroxide relaxer, bowl and brush.

- Wash and sanitize your hands; drape the client for a chemical service; perform analysis of hair and scalp; wear protective gloves and chemical apron; review previous client record card, if applicable.

- **Do not pre-shampoo the client's hair.**

- Section the hair into 4 or 5 sections, base the hairline, ears and scalp.

- Begin the application of the relaxer at the most resistant area. Use 1/4" (.75 cm) partings and apply the relaxer 1/4" (.75 cm) to 1/2" (1.25 cm) or farther away from the scalp up to the porous ends.

- Complete the entire head and follow manufacturer's directions for processing.

- Apply relaxer to the scalp area and ends, if necessary. Smooth each parting with back of the comb using a light to moderate smoothing action from scalp to ends.

- Perform comb test. If minimal indentation occurs, continue smoothing to achieve desired texture pattern. If strong indentation occurs, proceed to rinsing.

- Rinse thoroughly with warm water, and without scalp manipulations, until water runs clear. Direct the water spray away from the client's face. Follow with neutralizing shampoo.

- Condition the hair. Then you may wish to cut the hair wet or dry. Style the hair as desired.

- Complete client record card; offer your client a rebook visit; recommend retail products that will enhance or maintain the relaxer service; disinfect implements, discard non-reusable supplies and clean your work area.

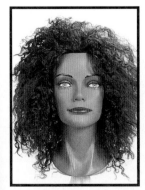
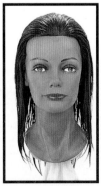
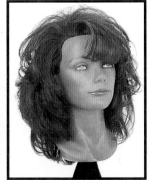

Virgin Thio Relaxer

When you are working with a thio relaxer, the first-time application is applied to the most resistant area and 1/4" (.75 cm) to 1/2" (1.25cm) away from the scalp out to the porous ends. Additional product may then be applied at the base (scalp area) if necessary. **Product is applied to the base last since the hair near the scalp will process more quickly due to body heat.** A non-alkaline shampoo is recommended after the chemical relaxer has been rinsed from the hair. The natural oils that are removed during the chemical relaxing process are replaced with a conditioning treatment. In this exercise a thio relaxer is used within five sections. Horizontal partings are used for the back, side and top sections. A bowl and brush method is used.

The above application procedure is a guideline. However, other application techniques are also acceptable. For example:

- You may begin the application at the ridge of the first curl, which may be farther from the scalp.
- To equalize processing time on long hair, you may begin application farther away from the scalp to avoid over processing the hair.

Your instructor may have additional guidelines that are equally acceptable for you to follow.

Virgin Thio Relaxer Preparation

As with any professional service, it is important to have your area, products, implements and equipment in proper order. Before performing a virgin thio relaxer service, be sure to satisfy the following points:

- Perform analysis of hair and scalp
- Perform strand test and elasticity test
- Clean work station with disinfectant
- Arrange implements/supplies including sectioning clips, non-metal tail comb, gloves, base, relaxer, bowl and brush
- Wash your hands with liquid antibacterial soap
- Ask the client to remove jewelry and store in a secure place
- Drape your client for a chemical service
- **Shampoo client's hair lightly; do not sensitize the scalp**

Virgin Thio Relaxer Procedure

- Section hair for control
- Apply base (protective cream) around hairline and ears
- Begin at back top section or where hair is most resistant
- Use 1/4" (.75cm) horizontal partings
- Apply relaxer 1/4" (.75 cm) to 1/2" (1.25 cm) away from the scalp to both sides of the strand up to the porous ends
- Work from top to bottom of each section and complete back sections
- Move to back of top section
- Complete top section

- Move to sides and repeat same techniques

- Complete sides

- Comb, then smooth each section with back of comb using smooth, light, even strokes from scalp to ends

- Comb and smooth all sections

- Perform comb test

- If an indentation occurs, continue smoothing

- Follow manufacturer's directions for processing

- Once the hair has reached desired degree of relaxation, rinse relaxer from the hair until water runs clear

Virgin Thio Relaxer

1-2. Section the hair into five sections for control. Subdivide the back in half. Subdivide the front into three sections, top and sides. **Apply base (protective cream) to the entire hairline and ears.**

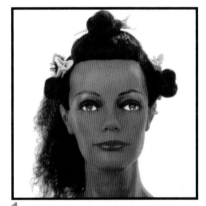
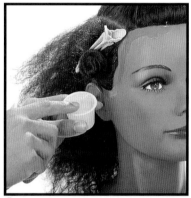

3-4. Begin at the back top section or where the hair is the most resistant. Use 1/4" (.75) horizontal partings. Apply relaxer 1/4" (.75 cm) to 1/2" (1.25 cm) away from the scalp up to the porous ends to both sides of the strand. Do not touch the scalp with the tail of the comb or brush while parting. **Work from the top to the bottom of each section.** Then bring each parting down. **Complete the back sections using the same techniques.**

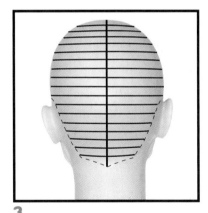
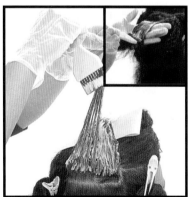

Optional

Application methods for a virgin thio relaxer may vary. Product may be applied directly from the scalp to the ends. Follow manufacturer's directions and your regulating agency for specific guidelines. And remember, always do a complete hair/scalp analysis prior to beginning a relaxer service.

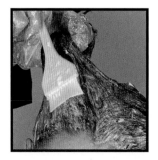

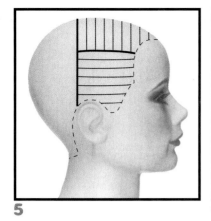
5

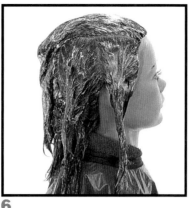
6

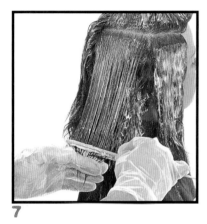
7

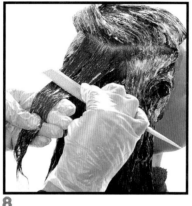
8

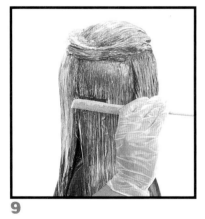
9

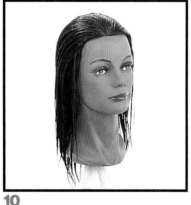
10

5-6. **Move to the back of the top section.** Apply the relaxer using the same techniques. **Complete the top section. Move to the sides and apply the relaxer from horizontal partings using the same techniques. Complete the sides.**

7-8. **Comb, then smooth each section with the back of the comb using smooth, light, even strokes from scalp to ends.** Reapply product if necessary near the scalp. **Comb and smooth all sections.** Close up the sectioning lines by combing the hair between the major partings.

9-10. **Perform comb test.** If an indentation occurs, continue smoothing. Follow manufacturer's directions for processing. Once the hair has reached the desired degree of relaxation, approximately 85%, rinse the relaxer from the hair until the water runs clear. Then shampoo the hair with a non-alkaline (neutralizing) shampoo. Condition and finish the hair as desired.

Optional: An alternative application method includes applying product to one side of the strand only as shown on the DVD. Therefore, be guided by your instructor and regulating agency.

Virgin Thio Relaxer Completion

- Complete client record card
- Offer a rebook visit to your client
- Recommend retail products to your client
- Discard non-reusable materials, disinfect implements and arrange work station in proper order
- Wash your hands with liquid antibacterial soap

Relaxer Retouch

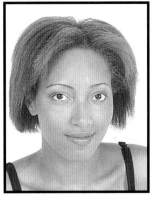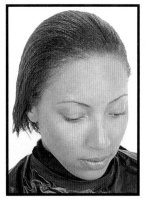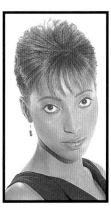

A retouch should be performed when there is a sufficient amount of new growth, generally not more than one inch (2.5 cm), to avoid overlapping the product onto the previously straightened hair. All the same procedures are followed as with the virgin application except that the relaxer is applied to the new growth only. The retouch application is performed with the same product that was used for the previous application. The product is applied slightly away from the scalp up to the previously relaxed hair. Applying the product beyond the new growth, onto the previously relaxed hair, is known as overlapping. Overlapping can cause breakage to the hair. In this exercise, horizontal partings within five sections are used throughout. The relaxer is applied to the new growth only. A protective cream is applied to shield the previously relaxed hair from relaxer and product run off during rinsing.

Relaxer Retouch Preparation

As with any professional service, it is important to have your area, products, implements and equipment in proper order. Before performing a chemical reforming service, be sure to satisfy the following points:

- Perform analysis of hair and scalp
- Perform strand test and elasticity test
- Clean work station with disinfectant
- Arrange implements/supplies including sectioning clips, tail comb, gloves, base, relaxer, protective cream, bowl and brush
- Wash your hands with liquid antibacterial soap
- Ask the client to remove jewelry and store in a secure place
- Drape your client for a chemical service

> • Note:
> For a thio retouch application, pre-shampoo the hair lightly without scalp manipulations; do not base scalp
> For a sodium hydroxide retouch application, do not pre-shampoo the hair; base the scalp

Relaxer Retouch Procedure

- Section hair for control
- Apply protective cream to previously relaxed hair
- Begin at top back section or most resistant area
- Use 1/4" (.75 cm) horizontal partings
- Apply product slightly away from scalp up to previously relaxed hair to both sides of the parting
- Complete back sections
- Complete remaining sections using the same procedures
- Follow manufacturer's directions for processing
- Smooth each section with back of comb
- Follow manufacturer's directions for processing and perform comb test
- Rinse the hair until water runs clear after you have reached the desired degree of relaxation
- Shampoo hair with a neutralizing shampoo

1
2

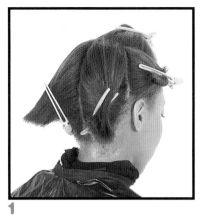

1

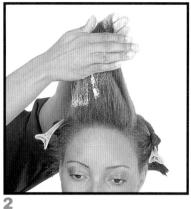

2

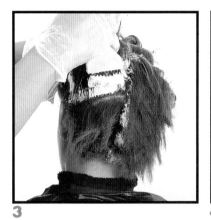

3

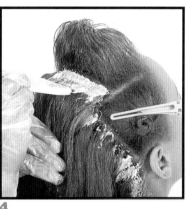

4

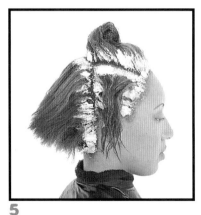

5

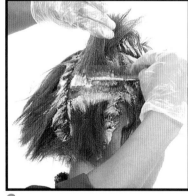

6

Sodium Hydroxide Relaxer Retouch

1. Section the hair into five sections for control. Divide the back from the front. Subdivide the back in half. Subdivide the front into three sections, top and sides. Apply base around the entire hairline. Apply base to the scalp using a checker-board pattern.

2. Apply a protective cream to the previously relaxed hair. The protective cream will protect the previously treated hair from the chemical product.

3. Begin at the top back section or the most resistant area and use 1/4" (.75 cm) horizontal partings. Apply product slightly away from the scalp up to the previously relaxed hair to both sides of the parting. Work from the top to the bottom of each section. Do not touch the scalp with the tail of the comb or brush. Do not apply the product directly onto the scalp. **Complete back sections.** As you complete each section, bring the hair down.

4. Move to the top section. Use the same procedures from horizontal partings. Work from the back of the section to the front hairline.

5. Complete remaining sections using the same procedures. Use horizontal partings at the sides. **Follow manufacturer's directions for processing.**

6. Smooth each section with the back of the comb using the same parting pattern. Follow manufacturer's directions for processing and perform comb test. Rinse the hair until the water runs clear after you have reached the desired degree of relaxation. Shampoo the hair with a neutralizing shampoo. Condition and finish the hair as desired.

Optional: An alternative application method includes applying product to one side of the strand only as shown on the DVD. Therefore, be guided by your instructor and regulating agency.

Relaxer Retouch Completion

- Complete client record card
- Offer a rebook visit to your client
- Recommend retail products to your client
- Discard non-reusable materials, disinfect implements and arrange work station in proper order
- Wash your hands with liquid antibacterial soap

Home Maintenance

Because chemical relaxers are caustic, it is important to maintain the health of the hair on a regular basis. Recommend that your client return to the salon for conditioning treatments to help restore the hair to its optimal condition.

If the client prefers to maintain her hair at home, retail the proper shampoo, conditioner and styling aids to use between in-salon relaxer services. Educate your client about how to use these products for successful maintenance of healthy hair. Take the time to share a few easy styling techniques. Be sure to point out that regular maintenance prepares the hair for future chemical services.

CURL REFORMING

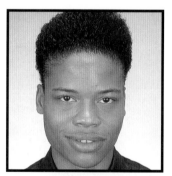

You are now ready to consider the third kind of chemical texturizing service, Curl Reforming, which combines the knowledge you gained in the "Perming" and "Relaxing" sections. The curl reformation process was introduced in the 1970s as demand grew for a wider range of styling options and more control over natural, overly curly hair. This new procedure used milder chemicals that did not dry or break the hair, while offering new choices for the client with overly curly hair. It was also an option for clients with color-treated hair or hair too fine to withstand the negative effects of sodium hydroxide relaxers.

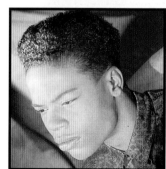

Curl Reforming, also known as soft curls, reformation curls or, in technical terms, a double-process perm service, is a chemical service designed to change overly curly hair to curly or wavy hair. The hair is first relaxed to reduce the curl pattern and then permed to create a new curl pattern.

Curl Reforming Theory

The curl reformation process involves three steps:

- Reduction, which reduces the existing curl pattern
- Reforming, which forms a new curl pattern around rods
- Rebonding, which bonds (neutralizes) the chemical bonds to complete the new curl

Reduction

In the first step, reduction, the natural curl is reduced by applying a product known as a rearranger. The rearranger is applied 1/2" (1.25 cm) away from the scalp and out to the porous ends. Next, the product is applied to the scalp area if necessary and the hair is smoothed from the scalp to the ends.

Ammonium thioglycolate (thio) is the main ingredient found in rearrangers. The rearranger is applied to the hair using the same application procedures as in chemical relaxing. It is important not to over-relax the hair because it must maintain enough bonds to create a successful curl pattern in the next step. The rearranger is only rinsed but not shampooed from the hair prior to proceeding to the reforming step.

Since you are working with hair that will have some natural texture remaining, thinner partings are used while wrapping the hair. Also, when performing a curl reformation service, the rod diameter chosen is generally at least two times larger than the diameter of the natural curl pattern.

Thio is an alkaline chemical available in cream, lotion or gel, with a general pH of 9.6. It is called a chemical rearranger because it shifts and rearranges the polypeptide chains and disulfide bonds of the hair, the same as in perming. It is available in mild (pH 7) for fine hair, regular (pH 8) for average hair and super (pH 9) for very curly to resistant hair. Since the descriptions of strengths may vary between manufacturers, you should always read the manufacturer's directions carefully. For additional information on ammonium thioglycolate relaxers, refer to the "Chemical Relaxing" portion of this chapter.

Reforming

In the second step, reforming, the waving lotion, known as a booster, is applied to the hair and the hair is wrapped with the desired rod to begin forming the new curl pattern. A mild creamy form of ammonium thioglycolate is the main ingredient found in the booster. Once the hair is completely wrapped, additional booster is applied to the hair to ensure thorough saturation. Once the processing is complete, the hair is rinsed and towel blotted with the perm rods remaining in the hair.

Any perm wrapping pattern, such as the rectangle or bricklay pattern, may be used to wrap the hair. In the procedural part of this section, you will learn about a new wrapping pattern known as the contour pattern. Refer to the "Perming" portion of this chapter for further information on wrapping techniques

Rebonding

The third and final step, rebonding, involves neutralization. The neutralizer locks in the new curl pattern that was created in the reforming step. The neutralizer is applied to the rods and remains on the hair for the full processing time. Neutralizing with the rods in the hair will result in a firmer curl pattern. For a looser curl pattern, apply neutralizer to the rods, then remove the rods and apply additional neutralizer to the hair for the remaining processing time.

Application Techniques

There are two basic application techniques for a curl reforming service, virgin and retouch. With a virgin application, the chemical rearranger is applied 1/4" – 1/2" (.75-1.25 cm) away from the scalp and up to 1/2" (1.25 cm) away from the ends. The product is applied to the ends last, since this is the most porous area of the strand. A curl reforming retouch uses the same procedures as the virgin application, except that the rearranger is applied to the new growth only. It is important that the rearranger product not overlap with the previously treated hair, since overlap could cause breakage. Refer to the client's record card for documented information. Review the "Chemical Relaxing" portion of this chapter for more information.

Hair Analysis

It is important to give several preliminary tests before applying chemicals to determine the hair's porosity, elasticity, density, texture and type. The information learned from the hair analysis is necessary to help ensure successful results. Refer to the "Perming" and "Chemical Relaxing" portions of this chapter for further information.

Curl Reforming Essentials

To accomplish a successful curl reforming service, you need an organized selection of products, implements and equipment. Curl reforming products are produced by many different manufacturers, are disposable and must be frequently replaced. Refer to MSDS (Material Safety Data Sheets) for information on all salon products. Curl reforming implements are the hand-held tools you use, while curl reforming equipment includes furnishings and provisions necessary to provide a professional service.

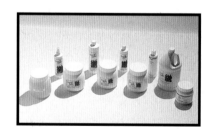

Curl Reforming Products

PRODUCTS	FUNCTION
Curl Rearranger	Reduces peptide bonds so hair can relax and become straight; thio-based product
Curl Booster	Assists hair to assume new shape of rod when wrapping hair in perm rods; milder form of thio

PRODUCTS	FUNCTION
Neutralizer	Fixes, locks in, restores bonds to make new shape of hair permanent; contains oxidizing agent
Shampoo	Cleanses/removes dirt and oils from scalp and hair
Protective Base Cream	Protects scalp, hair and ears from chemicals: petroleum-based product
Curl Activator	Helps new curl configurations retain their shape and provides moisture; applied frequently after every shampoo
Instant Moisturizer	Helps replace natural moisture and oils lost during chemical process
Protein/Moisturizing Conditioner	Restores protein and moisture lost during processing

Curl Reforming Implements/Supplies

IMPLEMENT/SUPPLIES	FUNCTION
Applicator Brush	Applies rearranger efficiently by having a tapered handle and a flat brush
Perm Rods (tools)	Determine the shape and size of the new curl; selected by shape, diameter and length
Towels	Absorb and remove water by blotting after rinsing rearranger, booster and neutralizer
Cotton Strips	Protect hairline, neck and area above ears from chemicals
Plastic Sectioning Clips	Hold hair in place in controlled sections before and during wrapping procedure
Bowl (non-metal)	Holds the product during application
Styling Comb	Parts and combs hair
Tail Comb	Parts out sections of hair for wrapping by using tapered end of comb
End Papers	Control the hair ends when wrapping; equalize porosity and absorbency during processing, rinsing and neutralizing
Spray Bottle with Water	Keeps hair damp and offers more control of hair
Protective Gloves or Cream	Protects stylist's hands from chemicals

IMPLEMENT/SUPPLIES	FUNCTION
Plastic Picks	Hold perm rods in position when placed under the rod band
Plastic Bag	Covers the hair during processing and sometimes during reconditioning treatments
Plastic Shampoo Cape	Protects client from chemicals; large, loose protective covering fastened at the neck area

Curl Reformation Equipment

EQUIPMENT	FUNCTION
Heat Equipment: Plastic Cap, Infrared Lamp, Hooded Dryer	Provides and captures heat as required by the manufacturer's instructions
Timer	Alerts stylist to check for maximum timing for product to be on hair and scalp; also used for neutralizing, as recommended by the manufacturer
Shampoo Bowl	Holds client's neck and hair during shampoo service; needed for rinsing rearranger, booster and neutralizer from hair
Styling Chair	Provides comfortable seating for client and adjustable working height for stylist

Infection Control and Safety

Practice infection control procedures by washing your hands with liquid antibacterial soap before beginning the procedure in order to prevent the spread of any harmful bacteria. Always use sanitized combs, brushes and cutting implements for every client every time.

Special Safety Considerations

1. Wear protective gloves to shield your hands from the harsh effects of chemicals.
2. **Examine the scalp for any irregular conditions, such as scratches, abrasions, irritations or cuts. If you discover any of these, do not proceed. Postpone and reschedule the curl reformation service when the scalp is healthy again.**
3. **Avoid brushing the hair before giving any chemical service to prevent scalp irritation.**
4. Apply protective base around the hairline and ears to prevent skin irritation.
5. Avoid chemical burns and irritation to the skin, eyes, ears and nose by keeping all products away from them. If chemicals accidentally get on the skin, flush the area with cool water. If the product gets into the eyes, flush them thoroughly with lukewarm water and consult a physician immediately.

12

6. Wrap cotton strips securely around the hairline before applying neutralizer to keep it off the skin. When the cotton becomes wet, replace it immediately.

7. Place a neutralizing bib around the hairline with the elastic bands on top of the cotton to prevent skin irritation or chemical burns. The neutralizing bib is optional and used for added protection.

8. Take special care with bleached hair. Most bleached hair is unable to receive chemical reformation services.

9. Cut off all hair that has been previously treated with sodium hydroxide if curl reforming is desired.

10. Strand test to determine the hair's competency. If the hair is dry, brittle or over-porous, recondition it first and/or cut off damaged ends to avoid overprocessing.

11. Never leave a client alone while the hair is processing.

Do not perform a curl reformation service on hair that has been relaxed with a sodium hydroxide or no-lye relaxer. Using thio-based products on hydroxide-treated hair will result in severe hair damage or breakage since these two chemicals are not compatible.

Draping for Chemical Services

Proper draping procedures for chemical services are of the utmost importance. It is essential to protect the client's clothing as well as take preventive measures to avoid skin irritations or burns caused by the chemicals you apply. Draping for a chemical service includes a towel under the cape and a towel on top of the cape. Refer to the "Perming" portion of this chapter for details on this draping procedure.

Testing for Metallic Salts

Color products that restore or progressively darken the hair (sometimes called hair restorers) contain metallic salts. These form a residue on the hair, which interferes with the chemical action. The results can be uneven curls, distinct discoloration, hair damage or breakage. To avoid such negative results, perform a test for metallic salts (also called a 1:20 test) prior to performing a perm service. Review the "Perming" portion of this chapter for details.

Preliminary Strand Testing

Preliminary strand testing is a good predictor of how your client's hair will react to the chemical rearranger, booster and neutralizer. Always take the time to test tinted, bleached, over-porous or damaged hair.

- Shampoo and towel dry the hair.
- Apply protective base cream on the scalp and hairline.

- Follow the manufacturer's directions and strand test the most delicate areas of the hair.

- Wrap a coil of cotton around the strand to isolate it from the rest of the hair.

- Apply chemical rearranger to the hair, smooth, rinse and blot it. Apply the booster and wrap the strand on a perm rod. Set a timer and process according to the manufacturer's directions.

- Pay close attention to the process and check the hair frequently.

- Unfasten a rod and carefully unwind the hair about 1.5 turns to check the test curl. Do not permit the hair to loosen or unwind from the rod completely. Hold the hair firmly by placing a thumb at each end of the rod. Turn it gently toward the scalp so that the hair falls easily into the wave pattern. Do not push the rod toward the head. Continue checking the rods until a firm curl pattern forms, equal to the rod's diameter.

- Process, rinse and neutralize the hair.

- Evaluate and document the results.

Shampoo only once before a curl reformation service to avoid sensitizing the scalp. Use light finger pressure and moderate water pressure with a mild temperature.

Client Consultation

Review the five steps of the consultation procedure, making sure to gather the client's chemical history and record it on the record card.

- Greet
- Ask, Analyze and Assess
- Agree
- Deliver
- Complete

Review the "Perming" and "Chemical Relaxing" portions of this chapter for more details on a successful client consultation.

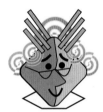

"The chemical service consultation is an essential element that will help you achieve the result you and your client desire."

Curl Reforming Service: Contour Wrap

A curl reformation service should not be considered a service by itself, but rather it should be regarded as part of a design that includes the haircut. The wrapping pattern you select should complement the shape of the haircut as well as your client's wishes.

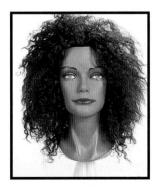
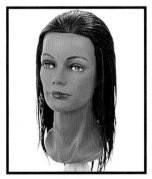
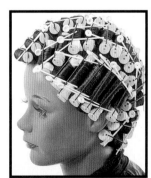
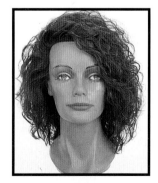

1 2

In this exercise, the contour wrapping pattern is used to create the new curl pattern. The contour pattern is a versatile wrapping pattern that adapts to the contour of the head. A center rectangle is positioned from the center front hairline to the center nape. Horizontal partings are used in the rectangle shape. The sides consist of two sections. The outer section, or the one next to the center rectangle, consists of a combination of diagonal and horizontal partings. Diagonal partings are used in the inner or last section.

Curl Reforming Preparation

As with any professional service, it is important to have your area, products, implements and equipment in proper order. Before performing a chemical reforming service, be sure to satisfy the following points:

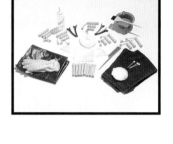

- Perform analysis of hair and scalp
- Clean work station with disinfectant
- Arrange implements/supplies including perm rods, picks, end papers, sectioning clips, non-metal tail comb, plastic cap, gloves, protective base cream, cotton, rearranger, booster, neutralizer, applicator bottle, bowl and brush
- Wash your hands with liquid antibacterial soap
- Ask the client to remove jewelry and store in a secure place
- Drape your client for a chemical service
- Shampoo hair lightly without scalp manipulations

Curl Reforming Procedure

- Apply protective base cream to hairline and ears
- Apply and smooth hair with curl rearranger, following the same procedures as for a virgin relaxer application
- Follow manufacturer's directions for processing
- Rinse and towel blot hair
- *Apply and distribute booster to each section as you wrap the hair
- Wrap first section
- Complete first section
- Wrap and complete remaining sections using the same procedures
- Follow manufacturer's directions regarding processing, plastic cap and text curl for "S" pattern
- Rinse booster and towel blot hair
- Apply neutralizer
- Follow manufacturer's directions for processing
- Rinse with low water pressure
- Remove rods
- Apply moisturizing conditioner
- Rinse conditioner
- Style the hair

*Note: You may follow one of three booster application procedures.
1. Apply and distribute booster to each section, wrap hair with tools.
2. Apply and distribute booster to entire head, then wrap hair with tools.
3. Wrap entire head, apply booster to top and/or bottom of each tool depending on texture.
Your choice may be governed by your wrapping speed. Be careful not to overprocess the hair.

Curl Reforming Service

1-2. Apply protective base cream to the hairline and ears. Apply the curl rearranger and smooth the hair following the same procedures as the virgin relaxer application. Follow manufacturer's directions for processing. Rinse and towel blot the hair.

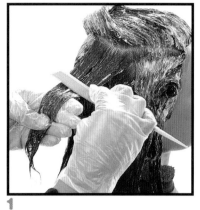
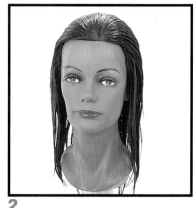

3-4. Apply and distribute the booster to each section as you wrap the hair. **Wrap the first section** or center rectangle. Use rods at least 2 times the diameter of the natural curl. Take partings 1/8" (.35 cm) smaller than the diameter of the tool. Use end papers to control the hair while wrapping. Position the tool half-off base. Use picks to control the rods. **Complete the first section** or center rectangle. Then wrap and complete the next section. Work from the front hairline to the nape using diagonal and horizontal partings.

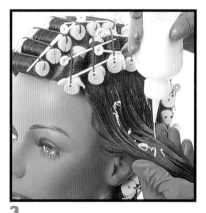
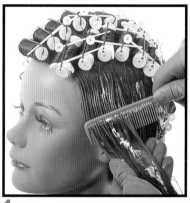

5-6. Wrap and complete the last section away from the face using diagonal partings.

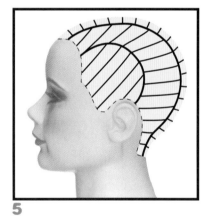
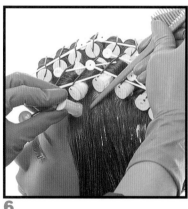

7. Wrap and complete the remaining sections using the same procedures. Follow manufacturer's directions regarding processing, plastic cap and test curl for "S" pattern. Rinse with tepid water and the tools in position. Towel blot the hair. Apply the neutralizer. Follow manufacturer's directions for processing. Rinse with low water pressure. Remove the rods and apply moisturizing conditioner.

8. **Style the hair** as desired or you may wish to cut the hair before styling.

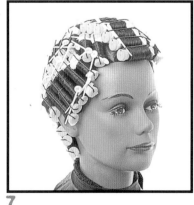
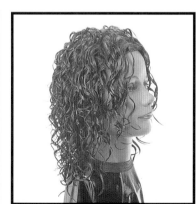

1
2

Curl Reforming Completion

- Complete client record card
- Offer a rebook visit to your client
- Recommend retail products to your client
- Discard non-reusable materials, disinfect implements and arrange work station in proper order
- Wash your hands with liquid antibacterial soap

Home Maintenance

The success of the curl reformation service depends largely on the client's home maintenance program. It is your responsibility to make sure that the client knows what to do for successful, easy-style maintenance.

- Ask the client to return in one week so that you can give the first shampoo and conditioning treatment. If there are any problems, you will see them immediately.
- Make sure the client uses a curl activator and moisturizer to maintain the needed moisture and oil balance. A lack of moisture will cause frizzy hair, limp curls and dryness.
- Advise the client that freshly shampooed hair usually takes a day or two to regain its oil-moisture balance. Covering the hair with a plastic cap immediately after applying the scalp oil, curl activator and instant moisturizer helps restore the oil-moisture balance.

Changing the texture of hair by offering perm, chemical relaxer or curl reforming services will be one of the many rewarding pursuits in your cosmetology career. Enhancing the client's image by freshening or vitalizing a hairstyle is considered a key element in a successful salon career. The powerful chemical services reviewed in this chapter lay the groundwork for your future.

Build Your Critical Thinking Skills

In this chapter you have prepared yourself to meet the following Industry Standards for entry-level cosmetologists:

- Provide styling and finishing techniques to complete a hairstyle to the satisfaction of the client.
- Perform hair relaxation and wave formation techniques in accordance with the manufacturer's directions.

It's Up to You to know what to do. Using your training to this point, review the following case scenario and think through how you would handle the challenge.

Your client has just shown you a photograph of a picture taken of herself at her son's wedding six months ago. The wedding was out of state and she had visited a different salon to have a perm and style prior to the wedding. Because she liked the style so much, she wrote down details of the service right down to the color of rods the stylist had used, the name of the perm product and the timing for processing. As you view the photograph and hear the details unfold, you realize the information has to be incorrect. The rod size indicated by the color she has given you is entirely too small and your salon does not carry the perm product used in the other salon. What would you do?

Chapter 13
HAIR COLORING

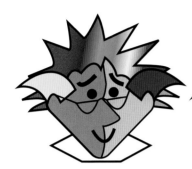

After studying this chapter you will be able to . . .

1. Define color and the law of color.

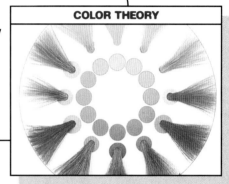

COLOR THEORY

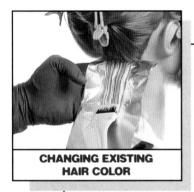

CHANGING EXISTING HAIR COLOR

3. Demonstrate and explain the procedures used to change existing hair color.

2. Idenfify the natural and artificial level, tone and intensity of hair color.

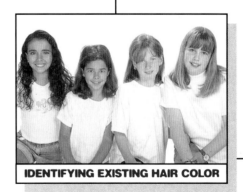

IDENTIFYING EXISTING HAIR COLOR

Whether it's a rainbow, a display of fireworks or a meadow filled with flowers, people have always delighted in color. Throughout the ages that delight has translated into the desire to color the human body, hair and clothing. You may already have a very developed eye for color when it comes to selecting and coordinating a wardrobe. Now you have the chance to apply that educated eye to the exciting world of hair color.

Having the ability to change a client's existing hair color will allow you to enhance the haircut or style you have selected for your client and therefore help the client maintain the best possible personal image and you the best possible professional image.

In the chapter on "Professional Development" you find information on "value-added" products and services, that little something extra like a prize in a cereal box. You can think of salon color services that way as well. They are not a little but a great VALUE you can add to your repertoire as a trusted and competent cosmetologist.

Understanding color, being able to identify the client's existing hair color and knowing how to change the client's existing hair color translates into a financial and professional reward for you as a stylist. Hair color is the second leading service in the salon.

To add the hair coloring skill to your resume, you need to focus on the BIG IDEA underlying color theory and its application to hair coloring and then practice the procedures you will learn in this chapter.

COLOR THEORY
What is Color?
The Law of Color

IDENTIFYING EXISTING HAIR COLOR
Melanin
Gray Hair
Identifying Natural Level and Tone
Identifying Artificial Level, Tone
  and Intensity
Additional Considerations

CHANGING EXISTING HAIR COLOR
Hair Color Chemistry
Hair Color Essentials
Hair Color Techniques
Infection Control and Safety
Client Consultation
Product and Application Overview
Temporary Color
Semi-Permanent Color
Oxidative Color: Darker Result
Oxidative Color: Lighter Result
Surface Painting
Partial Highlights: Slicing
Full Highlights: Weaving
Cap Highlighting
Double-Process Blonde
Tint Back
Hair Color Removal Techniques
Hair Color Problems and Solutions

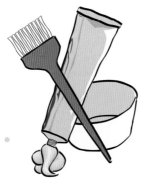

COLOR THEORY

As an artist uses paint to express artistic talents, a cosmetologist uses hair coloring. Color can define the lines and shape of a hair style, soften facial features, warm skin tones and accentuate a person's lifestyle and personality.

Hair coloring techniques have been used since antiquity. In ancient times, Cleopatra was said to have anointed her hair with henna. Roman women created concoctions of wood ash, unslaked lime and sodium bicarbonate to lighten their hair. Eventually it was discovered that the hair could be lightened by sitting in the sun. It wasn't until the mid 1800s when a German professor, Wilhem Hofman, and one of his students, William Henry Perk, accidentally discovered how to create permanent dyes. Their discovery eventually led to the synthetic hair colourants that are used today.

Hair color can be changed in one of two ways:

1. Temporarily by adding pigment that shampoos out
2. Permanently either by adding or removing pigment

Reasons for Getting Hair Color

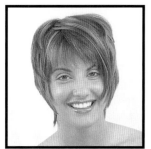 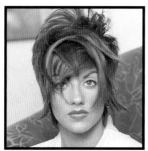

To create a fashion statement

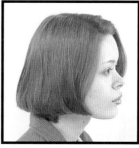 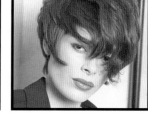

To enhance existing or natural
hair color

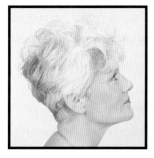 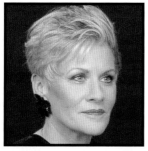

To cover or blend gray for a more
youthful appearance

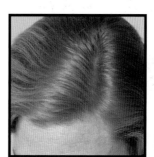 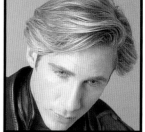

To mimic or correct the sun's
lightening effects

13

What is Color?

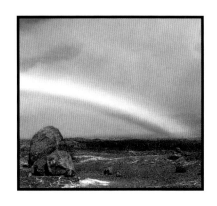

Color is a phenomenon of light. In other words, without light, there would be no color. Isaac Newton discovered this fact in 1676 when he passed white light through a prism and found that the light broke out into continuous bands of color, ranging from red to orange to yellow, then green to blue to indigo and finally violet.

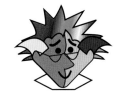

"When you want to remember the order of the colors of the rainbow, think of ROY G. BIV."

Each of these colors is a group of electromagnetic waves (also called wavelengths) traveling through space. Although many forms of electromagnetic waves, such as radio waves and infrared waves, are not visible to the eye, the waves that can be seen create color. These waves are known as "visible light."

These wavelengths cannot be seen unless they are reflected off an object. The brain then interprets these waves of light as color. For example, when white light shines on a red apple, the apple absorbs most of the light waves except the red ones. These reflected red light waves are interpreted by the eye as the color red.

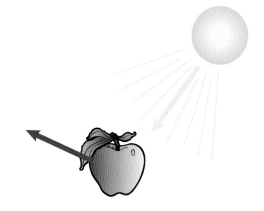

The Law of Color

As a hair colorist, you will recommend hair color options for your client. In order to do this, you will first need to become familiar with the law of color. **The law of color states that, out of all the colors in the universe, only three - yellow, red and blue, called primary colors - are pure.** That means they cannot be created by mixing together any other colors. Instead, when they are mixed together in varying proportions, these primary colors create all other colors. Keep in mind that **the name of a color is often referred to as tone.**

When the primary colors are mixed in equal proportions, they produce the three secondary colors, orange, green and violet. Orange contains equal amounts of red and yellow; green contains an equal mixture of blue and yellow, and violet contains equal proportions of red and blue.

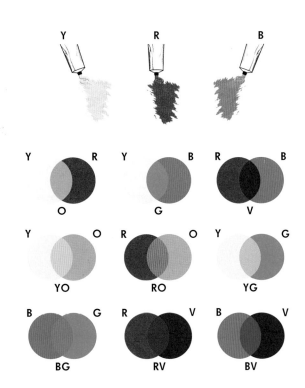

Tertiary colors are made by mixing primary colors with their neighboring secondary color in equal proportions. There are six tertiary colors, yellow-orange, yellow-green, blue-green, blue-violet, red-violet and red-orange. Colors such as browns and grays are made by mixing primary, secondary and tertiary colors in equal or unequal proportions.

Color Wheel

A color wheel is a tool in which the twelve colors, (three primary, three secondary and six tertiary) are positioned in a circle, allowing any mixed color to be described in relation to the primary colors.

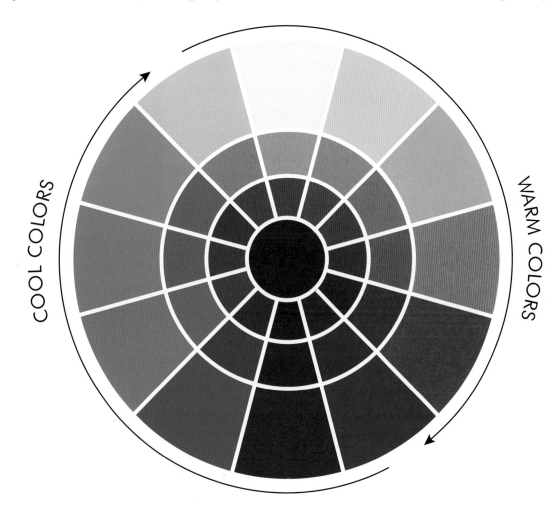

COOL COLORS

WARM COLORS

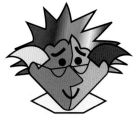

"Creating your own color wheel will help you understand the law of color so you can become a cool colorist! No pun intended. Use white yak hair and non-oxidative colors to create a color wheel out of hair!

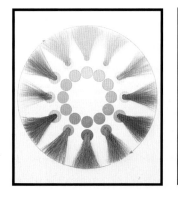

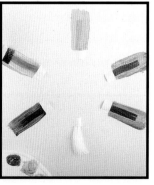

1
3

Warm and Cool Colors

On the color wheel, **colors can be classified as either warm colors (tones) or cool colors (tones).** Warm colors generally fall into the orange and red half of the color wheel (think of a sunset), while cool colors generally fall into the blues and greens (think of a mountain lake). Yellow-green and red-violet can be considered either warm or cool, depending on whether there's more pigment from the cool side of the color wheel or the warm side. Skin tones are also classified into these two categories. You can determine whether a person is in the warm or cool category by that person's skin and hair color. Knowing a client's skin tone is important in hair coloring in order to complement a client's natural coloring. For example, **if someone is classified as warm, this means his/her color falls into the yellow, red and orange category.** You would normally keep the hair color in this same range. The same would be true with a client who has cool undertones. Hair colors that lack warm tones would complement these skin tones.

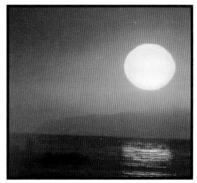

WARM COLORS

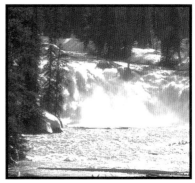

COOL COLORS

Why is a color considered warm or cool? Remember that colors have different wavelengths. The longer waves of the warm colors - red, orange, yellow and their combinations - strike the retina of your eye in a way that affects the focus of the lens and causes the blood pressure to rise slightly and the pulse to quicken. These reactions produce an overall warm feeling. It may not be physically obvious, but scientific studies have confirmed this phenomenon.

When you look at violets, blues, greens and their combinations, the opposite reaction takes place. These colors produce a calming effect by lowering the blood pressure and pulse rate and, in a sense, provide a "cooling off" effect.

Complementary Colors

Colors found opposite one another on the color wheel are referred to as complementary colors. In hair color they neutralize or cancel out one another when they are mixed together. This is important because complementary colors are often used to neutralize unwanted tones. For instance, in hair coloring, an application of a blue-based color would eliminate unwanted brassiness or orange tones. Mixing colors found opposite one another on the color wheel produces a neutral color, such as dark gray or brown depending on the proportions used.

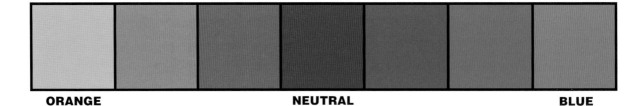

ORANGE   **NEUTRAL**   **BLUE**

Level of Hair Color

Every color has a degree of lightness or darkness, which is often described as level. You can understand level by thinking of a black and white photograph. In reality such a photo is seen in various shades of gray. If you added color to this photograph, you would notice that the color levels do not change. In hair color, these levels of lightness and darkness are identified on a scale of 1 to 10, with 1 being the darkest and 10 the lightest. For example, a level 5 red would be lighter than a level 3 red and darker than a level 7 red. It is important to note that **of the three pure primary pigments, blue is the darkest**, yellow is the lightest and red is considered medium.

Intensity of Hair Color

Intensity is another term used to describe and identify a hair color. It refers to the brightness or vividness of a color or the strength of the tone. Examples of words used to describe a color's intensity include deep red, rich blue and vibrant yellow. The intensity of a hair color, such as red or red-orange, can vary from mild to strong.

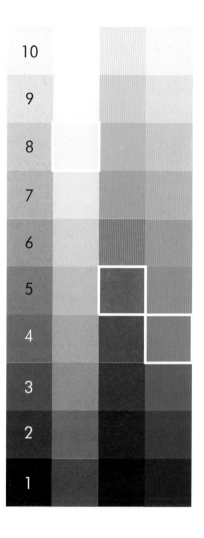

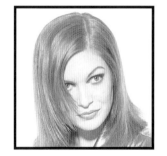 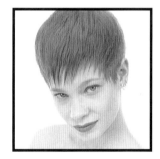

IDENTIFYING EXISTING HAIR COLOR

Identifying your client's natural or existing color is one of the first steps in a hair color service. Unlike painting a white wall, you as a hair colorist will apply color over natural or previously colored hair.

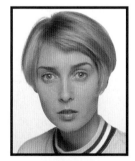 + 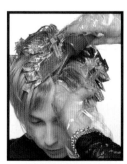 =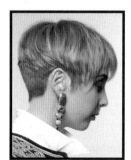

Natural Melanin + **Artificial Pigment** = **Final Color Result**

Melanin

Natural hair color is determined through genetic coding. Like eye and skin color, it is the color with which you are born. How does hair get its color? Think back to what you learned in the trichology chapter about the composition of the hair. A quick review of that material leads directly to the source of hair color.

You may recall that the three parts of the hair are the cuticle, the cortex and the medulla. Down in the hair bulb there are pigment-producing cells called melanocytes. These melanocytes produce small egg-shaped structures called melanosomes. Melanosomes are protein packets that surround pigmented granules called melanin. The melanin eventually becomes incorporated into the keratin protein of the cortex as the hair grows.

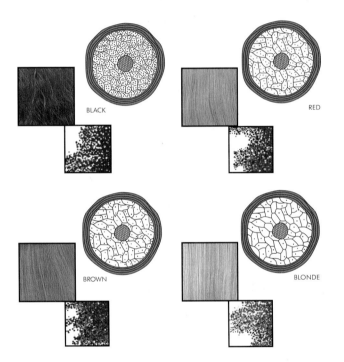

BLACK

RED

BROWN

BLONDE

The melanin created by the body is first developed at the bottom of each hair follicle. From here, the melanin becomes seated in the cortex of the hair shaft. As the hair grows from the follicle, it develops its color according to inherited characteristics.

There are two types of melanin found in the cortex of the hair, eumelanin (black pigment) and pheomelanin (red pigment). It is the type, amount and distribution of melanin that determines whether hair will be black, brown, red or blonde. A dense concentration of eumelanin will produce very dark hair. A small population of eumelanin will produce light blonde hair. A predominant amount of pheomelanin will create red hair.

Gray Hair

When the melanocyte cells slow down in their production of melanin (as is common in old age), each hair strand gradually loses its color and the result is white hair. There are many things that affect melanosome production but heredity is the primary cause. Since each hair is individual, it is not unusual to find a mixture of nonpigmented (white) and pigmented hair on the same head, thereby making the hair appear gray. As more and more melanocyte cells become inactive, there will be more white hair.

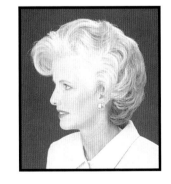

Different patterns of graying can occur with each individual. Some people gray around the front hairline and sideburn area, while others may begin to gray at the top or crown area first. In most cases, the back of the head or nape area is the last area to begin to gray.

Different percentages of gray can also occur from the front to the back. Prior to a color application it is important to determine the percentage of gray your client has, since you may need to use different color formulas to accommodate the different percentages of gray hair.

PERCENTAGES OF GRAY HAIR

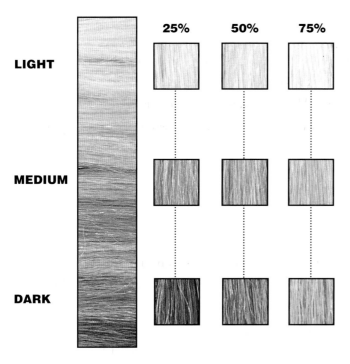

Gray hair is found in every field of hair color. Generally, gray hair can be categorized as 25%, 50% or 75% gray. With 25% gray hair, there is more pigmented hair and less nonpigmented hair. With 50% gray, there is an even mixture of pigmented and nonpigmented hair. If the client exhibits a very high percentage of gray (75-80%), the hair will appear lighter overall. When creating a color formula for a client with this type of hair, you may need to adjust your color formula by applying a color that is one level darker than the desired level. **If the client has approximately 25%-30% gray hair, apply a color one level lighter than the desired shade.**

It has been said that **gray hair is more resistant to color applications than pigmented hair.** This is not necessarily true. As the color molecules wash out or fade from sunlight, the hair looks lighter faster because there is no natural pigment or background color. **It has also been said that in some instances gray hair may be more coarse and less elastic, which can make it more resistant to chemical services than pigmented hair. Again, recent studies have shown that there is no difference between gray (nonpigmented) and pigmented hair. If you find that you are working with resistant hair, you may need to pre-soften or pre-lighten the hair first by mixing and applying a lighter shade to make it porous enough to receive the final color application.**

Identifying Natural Level and Tone

As you learned earlier in this chapter, the level of a hair color can be identified on a scale from 1-10, with 1 being the darkest and 10 being the lightest. This scale allows hair colorists to speak a common language.

These levels (which are often identified by a name such as "lightest blonde") fall into one of the three major fields of color. The major categories or fields of hair color are light,

medium and dark (or blonde, brown and black.) These categories can be further subdivided to medium light and medium dark.

As you look around, you will see a multitude of hair colors from the deepest blue black to the whitest white and all the various shades of browns and reds in between. It is interesting to note that the majority of the world's population falls under the dark category. Keep in mind that these names and numbers (levels) may vary slightly with each manufacturer.

NATURAL HAIR COLORS

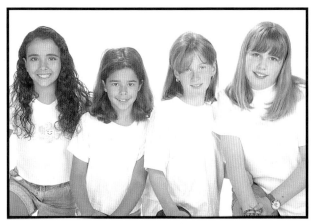

MAJOR FIELDS OF COLOR

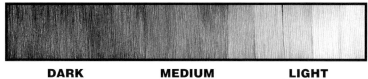

DARK	MEDIUM	LIGHT

LIGHT		10 Lightest Blonde 9 Very Light Blonde 8 Light Blonde
MEDIUM		7 Medium Blonde 6 Dark Blonde 5 Lightest Brown 4 Light Brown
DARK		3 Medium Brown 2 Dark Brown 1 Black

Before performing a color service, it is important to analyze your client's natural (existing) hair color in order to determine which techniques and products will give your client the best results. Once you have identified the level, you can further describe the natural tone of the hair color as either warm or cool. For example a level 8 blonde can further be described as a level 8 warm (golden) blonde or a level 8 cool (ash) blonde.

Identifying Artificial Level, Tone and Intensity

Manufacturer's identify and name their artificial hair colors in several ways. For example:

- By level and tone, such as level 5 red-violet
- By field and tone, such as medium red-violet
- By tone or name, such as red-violet or mahogany

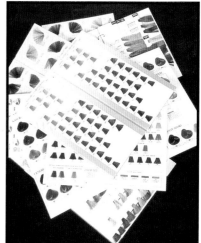

In artificial hair coloring, the tone or base color identifies the warmth or coolness of a color. Artificial warm colors such as yellow or orange may be described as gold or auburn. Artificial cool colors containing green or violet might also be described as ash or platinum.

The tone or base color of an artificial hair color is often abbreviated on hair color packages and swatch charts for easy identification. The following are some common names for artificial hair colors along with their abbreviations or base colors. These hair colors can be used alone or mixed together to create a wide array of tones. Note that these tones also come in a variety of levels and intensities.

Tones/Base Colors

Yellow (Y)

Red (R)

Blue (B)

Gold (G)

Violet (V)

Ash (A)

Neutral (N)

Green (GR)

Red-Orange (RO)

Red-Violet (RV)

Blue-Violet (BV)

Platinum (violet)

Golden Blonde (yellow or gold)

Ash Blonde (blue-violet)

Chestnut Brown (green)

Golden Brown (gold)

Copper Gold (orange)

Auburn (red-orange)

Burgundy (red-violet)

Mahogany (red-violet)

Plum Brown (red-violet)

Black Velvet (violet)

Blue Black (blue)

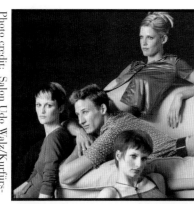

Photo credit: Salon Udo Walz/Kurfürstendamm, Berlin, PPS Studios, Berlin.

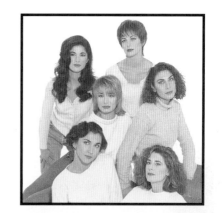

Intensity

When identifying artificial hair color, you'll also need to recognize its intensity. For example, when referring to a red-orange haircolor, you might describe it as a mild red-orange compared to a strong red-orange. Keep in mind that the intensity of an artificial hair coloring may be altered by adding a complementary color to neutralize or lessen the intensity. To intensify a color when formulating, a concentrated color such as yellow, red, blue, green or violet may be added. For example, a mild red-orange color may become stronger by adding a red concentrate to the formula. You will learn more about concentrates later on in this chapter.

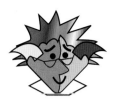

"Remember, level refers to lightness or darkness, tone to the name of the color. For example, a 9RO would be considered a level 9 red-orange."

Additional Considerations

Along with the hair's level and tone, it is important to consider the texture (diameter) and porosity of your client's hair. These considerations will greatly influence color absorption and processing time.

Texture

As you may recall from the trichology chapter, the degree of coarseness or fineness in the hair fiber is referred to as texture. Coarse hair may be resistant to lightening or it may appear to process slightly lighter than the intended level. On the other hand, fine hair, which has pigment grouped more tightly together and is generally less

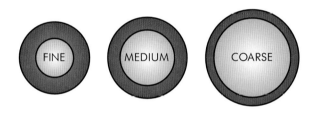

resistant, may appear to process darker when color is deposited. When lightening or removing pigment from fine hair, a mild lightener is usually recommended. Generally, medium textured hair has an average response to color products.

Porosity

Porosity refers to the amount of moisture the hair is able to absorb. This information is important in hair coloring because, depending on its porosity, the hair may absorb or not absorb enough color.

Some common factors that affect the porosity of the hair include sun exposure, alkaline shampoos and chemical products such as hair colors, lighteners, perms and relaxers. Even the heat from hair dryers and curling irons affects the porosity of the hair. The more the hair is exposed to these factors, the greater the porosity.

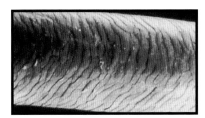

With **resistant porosity**, the cuticle layers are smooth, tightly packed and compact. Color absorption in this case may take longer or you may have to apply additional pigment to ensure color absorption.

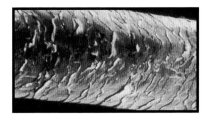

With **average or normal porosity**, the cuticle is slightly raised, thereby accepting color products easily.

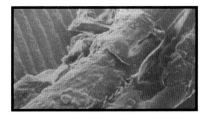

The condition in which the cuticle is lifted or missing is referred to as **extreme porosity**. With this type of porosity, the hair may accept the color intensely or it may fade quickly.

In many instances, you will note that a client has more than one type of porosity or what is called uneven porosity. Clients who have had previous chemical services offer examples of uneven porosity. They may exhibit extreme porosity on the mid-strand or ends and average porosity on the new growth. **Often clients with long hair may exhibit uneven or variations in porosity because the hair on the ends has been more exposed to environmental elements.** These elements coupled with repeated use of shampoo and styling products can leave the ends with extreme porosity. Uneven porosity happens not only along the hair strand but throughout the head as well. An example of this would be a client with highlighted hair. The hair that has been lightened may be one type of porosity, while the hair that is natural may be another type. **In cases of uneven or extreme porosity, a filler may be required to even out the porosity prior to the color service to ensure even color absorption.** You will learn more about fillers later in the chapter.

To determine porosity, select a small section of hair. Hold the ends and slide your thumb and forefinger along the hair strand toward the scalp. The more rough the hair feels and the easier the hair backcombs, the greater the porosity.

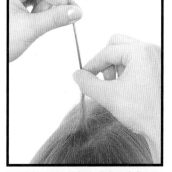

TESTING FOR POROSITY

1
3

CHANGING EXISTING HAIR COLOR

How can hair color be changed? As you may recall, hair color can be changed in one of two ways, either temporarily by adding pigment or permanently by adding and/or removing pigment. Deciding which method you will use will help you select the right products for the service.

When changing the color of the hair, the colorist should keep in mind that the final hair color is the combination of the melanin (existing pigment) and the new hair color (artificial pigment) applied to the hair. It is also necessary to determine the amount or density of pigment contained in the hair before determining how much color to add or subtract. This density or amount of pigment, as you may recall, is called the level of color. Remember, the darker the hair, the greater the concentration of pigment, the lighter the hair, the less concentration of pigment.

Use the following steps to create a new hair color, and remember,

Natural Melanin + Artificial Pigment = Final Color Result:

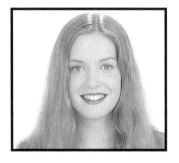

Natural Melanin

1. **Determine the client's existing level and tone.** Identify the actual hair color, which may be natural, gray, previously color-treated, brassy or lightened by the sun. Use your swatches or swatches provided by the manufacturer. Consider the porosity.

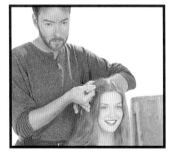

Artificial Pigment

2. **Determine the client's desired level and tone.** Use your swatches or swatches provided by the manufacturer. Consider the porosity. Determine whether you need to go lighter, darker or remain in the same level and just change the tone or intensity.

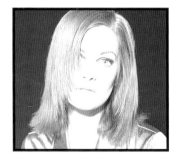

Final Color Result

3. **Choose the formula.** The formula may include color(s), developer and/ or lighteners.

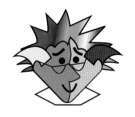

"When formulating a hair color, ask yourself:
- Where am I?
- Where do I want to go?
- How do I get there?"

Hair Color Chemistry

Manufacturers create an array of colors and lighteners that give the colorist the ability to create subtle to dramatic color changes. Listed below are the general categories of hair color products:

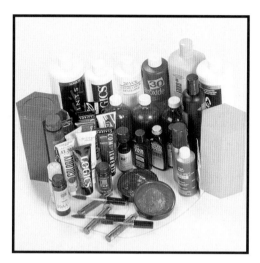

Nonoxidative Colors
- Temporary
- Semi-permanent

Oxidative Colors
- Long lasting semi-permanent (demi-permanent)
- Permanent
- Toners
- Fillers

Lighteners
- On-the-scalp
- Off-the-scalp

Developers

Other Color Products
- Vegetable
- Metallic
- Compound Dyes

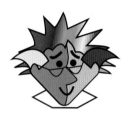

"Before you study this section, you may want to read or review the color section in the "Chemistry" chapter, especially the description of oxidants (developers)."

Nonoxidative Colors

Nonoxidative colors are not mixed with a developer (developers are explained in detail later in the chapter) and are applied directly to the hair. These types of colors create only a physical change to the hair by depositing colors that shampoo out.

Temporary

Temporary colors, as the name implies, are used to create temporary color changes that last from shampoo to shampoo. They are non-reactive, direct dyes, which means no chemicals are needed to develop them. They contain large color molecules that coat only the surface of the cuticle, thereby creating a physical (and not a chemical) change to the hair. There's nothing in the product that will lighten the hair and no chemical changes occur in the solution or in the hair. Therefore, they can neutralize unwanted tones, add tone to faded hair or add pigment to the hair without chemically altering the structure of the hair. These colors are called certified colors and are accepted by the Food and Drug Administration (FDA) for use in foods, drugs and cosmetics.

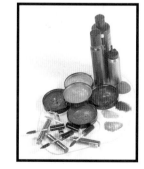

13

Temporary colors do not require a patch or predisposition test (test for allergic reaction), since they do not contain aniline derivative (coal tar) substances, which do require a patch test.

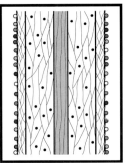

LARGE COLOR MOLECULES COAT CUTICLE

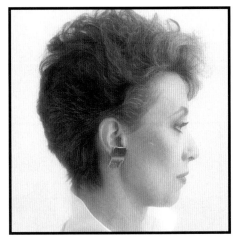

FINAL COLOR RESULT

Temporary colors are also known as weekly rinses, color mousses, color gels, color crayons, mascaras, color pomades, spray-on colors, color shampoos and rinses. Unlike other color products, once you apply temporary hair colors to the hair, you do not rinse the color. You simply dry and style as desired.

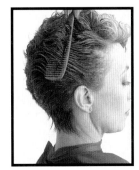

COLOR APPLICATION

Weekly rinses are generally applied at the shampoo bowl and are used to add tone to faded hair, neutralize unwanted tones or to temporarily add color to the hair without creating a chemical change.

A polymer is a chemical compound or mixture of compounds that consists of many molecules in a long chain-like structure. It is found in many products including nonoxidative and oxidative hair colors. It can add shine or conditioning qualities to the hair, or it can be used as a thickening agent in a hair coloring product. When applied to the hair, it acts as a coating.

Color mousses and gels come in a variety of colors and are used to brighten the existing color, tone gray hair and create dramatic effects. Since mousses are also designed to add volume to the hair, they aid in the styling process.

Color crayons and mascaras also come in a variety of colors and are used for a number of effects ranging from blending in the regrowth to creating fun, colorful designs.

Pomades also come in a variety of colors and, aside from adding shine to the hair, can add tone or create special color effects on the hair.

Spray-on colors come in an aerosol can, which may become flammable. Do not use this product around someone who is smoking or around an open fire. Spray-on colors come in a multitude of colors and are a quick and easy way to add color to the hair for special effects.

Color-enhancing shampoos and conditioners are used to maintain the existing color after a color service or to add tones to the hair. They are also used to eliminate unwanted tones.

Semi-Permanent

Semi-permanent colors use a direct-dye process. Direct-dye colors need no mixing and the color you see in the bottle is the color that is deposited on the hair. These colors are alkaline and generally last through several shampoos, depending on the porosity of the hair. They contain small and large color molecules. The small color molecules are able to penetrate the cuticle layer of the hair and enter the cortex, instead of just coating the hair strand as with temporary colors. **Since these colors do not use chemicals to alter the hair, they can only deposit color and cannot lighten the hair. Therefore, depending on the color chosen, these colors will fade, leaving no line of demarcation. Retouches are not required.**

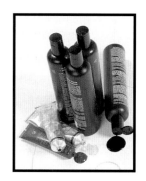

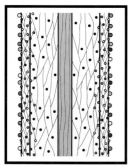

SMALL COLOR MOLECULES COAT CUTICLE, PENETRATE CORTEX

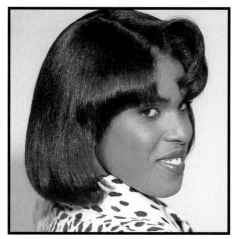

FINAL COLOR RESULT

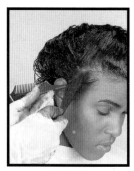

COLOR APPLICATION

A wide array of semi-permanent colors, referred to as glosses or color enhancers, are used to create subtle to dramatic color changes. They can add tone or deepen the existing color, tone prelightened hair, refresh a faded hair color or neutralize unwanted tones. They can cover small percentages of gray hair and are used for blending higher percentages of gray. **Although these types of haircolors are not mixed with a developer, a predisposition or patch test for allergic reactions, must be given if the product contains an aniline derivative ingredient.** This type of test is explained and outlined later in the chapter.

Depending on the ingredients in the product and the porosity of the hair, repeated applications of semi-permanent colors may alter the structure of the hair, especially when applied to previously chemically treated hair, such as permed hair. Therefore, be cautious when working with this type of product to avoid unwanted permanent results. You may wish to perform a strand test to preview the results on a small section of hair. This procedure is also outlined later on in the chapter.

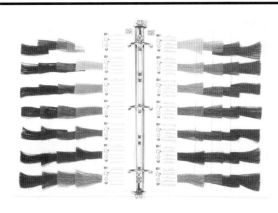

ACTIVITY:
Apply different manufacturer's nonoxidative color products on different hair color swatches and analyze the results. Note that these products cannot lighten the existing hair color. The resulting color is a combination of the color applied and the existing hair color.

Oxidative Colors

Oxidative colors are mixed with a developer to create a chemical change that has a longer lasting effect. Oxidative colors can deposit color only or lift (lighten natural melanin) and deposit color in a single process. Oxidative colors are generally applied to dry hair.

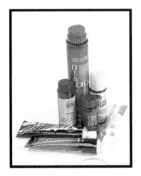

Long Lasting Semi-Permanent (Demi-Permanent)

Long lasting semi-permanent colors (sometimes referred to as demi-permanent, deposit only or oxidative without ammonia) use a low volume peroxide to develop the color molecules and aid in the color processing. They contain small color molecules. Once they enter the cortex, some of them join together, which prevents them from escaping. This process creates a longer lasting effect than can be achieved with nonoxidative color products. Peroxide alone does not lighten the hair. It needs an alkaline substance such as ammonia to create lift. **These products contain very little or no ammonia and are designed to deposit color or add tone to the hair. They are not designed to lift or lighten the existing hair color and generally last 4-6 weeks.** Long lasting semi-permanent colors are available in liquid, cream and gel forms and are generally mixed with a very low volume of developer. Since most long lasting semi-permanent colors contain aniline derivatives, a patch test is required.

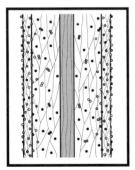

SMALL COLOR MOLECULES ENTER CORTEX SOME COUPLE TOGETHER

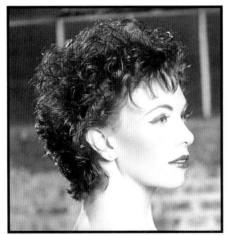

FINAL COLOR RESULT

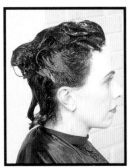

COLOR APPLICATION

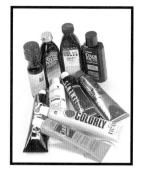

Permanent

Permanent hair colors are mixed with hydrogen peroxide and are capable of both lifting natural pigment and depositing artificial pigment in one process. They are sometimes called oxidative tints with ammonia or aniline derivative tints. Paraphenylenediamine (para-**PHE**-ni-line-i-**DIA**-min) and paratoluenediamine (para-tol-**U**-ene-i-**DIA**-min) are two types of dye intermediates, either one of which can be found in permanent tints. **Permanent hair colors contain small colorless molecules (para-dyes) that become colored when mixed with hydrogen peroxide. Once they are applied to the hair, the oxidative color swells the hair strand.** The small colored molecules enter the hair with the aid of an an alkaline substance (alkalizing ingredient), such as ammonia. Then, as they oxidize in the cuticle and the cortex, they link or couple together to form a permanent colored molecule. When this happens, they are permanently anchored in the hair. **It is the combination of the ammonia in permanent hair colors and hydrogen peroxide that allow for the lift and lightening of the hair's natural color.** The stonger the hydrogen peroxide, the greater the lift achieved. You will learn more about hydrogen peroxide later in this chapter.

Permanent hair colors, as the name implies, are permanent. In some instances, a color remover or dye solvent can be used to remove unwanted artificial pigment. Once you have removed the unwanted pigment, you may recolor the hair as desired.

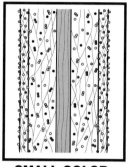

SMALL COLOR MOLECULES ENTER CORTEX SOME COUPLE TOGETHER

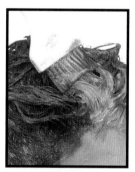

COLOR APPLICATION

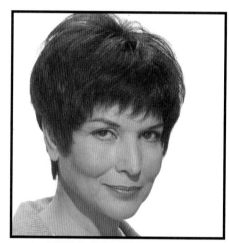

FINAL COLOR RESULT

Permanent hair colors have become one of the most popular color products used in the salon, since they offer the colorist a wide range of color possibilities. The colorist can choose from many levels and tones to create an infinite number of hair colors. **Permanent colors can add tone or darken the existing hair or lighten and deposit color in a single process.** They are mixed with various strengths of developer, depending on the desired amount of lift and/or deposit. Most permanent hair colors are mixed with 20 volume (6%) hydrogen peroxide. High-lift tints, (a type of permanent hair color) are designed to achieve lighter colors and are generally mixed with a double amount of 30 volume (9%) or 40 volume (12%) hydrogen peroxide. When mixing permanent hair colors, be sure to follow the manufacturer's directions since changing either the amount or the volume of the peroxide can affect the lift and deposit achieved.

1 3

As a general rule, 10 volume (3%) peroxide lifts one color level, 20 volume (6%) lifts two levels, 30 volume (9%) lifts three levels. The resulting color will be a combination of the pigment remaining (contributing pigment) and the artificial color that is deposited.

If you are not able to achieve the desired amount of lift using a single-process color, prelightening may be required. The lower the percentage of hydrogen peroxide, the less lift that will be achieved, the higher the percentage, the greater the lift that will be achieved.

Permanent hair colors come in three forms: liquid, creams and gels.

Liquid hair colors are thinner than creams and gels and are generally applied with a bottle. They may contain fewer conditioning agents and a greater ammonia content. These types of colors have a good penetration ability.

Cream hair colors are generally mixed with a cream developer and are applied with a bowl and brush technique. They have conditioners and thickening agents.

The consistency of **gel** colors is somewhere between that of a liquid and a cream. These colors are more penetrating than cream colors but have less conditioning agents. They have the same or more penetrating ability than a liquid, but more conditioning agents.

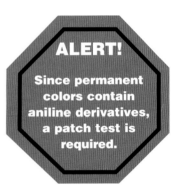

ALERT!
Since permanent colors contain aniline derivatives, a patch test is required.

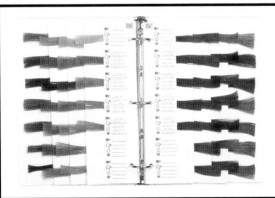

ACTIVITY:
Apply different manufacturer's oxidative color products on different hair color swatches and analyze the results. These products can tone or darken the existing level or lighten and deposit color in a single process.

Toners

Toners are light pastel colors used to tone prelightened hair. These tones are used to deposit color and neutralize unwanted pigment remaining after prelightening, such as brassy golds or yellows. Permanent toners are mixed with low volumes of developer, up to 20 volume (6%). Nonoxidative toners (not mixed with developer) can be used where there is a mixture of natural and prelightened hair, such as after a highlight service.

The level of prelightening will help determine the level of toner to be applied. (Refer to the lightener segment in this chapter.) All toners should be selected in relation to the law of color. As you know complementary colors (colors across from one another on the color wheel) will neutralize one another. For instance, a violet-based toner will produce a light neutral blonde on prelightened pale yellow hair. If the hair is lightened to yellow-orange (gold), a different color toner will be required. Remember, in order to predict results accurately, perform a strand test. Since toners contain aniline derivates, a predisposition test is also required.

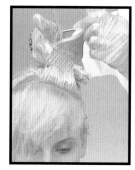
COLOR APPLICATION

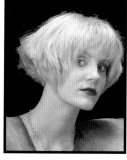
FINAL COLOR RESULT

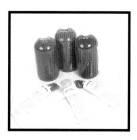

Fillers

Fillers provide an even base color by filling in porous, damaged or abused areas with materials such as protein or polymers. They equalize the porosity of the hair and deposit a base color in one application. Although fillers are not considered oxidative colors, they are designed to be used prior to or in conjunction with oxidative colors.

Fillers come in a variety of colors and are generally chosen to replace the missing primary color. There are two types of fillers: conditioning and color. Conditioning fillers are used to recondition damaged hair prior to a color service. The color is then applied right over the filler and they both process simultaneously. Color fillers are used on damaged hair and when there is a question as to whether or not the color will hold, such as with porous hair. Fillers have many advantages. They:

- Give more uniform color in a tint back (returning hair to its natural color)
- Deposit color on faded hair and ends
- Help hair hold color
- Prevent color streaking (uneven color absorption)
- Prevent off-color results
- Prevent a dull color appearance

Extremely damaged hair may absorb more color than normal, but it also has a hard time holding on to these color molecules.

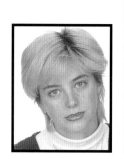
BEFORE

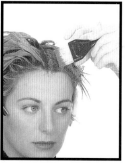
FILLER APPLICATION

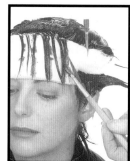
COLOR APPLICATION

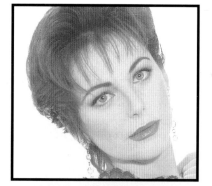
FINAL COLOR RESULT

1 3

Fillers can be applied directly to the hair before an oxidative color or they can be mixed with the color formula. Although filler products are available, fillers can also be made by mixing water and tint. Generally the intended color level is mixed with water and applied to the hair. Then the color formula is applied directly over the filler.

Concentrates, Intensifiers and Drabbers

Concentrates, intensifiers, pigments and drabbers are names given to products designed to increase the vibrancy of a color formula or to neutralize tones. They can be mixed into the color formula or they can be applied directly to prelightened hair to create a vibrant fashion statement. These products come in a variety of colors, including yellow, red, blue, orange, violet, green, silver and ash.

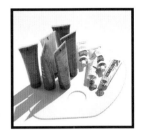

Lighteners

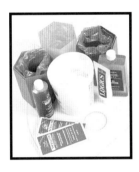

Lighteners, or bleaches, are used to remove or diffuse melanin. They can be used to create the final color result or create a new pigment on which to build the final hair coloring. Lighteners utilize ingredients, such as ammonia and peroxide, to facilitate the oxidation process. When this mixture is added to the hair, it penetrates the cortex, causing the melanin to break into smaller pieces before removing or diffusing the color. The longer this lightening solution remains in contact with the hair, the more the melanin changes. Lighteners are generally applied to dry hair.

Degrees of Decolorization

As the melanin changes, the hair goes through degrees (stages) of lightening or decolorization. Dark hair goes through approximately 10 levels. The main degrees to look for are red-orange, orange, yellow-orange (gold), yellow, pale yellow and palest yellow. Keep in mind that the **hair should never be lightened to white since this could cause extreme damage. If the hair is overlightened, a toner may make the hair appear ashy, gray or cool, since most of the warm tones will be missing.**

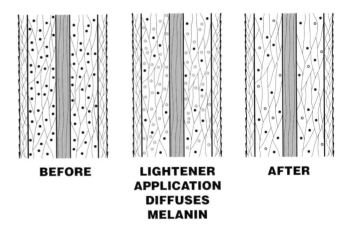

BEFORE   **LIGHTENER APPLICATION DIFFUSES MELANIN**   **AFTER**

BLACK   **DARK RED-BROWN**   **RED-BROWN**   **RED**   **RED-ORANGE**   **ORANGE**   **YELLOW-ORANGE (GOLD)**   **YELLOW**   **PALE YELLOW**   **PALEST YELLOW**

There are no established times for lightening hair to any given degree. Time always varies with the individual client because of the natural pigmentation and resistance of the hair. Different manufacturer's products may also have an effect on timing. The best way to find out the correct time (as well as determine if the hair is in proper condition for lightening) is to perform a preliminary strand test and follow manufacturer's directions.

If the desired color result is different from what can be achieved with decolorizing or lightening alone, color can be applied to recolorize the hair to the shade desired.

This process involves two steps:

1. The hair is decolorized (prelightened) to the desired degree, which is usually within two levels of the existing hair color. (This is sometimes called pigment foundation, contributing pigment or undertone.)

2. Hair color is applied to create the final color result. (This can be an oxidative or nonoxidative color or toner.)

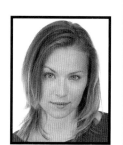
BEFORE

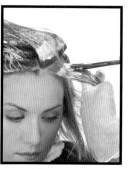
LIGHTENER APPLICATION DECOLORIZES

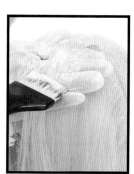
TONER APPLICATION RECOLORIZES

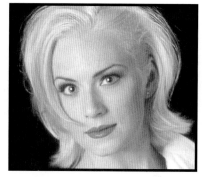
FINAL COLOR RESULT

On-the-Scalp Lighteners

There are two categories of lighteners: on-the-scalp and off-the-scalp. As the name implies, on-the-scalp lighteners can be applied directly on the scalp, since they are considered milder than off-the-scalp lighteners and are available in two forms: oil and cream. Both of these lighteners have a pH around 9 and can be mixed with an activator (accelerator, booster) to increase the speed of the oxidation process. The main difference between oil and cream lighteners is their consistency. Besides having a thicker consistency, which prevents the product from dripping, cream lighteners also contain conditioners.

Off-the-Scalp Lighteners

Off-the-scalp lighteners come in powder form and, when mixed with peroxide, become a strong lightening product. Because they have no added oils or creams, they can irritate the scalp, causing burns and blisters. This is why they are generally used for off-the-scalp procedures, such as painting. Keep in mind, however, that there are some powder lighteners that contain buffering agents and conditioners, which allow them to be used on and off the scalp. To ensure client safety, always read manufacturer's directions.

DECOLORIZING

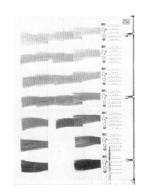

ACTIVITY:

Apply lightener to several swatches of dark hair and watch the hair decolorize. Remove the lightener when a swatch reaches a new decolorizing degree. The type of lightener you use, the length of time it remains on the hair and the strength of developer you use will all influence your results. Note that lighter fields of hair color go through fewer degrees of decolorization and will, therefore, take less time to reach the lighter shades.

RECOLORIZING

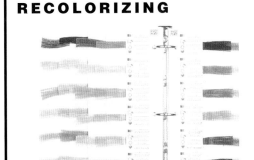

ACTIVITY:

Take the decolorization process one step further. Decolorize additional swatches then recolorize the hair with toners to achieve cool, neutral or warm color results. Remember, nonoxidative colors can be used on decolorized hair to achieve vibrant color results. On these charts, the original level is at the top followed by the decolorized degree without a toner. The remaining swatches were decolorized to the same degree, then recolorized to achieve various tonal results.

Developers

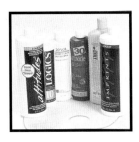

Developers are oxidizing agents used with demi-permanent and permanent colors, lighteners and toners. A developer may be referred to as a catalyst or conductor. **Hydrogen peroxide is the most commonly used developer (oxidizing agent) in hair coloring products. Its pH is between 2.5 and 4.5. It needs to be mixed with ammonia or other alkaline compounds to become active.**

In the United States developers are measured by volume, such as 10 volume, while in Europe they are measured by percentage, such as 3%. Volume refers to the amount of oxygen that would be removed from a peroxide solution if the molecules were broken into components. For example, hydrogen peroxide is a chemical compound consisting of hydrogen and oxygen. If the oxygen were set free, hydrogen peroxide would become water. To prevent the oxygen from escaping, it is important to immediately begin applying a color product that has been mixed with developer.

3%	= 10	vol.
6%	= 20	vol.
9%	= 30	vol.
12%	= 40	vol.

The strength of peroxide you choose for your color formula will depend upon the amount of lift or deposit you desire, as well as what the color manufacturer recommends. The lower the volume, the less lift that will be achieved, the higher the volume, the more lift that will be achieved.

Demi-permanent colors are designed to deposit color. Therefore, a low volume of developer (under 10 volume 3%) would be used to achieve minimal lift. On the other hand, a high-lift permanent tint may require 30 volume (9%) or 40 volume (12%) to achieve a greater amount of lift. Generally, 20 volume (6%) is used with the majority of hair coloring products.

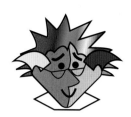

" Did you know that if you left the cap off your hydrogen peroxide antiseptic at home, you'd release all the oxygen and it would turn to water and other free radicals? The same is true for the stronger hydrogen peroxide you mix with hair color".

A hydrometer is used to measure the strength (volume) of hydrogen peroxide and allows you to dilute higher strengths to lower strengths. A hydrometer is also beneficial to determine whether hydrogen peroxide that has been stored for a long period of time is still potent.

Manufacturer recommendations will indicate shelf life (usually 3 years) of hydrogen peroxide and instruct that it be stored in a cool, dry place.

Developers come in different forms: clear, cloudy, creamy and gel. Hydrogen peroxide also comes in a dry form, which is used to increase the peroxide strength. **Mixing peroxide in a metal bowl may cause it to become to weak.** The metal ions in the metal bowl will have an adverse reaction with the hydrogen peroxide. Therefore, **always mix in a glass or plastic bowl.** Perform a strand test and follow manufacturer's directions to avoid any problems.

ALERT!

Increasing the strength of hydrogen peroxide in a formula beyond the manufacturer's recommendations may cause damage to the hair and chemical burns to the skin and scalp.

If lower volumes of developer are not available, you can dilute 20 volume (6%) hydrogen peroxide with zero volume (0%) hydrogen peroxide using the following guidelines:

15 vol (4.5%)	1-1/2 parts 20 vol H_2O_2 + 1/2 part 0 vol (0%)
10 vol (3%)	1 part 20 vol H_2O_2 + 1 part 0 vol (0%)
5 vol (1.5%)	1 part 20 vol H_2O_2 + 1-1/2 part 0 vol (0%)

Vegetable, Metallic and Compound Dyes

Vegetable, metallic and compound dyes are the least common types of hair coloring products used in the salon today. Although there are some areas of the world that use vegetable dyes in the salon, metallic and compound dyes are discouraged since they are unreliable and, sometimes, unsafe.

Vegetable Dyes

Vegetable dyes utilize natural products to color the hair. **The most common vegetable dye is known as henna, which, in its purest form, produces reddish highlights in the hair.** It is one of the oldest forms of hair coloring and is derived from the Egyptian privet plant. To create colors other than red, henna can be mixed with other substances, such as metals.

After a few applications henna can penetrate the cortex of the hair and build up. When this happens, the color is permanent since the molecules are anchored in the cortex. **Hair that has been colored with henna sometimes cannot be permed since the resulting build-up doesn't allow the neutralizing solution to penetrate evenly.** In addition, if a henna product contains metals, the product may react violently with other chemicals used in salon services. Since there is not a reliable product available to completely remove henna from the hair, it is usually best to wait until the hair has grown out to perform a chemical service. Refer to the end of this chapter for step-by-step procedures on how to remove as much henna as possible from the hair.

Chamomile is another vegetable product used in shampoos and rinses to color the hair. This product is used as a rinse after shampooing and is relatively harmless to the hair. Chamomile produces a yellow stain on the hair, which resembles golden highlights.

Metallic Dyes

Metallic dyes are known as progressive dyes because the hair turns darker with each application. These are not considered a professional product, since their use is not recommended. The reason metallic dyes are not recommended is because the metals in the product do not mix successfully with other salon chemical services, such as perms. The result of mixing these products can cause discoloration and breakage. To avoid any problems with chemical services, it is advisable to cut hair that has been colored with metallic dye.

Depending on the metals used, these dyes may fade into peculiar or unnatural shades. With exposure to the sun and chlorine, silver dyes may appear to have a green cast, lead dyes a purple cast and copper dyes a red cast. Another negative feature to this type of dye is that the metallic coating has a tendency to look and feel dry.

Compound Dyes

Compound dyes are a combination of metallic and vegetable dyes. Metallic salts are added to vegetable dyes to create a wider range of colors and a longer lasting color than achieved with vegetable dyes alone. Compound dyes tend to be unpredictable and they are incompatible with other chemical services in the salon.

Refer to "Infection Control and Safety" on page 523 to learn how to test for metallic salts.

Hair Color Essentials

To perform a professional color service, you need a selection of products, implements and equipment. Color service products are produced by many different manufacturers, are disposable and must be frequently replaced. Material Safety Data Sheets (MSDS) for all products used in the salon must be available. Color service implements are the hand-held tools you use. They must be disinfected or discarded after every use. Color service equipment includes the furnishings and provisions necessary to provide a professional color service.

Hair Color Products

PRODUCT	FUNCTION
NONOXIDATIVE	
Temporary	Adds tonal value or highlights to specific areas
Semi-Permanent	Adds tonal value and imparts shine, but does not lighten the natural melanin; gradually fades, lasting up to 4-6 shampoos; can have a longer lasting effect on porous hair or when heat is applied; can have a permanent effect on chemically relaxed and lightened hair
OXIDATIVE	
Long Lasting Semi-Permanent/ Demi-Permanent	Adds tone or darkens the existing color but does not lighten the natural melanin or previously colored hair; retouches may be required every 4-6 weeks
Permanent	Tones, darkens or lightens natural melanin in a single process; cannot lighten previously colored hair; remains on the hair until it is cut off or removed by chemical means such as with a lightener or color remover; retouches may be required every 4-6 weeks
LIGHTENERS	
On-the-Scalp Lightener	Lightens (decolorizes) melanin; used to achieve colors not attainable with a single process; gentle enough to be used on the scalp
Off-the-Scalp Lightener	Lightens (decolorizes) melanin; used for off-the-scalp techniques such as highlighting, surface painting, frosting cap or to achieve colors not attainable with a single process

1
3

PRODUCT	FUNCTION
Hydrogen Peroxide	Aids in the formation of color dye molecules; used as an oxidizing agent in hair coloring; available in different strengths
Fillers	Evens out the porosity of the hair or creates an even base color for the final color service; used before a color service; can be added to the color formula to help the hair hold color and prevent off-color results
Concentrates/Intensifiers/Drabbers	Intensifies or neutralizes colors; mixed into the color formula; used alone on prelightened hair to create a vibrant color statement
Protective (Barrier) Cream	Protects the client's skin from irritation and stains; used around the hairline
Talcum Powder	Allows gloves to be put on and taken off with ease; used inside gloves
Color Stain Remover	Removes color stains from skin

Hair Color Implements/Supplies

IMPLEMENT/SUPPLIES	FUNCTION
Glass or Plastic Bowl	Holds the color formula; some have an edge that can be used to rest the color brush and a rubber base that prevents the bowl from slipping; some also have a measurement guide that is used for accuracy for mixing; generally, a bowl and brush application is used when working with products that have a thick consistency
Color Brush	Consists of nylon bristles on one end that are used to apply the color and a pointed end on the other that can be used to part the hair; brushes come in a variety of shapes and sizes and are chosen according to the area you are working in and the effects desired
Plastic Applicator Bottle	Holds color formula; consists of a pointed end that is used to part the hair and apply (distribute) the color; marked with numbers that are used as a measuring guide; generally, a bottle application is used when working with products that have a thinner consistency
Measuring Device	Indicates the units of measurement in ounces (oz), milliliters (ml) or centimeters (cc); used to measure the formula
Foil/Thermal Strips	Isolates woven or sliced strands of hair from the untreated hair during a coloring service; also prevents colors from intermixing

IMPLEMENT/SUPPLIES	FUNCTION
Tail Comb	Used for combing and parting the hair; fine teeth on one end are used for combing the hair and pointed end is used for parting the hair
Wide-Tooth Comb	Combs in color for special effects and detangles the hair
Clip	Controls the hair while coloring
Protective Cape for Client	Protects the client and his/her clothing
Neck Strip	Protects the skin from coming into direct contact with the cape
Towels	Used as part of the draping procedure to protect the client's clothing; used for the shampoo service
Cotton Roll	Protects the client's eyes from product drips when positioned around hairline; used at the base in between partings to avoid product seepage during lightener applications; used to perform patch tests
Protective Apron/Smock for Stylist	Protects colorist's clothing from stains
Protective Gloves	Protect the hands during chemical services; in some areas, wearing gloves during any service, especially chemical services, is mandatory – check with your area's regulatory agency
Chemical Record Card	Documents client's personal and color information

Hair Color Equipment

EQUIPMENT	FUNCTION
Rollable Color/Product Table	Provides a place for laying out some color implements, supplies and products
Hydraulic Chair	Provides proper back support to the client during the color service; has a lever that can be used to adjust the height of the chair to ensure the proper level and comfort for the hair colorist
Timer	Allows colorist to keep track of processing time
Wet Disinfectant Container	Holds disinfectant for disinfecting implements such as combs
Hooded Dryer/Heated Lamps/ Accelerator Machines	Used to speed up the action of the color process
Shampoo Bowl/Area	Used to rinse and shampoo client's hair; holds shampoo and conditioning products

**1
3**

Hair Color Techniques

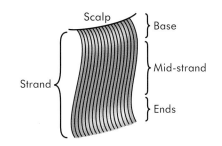

Now that you've become familiar with products that can change hair color, you are ready to learn some basic application techniques. You'll begin by identifying the areas of the hair strand, which are base, midstrand and ends.

Base to Ends (Darker Result)

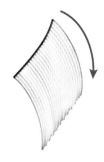
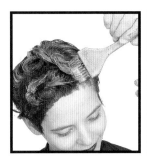
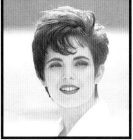

A base-to-ends application is used when you want to add tone to or darken the existing color. A base-to-ends application is also known as a virgin darker technique.

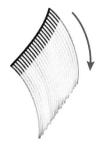
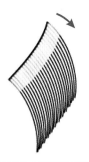

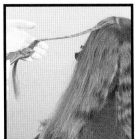
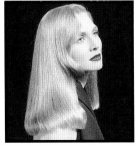

Midstrand to Ends Then Base (Lighter Result)

To lighten the existing color, the color or lightener is first applied to the midstrand, generally 1/2" (1.25 cm) away from the scalp, then up to but not including any porous ends. The product is applied to the base and porous ends later, since they will lighten faster. **The base area lightens faster for two reasons: First, the new growth is not fully keratinized and is more receptive to chemical processes and, second, the heat from the scalp will accelerate processing time.** If your client has porous ends, they will probably be lighter and not need as much processing time as the midstrand. The midstrand-to-ends-then-base application is also known as a virgin lighter technique.

Base (Retouch)

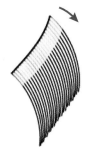
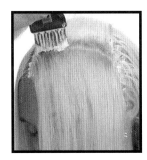
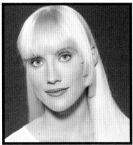

A base application is used for a retouch. Color or lightener is applied to the new growth only to match the existing color. To maintain a consistent color and to prevent breakage, avoid overlapping product onto the previously colored hair.

Special Effects Coloring Techniques

Special effects coloring techniques involve the positioning of lights and/or darks on the surface of the hair or to selected strands throughout the design.

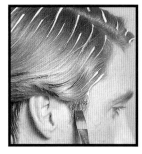
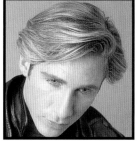

Freeform Painting

Painting is a technique in which a brush is used to strategically position color or lightener on the surface of the hair. Depending on the colors chosen, this can create a highlighted (lighter strands) or lowlighted (darker strands) effect.

Weaving and Slicing

Weaving and slicing techniques are generally used to add depth and dimension to the existing hair color. Lightener and/or color are used to create a highlighted or lowlighted effect. Keep in mind that the number and size of weaves/slices within a design and the color chosen will determine the degree of lightness or darkness achieved.

With the weaving technique, a tail comb is used to weave out selected strands in an alternating pattern. These strands are then positioned over a piece of foil or thermal strip and the lightener or color is then applied. The foil/thermal strip is then folded to isolate the selected strands and protect the untreated hair.

WEAVE

CHUNKY WEAVE

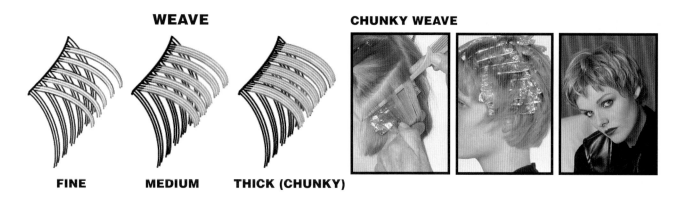

FINE   MEDIUM   THICK (CHUNKY)

With the slicing technique, the tail comb is used to part off a section of hair. This section is then positioned over a piece of foil or thermal strip and the lightener or color is then applied. The foil/thermal strip is then folded to isolate the selected strands to protect the untreated hair.

SLICE

FINE SLICE

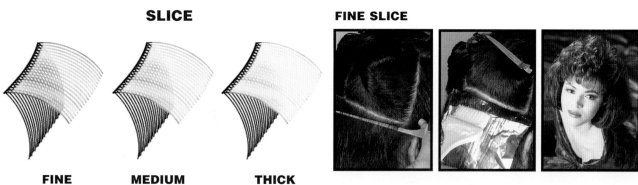

FINE   MEDIUM   THICK

13

Cap Method

Another way to create highlights is with a cap method. Selected strands are pulled through perforated holes in a rubber coloring cap with a crochet hook. The amount and the density of the strands will determine whether a light or heavy amount of highlights or lowlights will be achieved. Keep in mind that the fewer holes you pull hair through, the more subtle the effect, while the more holes you pull hair through, the more dramatic the effect.

Lightener or color is then applied to the selected strands. If lightener is used, a plastic cap or bag is positioned over the strands to aid with the processing time. Once the desired result has been achieved,

HIGHLIGHTS

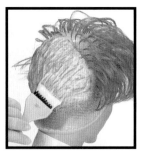 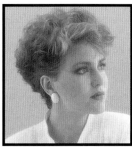

LOWLIGHTS

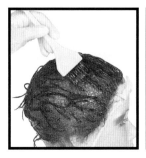 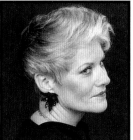

the product is removed with lukewarm water. If a permanent toner is used, shampoo and towel dry the hair with the cap in place. Then apply toner to the prelightened strands. Process and rinse. Remove the cap and shampoo. If a semi-permanent toner is used, you can remove the cap, shampoo, towel dry the hair and then apply toner to the entire head. Highlighting with the cap method is generally performed on shorter hair and can be ideal for the client who has a sensitive scalp, since the product doesn't come in contact with the scalp.

Infection Control and Safety

The following is a list of safety precautions that you must adhere to prior to and during a color service to protect the client and yourself. Always:

1. Practice infection control guidelines.

2. Protect yourself. Wear a cape and gloves.

3. Perform a patch test 24 hours prior to the application of an aniline derivative tint.

4. Protect the client's clothing with proper draping.

5. Perform the color service only if the patch test is negative and there are no metallic or compound dyes present.

6. Check the scalp for abrasions. Do not proceed with the service if there are any cuts or irritations.

7. Do not brush the hair prior to the color service. To do so will irritate the scalp.

8. Use sanitized applicator bottles, brushes and combs. Only use plastic or glass bowls to mix the color formula.

9. Once you've mixed the formula, use immediately and discard any leftover product.

10. Do not permit the product to come into contact with the eyes. If it does, rinse the eyes immediately with tepid water and refer the client to a physician.

11. During a retouch service, avoid overlapping the product especially with lightener. To do so may cause breakage.

12. Never leave the client unattended during a hair color service.

13. **Never color hair that has been colored with a product that contains metallic salts. To test for metallic salts, immerse a small strand of the client's hair in a solution of 1oz. 20 volume (6%) peroxide and 20 drops of 28% ammonia (mix in a glass container). Both of these ingredients are found in permanent tints, lighteners and permanent waves.**

    Check for results after 30 minutes. If the hair has an extreme coating, it may dissolve. The most common reaction is discoloration, a "gummy" feeling and/or a foul smell. Future chemical services cannot be performed unless the previously chemically treated hair is cut.

14. Rinse the hair with lukewarm or cool water, never hot.

15. **Do not use aniline derivative tints to color eyelashes or eyebrows. To do so may cause blindness.**

16. Complete client record card, noting any allergies or adverse reactions the client may have experienced.

ALWAYS FOLLOW MANUFACTURER'S DIRECTIONS AND READ MATERIAL SAFETY DATA SHEETS (MSDS).

Predisposition (Skin Patch) Test

According to the U.S. Federal Food, Drug and Cosmetic Act, **all permanent, aniline derivative tints require a predisposition (skin patch) test 24-48 hours prior to the hair color service.** This test will help determine if the client is sensitive or allergic to certain chemicals in the hair color product.

Once the predisposition test has been performed, it is important to analyze the results. **If the results are negative (no reaction), it means that the formula may safely be used. Positive results include redness, swelling, blisters, itching, burning of the skin and/or respiratory distress. If the predisposition test results are positive, do not proceed with the service and have the client seek medical assistance.**

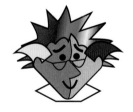

"Analine derivative products should not be used for coloring eyelashes or eyebrows."

1
3

Predisposition (Skin Patch) Test Guidelines

- Wash and sanitize hands.
- Cleanse test area (inside of the elbow or behind the ear).
- Apply intended formula with cotton swab.
- Leave undisturbed for 24 hours.
- Analyze results; determine a negative (no signs) or positive (signs of redness, swelling, blisters, itching or burning of the skin and/or respiratory distress) reaction.
- If reaction is negative, proceed with the service. If reaction to the predisposition test is positive, do not proceed with the service.
- Record results on client record card.
- Clean work area.

INSIDE ELBOW   **BACK OF EAR**

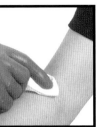 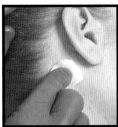

CLEANSE AREA

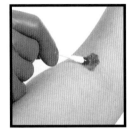 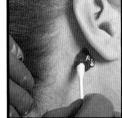

APPLY INTENDED FORMULA

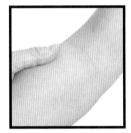 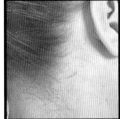

CHECK FOR RESULTS

Draping for Chemical Service

Proper draping is required in order to protect the client's skin and his/her clothing during hair color services. Keep in mind that draping for a chemical service is different from draping for a shampoo, cutting or styling service. Prior to draping the client, ask the client to remove neck jewelry, earrings or eyeglasses and store them in a safe place. To perform a proper draping procedure for a hair color service, you will need two towels and a plastic cape.

Draping for Chemical Service Guidelines

- Wash and sanitize hands.
- Have client remove jewelry.
- Clip client's hair out of the way.
- Turn the client's collar under.
- Cross towel over client's shoulders.
- Position cape over towel and fasten.
- Drape a second towel over cape.
- Detangle the hair and section according to the applicable service; avoid brushing the scalp.
- Apply barrier cream to entire hairline to prevent irritation and staining.
- Clean work area.

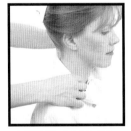 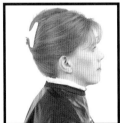 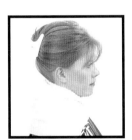

TURN COLLAR UNDER   **POSITION CAPE OVER TOWEL**   **DRAPE SECOND TOWEL**

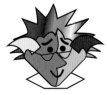

"Your instructor may prefer another draping procedure, which may be equally acceptable. In some cases, additional client protection can be added by having the client change into a gown for the service."

Preliminary Strand Test

A preliminary strand test is a color test that is performed (24-48 hours) before the actual hair color service. The important factors you'll discover by performing a strand test and analyzing the results prior to the service include:

- Correct formula and processing time to be used
- The reaction of the hair and what particular procedures may be needed to ensure proper color absorption (conditioning, filling, etc.)
- The possible presence of coating on the hair from previous applications that could be damaging or undesirable when new color is applied (metallic, henna, styling aid build-up, etc.)

The intended color formula is mixed and applied to a section of hair, preferably somewhere that is visible for the client to see as well, such as above the ear area. You may do as many strand tests as necessary. For example, if the hair has not reached the desired degree (level) of lightness, additional processing time would be required.

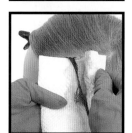

Preliminary Strand Test Guidelines

- Wash and sanitize hands.
- Analyze the patch test results; if negative, proceed with service.
- Drape client for chemical service.
- Wear protective gloves and stylist apron.
- Isolate a small section of hair at the crown or another area of your choice (preferably an area where the results are visible to the client).
- Apply the intended color formula.
- Set the timer.
- Rinse, shampoo and dry the hair.
- Make any necessary color formula adjustments. Analyze and document your results.
- Clean color service area.

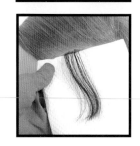

Strand Test (During Service) Guidelines

Strand testing during the color service will help ensure that color is processing properly. Therefore, you should perform strand tests in several areas, such as the most resistant area and the area of the initial application. Strand testing during processing is most often performed when you are working with oxidative colors and lighteners but can also be performed for nonoxidative colors. To perform a strand test, you will need a water bottle and white towel.

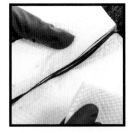

- Select a small section of hair.
- Position the selected strand on a towel.
- Spray water along the entire strand.
- Gently rub across the strand to remove the product thoroughly.
- Check results against a white towel.
- If results are desirable, rinse, shampoo and condition the strand.
- If results are not desirable, continue processing until proper results are achieved.

Client Consultation

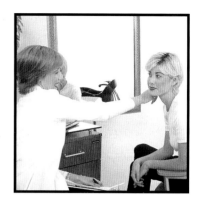

As with all hair services, consulting with your client prior to the actual service will ensure predictable results and will help you avoid any misunderstandings that may arise. Ensure client comfort by performing your consultation in a private area. To avoid any false color analysis, be sure the area is well lit, preferably in a room with a window. Proper lighting in the hair color area of the salon is essential for accurate analysis, color selection, application and final evaluation. Keep in mind that incandescent lighting generally makes the hair appear warmer, while fluorescent lighting makes the hair appear cooler. To create a more natural light reflection, use fluorescent lighting that is balanced for daylight. Ultimately, only sunlight gives a true color reflection!

During your consultation, be sure to use a technique that is know as *reflective listening*. **Reflective listening involves repeating what your client has said to you to avoid any misunderstandings.** Also, using hair color swatches, magazines and pictures while consulting with your client will help you reinforce the communication process and avoid misunderstandings.

To help you remember the important steps in the consultation process, remember: **Great Artists Always Draw Creatively**. Just change your focus to your client's hair color.

Greet

- Meet and greet the client with a firm handshake and a pleasant voice.
- Communicate to build rapport and develop a relationship with the client.

Ask, Analyze, and Assess

- Ask questions to discover client's needs and past color services. For example, ask questions such as, "What made you interested in a color service today?" Some responses may include, "I'd like to look more trendy like that actress from the new television series," or "I'd like to cover up my gray."

- Ask about clothing and lifestyle. Refer to Clothing and Lifestyle in the Design Decisions chapter for guidelines.

- Ask your client whether he/she will be able to maintain the new color and make him/her aware of the financial commitment.

- Analyze client's face, body shape, physical features, eye and skin tones. Refer to Considerations for Design Decisions in the Design Decision chapter for guidelines. Keep in mind that you can widen or lengthen face shapes with the proper placement of light and dark hair colors.

- Analyze the porosity and condition of the hair. Remember, you always want to maintain the best optimal condition of the hair.

- Assess the facts and thoroughly think through your recommendations. Use photos, magazines and/or hair color swatches to better understand your client's desires. Don't be afraid to let your client know if you are unable to perform a service. Remember, not all requests are possible even on healthy hair.

Agree

- Explain your recommended solutions and the price for today's service(s) and for future services as well.

- Return to step two (ask, analyze and assess) if your client is hesitant about your recommendation.

- Gain feedback and approval from your client.

Deliver

- Ensure client protection by draping the client with towels and a chemical cape.

- Ensure client comfort during service.

- Stay focused on delivering the service to the best of your ability.

Complete

- Request satisfaction feedback from your client.

- Escort client to retail area and show him/her at least two products you used.

- Recommend products to maintain appearance and condition of your client's hair color, such as color shampoos and conditioners.

- Invite your client to make a purchase.

- Suggest a future appointment time for your client's next visit.

- Offer appreciation to your client for visiting the school or salon.

- Record recommended products on client record card for future visits.

For more information on consultation, refer to the Design Decision chapter.

Client Record Card/Release Form

The key to successful client relationships and maintaining ongoing hair color services and consistent chemical results is to keep accurate records. The client record card contains information such as the client's name, address, and telephone number. The client record card also contains information about the condition of the hair and scalp, especially noting if the client is on any type of medication or taking vitamins. The client record card is used from the consultation period up until the client has left the salon.

A client release statement helps the school or salon owner avoid retribution from any damages or accidents and may be required by some malpractice insurance. However, it is not a legal document and may not absolve the hair colorist from any damage that may occur to the client's hair as a result of the chemical service.

Promoting and Retailing Hair Color Services

Today's clients are more sophisticated, educated, style conscious and demanding than ever before. They expect the same sophistication and professionalism from their stylist.

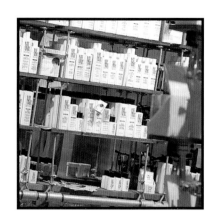

"Credibility" is the key to effective client communications. Therefore, you should become a personal advertisement for hair color services. In other words, having a good color design yourself will go a long way in selling that service. You must also be aware of basic color theory, use the best hair color products on the market and be able to communicate the value of hair color using current, professional terminology. Examples of professional terminology include:

- Lighten (versus bleach);
- Color (versus dye);
- Highlight or weaving (versus frosting or streaking).

Rule number one in merchandising is to display your products and services. However, since in the case of professional hair color it's impractical to display all your products, you can certainly display your hair color services. Here's how:

- Decorate with hair color pictures. Use posters and photos clipped from magazines.
- Put up signs at your work station advertising hair color techniques.

ACTIVITY:

Create your own hair color consultation binder by clipping photos of various color designs from magazines and books. Use your binder as you discuss color options with your clients.

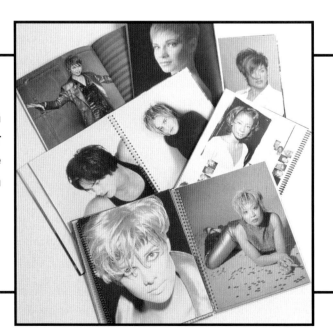

Product and Application Overview

In this portion of the chapter you will overview the hair color products and application techniques you will perform in the exercises that follow. These products and application techniques will help prepare you for the many hair color service possibilites you'll encounter in the salon.

Hair Color Products

CATEGORY	LASTING POWER	FUNCTION	APPLICATION METHOD
NONOXIDATIVE (not mixed with developer)			
Temporary	From shampoo to shampoo	Deposits color	Base to ends at shampoo bowl; combed on
Semi-Permanent	4-6 shampoos	Deposits color; adds shine; cannot lighten hair	Base to ends (heat may be required)
OXIDATIVE (mixed with developer)			
Demi-Permanent	Fades in 6-8 weeks	Deposits color, but usually does not lighten hair	Base to ends (darker result)
	Regrowth 6-8 weeks		Base only
Permanent (also known as single process tints)	Permanent	Lightens and deposits color	Base to ends (darker result)
			Midstrand to porous ends, then base and ends (lighter result)
	Regrowth 3-6 weeks		Base only
LIGHTENERS (mixed with developer)			
On-the-scalp	Permanent	Lightens existing hair color (safe enough to be used on scalp)	Midstrand to porous ends then, base and ends (lighter result)
	Regrowth 3-6 weeks		Base only
Off-the-scalp	Permanent	Lightens existing hair color (used off the scalp for special effects, i.e., highlighting, painting, etc.)	Slightly away from the scalp to the ends (lighter result)
	Regrowth 12-16 weeks		Base only

Hair Color Application Techniques

By understanding the following hair color application techniques, you will be able to create an endless array of hair color designs on your clients. Here we've used a color quadrant mannequin to show the four basic application techniques you will need to learn. Note that by practicing these application techniques on a smaller area first, you will more easily acquire the skills you need to work on an entire head.

BASE TO ENDS (DARKER RESULT)

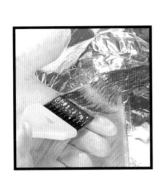
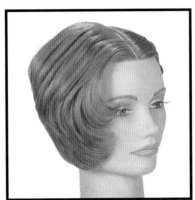

MIDSTRAND TO ENDS, THEN BASE (LIGHTER RESULT)

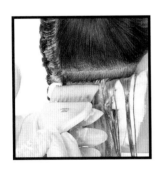
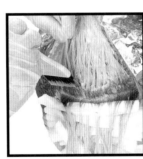
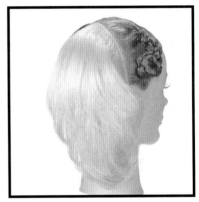

BASE ONLY (RETOUCH)

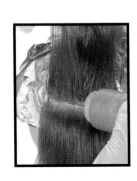
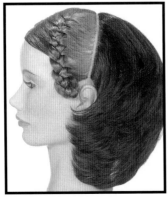

AWAY FROM SCALP (HIGHLIGHTS)

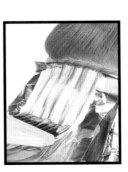
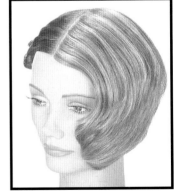

Temporary Color

Temporary colors, also known as color rinses, are usually applied to clean, towel-blotted hair and remain on the hair until the next shampoo. These colors are generally applied at the shampoo bowl with an applicator bottle because of their liquid consistency. Read the manufacturer's directions for application procedures. Listed below are general guidelines to follow for a temporary color rinse application.

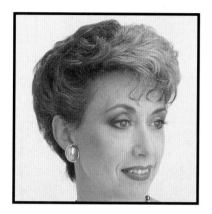 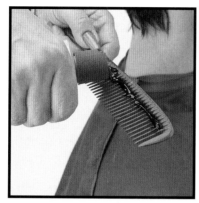 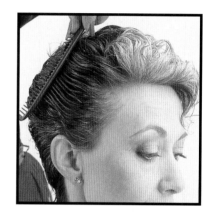

Temporary Rinse Guidelines

- Wash and sanitize hands; gather and assemble implements/supplies; wear protective gloves and apron; drape the client for a chemical hair service.

- Shampoo and towel-blot the hair thoroughly.

- Apply color with an applicator bottle from scalp to ends for all-over coverage, or comb the the color on for a blended effect.

- Blot excess color to prevent dripping; do not rinse the hair.

- Proceed with styling.

- Record the results on the client record card; organize materials; clean work space.

Semi-Permanent Color

Semi-permanent colors, also known as glosses or color enhancers, penetrate the cuticle and enter the cortex. These colors gradually fade with each shampoo. For application and processing procedures, read manufacturer's directions, which may vary. Semi-permanent colors are usually applied to shampooed, towel-dried hair with a bottle or bowl and brush. Semi-permanent colors that contain aniline derivatives require a predisposition (skin patch) test, in which case, perform the predisposition test 24-48 hours prior to the color service.

13

For this technique you will apply color on dark field hair for a tonal effect. One-inch (2.5 cm) partings are used from horizontal and diagonal back partings. Application timing for semi-permanent color should not exceed 15 minutes.

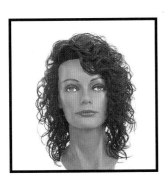
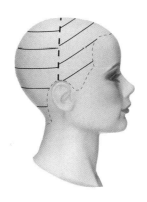
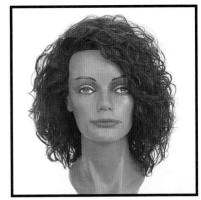

Semi-Permanent Color Preparation

As with any professional service, it is important to have your area, products and equipment in proper order. Before performing a semi-permanent color service, be sure to satisfy the following points:

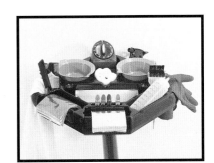

- Perform a predisposition test

- Disinfect color table

- Arrange implements/supplies, including semi-permanent color(s), bowl, brush, gloves, large-tooth comb, sectioning clips, barrier cream, cotton, plastic cap

- Wash and sanitize hands; drape the client for a chemical service; perform hair and scalp analysis; wear protective gloves and color apron; perform preliminary strand test if needed

- Review previous client record card, if applicable

Semi-Permanent Color Procedure

- Part the hair into four sections
- Apply barrier cream
- Pour color into bottle
- Outline first back section
- Take 1" (2.5 cm) horizontal partings in back
- Apply color from base to midstrand, omitting porous ends
- Complete first back section
- Complete other back section
- Outline front sections, then apply color to these sections from diagonal partings

- Apply color to remaining midstrand and ends
- Work color through for even saturation
- Apply cotton around hairline
- Place plastic cap over hair
- Position client under pre-heated dryer if applicable
- Set timer
- Perform strand test if desired
- Rinse, shampoo and remove any color stains
- Condition and finish hair as desired

Semi-Permanent Color

1-2. Part the hair into four sections, from forehead to nape and ear to ear, to create a working pattern. **Apply barrier cream** around the hairline.

3. Pour color into bottle. Here a medium red-violet and a medium dark red-violet formula is used.

4. Outline the first back section.

5. Take 1" (2.5cm) horizontal partings in the back. Begin at the top of the section. **Apply the color from the base up to midstrand, omitting the porous ends.** Subdivide the parting for control. Work toward the hairline to **complete the first back section,** then bring the hair down to allow for air oxidation.

6. Outline the next back section and repeat the same procedures. **Complete the other back section.**

7-8. Outline the front sections, then apply color to these sections from diagonal partings using the same procedures.

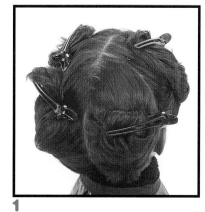

1

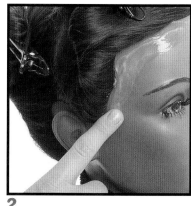

2

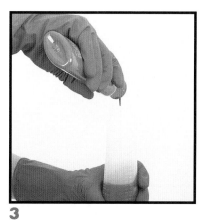

3

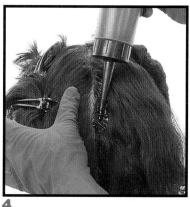

4

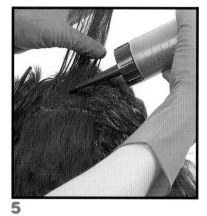

5

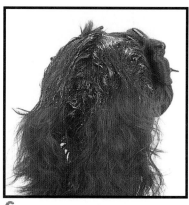

6

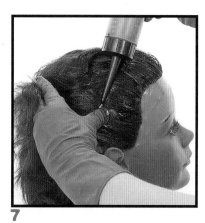

7

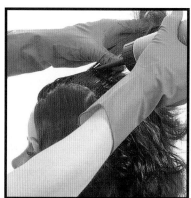

8

1 3

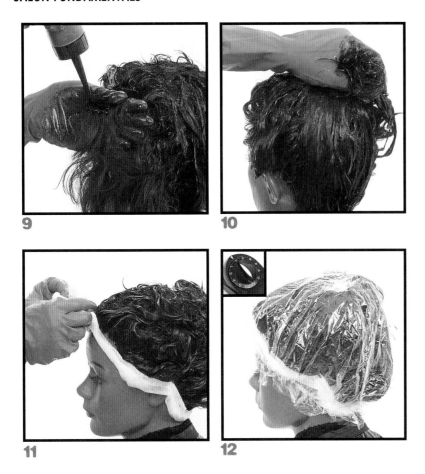

9

10

11

12

9-10. Apply the color to the remaining midstrand and ends. Work color through for even saturation.

11-12. **Apply cotton around the hairline.** This will prevent the product from dripping onto the client's face and neck. **Place a plastic cap over the hair** to allow for better color penetration. **Position client under pre-heated dryer if applicable. Set the timer** according to manufacturer's directions. **Perform strand test if desired** for color development. **Rinse, shampoo and remove any color stain. Condition** and **finish the hair** as desired.

Semi-Permanent Color Completion

- Complete the client record card
- Offer your client a rebook visit
- Recommend retail products, such as shampoos and conditioners for color-treated hair

Semi-Permanent Color Retouch

Since semi-permanent colors gradually fade from your client's hair, a regrowth area will not be very evident. Retouches are scheduled whenever the color needs refreshing. An average is every 4 to 6 weeks, but it is influenced by how frequently your client shampoos as well has how porous the hair is. When semi-permanent color needs refreshing, it is applied from base to ends, just like the original color application.

Oxidative Color: Darker Result

When applying an oxidative color for a darker result, color is applied from base to ends using a bowl and brush or an applicator bottle, depending on the consistency of the product and personal preference. If the ends are porous, you may apply a filler to them first or delay application of color to the porous ends until later. This application technique is also called a virgin darker when it is performed for the first time. Retouches are applied to the base area only.

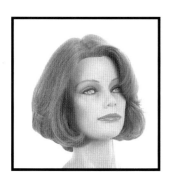
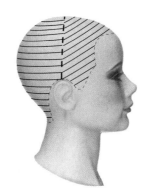
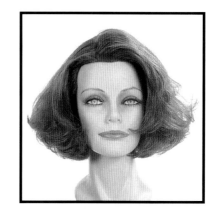

In this exercise, a medium dark, warm brown color is applied to darken the medium light field of this graduated form. Horizontal and diagonal partings are used within four sections, with a base-to-ends technique. A base-to-ends color application should not exceed 15 minutes.

Oxidative Color: Darker Result Preparation

As with any professional service, it is important to have your area, products, implements and equipment in proper order. Before performing an oxidative hair color service, be sure to satisfy the following points:

- Perform predisposition test 24-48 hours before service (be guided by manufacturer's directions); if negative, proceed with hair color service

- Disinfect color area; arrange implements and supplies, including color bowl and brush, gloves, large-tooth comb, tail comb, sectioning clips, long lasting oxidative hair colors, developer and protective creme

- Wash and sanitize hands; drape the client for a chemical service; perform hair and scalp analysis; wear protective gloves and color apron; perform preliminary strand test

- Review previous client record card, if applicable

Oxidative Color: Darker Result Procedure

- Subdivide the hair into four sections

- Apply barrier creme

- Measure and mix color formula

- Outline first front section

- Apply color from base to ends using 1/4" (.75 cm) diagonal back partings

- Work from top of section to bottom

- Complete this section, then outline hairline

- Bring hair down

- Repeat color application on other front side

- Position protective strips along hairline, if desired

- Move to back and repeat same procedures from horizontal partings

- Crosscheck

- Set timer

- Perform strand test

- Rinse, shampoo and remove any color stains

- Condition and finish hair

1
3

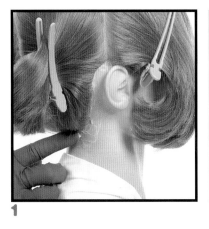

1

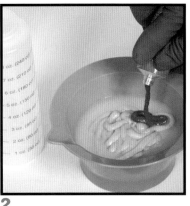

2

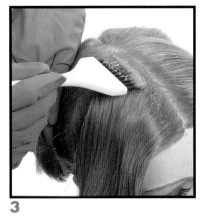

3

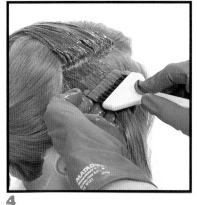

4

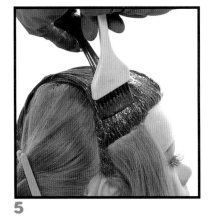

5

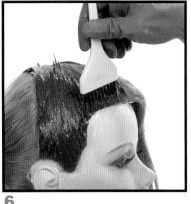

6

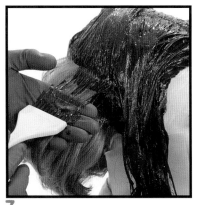

7

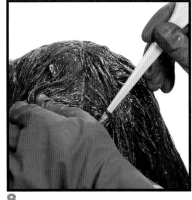

8

Oxidative Color: Darker Result

1-2. **Subdivide the hair into four sections,** from forehead to nape and ear to ear, to create a working pattern. **Apply barrier cream** around the entire hairline. **Measure and mix the color formula.** Here, an equal proportion of a level 4 red brown and level 4 neutral brown are mixed with equal parts of a catalyst.

3-4. **Outline the first front section. Apply the color from base to ends,** using 1/4" (.75 cm) diagonal back partings. Omit the ends until later if porous. **Work from the top of the section to the bottom.**

5-6. **Complete this section,** then outline the hairline to ensure coverage. **Then bring the hair down**, lifting it at the base to allow for oxidation, as you complete each section. **Repeat the color application on the other front side.**

7-8. **Move to the back and repeat the same procedures** along horizontal partings. **Position protective strips along the hairline** to protect the client and to prevent their skin from staining. **Cross-check** throughout to ensure complete coverage. Protect the skin from staining by directing hair off the face or using a protective barrier.

9-10. Set the timer according to the manufacturer's recommendation. **Perform a strand test** to determine color development. **Rinse, shampoo and remove any color stains** once the color has processed. **Condition and finish the hair** as desired.

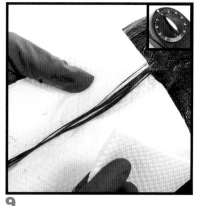
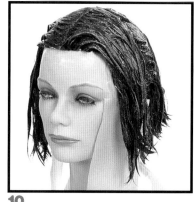

9

10

Oxidative Color: Darker Result Completion

- Complete the client record card
- Offer your client a rebook visit
- Recommend retail products such as shampoos and conditioners for color-treated hair
- Disinfect implements, discard non-reusable supplies and clean your work space
- Wash your hands with liquid antibacterial soap

Oxidative Color: Darker Result Retouch

Depending on how fast your client's hair grows, retouches are generally performed every 6-8 weeks. Apply color to the new growth only. Do not overlap onto the previously colored hair. If the previously colored hair has faded, apply a semi-permanent or demi-permanent color in a matching shade. Applying color over previously colored hair to refresh the color is sometimes referred to as color glazing. A soap cap, which is created by mixing remaining color with shampoo, is another way to refresh faded ends. Retouch color applications should not exceed 10 minutes.

Oxidative Color: Lighter Result

When permanent colors are mixed with higher strengths of developers, they have the ability to lighten and deposit color in a single process. Hair colors that are lighter than your client's hair, as well as high lift tints, fall into this category. When lightening your client's hair for the first time (virgin), the color is applied from the midstrand out to the porous ends first. The color is applied to the base area last, since the lightening action there is accelerated due to incomplete keratinazation of the new growth as well as additional body heat at the base area. Very porous ends may also process faster and, therefore require less processing time. The retouch application is at the base area only. The application of oxidative color for lighter result should not exceed 15 minutes.

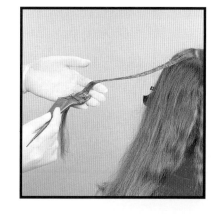
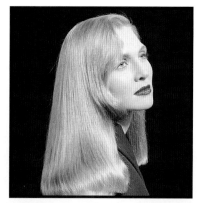

1
3

Oxidative Color: Lighter Result Guidelines

- Perform predisposition test 24-48 hours before service (be guided by manufacturer's directions); if negative, proceed with hair color service.

- Disinfect color service area; arrange implements and supplies, including color bowl and brush, gloves, large-tooth comb, tail comb, sectioning clips, oxidative hair color(s), developer and protective crème.

- Wash and sanitize hands; drape the client for a chemical service; perform hair and scalp analysis; wear protective gloves and color apron; perform preliminary strand test; review previous client record card, if applicable.

- Part the hair into four sections, apply protective creme around the hairline.

- Measure and mix the formula.

- Begin the application in the most resistant area. Use 1/4" (.75 cm) partings and apply the color product 1/2" (1.25cm) away from the scalp on both sides of the strand, out to the porous ends. If the ends are not porous, apply the color to the ends. Move to remaining sections, working from the top of the section to the bottom.

- Crosscheck to ensure even coverage and set the timer. Perform a strand test to determine development.

- Apply newly mixed color product to the base and ends when the hair has reached 50% of the desired level. Use the same parting pattern.

- Set the timer and perform a strand test to determine development.

- Rinse the hair thoroughly when the hair has reached the desired level. Shampoo, condition and finish the hair as desired.

- Complete the client record card; offer your client a rebook visit; recommend retail products that will enhance or maintain the color service; disinfect implements, discard non-reusable supplies and clean your work area.

Oxidative Color: Lighter Result Retouch

Regrowth is more visible on lightened hair and generally requires more frequent retouches. Depending on the contrast between lightened and natural hair, some clients will need to schedule retouch-es every 3-6 weeks. Color is applied to the base area, avoiding the previously colored hair. If the remaining hair has faded, apply an oxidative product without ammonia in a matching tone to refresh the color. Retouch lighter applications should not exceed 10 minutes.

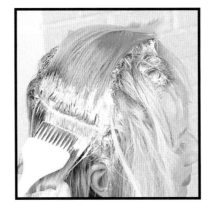
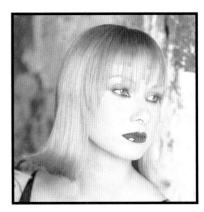

Surface Painting

Surface painting techniques are performed on the surface of the hair to create subtle to dramatic highlighted or lowlighted color effects. Surface painting techniques are performed to imitate the sun's natural lighting abilities or to create textural qualities on the hair. Although the color can be painted on in any way desired, usually a color or paint brush is used to paint the color vertically on the hair in an alternating pattern. Pale yellow highlights have been introduced to this medium light field solid form. Surface painting techniques are also known as freeform or freehand painting.

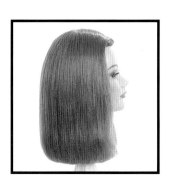 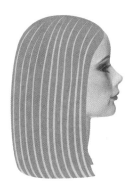 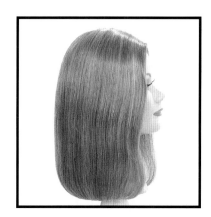

Surface Painting Preparation

As with any professional service, it is important to have your area, products, implements and equipment in proper order. Before performing a surface painting hair color service, be sure to satisfy the following points:

- Perform a predisposition test (if a toner is going to be used)

- Disinfect color table

- Arrange implements/supplies, including off-the-scalp powder lightener, developer, color bowl, brush, gloves, large-tooth comb and tail comb

- Wash and sanitize hands; drape the client for a chemical service; perform hair and scalp analysis; wear protective gloves and color apron; perform preliminary strand test

- Review previous client record card, if applicable

Surface Painting Procedure

- Mix the formula

- Comb the hair as it will be worn

- Dip brush in bowl

- Apply lightener vertically, slightly away from base to ends

- Work from front hairline to center back

- Repeat application on opposite side

- Follow processing directions

- Rinse, shampoo, condition and finish hair

1
3

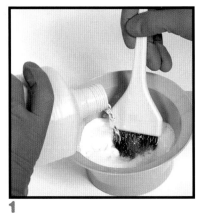

1

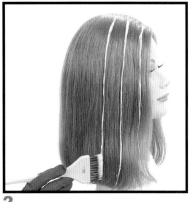

2

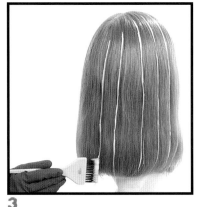

3

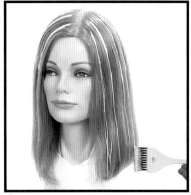

4

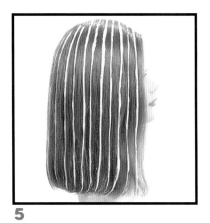

5

Surface Painting

1-2. Mix the formula, which, for this design, is an off-the-scalp lightener mixed with 20 volume (6%) developer. **Comb the hair as it will be worn. Dip the brush in the bowl** and then **apply the lightener vertically, slightly away from the base to the ends** to achieve a natural grown-out effect.

3-5. Work from the front hairline to the center back. Dip the brush in the bowl as often as necessary to obtain the required product. **Repeat the application on the opposite side.** Once you have finished the application, you may wish to add more highlights in various sizes and positions as needed. **Follow the processing directions. Then rinse shampoo, condition and finish the hair as desired.**

Surface Painting Completion

- Complete the client record card
- Offer your client a rebook visit
- Recommend retail products for your client
- Disinfect implements, discard non-reusable supplies and clean work space
- Wash your hands with antibacterial soap

Surface Painting Retouch

Surface painting techniques are a great way to introduce clients to color services. Retouch services are not always required since surface painting is a technique in which only selected areas are colored to achieve a special or natural highlighted effect. However, to maintain the effect, retouch applications will vary depending upon the degree of contrast between the color-treated hair and the nontreated hair and the rate at which the hair grows. Retouch applications are performed from the base up to the previous color-treated hair, anywhere from 3-8 weeks or depending on the desired effect.

Partial Highlights: Slicing

Partial highlighting techniques are used to create an alternation of colors beyond the surface of the hair. Partial highlights are generally positioned in the fringe area for a face-framing effect or throughout the top for an illusion of an allover highlighted effect. Color or lightener is applied to selected strands, which are then isolated in foil or thermal strips to protect the untreated hair. Here, to add lightness and brightness around the face, golden highlights are introduced to the fringe area of this medium light field increase-layered form. A fine slicing technique is used within a triangular shape to create an alternation of highlights that gradually diminish for a blended appearance.

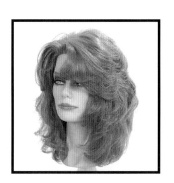 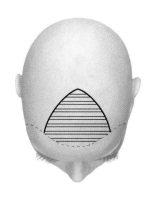 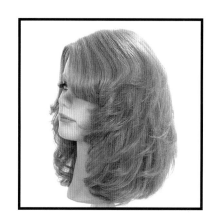

Partial Highlights: Slicing Preparation

As with any professional service, it is important to have your area, products implements and equipment in proper order. Before performing a surface painting hair color service, be sure to satisfy the following points:

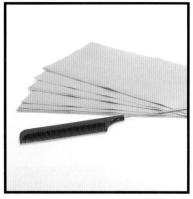

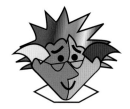

"Although thermal strips are used in this exercise, foil may be used instead."

- Perform a predisposition test (if an aniline derivative tint will come in contact with the scalp)

- Disinfect color table

- Arrange implements/supplies, including off-the-scalp powder lightener, color (optional), developer, thermal strips or foil, color bowl, brush, gloves, large-tooth comb, tail comb and sectioning clips

- Wash and sanitize hands; drape the client for a chemical service; perform hair and scalp analysis; wear protective gloves and color apron; perform preliminary strand test

- Review previous client record card, if applicable

13

Partial Highlights: Slicing Procedure

- Create a triangle section at fringe area
- Mix formula
- Begin at large end of triangle
- Make a horizontal parting and part off a fine slice from top of parting
- Position thermal strip underneath slice
- Apply lightener in a zigzag pattern away from scalp out to ends
- Fold thermal strip in half
- Release a section to remain natural
- Continue to alternate between highlighted and natural sections
- Work toward narrow end of triangle
- Clip highlighted section upward
- Set timer and follow processing directions
- Strand test
- Remove thermal strips
- Rinse, shampoo, condition and finish hair

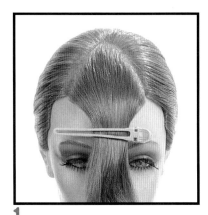

1

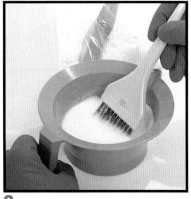

2

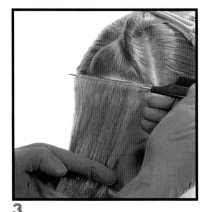

3

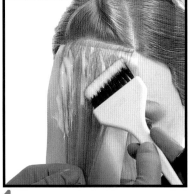

4

Partial Highlights: Slicing

1-2. Create a triangle section at the fringe area. This section will be highlighted. **Mix the formula.** For this exercise, off-the-scalp powder lightener and 20 volume (6%) developer is used.

3-4. Begin at the large end of the triangle. Make a horizontal parting and part off a fine slice from the top of the parting. The hair left natural is double the density of the fine slice. **Position the thermal strip underneath the slice** and **apply the lightener in a zigzag pattern away from the scalp up to the ends** to create a natural, grown-out effect.

5-6. **Fold the thermal strip in half** to cover the product and to avoid seepage. **Release a section to remain natural** and **continue to alternate between the highlighted and natural sections. Work toward the narrow end of the triangle,** adjusting the density of highlights as desired.

7-9. Complete the highlights. **Clip the highlighted section upward** to protect the eyes. **Set the timer and follow the processing directions. Strand test** until the degree of decolorization has been achieved. **Remove the thermal strips** or foils when hair has reached the desired degree of lightness. **Rinse the lightener from the hair,** then **shampoo, condition and finish the hair** as desired. Note the alternation of highlights.

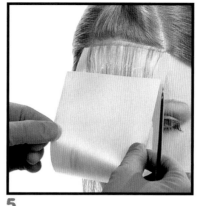

5

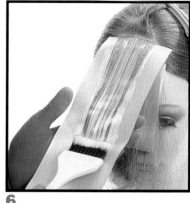

6

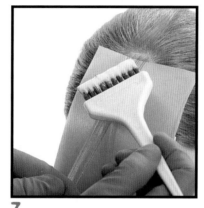

7

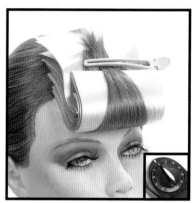

8

Partial Highlights: Slicing Completion

- Complete the client record card
- Offer your client a rebook visit
- Recommend retail products for your client
- Disinfect implements, discard non-reusable supplies and clean work space
- Wash your hands with liquid antibacterial soap

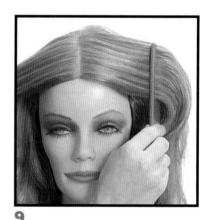

9

Partial Highlights: Slicing Retouch

Scheduling a retouch service for partial highlights depends on how the hair looks as it grows out. Sometimes highlights look good as much as three months later. On average, retouch appointments are booked every 10 to 12 weeks. Retouches may consist of introducing new highlights into the

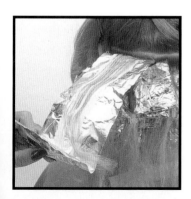

same area or applying lightener to the base area of previously lightened strands. If you select previously lightened strands, apply lightener to the base area (regrowth) only and remove the ends from the foil before folding. With shorter hair, fold the foil upward just enough to cover the untreated hair. Then fold the foil again to cover the product. This folding method will prevent the untreated hair from coming into contact with the product.

13

Full Highlights: Weaving

For a full highlighting procedure, selected strands are lightened to create an alternation of lighter tones throughout the entire design. Generally, foil or thermal strips are used to isolate the selected strands to protect the untreated hair. With foil applications, the foil is usually folded upward once or twice, then the sides are folded inward. For thermal strip applications, the thermal strip is folded upward in half, making sure the product is completely covered.

Performing a full head of highlights can take up to 45 minutes. To equalize the processing time, you may wish to begin with a lower volume of developer and gradually increase it as you work. Once you have finished the application, it is necessary to strand test for color development or degree of decolorization. If areas process quicker, you can spray them down with water to delay processing. Keep in mind, however, that these areas are still lightening. To completely stop the process, you may need to take the client to the shampoo bowl and completely rinse and shampoo the lightened strands that have reached the desired degree of lightness.

When you select foil or thermal strips for this procedure, you will want to make sure they are wider and longer then the section you are weaving. For this exercise, the woven section is approximately 2" (5 cm) wide. Keep in mind that if the sections become too wide, the hair product may seep out of the foil and cause "bleeding" or "spotting" on the untreated hair. If this happens, you can apply a darker color to the spotted hair to return it to the appropriate color.

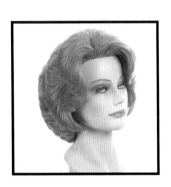 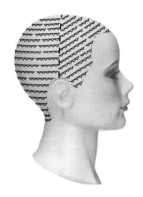 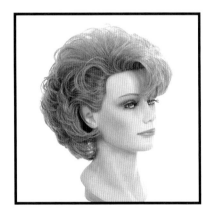

Here, an alternation of pale yellow highlights is introduced throughout this medium light field. A fine weaving technique is used throughout this uniformly layered form. A bricklay pattern is used in the back with horizontal partings, while diagonal back partings are used at the front. In this exercise foil is used to isolate the selected strands. A tail comb is used for the weaving technique and a small color brush is used to apply lightener.

Full Highlights: Weaving Preparation

As with any professional service, it is important to have your area, products, implements and equipment in proper order. Before performing a weaving hair color service, be sure to satisfy the following points:

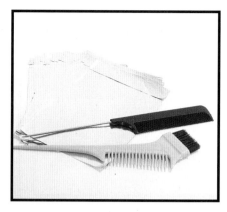

- Perform a predisposition test (if an aniline derivative tint is going to be used for toning the hair)

- Disinfect color table

- Arrange implements/supplies, including off-the-scalp powder lightener, color, developer (at least 2 different strengths), color bowls, brushes, foil, gloves, large-tooth comb and tail comb

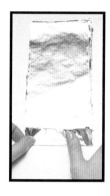

- Wash and sanitize hands; drape the client for a chemical service; perform hair and scalp analysis; wear protective gloves and color apron; perform preliminary strand test

- Review previous client record card, if applicable

Full Highlights: Weaving Procedure

- Section hair into 4 basic sections
- Mix formula
- Begin at nape
- Take a horizontal parting and weave out selected strands
- Position prefolded edge of foil underneath woven strands
- Apply lightener from edge of foil to ends
- Fold foil upward twice
- Fold sides of foil inward
- Create a bricklay pattern
- Alternate between natural and highlighted sections
- Complete back section
- Continue weaving from diagonal back partings, using a bricklay pattern at front side

- Complete other side
- Set timer
- Perform strand test
- Remove foils
- Rinse, shampoo and dry hair
- Mix toner
- Apply toner using a base-to-ends technique from diagonal back and horizontal partings
- Set timer
- Perform strand text
- Rinse, shampoo and finish the hair

13

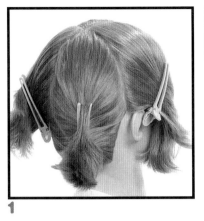

1

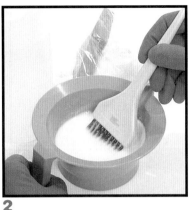

2

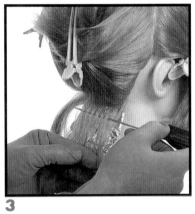

3

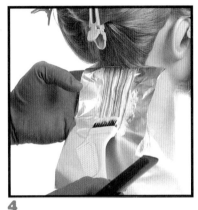

4

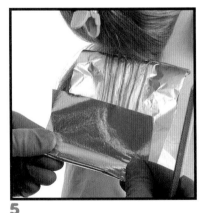

5

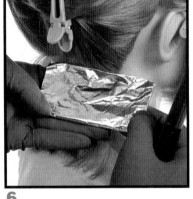

6

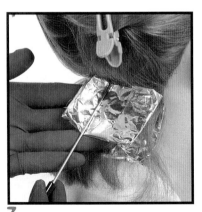

7

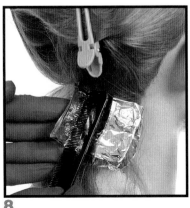

8

Full Highlights: Weaving

1-2. Section the hair into 4 basic sections. To ensure equal processing, the percentage of developer can be adjusted as you work from the back to the front. **Mix your formula.** In this exercise, off-the-scalp powder lightener is mixed equally with 10 volume (3%) developer for the back, while 20 volume (6%) is used at the front.

3-4. Begin at the nape. Take a horizontal parting and weave out selected strands, using the tail of the comb. **Position the prefolded edge of a foil underneath the woven strands.** Note that the index finger is positioned within the fold of the foil near the scalp so that you can apply the product as close to the scalp as possible without getting product on the scalp. **Apply the lightener from the edge of the foil to the ends.**

5-6. Fold the foil upward twice. Be sure to cover the product completely to avoid spillage.

7-8. Fold the sides of the foil inward with the tail or teeth of the comb. Folding the sides of the foil inward forms a little packet, which helps to prevent the foil from slipping and the product from seeping.

9-10. **Create a bricklay pattern.** As you work upward, **alternate between the natural and highlighted sections.** At the wider areas of the head, release a horizontal parting all the way across. Work from the center to one side, then to the other.

11-12. **Complete the back section.**

13-14. **Continue weaving from diagonal back partings, using a bricklay pattern at the front side.** Work from the hairline to the top.

15-17. **Complete the other side** using the same procedures. **Set the timer** according to manufacturer's directions. **Perform strand test** for desired degree of lightness. Once you have reached the desired degree of lightness, **remove the foils. Then rinse, shampoo and dry the hair** according to manufacturer's directions.

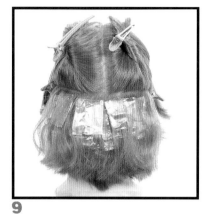
9

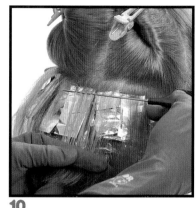
10

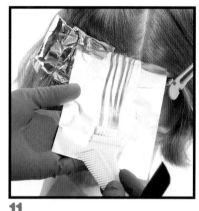
11

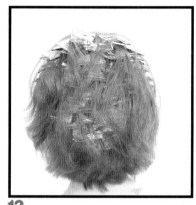
12

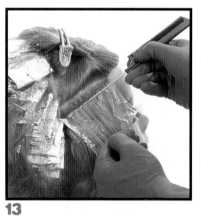
13

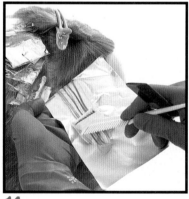
14

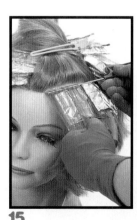
15

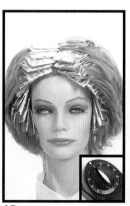
16

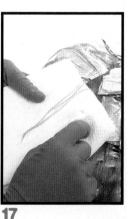
17

1 3

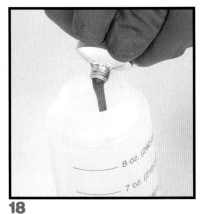

18

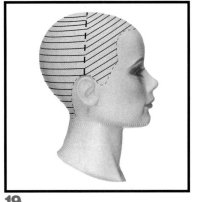

19

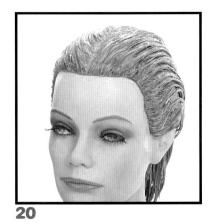

20

18-20. If needed, **mix a toner.** Be sure to have performed a patch test prior to the service. Here, a level 10 violet base is mixed with equal proportions of catalyst. This mixture will tone the highlights and add shine to the non-highlighted hair. **Apply the toner using a base-to-ends technique from diagonal back and horizontal partings.** Set the timer according to manufacturer's directions. **Perform strand test.** Then **rinse, shampoo, condition and finish the hair** as desired.

Full Highlights: Weaving Completion

- Complete the client record card
- Offer your client a rebook visit
- Recommend retail products for your client
- Disinfect implements, discard non-reusable supplies and clean work space
- Wash your hands with antibacterial soap

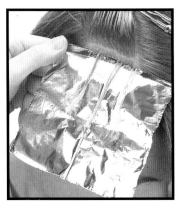

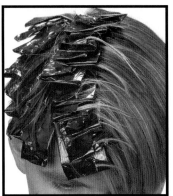

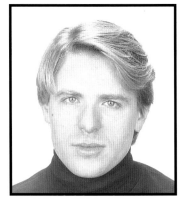

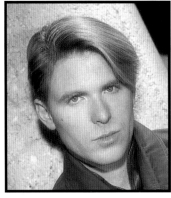

Full Highlights: Weaving Retouch

A full head of highlights requires a retouch service every 12 to 16 weeks. Heavier concentrations of highlights may require a retouch more often since the regrowth area may have more contrast. Record the pattern and the density of the strands selected on your client's record card so that you can repeat the service or adjust it as necessary. For instance, a fine weave with a light density will produce a very different result than a thick weave with a heavy density. Whether you are retouching a full or partial head of highlights, be sure to apply the product to the regrowth area only. Leave the previously lightened strands out of the foil to avoid overlapping the product.

Reverse Highlighting

Follow the directions given for the weaving procedure earlier. Use a color that blends with the client's natural color. Weave out some of the previously highlighted hair strands and apply color primarily to these strands.

Cap Highlighting

The cap highlighting technique is generally performed on short hair, no longer than 6" (15 cm). A crochet hook is used to pull strands through a perforated cap. Color or lightener is then applied to the hair. Some manufacturers may recommend that a plastic bag or cap be positioned over the color-treated hair to facilitate processing and keep the product moist since the cap reduces available body heat.

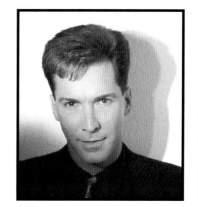
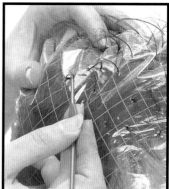
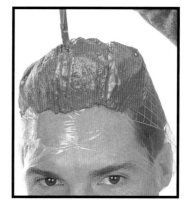
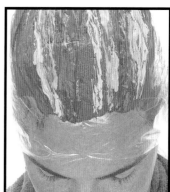

If a lightener is used to decolorize the hair, a toner may be required afterward to achieve the desired results. Note that since the lightener will not come into contact with the scalp, a powder or off-the-scalp lightener may be used. Also keep in mind that the highlighting cap may be used with on-the-scalp lightener or color to achieve the desired results.

Cap Highlighting Guidelines

As with any professional service, it is important to have your area, products, implements and equipment in proper order. In addition to following the same preparation procedures as outlined in the highlighting section, be sure to assemble a color cap, crochet hook, lightener, toner, developer and plastic bag.

- Gently remove tangles with a wide-tooth comb and comb hair straight back and close to head.

- Place color cap on client's head and, when applicable, tie the cap.

- Using a fine crochet hook, gently pull strands of hair through the perforated holes in the cap just behind the front hairline. Repeat on the sides, then move to crown and finally, the back or nape.

- Apply lightener or color to the strands and place a plastic cap over the color-treated hair to keep the product moist while processing. Process and strand test according to manufacturer's directions.

- After the hair has reached the desired degree of lightness, remove the plastic cap. Rinse and shampoo the hair with the color cap in place.

1
3

Option A:

- Remove the color cap during the shampoo. Complete shampoo and apply toner to entire head.

Option B:

- Leave the color cap in place and complete shampoo. Apply the toner to the highlighted strands only.
- Set the timer and allow the toner to process. Strand test.
- Remove the cap, rinse, shampoo and condition the hair.

Pulling a few strands through the cap will produce a light highlighted effect, while pulling many strands through the cap will produce a heavier highlighted effect. The number of holes you pull hair through, the degree of lightness desired and the color chosen will all determine the final result.

Double-Process Blonde

A double-process technique is a two-step process that involves lightening (decolorizing) the hair first and then recoloring the hair to the desired tone. The first time the hair undergoes a double-process technique (also known as virgin lighter) the **lightener is first applied 1/2"** **(1.25 cm) away from the scalp out to the porous ends.** Once the color has reached approximately 50% of the desired lightness, a fresh mixture is applied to the base.

If the ends are very porous, you will want to delay application of the lightener until after the base application, since they may develop quicker. In this double-process exercise, the product was applied midstrand to ends due to the shorter hair length and even porosity. Once the medium light field was decolorized to a very light blonde, a base-to-ends technique was used to tone the hair.

For this design 1/8" (.35 cm) horizontal partings are used throughout. This exercise is performed on a combination form. Application of the lightener to the midstrand and ends should not exceed 15 minutes. Application of lightener to the base should not exceed 5 minutes.

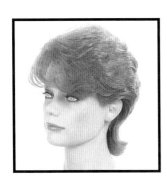
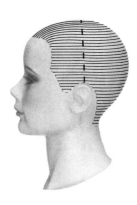
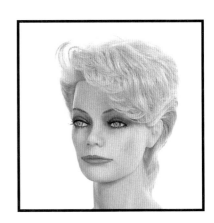

Reminder: With a double-process technique, the product is not applied immediately to the base because the body heat and incomplete keratinization at the base will cause the hair to lighten quicker, resulting in an uneven color formation.

Double-Process Blonde Preparation

As with any professional service, it is important to have your area, products, implements and equipment in proper order. Before performing a double-process hair color service, be sure to satisfy the following points:

- Perform predisposition (skin patch) test 24-48 hours prior to service

- Disinfect color area

- Arrange implements/supplies, including on-the-scalp lightener, developer, toner, catalyst, color bowl, brush, color applicator bottle, cotton strips, gloves, large-tooth comb, tail comb, sectioning clips and barrier cream

- Wash and sanitize hands; drape the client for a chemical service; perform hair and scalp analysis; wear protective gloves and color apron; perform preliminary strand test

- Review previous client record card, if applicable

Double-Process Blonde Procedure

- Section hair into four sections
- Apply barrier cream
- Measure and mix formula
- Release 1/8" (.35 cm) horizontal partings at the crown
- Apply lightener 1/2" (1.25 cm) away from scalp through to ends on both sides of the strand. If ends are porous, delay application of lightener until after base application.
- Place cotton at base
- Work downward to complete each section; lift and bring each parting down for air oxidation
- Move to sides and use same procedures
- Set timer

- Perform strand test
- Remove cotton and apply newly mixed lightener to base only, beginning at top of back
- Outline each section
- Bring down each section
- Perform strand test periodically
- Rinse hair with cool water, shampoo and towel dry
- Re-examine scalp
- Mix and apply toner from diagonal back and horizontal partings
- Set timer
- Perform strand test
- Rinse, shampoo, condition and finish the hair

1
3

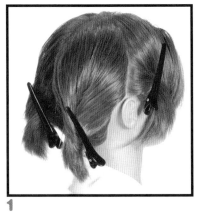

1

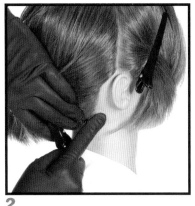

2

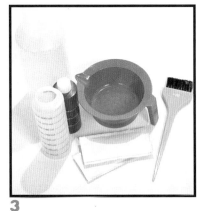

3

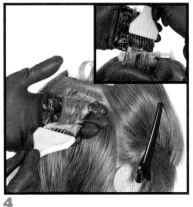

4

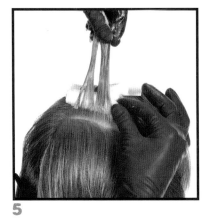

5

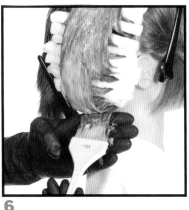

6

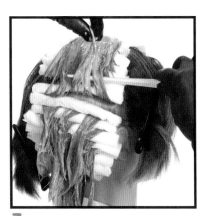

7

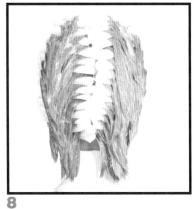

8

Double-Process Blonde

1-2. **Section the hair into four sections,** from forehead to nape and ear to ear. **Apply barrier cream** around the entire hairline.

3. **Measure and mix the formula** using an on-the-scalp lightener. Here, two activators are mixed with 2 oz. (60 ml) cream lightener and 4 oz. (120 ml) of 20 volume (6%) developer.

4. **Release 1/8" (.35 cm) horizontal partings at the crown. Apply the lightener 1/2" (1.25 cm) away from the scalp through to the ends on both sides of the strand.***

5. **Place cotton at the base,** in between partings, to prevent seepage.

6. **Work downward to complete the back section,** using the same procedures.

7-8. **Lift and bring each parting down to allow air oxidation. Complete the back** using the same procedures.

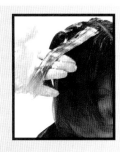

*If ends are porous, delay application of lightener until after base application.

Check the application to ensure even coverage. Keep the lightener moist during development time by reapplying newly mixed product if necessary.

9-10. Move to the sides and use the same procedures.

11-12. Set the timer according to manufacturer's directions. **Perform strand test** for desired degree of lightness.

13-14. Remove cotton and apply newly mixed lightener to base only, beginning at top of back. Then outline each section to ensure even coverage. Be extremely careful when you outline the front hairline. Bring each section down to allow for air oxidation.

15-16. Perform strand test periodically. Rinse the hair with cool water, shampoo and towel dry when you reach the desired degree of lightness. Re-examine the scalp for abrasions and any irritations.

Optional: An alternative application method includes beginning at the nape and applying the product to one side of the strand only as shown on the DVD. Therefore, be guided by your instructor and regulating agency.

The area along the hair strand where two colors meet (i.e., the area where the new growth meets the previously colored hair) is known as the line of demarcation. It is important to avoid overlapping the product, especially with a lightener retouch service, since it could cause breakage.

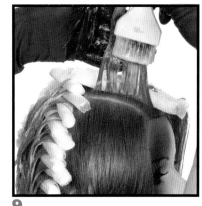

9

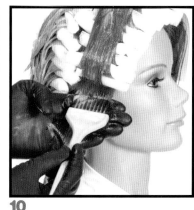

10

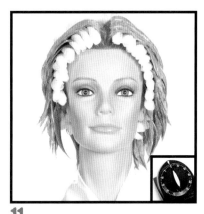

11

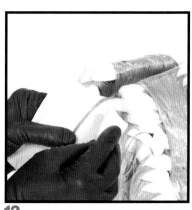

12

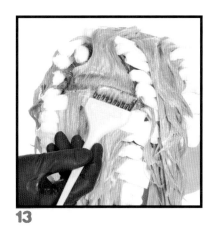

13

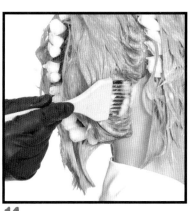

14

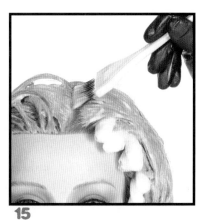

15

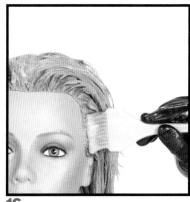

16

1 3

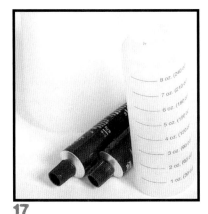

17

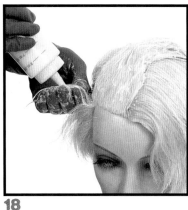

18

17-18. Mix and apply toner. Here a level 10 ash (pearl blonde) was mixed with equal proportions of clear and 20 volume (6%) developer. **Apply the toner from 1/4" (.75 cm) diagonal back partings at the sides and horizontal partings at the back** using a base-to-ends application.

19. Set the timer according to the manufacturer's directions. **Perform strand test** for color development. **Rinse, shampoo and condition the hair** once the color has developed. **Finish the hair** as desired.

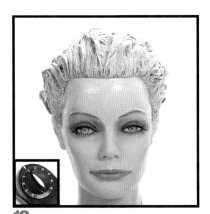

19

Double-Process Blonde Completion

- Complete the client record card
- Offer your client a rebook visit
- Recommend retail products for your client
- Disinfect implements, discard non-reusable supplies and clean work space
- Wash hands with antibacterial soap

Double-Process Blonde Retouch

Retouch applications are performed every 3-6 weeks depending on the rate of regrowth and degree of contrast. **Lightener is applied to the new growth only.** Use 1/8" (.35 cm) partings to ensure consistent application. **Do not overlap the product onto the previously treated hair, since this may cause over-processing and breakage. Finally, a color may be applied over the hair to tone or blend the color.**

Depending on the consistency of the product and personal preference, the product may be applied with a brush or applicator bottle. To ensure even color, it is very important to decolorize the new growth to the same degree as the previously lightened hair. Once the lightener is

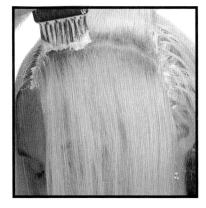

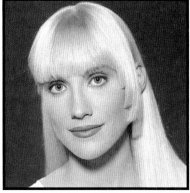

shampooed from the hair, towel-dry the hair and apply the toner to the new growth. If the mid-strands and ends need refreshing, distribute diluted color formula or a matching, non-ammonia hair color through the ends for the last few minutes of processing.

Tint Back

Coloring the hair back to its natural color (tint back) is a service that utilizes all your hair coloring skills and knowledge. The use of a color filler is generally recommended to provide an even base from which to work and to replace a missing primary color. The degree of porosity, the number of levels you are coloring back to and the color you wish to achieve will determine whether you will apply the filler directly to the hair prior to the color application or whether you will mix it into the color formula. Follow manufacturer's directions and perform a strand test to ensure predictable results. Refer back to "Fillers" in this chapter for additional information.

Tint Back Guidelines

- Perform a strand test.

- Subdivide the hair into four sections. Apply filler to desired areas.

- Process according to the manufacturer's directions.

- Re-section the hair and apply the color formula from the line of demarcation out to the porous ends.

- Process and strand test for color development. Then apply to the porous ends. Process accordingly. Note that a diluted color formula may be applied to the remaining hair to blend into the line of demarcation.

- Rinse with lukewarm or tepid water, followed by a shampoo.

- Apply acid rinse to the hair and rinse and style as desired.

- Record formula results on chemical record card. Complete the service by recommending at-home maintenance products.

- Disinfect implements, discard non-reusable supplies and clean work area.

Hair Color Removal Techniques

Occasionally it may become necessary to remove artificial pigment from the hair. Some reasons for removing artificial pigment may include:

- Repeated overlapped applications of hair color have left the hair too dark, dull or have caused an uneven band of color along the hair strand

- The client wants to return to his/her natural color, which is a lighter shade

- A fashion color was used, but the client now desires a more natural color

- Incorrect formulas were used, resulting in unwanted shades

Fortunately, there are products available to the hair colorist that can be used to remove artificial pigment. However, extreme caution must be exercised by the hair colorist, since trying to remove the unwanted pigment can be very difficult and can damage the hair, resulting in breakage and extremely porous hair. In some instances, it may require a second application while in others it may simply be impossible to remove the artificial pigment because of the extreme build-up of color on hair.

13

Products known as color removers and dye solvents are designed to remove artificial pigment. These products are sometimes mixed with hydrogen peroxide for a stronger effect and with distilled water for a milder effect. Always read manufacturer's directions. Although not generally recommended, lighteners are sometimes used to remove artificial colors. Just like color removers, lighteners simultaneously remove some of the natural melanin from the hair.

As with most color services, performing a strand test first is always advisable to avoid damaging the hair and verifying whether or not the service can be performed.

Permanent Color Removal Guidelines

- Follow manufacturer's directions regarding shampooing the hair prior to the color remover application.
- Section the hair into four basic sections.
- Mix the product in a glass or plastic bowl.
- Begin the application in the darkest area and apply the product throughout the four sections.
- Complete the application and cover the hair with a plastic cap if applicable.
- Strand test frequently.
- Once the color is removed, rinse the product immediately.
- Gently and thoroughly shampoo the product from the hair.
- Towel dry and analyze the hair. It may be necessary to re-apply in some areas.
- Once the product has been shampooed out, condition and dry the hair if applicable.
- It is important to note that once the artificial color has been removed, the final hair color has not yet been achieved. Generally, the resulting color serves as a foundation for the final hair color. If no signs of scalp irritations are present, perform a strand test. If a filler is needed, choose one according to the missing primary color. (Refer to the Color Wheel). Then choose the appropriate color. Keep in mind that the hair has gone through several chemical services, leaving the hair porous. Therefore, a low volume developer mixed with the desired color formula is advisable.

ALERT!
Do not leave the client unattended while performing a Permanent Color Removal.

Henna Removal Guidelines

As you may recall, henna is a vegetable dye that coats the hair. Hair coated with henna is generally not compatible with other hair coloring or chemical services. To remove henna, follow the procedures on the next page.

- Apply 70% alcohol to the hair strand, avoiding direct contact with the scalp. Allow alcohol to remain for 5 to 7 minutes.

- Apply mineral oil directly over the alcohol, completely saturating each strand from scalp to ends.

- Cover the hair with a plastic cap and place the client under a preheated, hooded dryer for 30 minutes.

- Without rinsing, apply concentrated shampoo for oily hair and massage into the lengths. Allow shampoo to remain on the hair for three minutes.

- Massage the hair again and then add hot, but comfortable, water and rinse thoroughly.

- Shampoo again. (Several shampoos may be necessary).

Hair Color Problems and Solutions

The following are a few problems that may occur with hair color, along with some possible solutions.

Problem: The Color Faded Quickly

Cause: The correct percentage of developer was not chosen.

Solution: Use a lower percentage of developer that will give you less lift. Remember, higher volumes give you more lift.

Cause: Repeated chemical overlapping caused uneven porosity.

Solution: Choose a deposit-only color when necessary to refresh the midstrand and ends.

Cause: A filler was not used prior to the color application to equalize the porosity on overly porous hair.

Solution: Use or create a filler and apply it to the hair prior to the color application. Follow manufacturer's instructions.

Cause: Improper at-home maintenance.

Solution: Recommend a shampoo and conditioner for color-treated hair at the end of each color service.

Problem: The Color Result Is Too Light

Cause: The color formula chosen was too light.

Solution: Choose a color with a heavier concentration of pigment.

Cause: Improper analysis of the existing field.

Solution: Use swatches to determine the existing color.

Cause: The strength of developer was too high.

Solution: Use a lower percentage when more deposit is desired.

Cause: The formula was not mixed accurately.

Solution: Generally the color and developer are mixed in equal proportions or a 1:1 ratio. However, in some instances you may need to alter this, such as when a 1:2 ratio may be required. Follow manufacturer's instructions.

13

Cause: The hair was decolorized past the desired degree.

Solution: Remember to perform strand tests frequently to view and assess the decolorizing degrees.

Note: If the color result was too light immediately upon completion of the color service, you may wish to apply a nonoxidative or an oxidative color without ammonia throughout or add a few low-lights to create depth.

Problem: The Color Result Is Too Dark

Cause: The color formula chosen was too dark.

Solution: Choose a lighter color. Use swatches to determine the existing and desired field. Also take into consideration the porosity of the hair.

Cause: Too low of a developer volume was chosen.

Solution: Adjust the developer strength according to the lift and deposit desired.

Cause: Improper analysis of the type of porosity was made.

Solution: Check the porosity of the hair prior to color application. Remember, with extreme porosity, the color may at first take quite intensely and then gradually fade with each shampoo. If this is the case, then wait about a week (after repeated shampoos have been performed) before re-evaluating.

Note: If the hair was too dark immediately upon completion of the color service, you may wish to use the following as a guideline to correct the situation: Additional shampooing may remove some of the unwanted pigment. If the color is still too dark, adding a few highlights to add brightness and lightness to the design may be enough. However, in extreme cases, lightener or a color remover may need to be used.

Problem: Insufficient Gray Coverage

Cause: The proper formula was not chosen.

Solution: Be sure to include all three primary colors in your formula or choose a natural series that was designed for gray coverage.

Cause: The color selected was too light.

Solution: Choose a color with a heavier concentration of pigment. Remember that very light hair colors may not contain enough warm pigment.

Cause: The proper analysis for percentage of gray was not made.

Solution: Although an accurate analysis may be difficult, use the following as a guide: Determine whether the hair looks more or less than 50% gray. Then, approximate from that point. For very high percentages of gray, use a lower level than the desired level and add warmth to the formula for a natural effect. If the gray is hardly noticeable, do not adjust the color formula.

Cause: Insufficient processing.

Solution: Process for the recommended amount of time, generally between 30-45 minutes.

Cause: A very high percentage of developer was used.

Solution: Generally, 20 volume (6%) developer is used in equal proportions. Follow manufacturer's directions.

Cause: Color was not applied evenly.

Solution: Be sure to apply the color evenly from a consistent parting pattern. Always double-check the hairline.

Note: If the situation arises immediately upon the completion of the color service, reformulate using all three primary colors and apply the color throughout.

Problem: The Ends Are Too Dark

Cause: Color was applied to the ends too soon or when not necessary.

Solution: Delay the application until the last 5-15 minutes of the processing time, depending on the porosity of the hair. Once the retouch is completed, apply color to the ends only if they are faded. Then reformulate with an oxidative color without ammonia.

Note: If the ends became too dark immediately upon the completion of the color service, try to remove some of the unwanted pigment by reshampooing the hair. In an extreme case you may need to use a lightener or color remover.

Problem: The Ends Are Too Light

Cause: Color was applied too late to the ends. Not enough development time was allowed.

Solution: Apply the formula sooner or adjust the color formula with a very low volume of developer.

Cause: Improper analysis of porosity was made.

Solution: If the ends are porous, use a filler on the ends prior to color application.

Cause: Improper at-home maintenance.

Solution: Recommend a shampoo and conditioner for color-treated hair to be used in between salon visits.

Note: If the ends are too light immediately upon the completion of the color service, reformulate using a very low volume of developer and apply the color to the ends.

It wasn't too long ago that many people approached the field of hair color with fear. Perhaps they had heard stories or had memories of coloring mishaps. Wonderful advances in coloring techniques and products have gone far to reduce that fear. After all, mistakes in hair cutting are often harder to remedy. A client may have to wait for the hair to grow back. Most color problems can be corrected immediately. For example, if the color is too light, you can add a few lowlights, if too dark, a few highlights.

Today a more common situation is the colorist who wants to give everyone a bold look. Many clients strive for a subtle, natural look. That is where your communication and consultation skills complement your ability to color. As your comfort and skill levels grow, your color work will take on an artistry of its own, defining the lines and shape of a cut or style, softening and warming a face, accentuating a client's lifestyle and personality. In the end, these skills will make you a sought-after and highly valued stylist.

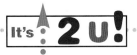

Build Your Critical Thinking Skills

In this chapter you have prepared yourself to meet the following Industry Standards for entry-level cosmetologists.

- Conduct a color service in accordance with a client's needs and expectations
- Conduct services in a safe environment and take measures to prevent the spread of infectious and contagious disease
- Take necessary steps to develop and retain clients
- Interact effectively with co-workers as part of a team
- Manage time to provide efficient client service

It's Up to You to know what to do. Using your training to this point, review the following case scenarios and think through how you would handle each challenge.

1. Your client has medium brown hair and is 30% gray. She has come to your salon for a corrective color. Her problem is that the last stylist did not use a color that covered the gray very well and the application was very poorly performed. Sections of the hair were missed completely, while other areas were spotty. What would you do?

2. A very busy executive who visits the salon every four weeks for a haircut has just mentioned to you that he is starting to notice his hair turning gray at the sides and crown. You have just mentioned the possibility of hair color and he appears to be interested but hesitant. What would you do?

Chapter 14

THE STUDY OF NAILS

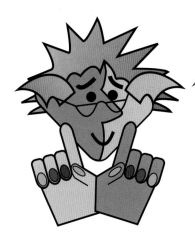

After studying this chapter you will be able to . . .

1. Describe the structure, growth, diseases, disorders and conditions of the nail.

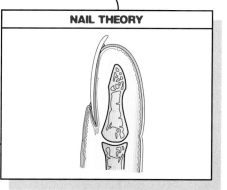

NAIL THEORY

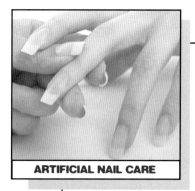

ARTIFICIAL NAIL CARE

3. Explain and demonstrate the services reviewed for artificial nail care.

2. Explain and demonstrate the services reviewed for natural nail care.

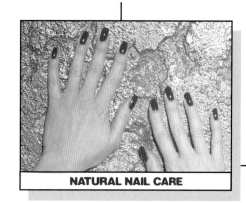

NATURAL NAIL CARE

Next to the face, the human hand is a person's most expressive feature. Just look at the way my hands in this chapter are a beautiful continuation of my face! Hands nurture, caress, instruct. You want to care for the hands of your clients as well as their feet so that they can continue to take their places in the world with confidence and composure and you can continue to take your place as an outstanding and caring professional.

MANI = hand + CURE = care
PEDI = foot + CURE = care

Providing specialized nail services for your clients will help improve their total image and in turn assist you in retaining more loyal clients.

Isn't it amazing that as you help improve your client's total image, you improve your own! A value-added service to the client brings VALUE to your life as well.

Knowing the theory behind nails plus the procedures for natural and artificial nail care prepares you to meet your client's total image needs.

To transform this chapter's BIG IDEA into action, I have a careful, three-point plan for you that once again helps you protect the health and safety of your clients at the same time as you enhance their total image.

NATURAL NAIL CARE
Nail Shapes
Nail Essentials
Infection Control and Safety
Client Consultation
Basic Manicure
Male Manicure
Pedicure Essentials
Basic Pedicure
Special Nail Services

ARTIFICIAL NAIL CARE
Artificial Nail Essentials
Infection Control and Safety
Nail Tips
Tips with Acrylic Overlay
Sculptured Nails
Additional Artificial Nail Services

NAIL THEORY
Nail Structure
Nail Growth
Nail Diseases, Disorders and
    Conditions

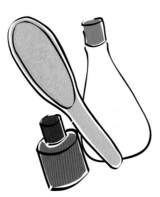

NAIL THEORY

Like the hair, the nail is an appendage of the skin. The technical name for the nail is onyx (**ON**-iks) just like the gemstone of the same name. The study of the structure and growth of the nails is called onychology (on-ih-**KOL**-o-gee).

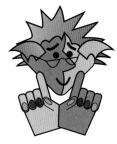

"You already know from Ch. 2 that ology means the study of something. If you add onyx + ology, PRESTO! You get onychology, one of those words in which the x changes to ch to make it easier to pronounce."

Nail Structure

The best way to learn nail structure is to examine a detailed diagram of the nail.

1. The **Free Edge** is the part of the nail that extends beyond the end of the finger and protects the tips of the fingers or toes.

2. The **Nail Body** (nail plate) is the visible nail area from the nail root to free edge. Made of layers. No nerves or blood vessels can be found here.

3. The **Nail Wall** is the folds of skin on either side of the nail groove.

4. The **Lunula** is the half-moon shape at the base of the nail, which appears white due to a reflection of light at the point where the nail matrix and nail bed meet.

5. The **Eponychium** (ep-o-**NIK**-ee-um) is the cuticle that overlaps the lunula at the base of the nail.

6. The **Cuticle** is the loose and pliable overlapping skin around the nail.

7. The **Nail Matrix** is the active tissue that generates cells, which harden as they move outward from the root to the nail.

8. The **Nail Root** is attached to the matrix at the base of the nail, under the skin and inside the mantle.

9. The **Mantle** is the pocket-like structure that holds the root and matrix.

10. The **Nail Bed** is the area of the nail on which the nail body rests. Nerves and blood vessels found here supply nourishment. Ligaments attach the nail bed to the bone.

11. The **Nail Grooves** are the tracks on either side of the nail that the nail moves on as it grows.

12. The **Perionychium** (**PER**-i-o-nik-ee-um) is the skin that touches, overlaps and surrounds the nail.

13. The **Hyponychium** (heye-poh-**NIK**-ee-um) is the skin under the free edge.

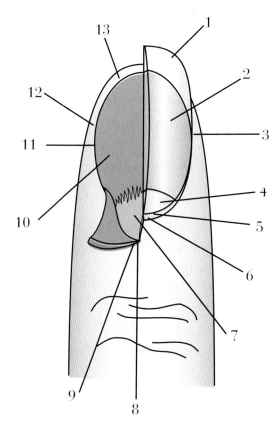

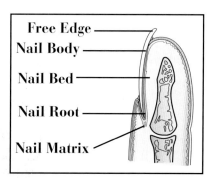

Free Edge
Nail Body
Nail Bed
Nail Root
Nail Matrix

Side view, cross section of finger

14

Nail Growth

Like the hair, the nail is made of keratin (hardened) protein. Although nail protein is much harder than the protein of hair, its growth is similar to the growth of hair. You already know that hair grows from a pocket-like structure called the follicle, originating from a row of reproducing cells called the germinal matrix. As these cells multiply, they are pushed upward and keratinize into the layers of the hair (cuticle, cortex, medulla). By the time the hair reaches the skin's surface, it is hardened and takes the shape of a hair strand. The same is true for nails.

Nail growth originates from active tissue known as the matrix, located in the mantle. The matrix contains lymph, blood vessels and nerves that create cells, which are pushed outward from the nail root. These cells keratinize (harden) as they continue toward the nail body (plate) and become fully hardened by the time they reach the eponychium. These hardened cells form the visible nail body (plate) that curves on the sides and travels in tracks found on the side of the nail called nail grooves. The nail plate can be thin, normal or thick, depending on the rate of production of cells in the matrix. **Under normal circumstances, growth of a new nail plate takes about four to six months.** The nail bed on which the nail body (plate) rests contains many nerves, as well as blood vessels for continuous nourishment.

Nails grow at an average rate of 1/8 inch (.35 cm) per month in adults. Nails grow more rapidly in younger people because general cell reproduction is occurring at a faster rate. Thus, as one ages, the growth of nails slows down.

Nail growth is faster in summer than in winter, and can be affected by nutrition, health or disease. The thumb nail grows slowest, while the nail on the middle finger grows fastest. Toenails are harder and thicker than fingernails but grow more slowly.

Injuries to the nail can result in shape distortions or nail discoloration. Most nail injuries are minor and resulting distortions and/or discoloration are temporary. Permanent distortions can occur when:

- **A nail is lost due to trauma and, without the protection of the nail plate, the nail bed or matrix is injured.**
- **A nail is lost through disease or infection. The regrown nail, in these circumstances, is often distorted in shape.**

Nail Diseases, Disorders and Conditions

Any disease, disorder or condition of the nail is called an onychosis (on-i-**KO**-sis).

- **If a disease is present, no nail service can be performed; the client must be referred to a physician.**
- **If a disorder is present, nail services may be done with care; the client may want to consult a physician for help and information.**

- **If a condition is present, nail services can be performed, and the condition should improve with correct techniques, products or improved nutrition.**

A study of onychosis considers four factors:

1. Identification of the disease, disorder or condition.

2. **Etiology** (e-te-**OL**-o-je) **or cause of the disease, disorder or condition.**

   a) Systemic (meaning throughout the system) causes are internal. They are related to illness, nutrition or heredity.

   b) Environmental causes include nail services or products (chemicals) that have adversely altered the skin or nail.

   c) Disease-related cause is often invasion of the skin or nail tissues by an agent like bacteria or fungi. These agents are contagious and spread by contact.

3. Diagnosis, the identification of an onychosis by the symptoms, and Prognosis, the outlook for recovery.

4. In-Salon Treatments:

   a) Products used and recommended for home care.

   b) Techniques used and taught to the client.

Hand and Nail Examination

To discover problems associated with the hands, nails or growth of nails, begin with a hand and nail examination. During a medical exam, a physician may look at a patient's hands, since they indicate the health of the body. As a cosmetologist, you observe the hands and nails to determine the type of services that should be performed to improve their condition and appearance. **There are six signs of infection in the nail and hands: pain, swelling, redness, local fever, throbbing and pus.** A healthy nail is smooth, curved, and without hollows or wavy ridges. It is flexible, translucent and pinkish in color.

Before performing an examination, wash and sanitize your hands and your client's hands. Then, hold the client's hands and turn front and back while observing:

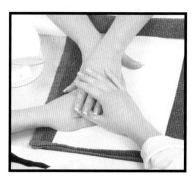

- Temperature of skin (coldness may indicate poor circulation; heat may indicate infection)

- Skin texture/feel (may indicate need for moisture)

- Inflammations/redness on hand or nails (may indicate need for moisture/possible diseases or disorders)

- Color/condition of nail bed (may identify visible injuries, disease and/or indications of poor circulation)

- Condition and length of free edge (may identify nail biter or "picker")

- Tenderness or stiff joints (special massage techniques may be required)

- Shape and thickness of nail plate (indicates how to properly file)

1 4

On determining that a special condition exists, explain it to the client and suggest products and care techniques to help overcome the condition. **Certain nail irregularities (often disease-related), however, must be referred to a physician for diagnosis or treatment and no nail service performed until the condition is alleviated.** When in doubt, refer your client to a physician.

Nail Diseases

Clients with nail diseases must be referred to their physician for treatment before nail services can be provided. A few of the irregularities shown below may have a disease-related or systemic cause. Identification of nail diseases is important to protect the health of the client and yourself.

Onychomycosis (o-ni-ko-mi-**KO**-sis) or **tinea unguium** (**TIN**-ee-ah **UN**-gwee-um) or **unguis** (**UN**-qwees) **is ringworm of the nail.**

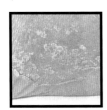

Cause: Fungus, disease-related, can result from a nail injury invaded by fungus.

Prognosis: Nail becomes thick and discolors from black to brown or beige to white; can develop white scaly patches with yellow streaks under nail plate; deformed nail may fall off; must be diagnosed and treated by a physician.

Treatment: No service may be performed.

Tinea (**TIN**-e-ah) **Manus is ringworm of the hand.**

Cause: Fungus, disease-related.

Prognosis: Appears as rings containing tiny blisters, dark pink to reddish in color; can have dry flakes; can be confused with eczema or contact dermatitis; can spread to nails, scalp, feet or body. Must be diagnosed and treated by a physician.

Treatment: No service may be performed.

Tinea Pedis (**TIN**-e-ah **PED**-is) **is "athlete's foot" or ringworm of the feet.**

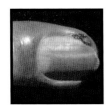

Cause: Fungus, disease-related; thrives in dark, moist places.

Prognosis: Itching and peeling of the skin on feet; blisters containing colorless fluid form in groups or singly on sores and between toes, leaving sore or itchy skin on one or both feet; must be diagnosed and treated by a physician.

Treatment: No service may be performed.

Paronychia (par-o-**NIK**-e-a), **or felon, is inflammation of skin around the nail.**

Cause: Bacterial infection, disease-related condition of the tissue surrounding the nail can occur if a hangnail gets infected. Prolonged exposure of hands to water can create conditions favorable for paronychia to develop.

Prognosis: Red, swollen, sore, warm to touch, can lose the nail; must be diagnosed and treated by a physician; healing takes 4 weeks; nail may grow out deformed but can recover shape.

Treatment: No service may be performed.

Onychoptosis (o-ni-kop-TO-sis) refers to shedding or falling off of nails.

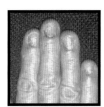

Cause: Disease and injury related.

Prognosis: If the disease causing the problem is cured, the nail will regrow; may occur on only one or two nails; nail bed will be sensitive and should be protected while nail regrows.

Treatment: No service may be performed on affected nails.

Onychia (o-NIK-e-a) is inflammation of the nail matrix.

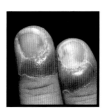

Cause: Bacterial infection, disease-related.

Prognosis: Inflammation of the nail matrix, pus formation; red, swollen and tender; nail may stop growing, and plate may detach; nail may not grow back; if it does, it will probably be deformed; must be diagnosed and treated by a physician.

Treatment: No service may be performed.

Onychatrophia (o-ni-ka-TRO-fe-a) is atrophy of the nail or wasting away of nail.

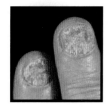

Cause: Injury or systemic disease.

Prognosis: Nail shrinks in size and may separate from nail bed; if illness-related, may not improve if matrix is damaged; the nail may improve in 3-6 months.

Treatment: No service may be performed.

Onycholysis (o-ni-KOL-i-sis) refers to a loosening or separation of the nail.

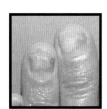

Cause: Internal disorder, infection or drug treatment; systemic, disease-related.

Prognosis: Loosening of the nail plate starting at the free edge and progressing to the lunula; nail doesn't come off; stays attached at root area; must be diagnosed and treated by a physician.

Treatment: Do not touch. No service may be performed.

Nail Disorders

Unless infection is present, clients with nail disorders may receive modified nail services.

Blue Nails appear bluish in color.

Cause: Systemic problems of the heart, poor circulation or injury.

Prognosis: "Blue" color in skin under nails; can be solved if cause is eliminated; common in older people.

Treatment: Make client aware of problem and possible causes; suggest seeing a physician; manicure with caution, using light pressure.

Eggshell nails are very thin, soft nails.

Cause: Hereditary or nervous condition

Prognosis: Thin nails, almost see-through, transparent

Treatment: Regular application of top coat, nail strengtheners or artificial nails as well as good dietary practices.

1
4

Corrugations (kor-u-GA-shuns) are horizontal wavy ridges across the nail.

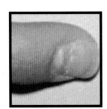

Cause: Injury, systemic conditions; uneven growth.

Prognosis: Easily recognizable; if injury-related, it may grow out and disappear; systemic conditions may cause permanent ridges.

Treatment: Lightly buff to level the nail surface; apply a base coat or ridge filler to protect and even surface. Avoid overbuffing, since it is easy to thin the nail plate.

Kolionychia (kol-e-o-NIK-e-a) or Spoon nails are nails with a concave shape.

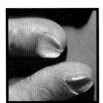

Cause: Systemic or long-term illness or nerve disturbance.

Prognosis: Unusual nail shapes; unlikely to disappear.

Treatment: File carefully; apply no pressure to nail plate; use polish to harden and protect nails.

Furrows are indented vertical lines down the nail plate.

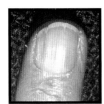

Cause: Injury to matrix that causes cells to reproduce unevenly; can be nutrition, injury or illness-related; pushing too hard with pusher during nail service or exposure to harsh chemicals.

Prognosis: Easily recognizable; may grow out; may be permanent.

Treatment: Lightly buff; apply base coat or ridge filler to protect and even out surface; perform nail service as usual.

Onychogryposis (o-ni-ko-GRI-po-sis) also called "claw nails" represent an increased curvature of the nails.

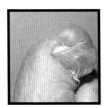

Cause: Systemic.

Prognosis: Increased thickness and curving of the nail that may occur with age or injury to nail; most often occurring in the big toe; physicians may remove if severely deformed or difficult to keep clean.

Treatment: Look for signs of infection; clean well under free edge; file with emery board and keep nails short; only a podiatrist should trim.

Onychocryptosis (o-ni-ko-KRIP-to-sis) are ingrown nails.

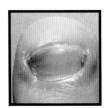

Cause: Environmental or poor nail trimming practices; can become infected.

Prognosis: If the nail grows into the edge of the nail groove cutting the skin or becomes deeply embedded and/or infected, refer client to a physician who will remove the skin or portion of nail causing the problem. It may also occur on toes if shoes are too tight, or if the toenails are filed too deeply on sides.

Treatment: Thoroughly soften skin, trim nail straight across to prevent pressure on the nail groove. If infection has occurred, DO NOT perform service. Refer to a physician.

Onychauxis (o-ni-**KOK**-sis) or **Hypertrophy is a thickening of the nail plate or an abnormal outgrowth of the nail.**

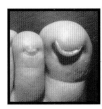

Cause: Injury to nail or systemic.

Prognosis: Easily recognizable; likely to disappear.

Treatment: Can be lightly buffed to even out the nail plate.

Nail Conditions

Nail conditions are generally minor irregularities that allow the client to receive either full or modified nail services.

Agnails (hangnails) are split cuticles; loose skin partially separated from the cuticle.

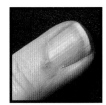

Cause: Cuticle is overly dry and splits; environmentally caused.

Prognosis: Skin breaks at corners of nails; can be trimmed with cuticle nippers and may heal in 2-3 days; can be reoccurring.

Treatment: Trim only separated hangnail skin completely; moisturize and avoid massaging the area. Instruct the client to use cuticle oil daily. Hangnails may become infected if not properly treated.

Bruised Nails (also called splinter hemorrages) show dark purplish discoloration under the nail.

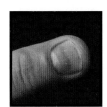

Cause: Trauma to nail; environmental; blood trapped under nails or small capillaries hemorrhage.

Prognosis: Discoloration under nail; normal nail growth will continue; bruised area will grow out with nail.

Treatment: No pressure on nail plate.

Leuconychia (loo-ko-**NIK**-e-a) **are white spots appearing in the nail.**

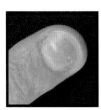

Cause: Injury to the nail, heredity, signs of systemic disorders or nutritional deficiency.

Prognosis: A small separation from the nail bed; grows out with the nail.

Treatment: Make client aware of possible cause; perform nail service as usual.

Pterygium (te **RIJ**-e-ge-uhm) **or pterygium unguis refers to overgrown cuticles.**

Cause: Cuticle sticks to the nail plate if not pushed back regularly.

Prognosis: Excess cuticle that splits and/or eventually tears.

Treatment: Soften and massage cuticles back into position with an orangewood stick; advise client to push cuticles back with a towel after bath or shower daily.

1 4

Onychophagy (o-ni-**KOF**-a-je) **refers to bitten nails.**

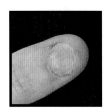

Cause: Nervous habit, stress related.

Prognosis: Easily recognizable; if biting stops, the nails will regrow; may be sensitive to touch; nail plate will appear flat and may be deformed until an entire nail has regrown from the matrix; can completely recover.

Treatment: Perform nail service weekly, apply polish to nails.

Onychorrhexis (o-ni-ko-**REK**-sis) **are split or brittle nails.**

Cause: Injury, improper filing, harsh chemical contact.

Prognosis: Easily recognizable; file with emery board carefully; may be a permanent condition.

Treatment: Soften nails well before trimming; do hot oil manicure; advise client to perform moisturizing treatments daily at home. Wear rubber gloves when hands are in water or chemicals.

Pigmentation Problems

Discoloration of the nail can indicate serious problems in the nail bed or nail plate. In general, all changes of color should be referred to a physician unless they can be removed by a cleansing agent like soap. Vitamin deficiencies, bacterial infections, fungal infestations, protein deficiencies, kidney or liver disorders or reactions to medications can all cause discoloration. They should not be ignored. **The condition of the hands and nails will often indicate the overall health of the body.**

> **Nail fungus or mold causes discoloration and is a very contagious vegetable parasite that is easily spread. Early stages are indicated by a yellow-green spot that eventually becomes black. At that stage the nail softens and smells bad. Refer clients with nail fungus to a physician.**

NATURAL NAIL CARE

Nail care, like hair design, is a science, a service and an art. Nail care can be an "extra" service you provide to your client or it can be a creative specialty. Nail specialists are called nail technicians.

Since women compose an ever-growing portion of the workforce, it is increasingly important that a woman's hands always look their best. Women, however, are not unique in their need for well-groomed hands. The well-dressed man conducting a business meeting during which attention is drawn, even inadvertently, to bitten, ragged, or dirty nails is conveying a subtle message of inconsistency or of failure to pay attention to detail. All people are at least initially judged by their appearance.

The purpose of a nail service is to improve the appearance of the hands and, in particular, the nails. A good nail service completes the picture begun by great looking hair and skin and carefully selected clothing.

Nail Shapes

Although nails grow in assorted shapes and sizes from convex to concave, wide to narrow, round to angular, **there are four basic nail shapes: pointed, oval, round and square.** Generally, the more square the nail shape, the stronger it is. It will be your job to enhance the natural shape of

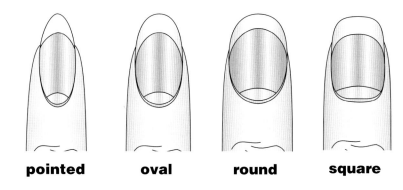

pointed   **oval**   **round**   **square**

your clients' nails, the shape of their fingers and the overall appearance of their hands. In choosing the nail length and polish color you'll recommend, consider the appearance of your clients' hands, what they do with their hands each day and, of course, your clients' wishes.

Nail Essentials

To perform a professional nail service, you need a selection of products, implements and equipment. Nail service products are produced by many different manufacturers, are disposable and must be frequently replaced. Material Safety Data Sheets (MSDS) for all products used in the salon must be available. Nail service implements are the hand-held tools you use. They must be disinfected or discarded after every use. Nail service equipment includes the furnishings and provisions necessary to provide a professional nail service.

Nail Service Products

PRODUCT	DESCRIPTION	FUNCTION
General Disinfectant	Liquid, effective bactericidal	Disinfects metal tools and implements
Antiseptic	Liquid or foam-based products	Reduces bacteria, viruses and fungus on skin
First Aid Cream or Styptic Powder	Antiseptic	Stops bleeding when applied
Polish Remover	Acetone or non-acetone	Dissolves polish
Cotton Balls or Pledglets	Absorbent; pledglets are cotton pads	Used to apply polish removers, powder feet, remove lotions from nail plate
Cuticle Remover Cream	Low percent hydrogen peroxide, sodium or potassium hydroxide	Loosens dead skin

14

PRODUCT	DESCRIPTION	FUNCTION
Nail Bleach	Lightener or high percent hydrogen peroxide	Removes stains and whitens nails
Soaking Solution	Liquid antibacterial soap used with warm water in finger bowl	Softens skin, loosens dirt, aids in pushing back cuticle
Cuticle Cream or Oil	Moisturizer	Softens cuticle skin, moisturizes brittle nails
Hand Lotion	Lubricant	Softens skin and aids when providing massage manipulations
Base Coat	Colorless polish	Evens out nail plate, holds nail color to nail, prevents pigments from penetrating nail plate
Liquid Polish	Colored polish, enamel	Creates a colored effect
Top Coat or Sealer	Colorless hard polish	Protects colored polish from chipping, fading and peeling
Speed Dry (Nail Dryer)	Drying agent; spray or polish applied over top coat	Aids in fast drying of polish; protects from stickiness or matte finish to polish
Nail Conditioner	Moisturizing ingredients	Applied to nails to avoid dryness
Nail Mend Fiber	Mending material; silk, paper, fiberglass	Repair splits or cracks on the nail
Nail Strengthener (Nail Hardeners)	Usually a clear polish applied prior to the base coat; may contain strengthening fibers	Prevents nails from splitting and peeling
Liquid Nail Wrap	Polish consisting of tiny strengthening fibers; more fiber than a nail hardner	Hardens and protects the nail

Nail Service Implements/Supplies

IMPLEMENT/SUPPLIES	FUNCTION
Emery Board	Shortens and shapes natural nails and smoothes rough edges by using sandpaper-like fine and coarse sides
Cuticle Pusher	Pushes cuticle; pointed ends should be used carefully
Orangewood Stick	Loosens debris and is used to apply creams and clean under free edge

IMPLEMENT/SUPPLIES	FUNCTION
Cuticle Nipper	Trims hangnails; check with your regulatory agency regarding usage
Nail and Cuticle Scissors	Cuts nails or trims mending fiber
Nail Brush	Cleans nails and removes debris before polishing
Tweezer	Manages detail work such as nail art
Block Buffer/3-Way Buffer	Smoothes surface of the nail; some states do not permit use
Cosmetic Spatula	Removes cream from jars in an effort to meet infection control guidelines
Finger Bowl	Allows comfortable soaking of nails
Towels	Dries hands and nails

Nail Service Equipment

EQUIPMENT	FUNCTION
Nail Service Table	Provides a place for all tools to be laid out; is the proper height for comfort; may have an attached light
Nail Service Stool	Allows easy access to all tools and the client because seat is adjustable
Client's Chair	Provides proper back support and comfort to client during nail service
Nail Service Cushion	Forms a cushion to rest client's arm during service while drying hands (towels may be used in the absence of a cushion)
Wet Disinfectant Container	Holds disinfectant for disinfecting implements under infection control guidelines
Electric Heater	Heats cream for specialized nail services
Glass Container	Holds absorbent cotton, cotton swabs and other accessories
Lamp	Lights the area for close detail work (most often purchased as part of the table or may be purchased separately and attached to table); generally uses a 40 watt bulb

1
4

Infection Control and Safety

Infection control and safety while performing nail services is essential in order to protect the health and well-being of you and your client. It begins with your conscientious efforts to keep your nail table clean and organized and continues throughout the service. Always:

- Wash your hands and have your client wash their hands with liquid antibacterial soap.

- Follow manufacturer's directions on all products being used.

- Avoid filing too deeply into the corners of the nails to prevent ingrown nails.

- Wash implements with soap and water then disinfect after every service; store in a dry, covered container and handle sharp-pointed implements carefully.

- Wear protective gloves during nail services, if required.

- Clean and disinfect nail service tabletop after every service.

- Check that all bottle tops and container lids are tightly sealed and labeled.

- Empty soaking solution from finger bowl. Disinfect and replace with fresh solution for every client.

- Clean the surface of the foot bath ensuring that all debris is removed from behind the drain screen; disinfect following manufacturer's directions.

- Arrange all products and implements in proper order.

- Handle all products carefully and avoid spillage. Use spatulas to remove creams from containers.

- Practice blood spill procedures if a blood spill occurs.

- Discard non-reusable materials such as emery boards in a closed (container) waste receptacle.

Blood Spill Procedure

If a blood spill should occur, use the following steps:

1. Stop the service and wash your hands.

2. Cover your hands with protective gloves.

3. Supply the injured party with styptic powder or spray and the appropriate dressing to cover the injury. If you are injured, cover the area with a finger guard or glove, as appropriate.

4. Do not allow containers, brushes, nozzles or styptic container to touch the skin or come in contact with the wound.

5. Disinfect implements and work station with a broad spectrum disinfectant.

6. Double-bag all blood-soiled (contaminated) articles and label the bag as hazardous waste or as directed by your area's regulating agency.

7. Remove your gloves and clean your hands with a liquid antibacterial soap.

8. Return to client and continue the service.

Client Consultation

To help you remember the important steps in the consultation process, remember: Great Artists Always Draw Creatively. Just change your focus to your client's nails.

Greet

- Meet and greet the client with a firm handshake and a pleasant voice.

- Communicate to build rapport and develop a relationship with the client.

Ask, Analyze and Assess

- Ask questions to discover client needs.

- Analyze client's nails and hands.

- Assess the facts and thoroughly think through your recommendations.

Agree

- Explain your recommended solutions, the products that will be used and the price of the service.

- Think not only of today's service, but future services also.

- Return to step two (ask, analyze and assess) if your client is hesitant with your recommendation.

- Gain feedback and approval from your client.

CLIENT NAIL RECORD CARD

Name: _____ Nail Technician: _____
Home Address: _____ Work Address: _____
_____ _____
_____ _____
Home Phone: _____ Work Phone: _____
Best hours for appointment are: _____

Client Profile
1. What type of work do you do? _____
2. Do you have any hobbies that require you to work with your hands? _____
3. Do you participate in sports activities? _____ If so, what type? _____
4. Do you use rubber gloves when doing housework? _____
5. How much time do you spend each week caring for your own nails? _____
6. How frequently do you have professional nail service(s)? _____

Medical Record
Do you have:__ Arthritis __ Heart Problems __ High Blood Pressure __ Cancer __ Diabetes
If you answered yes to any of the above questions, what kind of medication, if any, do you take?

Are there any other medical conditions or medications that we should be aware of?
_____

Deliver

- Ensure client comfort during service.

- Stay focused on delivering the service to the best of your ability.

- Teach the client how to perform home nail-care maintenance.

- Have a range of colors available and emphasize the importance of a base coat and a top coat.

Complete

- Request satisfaction feedback from your client.

- Escort client to retail area and show him/her at least two products you used.

- Recommend products to maintain appearance and condition of your client's nails.

- Inform client that you keep these products in stock for purchase at all times.

- Invite your client to make a purchase.

- Ask your client for referrals for future services.

- Suggest a future appointment time for your client's next visit.

- Offer appreciation to your client for visiting the school or salon.

- Record recommended products on client record card for future visits.

1
4

Basic Manicure

Manicure is the cosmetic care of the hands and finger-nails. The Latin word "manus" means hand and "cura" means care.

As with any professional service, it is important to have your area, products, implements and equipment in proper order prior to your client's arrival. Before performing a basic manicure service, be sure to satisfy the following client preparation points.

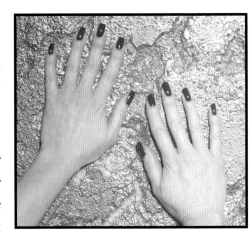

Basic Manicure Preparation

- Clean nail table with disinfectant

- Place fresh soaking solution to the left of the client on the nail service table, near technician

- Clean, disinfect and place nail service implements on the nail table

- Review and arrange products conveniently, in order of usual use

Basic Manicure Procedure

- Wash and sanitize hands*
- Perform visual examination of hands and nails
- Remove polish
- Analyze skin and nails thoroughly
- Consult with client
- File and shape nails
- Apply cuticle remover
- Place hand in finger bowl
- Repeat filing, shaping and cuticle care on opposite hand
- Pat first hand dry
- Push back cuticles
- Scrub hand and nails

- Clean under free edge
- Pat hand dry
- Repeat cuticle care and cleaning on opposite hand
- Apply massage lotion or cream
- Perform massage techniques
- Remove all traces of massage lotion or cream from nails
- Apply base coat
- Apply two coats of polish
- Apply polish at free edge
- Remove excess polish from skin
- Apply top coat and quick-dry product

*Wear protective gloves if required by your regulating agency.

Manicure

1. Wash and sanitize your own and your client's hands and nails and apply a topical antiseptic. **Perform visual examination of the hands and nails.** Continue if there are no noticeable diseases or disorders.

2. Remove polish from base to tip on the nails of both hands to prepare for the examination. Use polish remover and cotton, and wipe from the base of the nail to the tip to avoid leaving polish residue on the skin.

3. Analyze skin and nails thoroughly. Consult with your client about shape and length of nails desired.

Nail Prep

4. File and shape the nails with an emery board.

    a. Begin with the little finger on one hand and shape from the outer edge of the nail toward the center to avoid splitting.

    b. Use 2-3 short strokes on each side of the nail and one longer stroke per side to blend. Round the top of the nail gently.

Cuticle Care

5. Apply cuticle remover cream to one hand.

6. Place the hand in the finger bowl to allow cuticles to soften. **Repeat filing, shaping and cuticle care on the opposite hand.**

7. Pat the client's first hand dry with a towel, and place the other hand in soaking solution. Gently **push back the cuticle** on each finger on the first hand with a cotton-wrapped orangewood stick or cuticle pusher.

Manicure

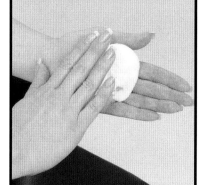

1

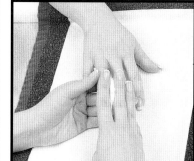

2

Nail Prep

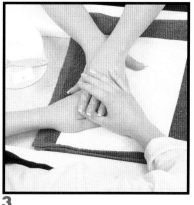

3

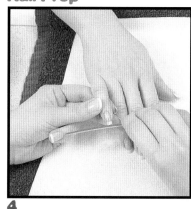

4

Cuticle Care

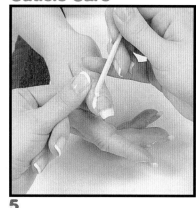

5

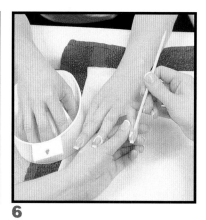

6

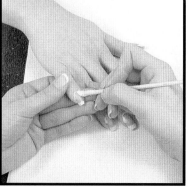

7

If you trim the cuticle, try to use a cutting method that utilizes removing the cuticle as one segment.

1
4

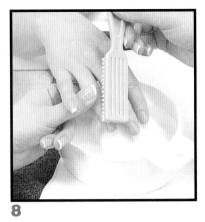

8

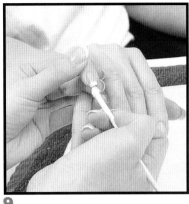

9

Massage

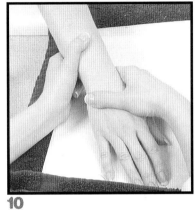

10

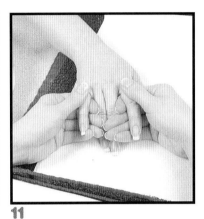

11

Polish

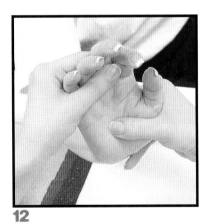

12

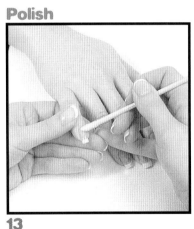

13

Reminder:

- Ensure the comfort of your client throughout the service

- Work neatly

- Maintain professional communication

Hangnails may be trimmed to the surface of the skin. Note that cutting or trimming cuticles is illegal in some areas. Check with your area's regulating agency.

8. **Scrub hand and nails** with a nail brush in a downward direction and then dry hand.

9. **Clean under the free-edge** of each nail with a cotton-wrapped orangewood stick. **Pat hand dry. Repeat cuticle care and cleaning on the opposite hand.**

Massage

The massage portion of the manicure is key to the relaxation and pampering of the client. The following are some basic techniques. Be guided by your instructor for additional manipulations.

10. Apply massage lotion or cream from elbow to forearm and down to the fingertips to prepare for the massage. **Perform massage techniques** on both hands using long rhythmic effleurage strokes. Rotate in a circular motion to loosen the wrist.

11. Massage fingers using a circular motion called joint movement.

12. Knead palm with petrissage, moving thumbs in a circular motion from wrist to fingers.

13. Remove all traces of massage lotion or cream from nails before applying polish. Use a cotton-wrapped orangewood stick soaked in polish remover underneath and on the surface of the nail.

Polish

14. **Apply base coat,** beginning with the little finger of one hand and working toward the thumb. Repeat on opposite hand.

15. **Apply two coats of polish,** using light, sweeping strokes from nail base to free edge. Polish middle of nails first, then the sides. Repeat the second coat when all ten nails are polished.

16-17. **Apply polish at the free edge** to help prevent chipping. **Remove excess polish from skin** with orange-wood stick, wrapped in cotton and saturated with polish remover. **Apply top coat and a quick-drying product,** which may be a spray, pump or polish.

Polish

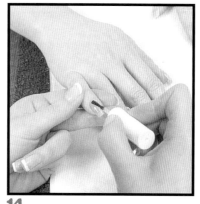
14

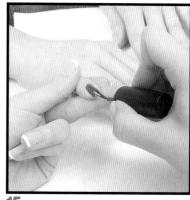
15

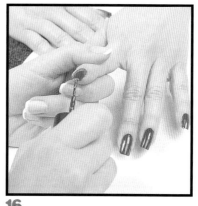
16

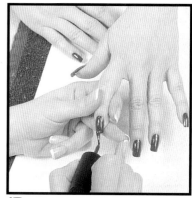
17

Basic Manicure Completion

Perform after every nail service:

- Offer a rebook visit to your client

- Recommend retail products to your client

- Discard non-reusable materials, replace used towels with fresh towels and arrange all products and implements in proper order

- Disinfect your nail service implements and the top of the nail service table

- Wash your hands with antibacterial liquid soap

Avoid causing air bubbles by rolling the nail polish bottle between your palms to mix. Shaking a polish bottle will cause the application to appear uneven.

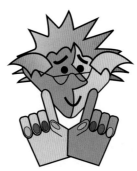

"Keep in mind that the techniques in the basic manicure are the foundation for all other nail services."

14

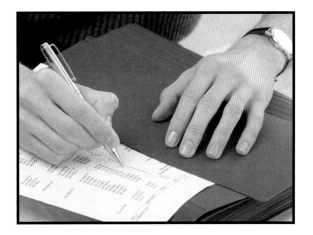

Male Manicure

The procedure for a male manicure is basically the same as the basic manicure just described. There are a few variations to keep in mind.

1. File men's nails short usually into either a round or square shape.

2. Apply a clear base coat and top coat only, if polish is desired.

3. Use a 3-way buffer to create a natural shine or proceed to step 4 for an oil buff. Use horizontal movements, working from the base of the nail to the free edge. Buff with the black side, then buff with the white side, and finally the gray side. Lift the buffer from the nail to break contact between strokes, which will avoid overheating the nail.

4. Apply oil to the nail before buffing with the gray side to create an oil buff. Buffing should be limited to every 2-3 weeks to avoid overthinning the natural nail.

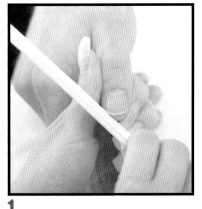

1

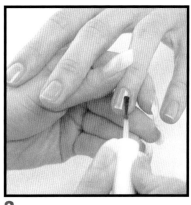

2

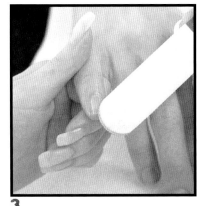

3

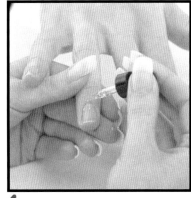

4

Pedicure Essentials

The following items are necessary to complete a pedicure service along with the items used for the basic manicure service.

Pedicure Service Products

PRODUCT	FUNCTION
Foot Soak	Cleans and softens the work area; antibacterial soap
Foot Spray	Removes germs from skin; acts as an antiseptic

PRODUCT	FUNCTION
Sloughing Lotion	Removes dead skin cells
Foot Lotion	Moisturizes and stimulates the feet
Foot Powder	Dries and deodorizes

Pedicure Service Implements/Supplies

IMPLEMENT/SUPPLIES	FUNCTION
Foot File	Softens and removes calluses; paddle with a gritty surface
Foot Brush	Cleans nails and removes debris; stiff brush
Toenail Clipper	Shortens toenails
Toe Separators	Separates toes during polish technique; made of foam, rubber or cotton
Slippers	Protect feet while polish dries

Pedicure Service Equipment

EQUIPMENT	FUNCTION
Pedicure Table	Holds and stores all equipment, products and implements
Pedicure Foot Rest	Props up the client's feet for the service
Pedicure Chair	Provides comfortable chair for clients
Foot Bath or Tub	Serves as basin to soak feet

Basic Pedicure

Pedicuring is the cosmetic care of the feet and toenails. The Latin word "ped" means foot and "cura" means care.

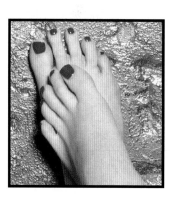

Basic Pedicure Preparation

Preparation for a basic pedicure is similar to that for a manicure along with the guidelines listed below:

- Clean and disinfect implements

- Set up equipment and lay out tools on sanitized table

- Review and arrange products conveniently, in order of use

- Gather products and solutions needed from the dispensary

- Prepare the foot bath with enough sanitizing solution to cover both feet

- Wash your hands with liquid antibacterial soap

1
4

Basic Pedicure Procedure

- Wash and sanitize hands*
- Sanitize client's feet
- Perform a visual examination
- Soak and dry feet
- Remove nail polish
- Examine feet
- Trim and file nails
- Apply cuticle remover cream
- Push back cuticles
- Apply sloughing lotion and massage to remove dead skin cells
- Repeat trimming, filing and cuticle care on opposite foot

- Soak and scrub both feet with brush to remove debris
- Dry thoroughly
- Massage with lotion
- Remove excess lotion from nail surface
- Apply powder and position toe separators
- Apply base coat
- Apply two coats of polish
- Apply top coat, followed by quick-drying product
- Allow drying time
- Remove toe separators when dry

*Wear protective gloves if required by your regulating agency.

Pedicure

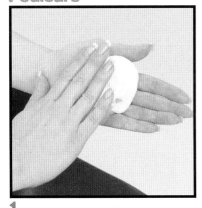
1

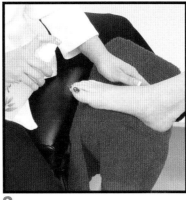
2

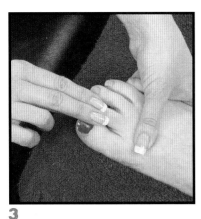
3

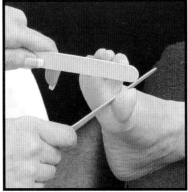
4

Pedicure

1. Wash and sanitize hands by washing and applying antiseptic. Waterless or foam antiseptics are easy to use.

2. Sanitize your client's feet by spraying each foot with an antiseptic. **Perform a visual examination.** If there is no sign of disease or disorder, place client's feet in the foot bath and allow to **soak** according to manufacturer's directions, usually 5-10 minutes.

3. Remove client's feet from the foot bath, **dry** them and place on the foot rest. **Remove nail polish**, if any.

4. Examine the feet for any abnormalities. Use disposable spatulas to separate toes. If there are no problems, continue service.

5. Trim and file nails. If nails are too long, use a toenail clipper. Position the clipper horizontally.

6. File straight across, softening the corners to avoid ingrown toenails. Avoid clipping or filing too deeply into the corners.

7. Apply **cuticle remover cream** to each toe. **Push back cuticles** with a cotton-wrapped orangewood stick.

8. Apply **sloughing lotion** to entire foot and **massage to remove dead skin cells.** If needed, use a foot file or paddle. **Repeat trimming, filing and cuticle care on the opposite foot. Scrub both feet with brush to remove any debris** and clean under toenails. Remove each foot from bath and **dry thoroughly**.

Massage

Foot massage is very similar to hand massage, but your movements can be firmer and larger. A benefit of foot massage is the prevention of foot and leg problems. In order to maintain relaxation, do not drop the foot or break contact during massage manipulation.

9. Massage with lotion. Use effleurage strokes to apply lotion to foot and calf.

10. Then, use circular kneading movements, beginning at the knee and going down to the ankle and back up to knee avoiding the shinbone and area above the knee. Apply pressure to the muscular tissue on either side of the shinbone. Repeat three times.

11. Massage top of each foot and toe.

12. Knead (petrissage) the sole, using circular movements.

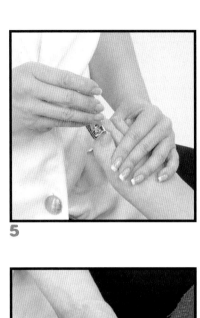
5

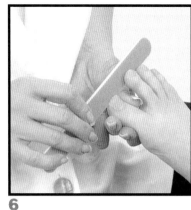
6

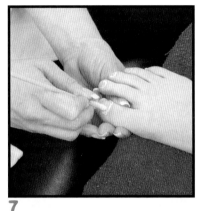
7

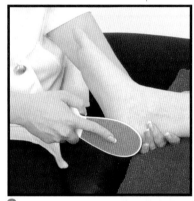
8

Massage

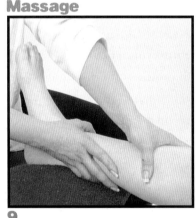
9

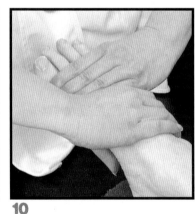
10

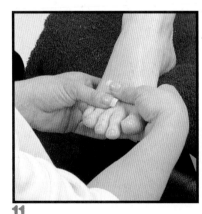
11

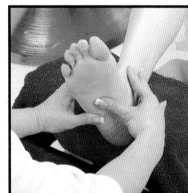
12

1
4

Polish

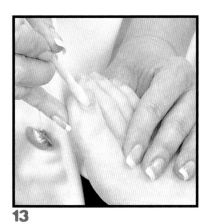
13

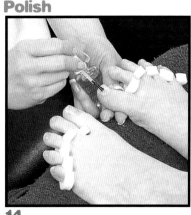
14

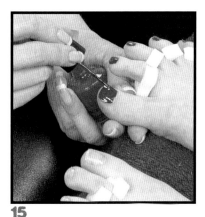
15

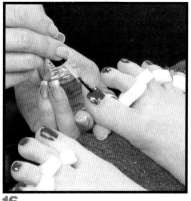
16

13. **Remove excess lotion from the nail surface** with a cotton-wrapped orangewood stick soaked in polish remover.

Polish

14. **Apply powder** with cotton to the feet, then **position toe separators.** If desired, slippers may be put on prior to the toe separators. **Apply base coat** to the nails of both feet. Start at the little toe and work to the big toe.

15. Apply two coats of polish.

16. **Apply top coat,** followed by a quick-drying product. **Allow drying time** up to one hour. **Remove the toe separators when polish is dry.**

Basic Pedicure Completion

- Offer a rebook visit to your client
- Recommend retail products for your client
- Discard non-reusable materials, replace used towels with fresh towels and arrange all products and implements in proper order
- Disinfect your pedicure service implements and equipment
- Wash your hands with liquid antibacterial soap

Special Nail Services

Additional services may sometimes be required to accommodate your client's special needs. Five of these special services will be described here.

French Manicure

A French manicure is similar to the plain manicure with two exceptions:

- White polish is applied on the free edge.
- Pink or peach polish is applied to the entire nail.

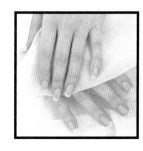

Nail Repair (Mending with Silk)

Along with the products used for the basic manicure procedure, you will also need the following items for repairing nails: adhesive accelerator, silk, dehydrant and an adhesive. Split or broken (cracked) nails can be repaired to a smooth surface appearance using the steps on the following page:

Nail Repair Guidelines

1. **Smooth the surface of the nail gently over the broken or split area** with the black side of a 3-way buffer to remove surface oil.

2. **Apply dehydrant** to the nail.

3. **Cut a small piece of** (silk) **fiber**, sized slightly larger, to cover split or break.

4. **Apply adhesive** to split or broken area of the nail. Do not touch skin or cuticle with adhesive.

5. **Place silk**, using tweezer, over split or broken portion of nail. Cut away any uneven edges.

6. **Smooth repaired area** with orangewood stick.

7. **Apply second layer of adhesive** to seal. Avoid touching the skin. You may apply adhesive accelerator to speed drying time.

8. **Allow to dry** thoroughly.

9. **Buff smooth** with 3-way buffer.

10. **Soak and scrub** nail repair area.

11. **Continue** with nail service.

Hot Oil or Cream Manicure

These nail services involve the use of an electric heating device. Instead of placing a client's hand in a warm water soaking solution, the hand is placed in warmed oil or cream. All other procedures for this nail service are the same as in a basic nail service. This procedure is helpful for very dry, aging or abused hands and on ridged or brittle nails.

Electric Nail Services

Special electrically powered tools can perform the same procedures as a basic nail service. Emery discs file the length of the nails, vibrating devices aid in pushing cuticles, spinning nail brushes remove debris, and coarse sandpaper discs act like an abrasive on calluses. Nail buffing discs can not be used in certain areas. Take precautions to avoid heat friction and overthinning of nail plates when using any electric equipment on natural nails. Nail drills should be used only on artificial nail applications. Check with your area's regulating agency. No matter what electric nail services you offer, always perform the service in a caring and personal manner.

Nail Art

Nail art is an additional service that some salons offer their clients. With this service, your creativity can be expressed in many different ways. Nail art can range from simple patterns to detailed landscape scenes, or even character faces. Flat nail art is created by using nail paints and stripping tape. Three-dimensional nail art is created with rhinestones, feathers, painted acrylic beads, etc. Airbrush nail art is applied with an airbrush gun and airbrush paints. Nail jewelry is also a popular option.

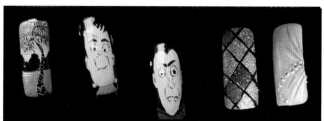

Nail art by Dora Brooks

1
4

ARTIFICIAL NAIL CARE

Artificial nails are used to improve the appearance of one's nails and help to conceal broken nails. There are several types of artificial nail products currently available for use in the salon. Each has special procedures individualized by the manufacturer of the product. Since each brand of artificial nails can vary greatly in application procedure, your review in this text will be centered around the basic product ingredients and procedures.

Some nails are too thin or weak to grow to the length the client may desire. These clients are no longer doomed to wearing their nails short forever. In offering your clients the alternative of wearing artificial nails, you're offering them something they may have thought they'd never have–the opportunity to have truly lovely hands!

Artificial nails can be applied over a plastic tip or created directly on the nail. Prior to an artificial nail service, a basic manicure should be performed up to but not including the base coat.

There are three general product systems by which artificial nails can be created, which are:

1. Powder and Liquid Acrylic
2. Wraps and No-Light Gels
3. Light-Cured Gels

In the past, a discoloration found between the nail plate and an artificial nail was referred to as a mold, but was actually a bacterial infection caused by pseudomonas aeruginosa, a bacteria occurring naturally on the skin. In favorable conditions, such as a lack of oxygen, the bacteria grows unrestrained and causes an infection which leads to discoloration of the nail.

In this chapter you will learn the procedures for the most common applications: Nail Tips, Tips with Acrylic Overlays and Sculptured Nails. You will also be introduced to Fiberglass Wraps and Light-Cured Nails.

Artificial Nail Essentials

Just like natural nail manicure and pedicure services, artificial nail services require a selection of products and implements. The following items are necessary to complete an artificial nail service along with the items used for the basic manicure service. Each is described by name, description and/or function.

Artificial Nail Service Products

PRODUCT	FUNCTION
Monomer	Mixes with the powder to form an acrylic nail; liquid in form
Polymer	Mixes with the monomer to form an acrylic nail; powder in form
Primer	Ensures adhesion of acrylic product to nail
Nail Tips	Adhere to nail; they have a hollowed area on one end called the nail well, which is attached to the natural nail; plastic extension

PRODUCT	FUNCTION
Nail Form	Forms an acrylic extension to the natural nail; plastic, paper or metal templates
Adhesive	Bonds a plastic tip to a natural nail; specially formulated for the nail industry; tacky (sticky) substance
Dehydrant (Antiseptic)	Reduces the amount of moisture in the nail when brushed over the nail plate; allows better adhesion of nail enhancements and reduces growth of fungus
Brush Cleaner	Removes any residual nail enhancement product from the bristles of a brush

Artificial Nail Service Implements/Supplies

IMPLEMENT/SUPPLIES	FUNCTION
Dappen Dish	Holds monomer and polymer separately
Acrylic Brush	Builds the acrylic nail; may be flat, oval or rounded in shape and is made from natural hair, such as sable
Nail File	Shortens, files and shapes artificial nails; coarse-grit
Block Buffer	Smoothes nails; rectangular abrasive block
Eyedropper	Removes acrylic liquid from container to dappen dish

Infection Control and Safety

1. Wear protective goggles when using adhesive and filing acrylic nails.
2. Keep all lids on product containers tight to prevent vapor leakage.
3. Insure that ventilation is adequate and provides an intake of outside air and a return of salon air.
4. Avoid allowing primer (hydrant) to come in contact with skin since it may cause burning.
5. Dispose of all monomer and polymer together in a sealed plastic bag. Do not pour monomer or any nail liquid, including polish remover, down a drain.
6. Clean up any product spills immediately and dispose of in a covered container.
7. Avoid unnecessary pressure at base of nail when filing. Nail root or matrix damage could result.
8. Follow manufacturer's directions exactly. Do not mix and match chemicals from different manufacturers.
9. Avoid overheating nail during buffing.
10. Do not allow food or drink in the general area of acrylic nails.
11. Do not allow smoking in the salon, as vapors from nail products, such as adhesives, are flammable.
12. Keep all products organized and labeled, and maintain MSDS guidelines for all products.

14

ALERT!

While many clients can be allergic to many products, those containing MMA (Methyl Methacrylate) pose a higher risk. MMA is an ingredient that was used in early artificial nail products, but has since been prohibited by the FDA. MMA has been found to cause health problems ranging from skin allergies and loss of the nail plate to respiratory problems, as well as nose, liver and kidney damage.

Since MMA is prohibited, you are unlikely to find it on the ingredient label. Still, it is usually not difficult to tell if a product contains MMA. Here are three indicators to watch for:

1. Unusually strong or strange odor which doesn't smell like other acrylic liquids
2. Nail enhancements that are extremely hard and very difficult to file, even with coarse abrasives
3. Nail enhancements that will not soak off in solvents designed to remove acrylics

Nail Tips

The length of your client's natural nail can be extended through the use of plastic nail tips. These come in sizes often numbered from 1-10 with number 1 the largest and 10 the smallest. Selecting the right size for each of your client's nails is a critical factor in the success of these extensions. Nail tips are reasonably strong and can be cut, filed and polished. Avoid damaging plastic nail tips by using non-acetone polish remover.

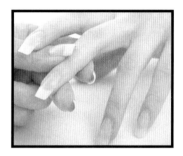

Nail Tips Preparation

In addition to following the same preparation procedures as outlined in the "Basic Manicure" section of this chapter, be sure to assemble the following products and implements:

- Nail tips
- Dehydrant
- Adhesive glue
- 3-way buffer

Nail Tips Procedure

- Wash and sanitize hands*
- Perform visual analysis
- Remove nail polish
- Perform thorough hand and nail examination and consultation
- Select correct size of nail tips
- File and shape natural free edge
- Buff nail surface gently
- Apply dehydrant to nail surface
- Apply first drop of adhesive to well of plastic tip

- Roll tip onto natural nail slowly
- Hold nail for 15-30 seconds
- Apply second drop of adhesive on top of seam
- Spray with adhesive accelerator
- Trim free edge of nail tip
- Measure length of all nails
- File free edge
- File and buff top of seam
- Buff to shine or polish
- Blend and smooth imperfections

*Wear protective gloves if required by your regulating agency.

Nail Tips

Wash and sanitize your hands and your client's hands. Perform visual analysis for signs of disease or disorder. If none are present, **remove nail polish.** Next, continue to **perform a thorough hand and nail examination and consultation.**

Sizing

1-3. Select correct size of nail tips to fit client's fingers. Match the width of each nail. If they are too wide or too small, they may loosen. They must fit sidewall to sidewall. They should cover no more than 1/3 to 1/2 of the nail bed and extend 1/3 to 1/2 the length of the free edge. Bevel the well of the nail tip with a file to reduce the amount of filing after initial adhesion.

Nail Prep

4. File and shape natural free edge and **buff the nail surface gently** to remove oil and prepare the natural nail.

5. Apply dehydrant to the nail surface to help remove moisture and oil, prevent fungus growth and maximize adhesion.

Adhering Nail Tips

6. Apply first drop of adhesive to the well of the plastic tip. This helps to avoid air bubbles under the tip and excess adhesive, which sometimes occurs if you apply the adhesive to the natural nail. **Roll tip onto the free edge of the natural nail slow**ly so you can see the adhesive moving up the natural nail.

7-8. Hold the nail for 15-30 seconds. Do not force nail on. If it has to be forced, it probably does not fit correctly.

Nail Tips

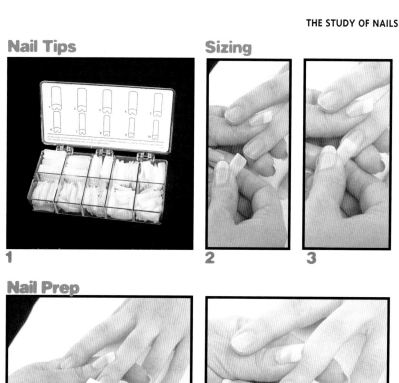

1

Sizing

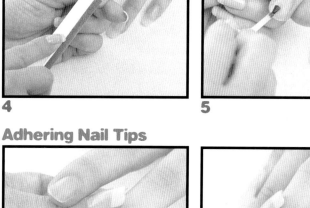

2
3

Nail Prep

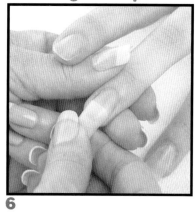

4
5

Adhering Nail Tips

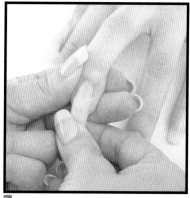

6
7

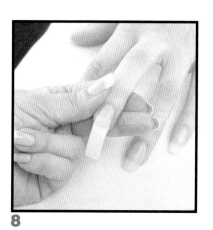

8

1 4

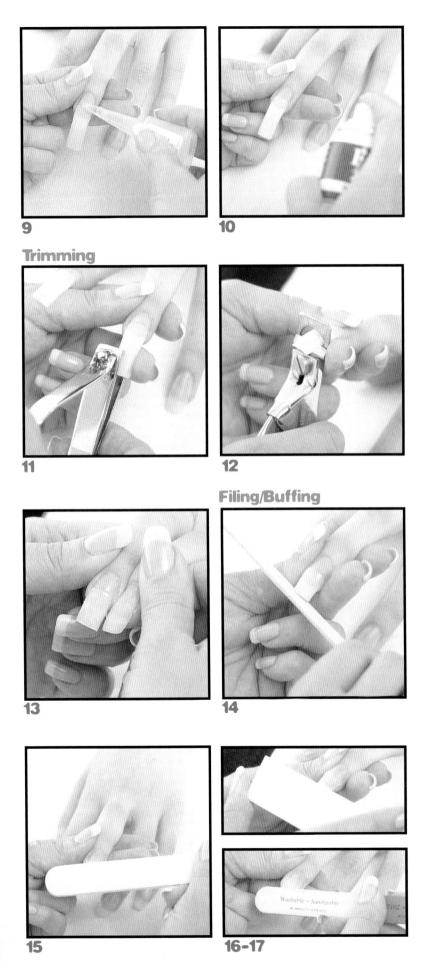

Trimming

9
10
11
12

Filing/Buffing

13
14
15
16-17

9. **Apply a second drop of adhesive on top of the seam** along the tip and natural nail. Apply the drop at the center and spread side to side.

10. **Spray with an adhesive accelerator** to help set the adhesive quickly.

Trimming

11. **Trim the free edge of the nail tip** with toenail clippers to the desired length. Always cut from the sides to the center.

12. You can also use a one-cut tool designed for this purpose. Do not use scissors, since it will cause lifting on one side of the tip and undue stress to the nail tip.

13. **Measure the length of all nails** and strive for symmetry.

Filing/Buffing

14. **File the free edge** to the shape desired.

15. **File and buff the top of the seam** to create a smooth finish. Keep the file flat on the nail tip to avoid filing into the natural nail. Be careful not to overheat the nail with constant buffing. Periodically, check the seams with your fingers for smoothness and temperature. Continue with each nail.

16-17. **Buff to a shine or polish. Blend and smooth imperfections** between the tip and natural nail with a buffer block. Use a 3-way buffer to add shine. Buff with the black side, then white and finally the gray side. Note: nail tips can be overlayed with acrylic for strength, as seen in the next procedure.

Nail Tips Completion

- Offer a rebook visit to your client
- Recommend retail products for your client
- Discard non-reusable materials, replace used towels with fresh towels and arrange all products and implements in proper order
- Disinfect your nail tips service implements and equipment
- Wash your hands with liquid antibacterial soap

Tips with Acrylic Overlay

To create a more durable extension and a longer lasting service, acrylic material can be applied over the nail tip. The overlay is created with a combination of acrylic powder called a polymer and a liquid called a monomer. A sable brush is dipped first into the liquid and then into the powder to combine the two ingredients and create "beads or balls" of acrylic on the end or side of the brush. These beads are then deposited onto the nail and nail tip to create the overlay. The parts of the sable brush you should know are identified in the illustration below.

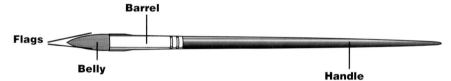

Barrel

Flags

Belly

Handle

Tips with Acrylic Overlay Preparation

In addition to following the same preparation procedures as outlined in the "Basic Manicure" section of this chapter, be sure to assemble the following products and implements:

- Sable brush
- Liquid in dappen dish
- Nail adhesive
- Regular nail implements and products
- Acrylic liquid and acrylic powder in dappen dish
- Nail tips
- Dehydrant and primer

Tips with Acrylic Overlay Procedure

- Wash and sanitize hands*
- Perform visual analysis
- Remove nail polish
- Perform thorough hand and nail examination and consultation
- Prepare natural nail–buff, dehydrate, prime
- Apply tips
- Buff nails and tips
- Form bead on side or tip of acrylic brush
- Apply acrylic at free edge (zone 1)
- Pat and press with belly of brush to blend
- Blend acrylic toward middle of nail plate (zone 2)
- Place second acrylic bead in middle of nail plate (zone 2)
- Pat and press toward free edge
- Place third acrylic bead at cuticle area (zone 3)
- Pat and press toward middle of nail plate (zone 2)
- File and shape nail
- Buff to smooth finish

*Wear protective gloves if required by your regulating agency.

1 4

Tips with Acrylic Overlay

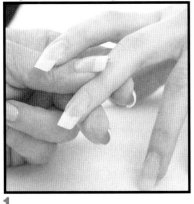
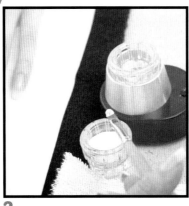

1

2

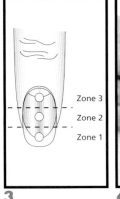

Zone 3
Zone 2
Zone 1

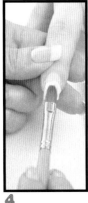
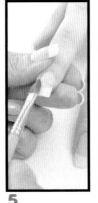
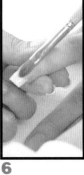

3   4   5   6

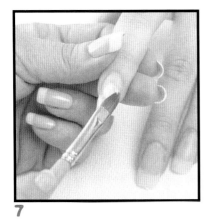
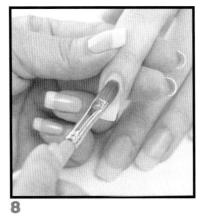

7   8

Tips with Acrylic Overlay

1. Wash and sanitize your hands and your client's hands. Perform visual analysis for signs of disease or disorder. If none are present, **remove nail polish.** Next, continue to **perform a thorough hand and nail examination and consultation. Prepare natural nails by buffing, applying dehydrant and primer. Apply tips** as shown under nail tips procedure. **Buff nails and tips.**

Acrylic Overlay

2. Form a bead on the side or tip of your acrylic brush by dipping flags into liquid and laying or dragging the brush through the acrylic powder.

3. Think of the nail as subdivided into 3 zones to help build the overlay.

4-6. Apply acrylic at free edge (zone 1). This should be medium in size. **Pat and press with the belly of the brush to blend** from side to side. **Blend acrylic toward the middle of the nail plate (zone 2)** by stroking gently.

7. Place a second acrylic bead in the middle of the nail plate (zone 2) and spread from side to side. This bead should be medium sized. **Pat and press toward the free edge,** blending the acrylic with zone 1. The consistency you create is very important. The bead should melt a little but not touch the sides of the nail wall.

8. Place a third acrylic bead at the cuticle area (zone 3) and spread it from side to side. This should be the smallest and most moist of all beads. **Pat and press toward the middle of the nail plate (zone 2)** blending over this zone. Take care that the acrylic in zone 3 is kept thin and off the skin.

Filing/Buffing

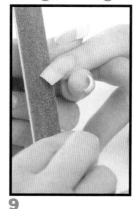
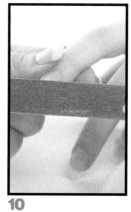
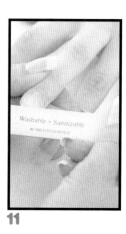

9   10   11

Keep all acrylic and products off the skin and cuticle. Contact could cause the acrylic to lift and/or produce an allergic reaction.

To determine when the acrylic is dry enough to file, tap it with the barrel of your brush, which should produce a clicking sound.

Filing/Buffing

9-10. File and shape the nail when the acrylic is dry. Hold the skin out of the way when you are filing. For the best leverage hold 1/3 of the file and use the remaining 2/3 of the file length.

11. Buff to a smooth finish with a 3-way buffer.

Nail Tips with Acrylic Overlay Completion

- Offer a rebook visit to your client
- Recommend retail products for your client
- Discard non-reusable materials, replace used towels with fresh towels and arrange all products and implements in proper order
- Disinfect your acrylic overlay service implements and equipment
- Wash your hands with liquid antibacterial soap

Sculptured Nails

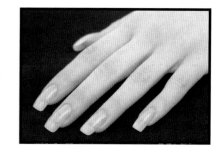

Sculptured nails produced with a nail form rather than a tip can be applied faster and used as an alternative to tips and overlays. Sculptured nails are created by combining two ingredients, which are the polymer and the monomer. A powder acrylic is mixed with a liquid containing both a plasticizer, which keeps the mixture flexible while drying, and a catalyst, which creates a chemical reaction that causes the acrylic and plasticizer to dry. Since you control the mixing, success is based on creating a consistent combination of ingredients on each nail.

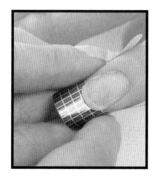

This mixture is applied to a nail form that extends the length of the nail plate and may extend beyond the free edge of the natural nail. After drying, the form is removed and the new nail is shaped, filed and polished. As the natural nail grows out, a "fill-in service" (referred to as re-balancing) is needed every two weeks. Because it is very difficult to remove properly applied sculptured nails, it is suggested that a client try wearing one before having an entire set created. Also, only non-acetone polish removers should be used with sculptured nails. The problem reported most often by clients who wear sculptured nails is the formation of fungus under the artificial nail. Applying a dehydrating product to the nail and making sure the nail

1
4

is completely dry before performing a sculptured nail service will help avoid trapping moisture and the occurrence of fungus. In addition, since most acrylic primers contain ingredients to help prevent the growth of fungus, avoid touching the nail with your hands after the primer has been applied.

Sculptured Nails Preparation

In addition to following the same procedures as outlined in the "Basic Manicure" section of this chapter, be sure to assemble the following products and implements.

- Acrylic liquid and acrylic powder in dappen dishes
- Liquid in dappen dish
- Dehydrant and primer (if required)
- Sable brush
- Regular nail implements and products
- Nail forms (plastic, paper or metal)

Sculptured Nails Procedure

- Wash and sanitize hands*
- Perform visual analysis
- Remove nail polish
- Perform thorough hand and nail examination and consultation
- File free edge
- Buff surface of nail lightly
- Remove filing residue
- Apply dehydrant
- Apply nail form
- Apply primer if directed
- Measure out required amount of acrylic powder
- Form bead on side of brush
- Apply acrylic bead to form to create free edge (zone 1)

- Rotate brush
- Pat and press toward edges of nail form
- Define shape and length of free edge
- Create second acrylic bead
- Place second bead in middle section (zone 2)
- Pat, press and stroke acrylic into place
- Place smallest bead just below cuticle (zone 3)
- Pat, press and stroke acrylic down to base of nail
- Apply fourth bead (optional)
- Remove form
- File
- Remove nail dust and filings

*Wear protective gloves if required by your regulating agency.

Sculptured Nails

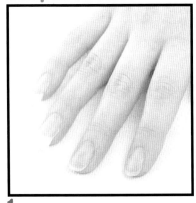

1

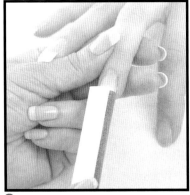

2

Sculptured Nails

1. Wash and sanitize your hands and your client's hands. Perform visual analysis for signs of disease or disorder. If none are present, **remove nail polish.** Next, continue to **perform a thorough hand and nail examination and consultation.**

2. File the free edge and **buff the surface of the nail lightly** using a 3-way buffer to prepare the natural nail. **Remove filing residue** with cotton.

3. **Apply dehydrant** to the natural nail.

Nail Form

4. **Apply the nail form** by sliding the nail form under the client's nail, and allowing the adhesive tabs to attach to the sides of the client's finger. Do not force the form under the nail as it may cut the hyponychium. Make sure the form fits snug under the edge, is positioned in a c-curve and is even with the client's nail.

Apply primer if directed by the sculpting brand you are using. Since most primers are acids, avoid any contact with the skin to prevent a burn or an allergic reaction. As you proceed with the application, use the art as a guide when determining the three zones.

5. **Measure out the required amount of acrylic powder** into the dappen dishes. **Form a bead on the side of the brush** by dipping the flags of the sable brush into the liquid, thoroughly moistening and laying or dragging the wet brush through the white acrylic powder. Avoid dipping the barrel of the brush as it will cause bristles to loosen. This should be the largest bead. More liquid in the brush allows you to draw more powder, producing a larger bead.

6. **Apply acrylic bead to the form to create a free edge** by placing the bead where the free edge meets the nail form (zone 1). **Rotate the brush** slightly as you deposit the acrylic bead. It will be formed into a half circle, often referred to as the smile line.

7-9. **Pat and press toward the edges of the nail form** with the belly of the brush spreading outward toward the edges of the nail form. **Define the shape and length of the free edge.** Some nail forms have a grid pattern on them, which will help you create symmetry.

Nail Form

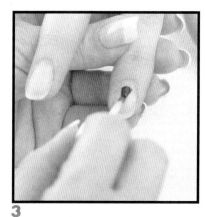
3

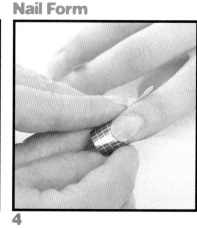
4

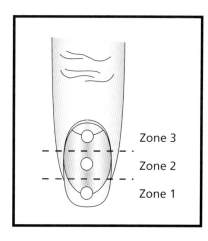

Zone 3
Zone 2
Zone 1

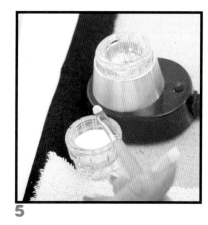
5

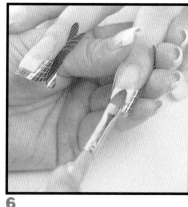
6

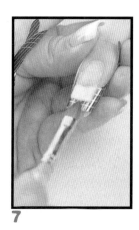
7

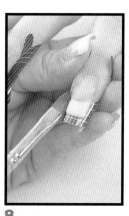
8

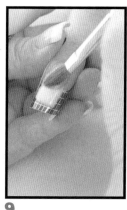
9

1
4

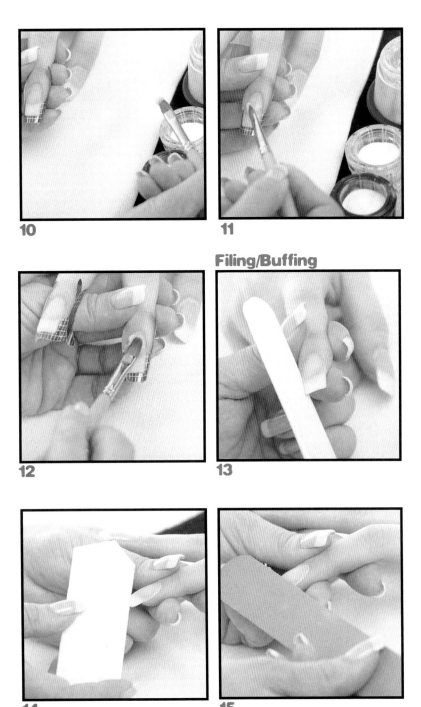

Filing/Buffing

10

11

12

13

14

15

10-11. **Create a second acrylic bead**, medium sized, by dipping your brush first into liquid than into the pink acrylic powder. **Place the second bead in the middle section (zone 2). Pat, press and stroke the acrylic into place**, gently overlapping zone 1.

12. **Place the smallest bead just below the cuticle (zone 3)**, just below the cuticle area. **Pat, press and stroke the acrylic down to the base of the nail.** Move out to the sides and past the point where the free edge meets the nail form, overlapping the acrylic material previously applied. **Apply a fourth bead for additional strength** across the stress area where the free edge meets the nail bed, if needed.

Filing/Buffing

13. **Remove the nail form** when acrylic is dry. **File** to create a smooth finish. **Remove the nail dust and filings.** Periodically break contact to reduce heat, check for smoothness and feel the temperature of the nail. Continue with each nail.

14-15. Buff with a buffer block and a 3-way buffer to create shine and a natural looking blend between the tip and the natural nail. Buff with the black side, then white and finally the gray side. Wash hands to remove nail dust. Sculptured nails can be left natural or polished.

Sculptured Nails Completion

- Offer a rebook visit to your client
- Recommend retail products for your client
- Discard non-reusable materials, replace used towels with fresh towels and arrange all products and implements in proper order
- Disinfect your sculptured nail service implements and equipment
- Wash your hands with liquid antibacterial soap

Fill-ins and Re-Balancing Acrylic Nails

Whenever you coat the entire surface of the nail with acrylic, the base of the nail (at the cuticle) will require fill-in services. These should be booked approximately every 2 weeks, when the nail has grown 1/16" (.156 cm). This is very important because otherwise as the natural nail grows, the artificial nail will lift, which can lead to trapped moisture and growth of fungus.

Fill-ins and Re-Balancing Guidelines

Preparation for the fill-in service is basically the same as the sculptured nails preparation other than the use of the nail form.

1. **Wash and sanitize your hands and your client's hands. Perform visual analysis** for signs of disease or disorder. If none are present, **remove all polish**, using a non-acetone polish remover and cotton. Next, continue to **perform a thorough hand and nail examination.**

2. **File the cuticle area** to remove any loosened acrylic material. **Blend the line of demarcation** by smoothing out the "edge" of acrylic material with your file in the new growth area. Be careful not to file the natural nail.

3. **Rebalance the shape of the entire nail** to keep it looking natural. Zone 1 should be thin, zone 2 should be thicker for strength and zone 3 should be thin. (See illustration to the right). **File and buff** to rebalance nail and blend remaining acrylic to new growth area.

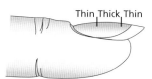
Thin Thick Thin

4. **Buff with the fine side of a block buffer** to gently buff any exposed surface of the natural nail.

5. **Cleanse nails** with antibacterial liquid soap and water; do not soak.

6. **Push cuticles back.**

7. **Apply dehydrant** to exposed natural nail only.

8. **Apply primer** to exposed natural nail only.

9. **Apply acrylic bead to new growth area.**

10. **Pat, press and stroke in place.**

> If you see signs of nail fungus, you may remove the artificial nail, but wear gloves and use proper disinfection procedures. Send the client to a physician for treatment. Do not perform further nail services until the fungus has cleared up.

11. **Apply acrylic bead to stress point** where the free edge meets the nail bed to complete.

12. **File entire nail smooth** with a file or 3-way buffer. Wash hands to remove nail dust.

13. **Apply base coat and polish** as desired.

Removing Nail Tips, Tips with Overlays and Sculptured Nails

To remove nail tips, tips with overlays and sculptured nails, soak nails in the product solvent recommended by the manufacturer. When adhesive is thoroughly softened, gently lift artificial nail product from natural nail. Cleanse entire nail using polish remover followed by cleansing solution.

Additional Artificial Nail Services

Additional artificial nail services include wrapped or fiberglass nails and light-cured or gel nails.

1
4

Wrapped or Fiberglass Nails

Fiberglass is a loosely woven mesh, thicker than silk, that adds strength to the nail. It can be applied over the natural nail or tips and is produced by applying a resin (thick adhesive) over the fiberglass. The resin is then hardened with a catalyst, which is usually in a spray form. The nail is then filed and buffed smooth to produce a natural-looking nail.

Care should be taken in applying resin. If the resin is applied too thick or the spray catalyst is sprayed too closely, it can cause a heat reaction.

Light-Cured or Gel Nails

This product is simply an acrylic gel that is applied to the nail plate, after which the hand is placed under a special light (ultraviolet or halogen) that creates a chemical reaction that causes the product to harden. This process is called "curing" the nail. This product is used to reinforce weak nails or can be used over tips to add sheen and strength. Manufacturers have created different gels to act as bonding agents for tips, nail builders or thickeners and nail glosses for shine. It is a fast and economical service for the client and an excellent way to help a client develop beautiful strong nails. Always follow manufacturer's directions carefully.

This chapter has provided you with a strong foundation in both natural and artificial nail care. Providing high quality nail services to your clients can be an added benefit to them, while offering you an opportunity for additional income.

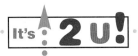

Build Your Critical Thinking Skills

In this chapter you have prepared yourself to meet the following Industry Standards for entry-level cosmetologists:

- Provide basic manicure and pedicure services
- Conduct services in a safe environment and take measures to prevent the spread of infectious and contagious disease

It's Up to You to know what to do. Using your training to this point, review the following case scenario and think through how you would handle the challenge.

1. A client scheduled for a sculptured nail service at 2:30 today is seated at your work station. You have washed and sanitized both your hands and your client's hands. You notice that the client has tiny rings with blisters that are reddish in color on several fingers. You also notice dry flakes of skin surrounding the area. The client is dismissing the area by saying that her hands always look that way when she has done a lot of dishwashing. What would you do?

Chapter 15
THE STUDY OF SKIN

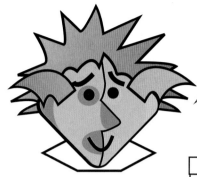

After studying this chapter you will be able to . . .

1. **Define the function, composition and types of skin and identify the difference between the disorders and diseases of skin.**

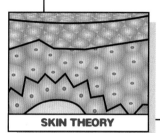

SKIN THEORY

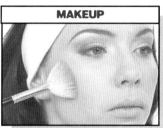

MAKEUP

4. **Explain the basic steps used during a makeup application.**

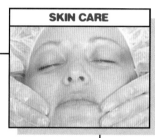

SKIN CARE

2. **Explain and demonstrate steps used during a basic facial, including massage techniques.**

HAIR REMOVAL

3. **Identify the difference between temporary and permanent hair removal and explain the techniques used for each.**

Have you walked through a pharmacy lately or even through the pharmaceutical section of your local grocery store? I've found literally dozens of products, more new ones every month it seems, with the word **DERM** in them. **DERM** means skin, by the way. More than ever before, people seem interested in healthy, beautiful skin - from the parent trying to lessen diaper rash to the teen desperate to hide acne to the adult hoping to remove unwanted hair to the older person wondering about age spots. Many of these same people will come to you as a trusted professional with concerns about their skin. That's why this chapter is so important to you.

In the profession of cosmetology your understanding of how to maintain and enhance the skin will allow you to provide services to help your clients look better and feel good.

Isn't it a great feeling to know that in addition to the hair services you offer, you can extend your VALUE to others through care of their skin? You can guess from the size of this chapter that there is a great deal to be learned, all focused on the BIG IDEA of skin maintenance and enhancement.

Healthy, glowing skin requires ongoing maintenance. In addition, many people choose to enhance their skin through carefully and creatively applied makeup.

My PLAN for you in this chapter, as you see, has four very different sections. Glance over them to get the total picture. As with nails, you start out with theory and move to care. Two very important sections complete your study of skin: hair removal and makeup. By the time you complete this chapter, you will have taken another major step toward your professional career.

HAIR REMOVAL

Hair Removal Essentials

Infection Control and Safety

Client Consultation

Temporary Hair Removal

Basic Waxing

Permanent Hair Removal

SKIN THEORY

Functions of the Skin

Composition of the Skin

Types of Skin

Skin Diseases and Disorders

SKIN CARE

Massage

Facial Masks

Skin Care Essentials

Infection Control and Safety

Client Consultation

Basic Facial

MAKEUP

Facial Shapes

Color Theory

Makeup Essentials

Infection Control and Safety

Client Consultation

Makeup Techniques and Products

Basic Makeup Application

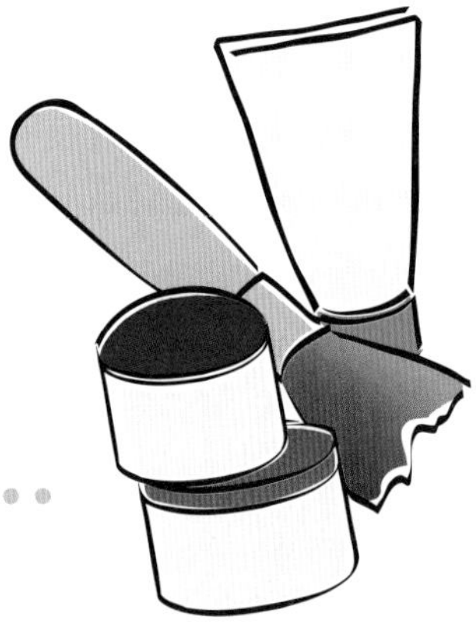

THE STUDY OF SKIN

SKIN THEORY

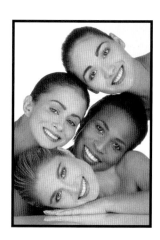

The skin is the largest – and perhaps most magnificent! – organ of the body. It is simultaneously sensitive and supremely durable and requires special attention and care to maintain its health, elasticity, color and vibrancy.

The study of the skin, its structure, functions, diseases and treatment is called dermatology. A dermatologist is a medical skin specialist. As a cosmetologist, it is important for you to have a basic understanding of skin and the skin care services offered in the salon. In the skin care industry, esthetics is known as the process of cleansing, toning, moisturizing, protecting, and enhancing the skin.

The skin, as the largest organ of the body, covers the entire body and protects it from invasion from outside particles. Except for the brain, the skin is the most complex organ of the body. Your skin is continuously working in its own efficient manner as an intermediary between your body and your environment, performing many functions. The skin and its layers make up the integumentary (in-teg-U-men-tary) system of the body.

Functions of the Skin

The skin has seven basic functions:

Sensation

Feelings generated by the nerve endings just under the outer layer of the skin make you aware of heat, cold, touch, pain and pressure. The reaction to a sensation is called a reflex.

Hydration

The skin contains water to keep itself soft and supple. It secretes perspiration and an oily, sebaceous fluid that maintains the skin's moisture balance.

Absorption

The skin permits certain substances like water and oxygen to pass through its tissues.

Regulation

The skin helps maintain the body's temperature.

Protection

The skin shields your body from the direct impact of heat, cold, bacteria and other aspects of the environment that could be detrimental to your health.

Excretion

The skin eliminates sweat, salt and wastes from the body, therefore helping remove toxins from the internal systems.

Respiration

The skin takes in oxygen through its pores and releases carbon dioxide.

Composition of the Skin

The skin has two main divisions:

1. **Epidermis, which is the outermost layer of the skin** (also referred to as cuticle or scarf skin)
2. **Dermis, which is the underlying, or inner, layer of the skin** (also called derma, corium, cutis or true skin)

Under the dermis layer is the sub-dermis or subcutaneous division, composed of fatty tissue.

Epidermis

The epidermis makes up the outer layers of the skin. It's almost like a bag that covers you and protects you from the environment. **The epidermis is composed of five layers of cells with differing characteristics and contains no blood vessels.**

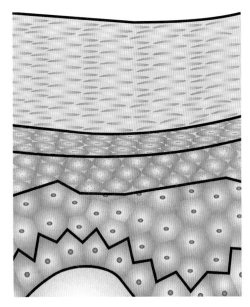

Stratum Corneum (**KOHR**-nee-um)

Stratum Lucidum (**LOO**-si-dum)

Stratum Granulosum (gran-yoo-**LOH**-sum)

Stratum Spinosum (spye-**NO**-sum)

Stratum Germinativum (jur-mih-nah-**TIV**-um) or Stratum Basale (Basal Layer)

Stratum Germinativum

At the lowest level of the epidermis you will find the stratum germinativum. It begins with the stratum basale, or basal cell layer, which is a single layer thick. **It is here where skin cell growth occurs through mitosis or cell division.** Basal cells are constantly dividing and producing new cells that are pushed toward the surface of the skin to replace cells that have been shed. Keratinization, the chemical conversion of living cells into dead protein cells, begins when the newly produced cells are pushed toward the surface. As the newly produced cells move toward the surface and farther away from the stratum germinativum, they flatten out, lose most of their water, die and, as keratinized cells, are finally shed. This process takes from 25 to 28 days, depending mostly on the area of the body, age and/or health of the individual. **Melanocytes are also found in the stratum germinativum.** These cells produce the melanosomes or pigment granules containing melanin that give color to the skin. **The amount of melanin present will determine the skin's color.** Brown skin contains a large amount of melanin while skin with little melanin will appear pale or pinkish. Melanin protects the skin, particularly in layers closest to the surface, by screening out harmful ultraviolet rays.

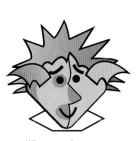

"The word stratum means layer."

Stratum Spinosum

The **stratum spinosum** is the next layer up and is sometimes considered to be part of the stratum germinativum. It includes cells that have absorbed melanin to distribute pigmentation to other cells. The cells then become irregularly shaped and have a "spiny" appearance.

Stratum Granulosum

The next layer is the **stratum granulosum**. In this layer the cells become more regularly shaped and look like many tiny granules. This layer of the epidermis gets its name from these granules. These granules (almost dead cells) are on their way to the surface of the skin to replace cells that are shed from the stratum corneum.

Stratum Lucidum

On the palms of the hands and the soles of the feet only, (where there are no hair follicles), there is another skin layer that is called the stratum lucidum. The cells in this layer are even more flattened and transparent (clear). They are called squamous (**SQUAW**-mus) cells due to their flat, scale-like appearance, thus making the skin thickest on palms of hands and soles of feet.

Stratum Corneum

The uppermost layer, the **stratum corneum** sometimes called the horny layer, is the toughest layer of the epidermis and is composed of keratin protein cells that are continually shed and continually replaced by new cells from below. Unlike the hard keratin found in nails and hair, the keratin produced by the skin remains soft throughout the keratinization and shedding process. The stratum corneum acts as a protective layer for the layers below it. It protects the skin's moisture balance by acting as a barrier to moisture loss. It, in turn, is protected by an acid mantle, a mixture of oil, secreted by sebaceous oil glands, and water secreted by sweat glands. The pH of the acid mantle averages 4.5 to 5.5.

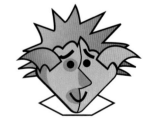

"According to some authorities, you have up to a hundred trillion cells in the body! You shed some five billion cells daily!"

The entire epidermis protects the dermis and the subcutaneous division below the skin. Since the skin cells are constantly being sloughed off at the stratum corneum, the replacement of the cells is a continuous process.

Dermis

The dermis layer is made up of connective tissues. Connective tissues are composed of a semifluid substance containing collagen protein and elastin fibers, both of which lend support to the epidermis and give the skin its elastic quality. Collagen protein fibers are strong and flexible while the elastin fibers are soft and pliable. It is in this layer that the collagen and elastin fibers deteriorate, causing the skin to sag and wrinkle during the aging process. Also found in the dermis are the sweat glands called sudoriferous (soo-dohr-**IF**-er-us) glands, oil glands called sebaceous (sih-**BAY**-shus) glands, sensory nerve endings and receptors, blood vessels, arrector pili muscles and a major portion of each hair follicle. Remember that hair is an appendage of the skin, as are the nails and sweat and oil glands.

The dermis is also called the 'true skin' or corium (KOH-ree-um).

Sudoriferous Glands

The sudoriferous (sweat) glands are controlled by the nervous system of the body. Each gland consists of a coiled base and tube-like duct opening on the surface of the skin to form a sweat pore. **The sweat glands have three major functions:**

1. **Control and regulation of body temperatures**

   When the body becomes overheated, large quantities of sweat are secreted onto the skin's surface. This allows for rapid evaporation, which cools the skin and maintains the body temperature at 98.6°F (37°C).

2. **Excretion of waste products**

   Waste materials, such as salt and other chemicals, are easily eliminated as sweat is produced.

3. **Helping to maintain the acidic pH factor of the skin**

   A mixture of sweat and oil (called the acid mantle) keeps the surface of the skin slightly acidic, which helps prevent bacteria from entering the body.

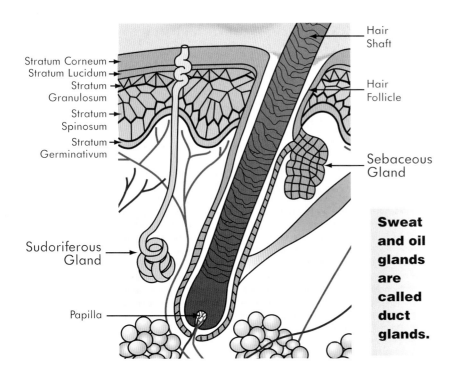

Stratum Corneum
Stratum Lucidum
Stratum Granulosum
Stratum Spinosum
Stratum Germinativum

Hair Shaft

Hair Follicle

Sebaceous Gland

Sudoriferous Gland

Papilla

Sweat and oil glands are called duct glands.

Sweat (also called perspiration) is a weak salt solution, the amount of which varies with your body temperature and activity. Besides water and salt, sweat contains other substances including lactic acid and uric acid, both of which help create the acidic pH of sweat.

The sudoriferous glands, also called eccrine glands, are widely distributed over the body surface. They are found in the greatest concentration on the palms of the hands, soles of the feet, scalp and forehead, underarms, anterior trunk and genital region.

Sebaceous Glands

Sebaceous, or **oil**, **glands** are partially controlled by the nervous system and are sac-like glands that are attached to hair follicles. These glands are 2-3 times larger around facial hair follicles than they are around scalp follicles. **When sebaceous glands produce an over-abundance of sebum, the result is "oily skin." No oil glands are found on palms of hands or soles of feet.**

Sebum is a complex secretion containing a high percentage of fatty, oily substances. The sebum mixes with the secretion of the sweat glands and spreads over the surface of the skin. It is this layer of oil and moisture that is called the acid mantle. **The acid mantle keeps the skin smooth, prevents dirt and grime from entering the outer layer of the epidermis, and also prevents the**

skin from drying or chapping. When we measure the pH of the skin, we are actually measuring the pH of the acid mantle.

The acid mantle is naturally acidic, ranging from a pH of 4.5 to 5.5 for most people. This is mainly due to lactic acid and sodium salt. The mantle protects against bacterial invasion by providing a hostile (acidic) environment for bacterial growth. Most of the problems encountered with skin are caused by the sebaceous gland, whether by underactivity or overactivity or blockage of the duct. The sebaceous glands are attached to the upper third of the hair follicles, and the oil (sebum) is secreted onto the surface of the skin by way of the papillary (**PAP**-e-lairy) canal.

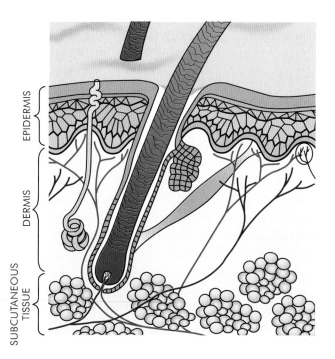

Subcutaneous

Below the dermis of the skin is a fatty layer called the subcutaneous tissue. **The subcutaneous tissue is a protective cushion for the skin.** It acts as a shock absorber to protect the bones and to help support the delicate structures such as blood vessels and nerve endings. This layer gives contour and shape to the body and acts as an emergency reservoir of food and water.

It is composed of adipose (fatty) and loose, connective tissue. The collagen and elastin fibers that run in all directions are continuous with those in the dermis. Depending upon genetics, nutrition, exercise and general health of the body, varying amounts of fat cells are found in the subcutaneous tissues. This fatty tissue provides insulation, acts as padding and stores energy for the body. Subcutaneous fat storage is partly under the control of sex hormones, which account for some of the differences in body contours between males and females.

The subcutaneous layer contains large blood vessels that transport nourishment to the skin and nerves. Also in this layer are the glandular parts of some of the sudoriferous glands and some sense organs for touch, pressure and temperature. Nerves of the skin are found in the subcutaneous layer and in the lower epidermis layer. Nerve bundles found in the subcutaneous tissue branch into the stratum granulosum layer and respond to pain. Cold, heat and touch affect other nerves, located in lower levels of the epidermis.

Skin Pigmentation

As previously mentioned, melanin-producing cells (melanocytes) are located in the basal layer of the epidermis. These cells, loaded with melanin, move toward the surface at a faster rate than other cells. **Melanin is distributed throughout all epidermal cells and forms an effective barrier from the penetration of ultraviolet rays to the deeper layers of the skin.**

Melanin tans the skin to protect it from the burning rays of the sun. Light and dark skin do not differ in the number of melanocytes they contain. They differ, rather, in the rate and amount of melanin produced. Dark skin contains more melanin, which serves as a more effective barrier to the damaging rays of the sun than is seen in light skin. Skin with little melanin present is light, pale or may appear slightly pink. The "pink" tone visible in pale skin is the reflection of red blood through the epidermis. Carotene, a yellow pigment located primarily in the top layer, can give skin a sallow or yellowish cast. No matter what color, all skin needs protection from the ultraviolet rays of the sun.

Ultraviolet rays of the sun speed up the production of melanin, making your skin darker. The stimulation of the production of melanin and the tanning of the skin that results protect the dermis layer of the skin by absorbing these ultraviolet rays. Overexposure to the sun can cause damage to the skin, such as burning, peeling, wrinkling and even skin cancer.

Many products have been developed to further help the skin from absorbing ultraviolet rays. One such product is sunscreen, which comes in various SPF (sun protection factor) strengths. This rating system allows you to determine how long you can stay out in the sun without burning. For instance, if your skin normally burns in one hour without sunscreen, an SPF 2 sunscreen might allow you to stay in the sun twice as long, or two hours, without burning.

The American Academy of Dermatology recommends the following tips to reduce the sun's harmful effects:

- Try to keep out of the sun between 10:00 am and 4:00 pm.
- Apply a sunscreen with Sun Protection Factor (SPF) of at least 15, and re-apply every two hours.
- Wear protective, tightly-woven clothing.
- Stay in the shade whenever possible.
- Avoid surfaces, such as water, that can reflect up to 85% of the sun's damaging rays.
- Protect children by keeping them out of the sun and, beginning at six months of age, minimize risk by applying sunscreen.

Studies show 90% of wrinkles are caused by excessive exposure to the sun, and only 10% by the natural aging process.

If you have had repeated sunburns, examine your skin monthly. If you see a change in the size, shape or appearance of a mole, see your dermatologist.

Types of Skin

Skin has a personality, just as does the individual it covers. If the skin is constantly abused, side effects such as blemishes, wrinkles, flakiness, roughness and a general lack of healthy color may appear. The skin requires a certain amount of care and attention on a daily basis to stay healthy and attractive. The thinnest skin occurs on eyelids, so be gentle on them when cleansing or applying make-up.

Although the structure of each person's skin is basically the same, the functioning of the various glands and the reactions of the skin to its environment can vary greatly. From a cosmetologist's point

of view, **the surface of the skin falls into four basic types: dry, oily, normal and combination.**
It is important for you to be able to recognize these four types so that the proper cleansing and moisturizing regimen can be recommended for each client.

Dry Skin

Dry skin is characterized by signs such as peeling and flaking. It chaps easily and has a general all-over taut feeling. Dry skin has fewer blemishes and is not prone to acne.

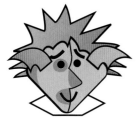

*"To keep your skin in its
optimum condition, you
should drink half your body
weight in ounces of water
per day."*

There are two types of dry skin: oil dry and moisture dry. Oil dry skin
lacks sebaceous activity, while moisture dry skin lacks water.
Although dry skin is often associated with more mature skin, it can be
found on a younger person as well. Dry skin can be caused by many
factors, including a systemic malfunction of the sebaceous glands,
diet, hormones or a combination of these conditions.

A good treatment program is essential for dry skin to supply moisture,
emollients and lubricants necessary for healthy, soft, smooth skin.

Oily Skin

Oily skin usually has an all-over shiny look and/or a rough texture with blackheads and enlarged
pores. The oily residue most often appears on the chin, nose, nasal-labial groove and forehead, which
is commonly called the "T" zone. In a young person, oily skin is prone to acne, but the cause of acne
or whiteheads cannot be attributed solely to oily skin. Any combination of conditions may be responsible, such as improper cleansing, hormonal imbalance, nervous problems, poor diet and even humid
weather.

A good treatment program is very important for this skin type. It must be kept in an "acid-balanced"
condition (pH 4.5 to 5.5). Maintaining the skin in an acid-balanced state aids in inhibiting the invasion of pathogenic bacteria that can contribute to skin infection. It also maintains the skin in its
"natural" environment and, thus, causes less irritation to the skin than alkaline conditions.

Normal Skin

Normal skin is very rare and quite beautiful. It is easily recognized because it has a fresh and healthy
color, a firm, moist and smooth texture, freedom from blackheads and blemishes, and does not
appear oily. This skin type requires a simple but consistent skin care routine to keep it in this condition. The objective with normal skin is to maintain its natural acid-balanced condition.

Combination Skin

The most common skin type found is that of combination skin. It can be found on skin of most any
age and is recognized by the shiny "T" zone (forehead, nose, and chin), and the presence at the same
time of a noticeable dryness in the cheek, jaw line, and hairline areas. Blackheads and enlarged pores

are often evident on the nose and chin. Combination skin requires the most specialized skin regimen, as you are treating two totally different skin types at the same time—oily and dry. The goal to achieve with this skin type is to stabilize the oily areas and lubricate the dry areas.

Skin Diseases and Disorders

As a professional, you need to be familiar with skin disorders and diseases so that you can recognize any problems that would prevent you from performing a skin care service. Keep in mind that only a dermatologist or medical doctor should diagnose and treat skin diseases and disorders. **In this chapter certain conditions are accompanied by an asterisk (*), which indicates that skin care services may <u>not</u> be performed.**

Important Vocabulary

Common terms related to the study of diseases and disorders and their definitions include:

An **allergy** is a sensitivity that may develop from contact with normally harmless substances. Symptoms of an allergy may include itching, redness, swelling and/or blisters.

Inflammation is an objective symptom (one you see) characterized by redness, pain, swelling and/or increased temperature.

Chronic is a term used to identify conditions that are frequent and habitual.

Acute is a term used to identify conditions that are brief and severe.

A **contagious disease** is communicable by contact. It is also known as an infectious or communicable disease.

Seasonal disease is influenced by weather.

Etiology is the study of cause of diseases.

Pathology is the study of diseases.

Prognosis is a medical opinion of the future condition of illness.

Occupational disorders occur in certain types of employment. For example, cosmetologists may be susceptible to *dermatitis venenata* (**VEN**-eh-nay-tah), sometimes referred to as contact dermatitis, an allergic reaction to certain cosmetics or chemicals. Hands that are immersed in water and shampoo many times a day are at high risk. Symptoms may include redness, cracking skin and weeping sores. Protective creams are available to provide a barrier for the skin. Infection control practices establish standards regarding protective gloves, goggles, surgical masks, etc., to assist in avoiding occupational disorders.

The **symptoms** or signs of a disease are divided into two classifications:
- Subjective – those you feel
- Objective – those you see

In other words, signs of a disorder or disease may be felt but nothing may be visible. Itching, burning, pain or symptoms that are felt are examples of **subjective symptoms**. Pimples or inflammation are **objective symptoms** because they are visible. In some cases, both objective and subjective symptoms may be present. Avoid direct contact with open wounds and/or tumors.

There are six signs of infection: pain, swelling, redness, local fever (heat), throbbing, discharge. Always avoid performing services on skin that displays any of these symptoms.

Lesions

Diseases and disorders are often accompanied by skin lesions, which are any abnormal changes in the structure of an organ or tissue. There are three categories of lesions: primary, secondary and tertiary. As a salon professional, you need to recognize primary and secondary lesions.

Primary Skin Lesions

Primary skin lesions include the following:

Macules are a discoloration appearing on the skin's surface. They are flat areas and, although they are usually rounded and distinct, they may be oval, irregular or have an outline that gradually fades into surrounding tissues. They may vary in size but are generally less than one cm in diameter.

A *freckle* is an example of a macule. The technical name for freckles is lentigines (len-tih-**JEE**-nees).

Papules are hardened red elevations of the skin in which no fluid is present. These lesions normally vary in size from that of a pinhead to that of a pea. The actual shape and coloration of the lesions may vary. Consistency may vary from hard to soft. Papules may persist unchanged but they can, sometimes, proceed to other types of primary lesions. A large papule is known as a tubercle.

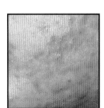

A *pimple* is an example of a papule.

Vesicles are fluid-filled elevations in the skin caused by localized accumulation of fluids or blood just below the epidermis. Vesicles may develop from macules, papules or poison oak or ivy and are generally short-lived.

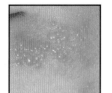

Herpes simplex*, also known as fever blisters, is a contagious, chronic condition characterized by a single vesicle or a group of vesicles on a red, swollen base. It usually appears on the lips, nostrils or other parts of the face.

*Indicates that services may <u>not</u> be performed.

Bulla are lesions, like vesicles, but larger. Found above and below the skin, they contain a clear, watery fluid. They occur in cases of second degree burns.

Pustules are small elevations of skin similar to vesicles in size and shape, but containing

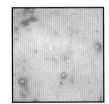

pus. They appear whitish or yellowish in color and may be surrounded by a reddish inflammatory border. They may develop from vesicles or papules.

A *pimple with pus* is an example of a pustule.

Wheals are a solid formation above the skin, often caused by an insect bite or allergic

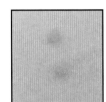

reaction. They are sharply defined and solid, rising above the skin (e.g., a mosquito bite). These lesions usually develop rapidly, disappear slowly and are accompanied by itching or tingling.

Hives*, also called Urticaria (ur-ti-**KAR**-e-uh), are an example of wheal lesions.

Tumors are solid masses in the skin. They are usually more than one cm in diameter. They may be soft or hard, depending upon their makeup, and may be fixed or freely movable. This classification often includes any new skin growths and any localized swelling, which may be elevated or deep. Skin tumors generally have a rounded shape.

A *nodule* is a small tumor.

A *cyst* (sist) is an abnormal membranous sac containing a gaseous, liquid or semi-solid substance.

Secondary Skin Lesions

Secondary skin lesions appear as a disease progresses into the later stages of development and need to be treated by a dermatologist or medical doctor.

Scales are shedding, dead cells of the uppermost layer of the epidermis. The epidermis normally undergoes constant exfoliation (removal) of small, barely perceptible flakes of skin. When the formation of epidermal cells is rapid or the normal process of keratinization is altered, one sees

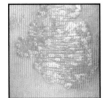

abnormal exfoliation of the epidermis, which results in scales. They may be dry, such as psoriasis, or oily, such as dandruff.

Psoriasis (soh-**REYE**-ah-sis) **is round, dry patches of skin, covered with rough, silvery scales. It is chronic and not contagious.**

*Indicates that services may <u>not</u> be performed.

Crusts are dried masses that are the remains of an oozing sore. The crusty material may contain blood, pus, sebum, epithelial tissue and bacterial debris.

The *scab* on a sore is an example of a crust.

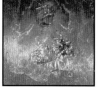

Excoriations are mechanical abrasions to the epidermis (or injuries to the epidermis). They appear bright to dark red, because of dried blood, and occur when an insect bite or a scab is scratched.

Scratches to the surface of the skin are considered excoriations.

Fissures are cracks in the skin. They usually appear as cracks or lines that may go as deep as the underlying dermis. They may be dry or moist. These lesions often occur when skin loses its flexibility due to exposure to wind, cold, water, etc.

Chapped lips are one example of a fissure.

Scars are formations resulting from a lesion, which extend into the dermis or deeper, as part of the normal healing process. Scars are permanent; however, they generally become less noticeable with time. A scar is also called a cicatrix (SIK-uh-triks).

The size and shape of a scar are dependent upon the extent of the original injury. *Keloids* are thick scars.

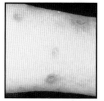

Ulcers* are open lesions visible on the skin surface that may result in the loss of portions of the dermis and may be accompanied by pus.

Hypertrophies (New Growth)

Hypertrophies are identified by an overgrowth or excess of skin.

Callus (sometimes called hyperkeratosis or keratoma) is a thickening of the epidermis, which occurs from pressure and friction applied to the skin.

Verruca* is a name given to a variety of warts. Warts are caused by a virus, can be contagious, and can spread all over the body. A dermatologist or medical doctor should be consulted for removal of warts. Warts are referred to as the most common tumor.

Skin tags are small elevated growths of skin, which can easily be removed by a physician.

*Indicates that services may <u>not</u> be performed.

Pigmentation Abnormalities

Pigmentation abnormalities describe conditions of too much color or too little color in a particular area of the skin.

Melanoderma

Melanoderma is the term used to describe any **hyperpigmentation** caused by overactivity of the melanocytes in the epidermis. It can be triggered by overexposure to sunlight, overactivity of the pituitary gland, circulation of hormones, disease and drugs. Some examples of melanoderma are chloasma and lentigines (freckles).

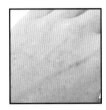

Chloasma (kloh-AZ-mah) is a group of brownish macules (nonelevated spots) occurring in one place. Chloasma is commonly called liver spots and often occurs on the hands and face.

Moles are small, brown pigmented spots that may be raised. Hair often grows through moles, but should not be removed, unless advised by a physician. If there is any change in appearance of a mole, seek medical advice. Melanotic sarcoma is a skin cancer that begins with a mole.

A naevus (NEE-vus) is a birthmark or a congenital mole. A birthmark may look like a stain on the face or other part of the body and is generally a reddish purple flat mark. The stain is caused by dilation of the small blood vessels in the skin.

Leukoderma

Leukoderma (Loo-ko-DUR-mah) describes hypopigmentation (lack of pigmentation) of the skin caused by a decrease in activity of melanocytes. Leukoderma is occasionally the result of a congenital defect such as albinism. However, hypopigmentation can be acquired, as in vitiligo.

Albinism (AL-bin-izm) is a congenital failure of the skin to produce melanin pigment. Persons with albinism have pink skin, white hair (it may sometimes be reddish) and pink eyes. They have a strong hypersensitivity to light and sun and skin that ages early. This skin must be protected from exposure to sunlight or ultraviolet lamps.

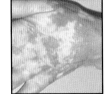

Vitiligo (vit-i-LEYE-goh) is characterized by oval or irregular patches of white skin that do not have normal pigment. Vitiligo is usually seen on the face, hands and neck as patches of hypopigmentation that may enlarge slowly. These patches of skin must be protected from exposure to sunlight or ultraviolet lamps.

Disorders of the Sebaceous Glands

Comedones (**KOM**-e-donz), **or blackheads, are masses of sebum (oil)** trapped in the hair follicles. Comedones can be removed with proper extraction procedures.

Milia (**MIL**-ee-uh), **or whiteheads, are caused by the accumulation of hardened sebum beneath the skin.** This disorder can occur on any part of the face, neck and chest.

Acne (**AK**-nee) occurs most often on the face, back and chest and is **a chronic, inflammatory disorder of the sebaceous glands.** Acne can be found in two stages: acne simplex or acne vulgaris. People with vulgaris (serious) acne should seek medical attention.

Rosacea* (ro-**ZA**-see-ah), **or acne rosacea, is a chronic inflammatory congestion of the cheeks and nose, observed as redness, with papules and sometimes pustules present.** Advise clients to avoid excessive heat, spicy foods and caffeine. Facials may be done under physician's approval.

Asteatosis (as-tee-ah-**TOH**-sis) is a condition of **dry, scaly skin with reduced sebum production.**

Seborrhea (seb-oh-**REE**-ah) is a condition caused by **excessive secretion of the sebaceous glands.** Seborrhea is commonly associated with oily skin types.

Steatoma (stee-ah-**TOH**-mah), **or sebaceous cyst or wen, is a subcutaneous tumor of the sebaceous gland, filled with sebum.** This disorder usually appears on the scalp, neck or back and ranges in size from a pea to an orange.

Furuncles* (fu-**RUN**-kel), **or boils, appear in the dermis and the epidermis and are caused by and acute staphylococcal infection.** They are localized infections of hair follicles.

Carbuncles* (**KAR**-bun-kel), **larger than furuncles, appear above and below the skin and are caused by acute staphylococcal infection of several adjoining hair follicles.** Carbuncles drain through multiple openings onto the skin's surface.

Disorders of the Sudoriferous Glands

Bromidrosis (broh-mih-**DROH**-sis) or **osmidrosis is foul-smelling perspiration.**

Anhidrosis (an-heye-**DROH**-sis) is a **lack of perspiration caused by fever or disease and requires medical attention.**

Hyperhidrosis (heye-per-heye-**DROH**-sis) is an **over-production of perspiration caused by excessive heat or general body weakness and requires medical attention.**

*Indicates that services may <u>not</u> be performed.

Miliaria rubra* (mil-ee-**AY**-re-ah **ROOB**-rah) or prickly heat is an **acute eruption of small red vesicles with burning and itching of the skin caused by excessive heat.** Milaria rubra is an inflammatory disorder of the sudoriferous glands.

Other Inflammatory Disorders

Dermatitis* (dur-mah-**TEYE**-tis) is an inflammatory disorder of the skin. The lesions come in various forms.

Eczema* (**EK**-see-mah) is characterized by **dry or moist lesions with inflammation of the skin and requires medical attention.** Eczema may be chronic or acute and should be referred to a physician for treatment.

*Indicates that services may <u>not</u> be performed.

SKIN CARE

In our culture, everyone recognizes the esthetic and hygienic reasons for caring for the skin. **Proper skin care is a combination of concerted efforts toward a good home-maintenance program, a well-balanced diet, proper intake of water, limited exposure to the sun, exercise, rest and professional skin care treatments and products.**

Keeping skin in good condition requires a minimum of three steps:

1. Cleanse thoroughly with a product that does not rob or strip the skin of its natural conditioners.

2. Tone the skin with an astringent or freshener.

3. Moisturize the skin to make up for the unavoidable losses it sustains from aging and exposure to the environment.

The skin should be cleansed daily with an appropriate skin-cleaning product. Ordinary soaps are not recommended for cleaning since they are generally alkaline and can strip the skin of its protective acid mantle.

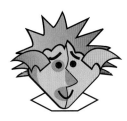

"You are familiar with a dehydrated grape. It's a raisin! Dehydration of human skin has the same effect. It shrivels and toughens the skin's outer layer."

Using astringents, toners or refreshers (sometimes called tonic lotions or skin refiners) helps to further cleanse the skin while bringing it to a normal pH.

The final step is moisturizing, which helps to keep the skin smooth. Moisturizers in a product operate in several ways. Some products, called humectants, attract moisture. Other products create a barrier that helps keep moisture in.

It is important to remember that oily skin needs moisturizing (hydrating) as much as dry skin. Excessive oil in skin does not replace loss of moisture. In fact, proper moisturizing can actually reduce the oily appearance because it contributes to a better balance of oil and moisture in the skin.

In addition to cleansing, toning and moisturizing, getting regular professional facial services helps keep your client's skin in optimum condition. Two of the steps generally performed in a facial include massage and facial masks.

Did You Know:
ONE CIGARETTE depletes the body of 25 mg. - 15 mg. of vitamin C. A deficiency of vitamin C in the body can contribute to cellular breakdown. Long term effects will speed up the aging and wrinkling process. Also, the ingestion of large amounts of caffeine, such as in coffee, tea or soft drinks, will affect not only the appearance but also the internal functioning of the skin. Research indicates that drinking a large amount of caffeine over a period of time will contribute to cellular aging.

Massage

Massage dates back to the Greeks, who used it as a cure for ailments. Women had their bodies massaged with vegetable and animal oils to keep their skin soft. **Massage is a scientific method of manipulation of the body by rubbing, pinching, tapping, kneading or stroking with the hands, fingers or an instrument.**

Massage is an excellent method for providing a restful, relaxing skin care treatment to a client. Every muscle and nerve has a motor point. Applying pressure to motor points soothes and stimulates the nerves and muscles. (See illustration.) There are many additional benefits of massage:

1. Increases circulation of the blood supply to the skin, causing blood vessels to dilate

2. Contracts the muscle when the movement is firm and rapid

3. Stimulates the glandular activities of the skin

4. Strengthens weak muscle tissue; relieves pain

5. Softens and improves the texture and complexion of the skin

6. Calms and relaxes the client and can relieve emotional stress and body tension

In most areas, stylists may massage the head, face, neck, shoulders, upper back, hands, arms and feet. For a complete body massage, some areas require that a client be referred to a licensed masseur (male) or masseuse (female). Refer to your area regulating agency.

The Five Basic Movements of Massage

1. **Effleurage (ef-LOO-rahzh) is a light, relaxing, smoothing, gentle stroking or circular massage.** It is used on the face, neck and arms and is often used as the movement that begins and ends a massage treatment. This method is carried out with the pads of the fingertips or with the palms of the hands.

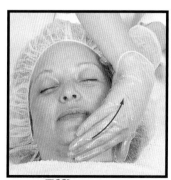

Effleurage

2. Petrissage (**PAY**-tre-sahzh) is a light or heavy kneading and rolling of the muscles. It is used on the face, the arms, the shoulders and the upper back. Petrissage is probably the most important of the massage movements, as it deeply stimulates the muscles, nerves and skin glands and promotes the circulation of blood and lymph. It is done by kneading the muscles between the thumb and fingers or by pressing the palm of the hand firmly over the muscles, then grasping and squeezing with the heel of the hand and the fingers.

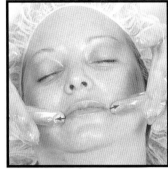

Petrissage

3. Tapotement (tah-**POHT**-mant), or percussion, is a light tapping or slapping movement applied with the fingertips or partly flexed fingers. The movement is usually carried out with the hands swinging freely from the wrist in a rapid motion. Tapotement increases blood circulation, stimulates the nerves and promotes muscle contraction. It should not be used when the client needs soothing. Hacking is a form of tapotement that is similar to a chopping movement with the edge of the hands used on the arms, back and shoulders.

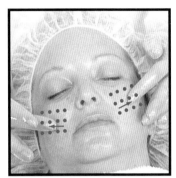

Tapotement

4. Friction (**FRIK**-shun) is a circular, deep rubbing movement with no gliding, usually carried out with the fingertips or palms of the hands. Friction is used most often on the scalp, hands or with less pressure during a facial massage.

5. Vibration is a shaking movement in the arms of the cosmetologist while the fingertips or palms are touching the client. Vibration should only be used in facial massage for a few seconds in one location, as it is very stimulating to the skin.

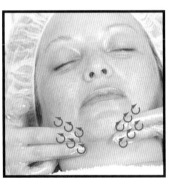

Friction

The following points should be kept in mind during the massage:

*   Massage should never be performed over an area exhibiting redness, swelling, pus, disease, bruises and/or broken or scraped skin.

*   Avoid massage if client has high blood pressure, heart condition or has had a stroke, since massage increases circulation and could present a risk for the client.

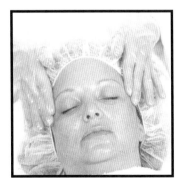

Vibration

*   Massage movements should be directed toward the origin of the muscles in order to avoid damage to muscle tissues.

*   When giving facial manipulations, an even tempo or rhythm is essential for the relaxation of the client. Do not remove the hands from the face once the manipulations have begun and, if it becomes necessary, feather the hands off the face and gently replace them on the skin with the same feather-like movements.

Facial Masks

Facial masks (or packs) have many different benefits, which include hydration (adding moisture), tightening of the pores and reduction of excess oil. Facial masks can be used in conjunction with facial services or they can be offered as a separate service. Facial masks are either applied directly to the skin or over a layer of gauze.

Masks should always be applied to clean skin. If a facial is desired, the facial manipulations are usually given before the mask is applied.

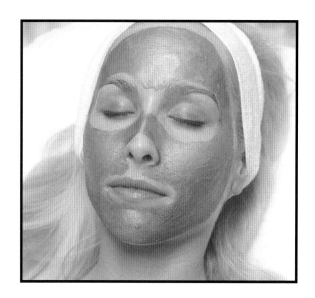

Types of Facial Masks

- **Clay packs** are usually recommended for normal or oily skin types.

- **Cream masks** are recommended for normal to dry skin.

- **"Siccative" masks** are drying masks. Most are made from a mineral powder base, such as clay, sand, zinc oxide or mud. This type of product is excellent when used on oily skin, as it will draw out oil and impurities from the pores. It is also good for acne-prone skin.

- **Paraffin (warm wax)** is heated and applied to the skin to rehydrate (moisturize) the skin's top layers. By coating the skin with warmth and blocking the skin's natural tendency to "breathe," the heat of a warm wax mask acts to draw oil and perspiration to the top layer of the skin. This mask is especially good for dry, wrinkled or dehydrated skin. It should be applied over a layer of gauze.

The Benefits of Facial Masks Include:

1. Increasing the firmness of the skin for a temporary period of time
2. Increasing the circulation of the blood in the areas treated
3. Absorbing and removing unwanted surface oil
4. Removing surface dirt
5. Absorbing and removing skin impurities
6. Softening and smoothing the skin
7. Relaxing and refreshing the client

Skin Care Essentials

As a cosmetologist, you will recommend the skin care treatments and products you will use during the service, as well as the products your client will take home. The following charts identify the products, implements and equipment you will use during a salon facial. Material Safety Data Sheets (MSDS) for all products used in the salon must be available.

Skin Care Products

PRODUCT	FUNCTION
Antiseptic	Aids in preventing the growth of bacteria on the skin
Cleansing Lotion	Removes impurities from the skin
Skin Astringent	Assists in cleansing skin and returns oily skin to a normal pH
Toner or Freshener	Assists in cleaning skin and returns normal to dry skin to a normal pH
Chemical Exfoliant	Removes dead skin cells by using enzymes and alphahydroxy acids
Manual Exfoliant	Removes dead skin cells by using a granular product manipulated on the skin; also called facial scrub
Massage Cream/Oil	Reduces friction and provides "slip" to the skin during massage
Dry Skin Masks	Add moisture to the skin
Oily Skin Masks	Absorb excess sebum and debris from the skin

Skin Care Implements/Supplies

IMPLEMENT/SUPPLIES	FUNCTION
Spatulas	Remove product from containers
Gloves	Protect hands
Fan Brush	Applies product on face or neck
Clean Sheets, Blankets	Provide warmth and comfort to client
Client Robe/Gown	Allows client to remove clothing to keep it clean
Towel	Cushions client's head; keeps hair protected; if wet and warm, removes mask product
Cotton Pads/Swabs	Remove product from face and neck
Facial Tissue	Removes lipstick or debris from extractions; blots face after toning; disposable
Head Band or Head Covering	Protects hair from the face and keeps product out of the client's hair

Skin Care Equipment

EQUIPMENT	FUNCTION	CAUTIONS
Magnifying Lamp	Provides thorough examination of skin's surface, using magnification and glare-free light; beneficial when analyzing the skin	Be aware of the electrical cord with floor-standing model
Facial Steamer	Uses warm, humid mist to open follicles for cleansing; softens dead skin cells for easier removal; causes increased blood circulation by making the blood vessels expand; improves cell metabolism	Water level should be in compliance with the manufacturer's directions; average distance from client's face is 16-18" (40-45 cm); adjust ventilating systems to avoid interfering with the flow of steam
Infrared Lamp	Provides a soothing heat that penetrates into the tissues of the body; relaxes the client, softens the skin to allow penetration of product and increases blood flow	Be aware of the electrical cord with floor-standing model; average distance from client is 30" (75 cm)
Wood's Lamp	Allows analysis of skin surface and deeper layers to aid in determining treatment by using deep ultra-violet light of the lamp; different colors will indicate various conditions	Do not allow the lamp to overheat; avoid direct contact between the lamp and skin; do not look directly at the bulb while it is being used
Suction	Acts as vacuum to give penetrating massage and increases blood circulation to the surface; helpful in deep-pore cleaning	Avoid use on skin with broken capillaries
High Frequency	Creates current that is thermal, or heat producing, and germicidal	Do not use on clients who are pregnant or who have high blood pressure or heart problems

Infection Control and Safety

Infection control and safety are essential while performing skin care services in order to protect the health and well-being of you and your client.

1. Disinfect the facial chair and table before and after every service with an approved broad-spectrum disinfectant.

2. Wash and sanitize your hands before and after every client.

3. Keep lids tightly closed on product jars to avoid spillage and contamination.

4. Remove all products from jars with a sanitized spatula.

5. Keep labels on all containers and store products in a cool place to protect shelf life.

6. Keep tools dry to avoid a short circuit when using electrical equipment.

7. Wear gloves during treatments, if required.

8. Discard any implements that cannot be disinfected.

9. Use eyepads to protect and soothe the eyes when analyzing the skin or applying masks.

10. Identify contraindications such as high blood pressure, heart problems, diabetes, pregnancy, pacemaker or metal implants and/or medications.

Client Consultation

To help you remember the important steps in the consultation process, remember: Great Artists Always Draw Creatively. Just change your focus to your client's skin.

Greeting

- Meet and greet the client with a firm handshake and a pleasant voice.
- Communicate to build rapport and develop a relationship with the client.
- Fill out consultation form with client (sample shown below).

SKIN CARE RECORD CARD

Name _____ Date _____
Address _____
City _____ State _____ Zip _____
Phone (H) _____ (B) _____
Occupation _____ Referred By _____

MEDICAL HISTORY
Age _____ Sex: Female / Male
Known Allergies _____
Are you under care of a Dermatologist? _____
Have you experienced any skin problems in the past 5 years? _____
If yes, please describe _____
Do you have any medical conditions such as:
High Blood Pressure _____ Heart Problems _____ Diabetes _____
Pregnancy _____ Wear Pacemaker _____ Are you on medication? _____
Others not listed above _____

DIETARY HISTORY
Are you currently dieting? _____
Do you take supplemental vitamins etc? _____
Do you exercise regularly? _____
Do you try to eat well-balanced meals? _____
Do you drink at least 8 glasses of water daily? _____

COSMETIC HISTORY
What is the purpose of this makeup application? Day / Evening / Bridal
Have you ever had a reaction from skin care products
  or makeup products? Yes No
Explain _____
Cosmetics now being used _____
Extent of facial care at home:
  Daily _____
  Weekly _____

SKIN EVALUATION

SKIN TYPE	CHARACTERISTICS	SKIN CONDITION /ELASTICITY
Normal _____	White Heads _____	Normal _____
Dry _____	Comedomes _____	Fair _____
Oily _____	Broken Capillaries _____	Poor _____
Combination _____	Discolorations _____	
_____	Blemishes _____	

SIGNS OF DEHYDRATION

None _____	Acne _____	How Long? _____
Moderate _____	Juvenilis _____	Vulgaris _____
Severe _____	Chronic _____	Cystic _____
Asphyxiated _____	Rosascea _____	Scars _____
(Blocked pores/follicles)		
Wrinkles _____	Remarks _____	

PRODUCT & TREATMENT RECOMMENDATIONS
Series Recommended: Corrective / Maintenance
Length of Time: (# of Weeks) 3 6 8 12

Treatment Date	Procedure	Esthetician

Remarks _____

Ask, Analyze and Assess

- Ask questions to discover client needs.

- Analyze client's face.

- Assess the facts and thoroughly think through your recommendations after reading completed client consultation form.

Agree

- Explain your recommended solutions, the products that will be used and the price of the service.

- Think not only of today's service, but future services also.

- Return to step two (ask, analyze and assess) if your client is hesitant with your recommendation.

- Gain feedback and approval from your client.

Deliver

- Ensure client comfort during service.

- Stay focused on delivering the service to the best of your ability.

- Teach the client how to perform home skin care regimen.

Complete

- Request satisfaction feedback from your client.

- Escort client to retail area and show them at least two products you used.

- Recommend products to maintain appearance and condition of your client's skin.

- Inform client that you keep these products in stock for purchase at all times.

- Invite your client to make a purchase.

- Ask your client for referrals for future services.

- Suggest a future appointment time for your client's next visit.

- Offer appreciation to your client for visiting the school or salon.

- Record recommended products on client record card for future visits.

Basic Facial

The benefits the client can derive from receiving a professional facial service include relaxing muscles, soothing nerves, correcting minor skin problems, improving circulation and enhancing healthy skin. Properly given, a facial service is a relaxing and pampering experience ... a service that almost always results in return clientele.

Many of the more common skin problems a cosmetologist may encounter (for example, oily skin prone to blackheads or whiteheads or overly dry skin) can be improved with weekly facial services and the correct home-care regimen you will recommend. Remember, the cosmetologist does not treat skin disease. Skin problems of a serious nature must always be referred to a physician.

Basic Facial Preparation

As with any professional service, it is important to have your area, products, implements and equipment in proper order prior to your client's arrival. Therefore, keep these points in mind:

- Disinfect facial service area
- Set up facial bed with clean blanket/sheet and arrange products
- Check equipment

Basic Facial Procedure

- Wash and sanitize hands*
- Drape client (cocoon wrap)
- Cleanse face
- Obtain cleansing cream
- Apply cleansing cream
- Remove cleansing cream
- Apply toner
- Place eyepads over client's eyes
- Analyze client's skin
- Apply exfoliant
- Remove exfoliant

- Apply toner
- Obtain massage cream
- Apply massage cream
- Perform massage movements
- Remove massage cream
- Apply toner
- Apply facial mask
- Allow mask to set
- Remove mask
- Apply toner
- Apply moisturizing cream

*Wear protective gloves if required by your regulatory agency.

Draping - Cocoon Wrap

Drape cotton blanket over facial bed and position white cotton sheet over blanket. Lay one flat towel and one folded towel at the top of the bed for client's head. Have client lay on top of the sheet.

1. Fold one edge of blanket/sheet combination toward middle of bed
2. Repeat with the other edge, overlapping at center
3. Wrap the end of the blanket/sheet under the client's feet
4. Tuck towel over top of cocoon wrap

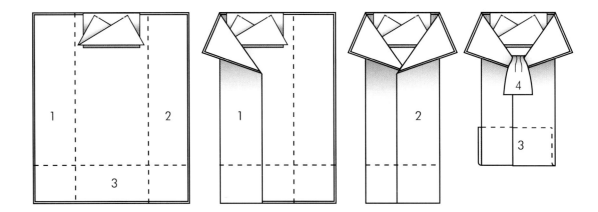

Basic Facial

1-2. Wash and sanitize hands. Ask client to put on gown for the service, **drape client** and position head band or covering to secure hair off the face. **Cleanse the face.** Using cotton and eye makeup remover, perform downward and inward strokes to remove eye makeup. Remove lipstick with tissue, beginning from the outer corner to the center on both sides of the lips.

3. Obtain cleansing cream with a spatula and apply to both hands.

4. Apply cleansing cream over the face and neck, using both hands and starting at the chin. Slide to the end of the jaw, from the base of the nose to the temple, along side of the nose, up over bridge of nose, between brows, across forehead, across to temples. Use smooth, sweeping strokes. Work under the eyes toward the bridge of the nose and out over the eyelid using the ring finger.

5. Remove cleansing cream using cotton pads and warm water. Start at the throat and follow the contour of the face, always working upward. Follow procedure until all cleansing cream has been removed.

6. Apply toner to skin surface with a piece of cotton. This restores pH and aids in cleansing.

Analyze

7. Place eyepads over client's eyes. Analyze client's skin using the magnifying lamp. Check for skin abrasions, excessive oil, flakiness or clogged pores. This will help you to determine skin type and to recommend additional services and retail products.

Basic Facial

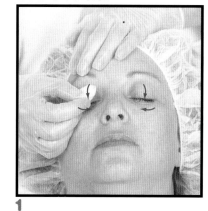
1

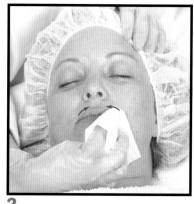
2

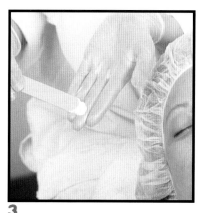
3

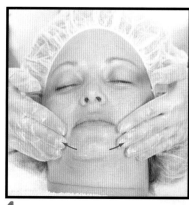
4

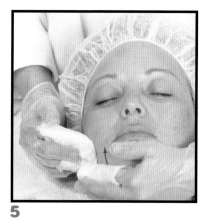
5

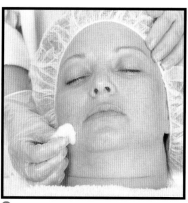
6

Analyze

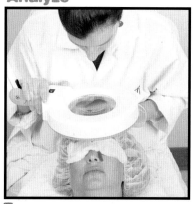
7

Exfoliate

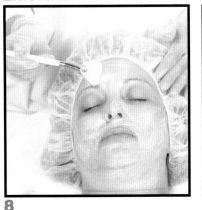

8

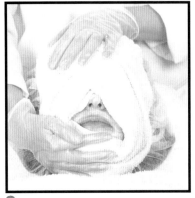

9

Massage

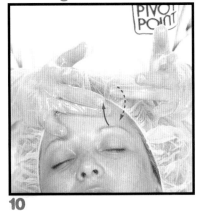

10

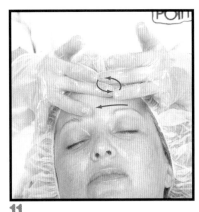

11

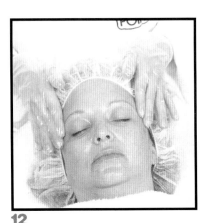

12

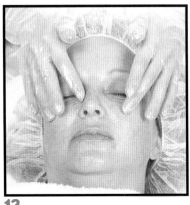

13

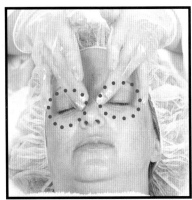

14

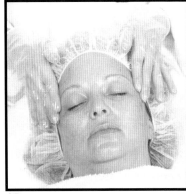

15

Exfoliate

8. Apply exfoliant product to the client's skin. If using a granular scrub, apply and massage in small circular movements. If using an alphahydroxy acid product, apply and let it stay on the skin for the given amount of time. If using an enzyme exfoliant, apply product and steam for approximately 10 minutes. Always follow manufacturer's directions.

9. Remove exfoliant using hot towel or cotton pads. If you use a hot towel, allow steam to release in order to avoid client discomfort or burning. **Apply toner** to close the pores.

Massage

Massage techniques and manipulations are varied. The procedures listed here are considered a foundation that you can build on. **Obtain the massage cream** from the container with a spatula. **Apply massage cream** to the face and neck.

10. Perform massage movements beginning at the forehead. Apply pressure to the forehead using a hand-over-hand movement and effleurage with the ring fingers. Cross the face, moving left to right and then right to left.

11. Slide the middle fingers of both hands over and under each other continuously, as you move across the forehead in half-circle movements.

12. Apply slight pressure at the temples.

13. Perform tapotement around the eyes.

14-15. Circle the outside of the eyes with the ring finger using light pressure. Pause at the temples.

16. Massage the outer corners of the nose, slide fingers up either side of the nose and apply pressure into the eye sockets. Repeat three times.

17. Perform scissor movements on the nose by creating a V-pattern with the index finger and middle finger, starting at the base of the nose and sliding up to the hairline three times.

18. Lift upward slightly on the corners of the mouth three times on each side.

19. Massage in a small circular motion around the mouth three times.

20. Perform scissor movements on the mouth by creating a V-pattern with fingers on both hands and slide across the mouth.

21. Repeat the scissor movement across the chin.

22. Massage upward on the jaw line in a circular movement with the thumb and index finger. Work upward to each earlobe.

23. Massage neck in a small circular motion using both hands.

Massage Tips:

- **Maintain contact with your client using a consistent rhythm**

- **Use up-and-out motions to prevent damage to underlying muscle tissue**

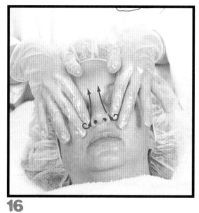
16

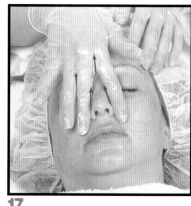
17

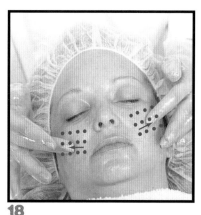
18

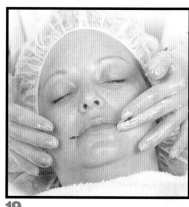
19

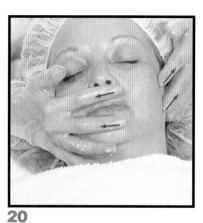
20

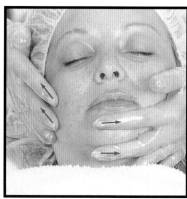
21

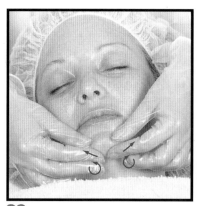
22

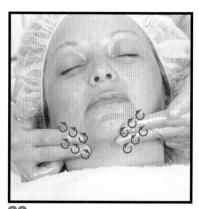
23

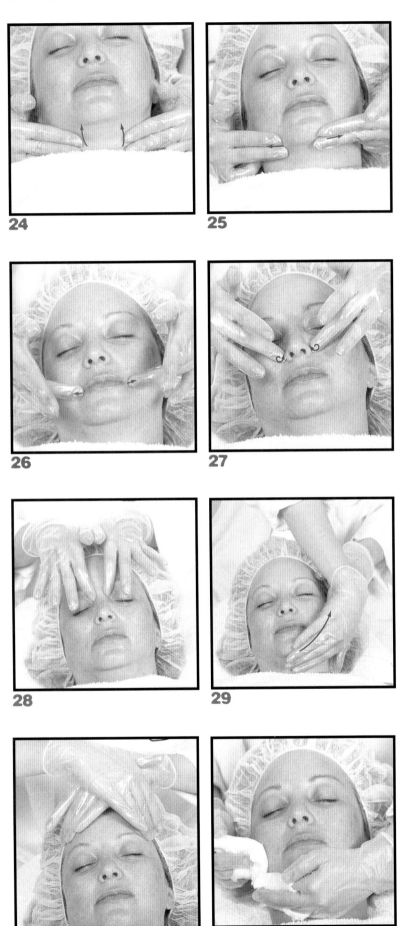

24 **25**

26 **27**

28 **29**

30 **31**

24. Use a hand-over-hand effleurage movement to follow through with the neck movement and bring you back to the chin.

25-28. Working in a continuous movement up the face, perform scissor movements at the chin. Glide to the sides of mouth and apply lifting movements. Then continue to the sides of the nose and perform circular movements. Glide up the sides of the nose and apply light pressure at the eye sockets.

29. Perform effleurage on both sides of the face. Finish the massage treatment by performing a feathering-off movement. This is done by starting at the cheek area with the right hand, followed by the left. Repeat on opposite cheek.

30. Continue by crisscrossing hands over forehead to each temple. Pause and release.

31. **Remove massage cream** from the face and then **apply toner.**

Massage Tips:
- **Pressure of massage must be effective, but not severe**
- **Use caution around the eyes and eyelids to avoid stretching sensitive skin**

Facial Mask

Facial Mask

32. **Apply a facial mask** to the entire face starting at the throat. Use a brush and long strokes.

33-34. **Allow mask to set** on the face for approximately 5-10 minutes, then **remove mask** with a hot towel and cotton pads. **Apply toner** to the skin.

35. **Apply a moisturizing cream** over entire face and neck, using effleurage movements. Conclude with massage around the neck and shoulder area to relieve client of any lingering tension or pressure.

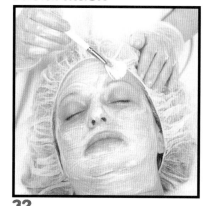
32
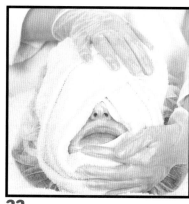
33
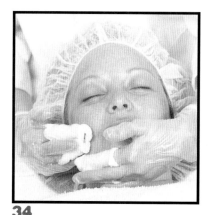
34
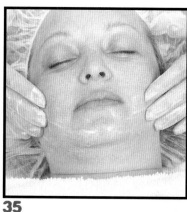
35

Basic Facial Completion

Perform after every facial service:

- Offer rebook visit to client
- Recommend retail products for client
- Throw away non-reusable materials used during the facial service, replace used towels with fresh towels and arrange all products and implements in proper order
- Disinfect your facial service implements and facial bed
- Wash your hands with liquid antibacterial soap

Many salons today are offering body treatments and spa services that cleanse, moisturize and pamper clients.

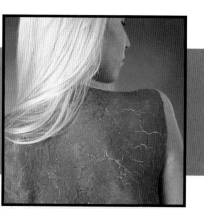
BACK MASK

15

HAIR REMOVAL

Society and personal preferences have long dictated a person's need or desire for removing unwanted or superfluous hair. **This condition of unwanted or superfluous hair is referred to as hyper-trichosis** (hi-per-tri-**KOH**-sis). It is up to you, as a professional cosmetologist, to recommend the best way to remove the unwanted hair or make it less visible.

There are two types of hair removal procedures: temporary and permanent. TEMPORARY procedures include shaving, the use of chemical depilatories, tweezing and waxing. PERMANENT hair removal requires the use of electricity. Most regulating agencies will not license a cosmetologist to perform permanent hair removal services without additional specialized training. An overview of permanent hair removal techniques is included at the end of this section.

If your client wants hair to be less visible without having it removed, consider lightening the hair. You can use a prepared product designed to lighten hair on the face or arms, or you can mix one part oil lightener with two parts hydrogen peroxide. Apply mixture to the area to be lightened and monitor until hair has lightened to the desired shade (15-60 minutes, depending on the hair's color and texture.) Thoroughly rinse off lightener and cleanse area. Apply a moisturizing cream.

Hair Removal Essentials

To perform a professional hair removal service, you need a selection of products, implements and equipment. MSDS guidelines for all products used in the salon must be available.

Hair Removal Products

PRODUCT	FUNCTION
Cleansing Gel	Removes dirt and oil
Antiseptic	Prevents bacteria growth
Wax	Removes unwanted hair
Wax Remover	Cleans wax residue
Soothing Lotion	Calms the skin after waxing
Powder (Talc)	Prevents wax from adhering to skin
Chemical Depilatory	Removes unwanted hair (cream formula generally)

Hair Removal Implements/Supplies

IMPLEMENT/SUPPLIES	FUNCTION
Brow Brush	Combs brow hair prior to shaping
Tweezers	Remove stray hairs
Removal Strips	Aid in removing stray hair; applied over wax
Wax Warmer (Pot)	Melts and holds wax
Spatulas	Remove wax from container/warmer; spread the wax
Gloves	Protect the hands
Sheet	Protects the facial bed
Plastic Bag	Holds garbage
Headband	Holds hair out of the way
Tissue	Aids in application of products

Hair Removal Equipment

EQUIPMENT	FUNCTION
Facial Chair	Holds client
Hand-Held Mirror	Allows client to view results

Infection Control and Safety

Infection control and safety while performing hair removal services are essential in order to protect the health and well-being of you and your client.

1. Always test the temperature of heated wax before applying by checking temperature on your forearm.

2. Keep wax and/or chemical depilatories away from client's eyes and any other areas from which you do not wish to remove hair.

3. Do not use wax over moles, warts, irritated or abraded skin, bruises or varicose veins.

4. Cleanse the skin prior to treatment.

5. Dispose of used wax after every client. Do not reuse wax.

6. Do not rewax sensitive skin or sensitive areas, such as eyebrows, within the same service time.

7. Use cold compresses, ice packs or aloe vera to soothe irritated skin.

8. Do not re-dip spatulas.

9. Do not apply wax if area is sunburned.

10. For 24 hours after waxing service, do not apply makeup following facial waxing or wear pantyhose following leg waxing.

11. Waxing vellus (also known as lanugo) hair is not recommended since it may cause the skin to lose its softness.

Client Consultation

To help you remember the important steps in the consultation process, remember: Great Artists Always Draw Creatively. Just change your focus to your client's hair removal needs.

Greeting

- Meet and greet the client with a firm handshake and a pleasant voice.

- Communicate to build rapport and develop a relationship with the client.

- Have client fill out consultation form.

Ask, Analyze and Assess

- Ask questions to discover client needs.

- Analyze client's skin where hair will be removed.

- Assess the facts and thoroughly think through your recommendations after reading completed client consultation form.

Agree

- Explain your recommended solutions, the products that will be used and the price of the service.

- Think not only of today's service, but future services also.

- Return to step two (ask, analyze and assess)if your client is hesitant with your recommendation.

- Gain feedback and approval from your client.

Deliver

- Ensure client comfort during service.

- Stay focused on delivering the service to the best of your ability.

Complete

- Request satisfaction feedback from your client.

- Ask your client for referrals for future services.

- Suggest a future appointment time for your client's next visit.

- Offer appreciation to your client for visiting the school or salon.

- Record recommended products on client record card for future visits.

CONSULTATION FOR WAXING PROCEDURE

Name _____ Date _____
Address _____ Phone _____
City _____ State _____ Zip _____

Area(s) being waxed: _____
Any adverse reactions to waxing in the past? _____
Any allergies? _____
Are you on any medications that may cause sensitivity to the skin? Yes ___ No ___
If yes, please list them: _____

Is your skin currently undergoing:
Retin-A	Yes ___	No ___	When _____
Retinol	Yes ___	No ___	When _____
Enzyme Peels	Yes ___	No ___	When _____
Glycolic Acid	Yes ___	No ___	When _____
Acutane	Yes ___	No ___	When _____
Alpha Hydroxy	Yes ___	No ___	When _____

Do you have or have you had:
Skin Cancer or Removal	Yes ___	No ___	When _____
Epilepsy	Yes ___	No ___	When _____
Heart Condition	Yes ___	No ___	When _____
Circulatory Condition	Yes ___	No ___	When _____
Swelling or Bruising	Yes ___	No ___	When _____
Rashes or Sores	Yes ___	No ___	When _____
Lesions or Cuts	Yes ___	No ___	When _____
Sunburn	Yes ___	No ___	When _____
Enlarged Varicose Veins	Yes ___	No ___	When _____
Hemophilia	Yes ___	No ___	When _____
HIV Positive	Yes ___	No ___	When _____
Psoriasis	Yes ___	No ___	When _____
Recent Scar Tissue	Yes ___	No ___	When _____
Raised Moles	Yes ___	No ___	When _____
Diabetes	Yes ___	No ___	When _____

I have answered the following questionnaire to the best of my ability and understand that this waxing procedure is done by a student under the supervision of a teacher. I realize that answering this questionnaire truthfully can only help the student assist me better. I understand, have read and completed this form correctly.

Signature _____ Date _____

Temporary Hair Removal

Depending on the type of technique used, hair can grow back in a matter of hours or days, such as with shaving, or in several weeks, as with waxing.

Shaving

The hair removal method most often used when unwanted hair covers large areas, such as women's legs, is shaving. Keep in mind that this service is usually performed by the client at home. Shaving can be performed using an electric shaver, clipper or razor. When using a razor, apply shaving cream before the service to make the skin softer and reduce the potential for skin irritations. Use moisturizing lotion or cream after the service to keep the skin soft and help eliminate dryness or flaking. As the hair grows back it may feel more coarse or thicker due to the blunt effect of the razor. Shaving unwanted hair at the nape hairline can be done with the clipper or razor. Be guided by your area's regulatory agency.

Chemical Depilatories

A chemical depilatory is a substance that dissolves the hair at skin level. Chemical depilatories are usually found in a cream, paste or powder form (which is designed to be mixed). The main ingredient of these products is a thioglycolic acid derivative, with an alkaline pH, that chemically softens and degrades the protein structure of the hair. An allergy test must be given to determine sensitivity to any depilatory product prior to use. A reaction, such as itching, burning or inflammation, is a negative indication to the use of the product. Always read and follow the manufacturer's instructions. To prepare for this hair removal service, assemble materials and prepare your workspace.

Chemical Depilatory Guidelines

- **Wash and sanitize** hands.
- **Drape client** after escorting to the hair removal service area.
- **Check patch test** area for reaction; if no signs are present, continue.
- **Cleanse** area to be treated.
- **Apply depilatory** with a spatula. Apply a thin, even coating. Avoid the mouth, eyes, and nose.
- **Start timing** (usually no more than 10 minutes). Keep room warm, since product works faster if the client's body is warm.
- **Wipe away depilatory** using a soft paper towel. After the manufacturer's recommended time, **reapply** if hair has not been removed.
- **Wash thoroughly** with a gentle soap and warm water. **Rinse.**
- **Apply moisturizer** to entire area. **Undrape and escort** client to reception area.
- **Offer rebook visit** to client.
- **Recommend retail products** for client.
- **Throw away non-reusable materials** used during the service. **Replace used towels** with fresh towels and **arrange all products and implements** in proper order.
- **Disinfect** your implements.
- **Wash your hands** with liquid antibacterial soap.

Tweezing

Tweezing is the hair removal method most commonly used to remove unwanted hairs from smaller areas, such as the eyebrows, chin or around the mouth.

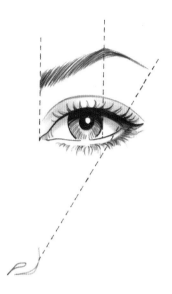

Eyebrow Guidelines

While the shape of your client's eyebrows needs to be customized for facial features, follow these general guidelines to achieve a well-arched eyebrow.

- The brow should begin over the inside corner of the eye.

- The peak, or highest point of the arch, should occur over the outside of the iris of the eye.

- Then imagine a diagonal line from the outside of the nose that extends past the outside of the eye. This point is where the brow should end.

A good brow design creates a frame for the face and "opens" the eye. A person with excessive hair may benefit from waxing instead of tweezing since it is faster and less irritating.

- **Assemble materials** and **prepare workspace**.

- **Wash and sanitize hands.**

- **Cleanse area** to be tweezed.

- **Analyze your client's brows** using the guidelines above. Consider the client's overall appearance before you determine how thick or thin the eyebrows should be. Note that this is outlined in more detail in the makeup section of this chapter.

- **Brush the hairs up** with a brow brush. This will allow you to see the base of the hairs and to remove them in neat rows, rather than at random.

- **Hold the skin taut** with one hand by stretching it between the thumb and index finger. **Tweeze the hairs in the direction of the hair growth,** using quick movements.

- **Tweeze stray hairs** that appear below the brow. To create a more pronounced arch, tweeze in an upward direction from just inside the beginning of the brow to the area you determined should be the highest point of the arch. Continue tweezing, sloping gently downward, toward the outer edge of the brow. The points you choose to begin and end your arch and the degree of slope you create will determine how pronounced the arch will be.

- **Complete one brow**, then the other, making sure they match.

- **Apply astringent** to the area, then apply a soothing cream.

- **Offer rebook visit** in a 4 - 6 week period.

- Return to service area and **perform necessary infection control procedures**.

Waxing

↑ Cold wax is for people who cannot tolerate Hot wax

Waxing is a procedure that is beneficial for temporarily removing hair from both large and small areas. **Waxing, using either hot or cold wax, is a service in which the hair is physically removed from the follicle by applying the wax, allowing the hair to firmly adhere to the wax and, finally, pulling off the wax/hair.** For clients who can't tolerate hot wax, which is outlined below, cold wax is an option. The application of cold wax is similar to a hot wax application, except that a thicker application of cold wax is used and strips are not used to remove the wax. Instead, the wax itself is pulled opposite the direction of the hair growth.

Basic Waxing

Waxing is a quick, easy way to temporarily remove hair around the eyebrow area. This procedure generally needs to be repeated every 4 to 6 weeks.

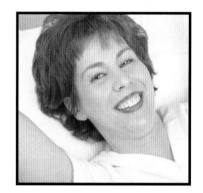

Basic Waxing Preparation

As with any professional service, it is important to have your area, products, implements and equipment in proper order prior to your client's arrival. Before performing a basic eyebrow or leg wax, be sure to satisfy the following points:

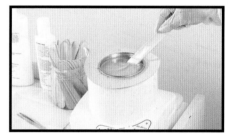

- Sanitize service area
- Place sheet on facial chair
- Pre-cut removal strips to be used
- Arrange pre-treatment cream/cleanser, powder, wax cleaner, soothing lotion, spatulas, tweezers, gloves and plastic bag
- Warm up wax at least 30 minutes before client arrives

Basic Waxing Procedure

Note that this procedure applies to both eyebrow and leg waxing.

- Wash and sanitize hands*
- Drape client
- Examine area to be waxed
- Cleanse area to be waxed
- Apply powder on area to be waxed
- Test temperature of wax
- Obtain wax
- Apply wax at a 45° angle in direction of hair growth
- Apply removal strip

- Press down
- Pull skin taut
- Remove strip quickly in opposite direction
- Apply pressure immediately
- Apply antiseptic
- Repeat procedure
- Apply and remove wax cleanser
- Apply soothing lotion
- Tweeze
- Show client results

*Wear protective gloves if required by your regulatory agency.

Eyebrow Wax

1. **Wash and sanitize hands. Drape client. Examine the area to be waxed. Clean area to be waxed** with an antiseptic gel.

2. **Apply powder on area to be waxed** to create a barrier for the skin against the wax.

3. **Test the temperature of the wax** on the back of your hand before applying. **Obtain wax** with clean spatula and **apply wax at a 45° angle in the direction of the hair growth**.

4. **Apply the removal strip. Press down** and **pull skin taut** holding the end of the strip in the direction of the hair growth.

5. **Remove the strip quickly in the opposite direction** of the hair growth. Do not pull upward.

6. **Apply pressure immediately** to minimize pain and redness. **Apply an antiseptic** if slight bleeding or irritation occurs. **Repeat procedure** for both eyes.

7. **Apply and remove a wax cleanser.**

8. **Apply a soothing lotion** with cotton.

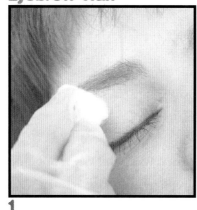
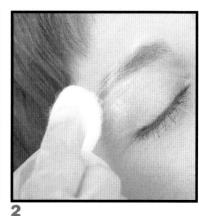
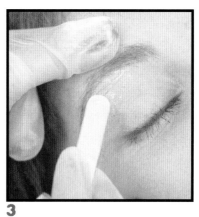
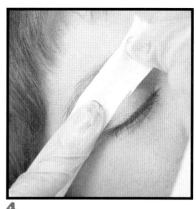
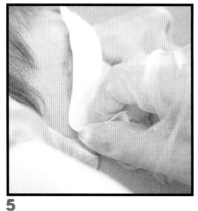
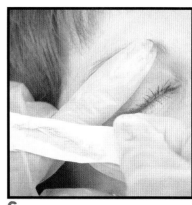
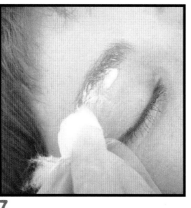
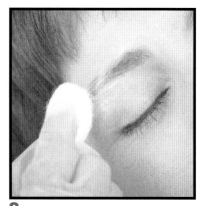

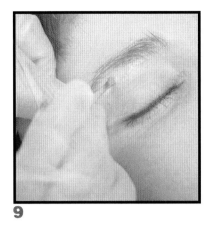

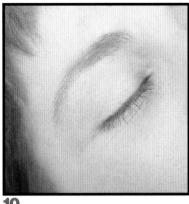

9

10

9. **Tweeze** to remove any stray hairs not picked up by the wax

10. **Show your client the results.** Undrape client and escort to reception area.

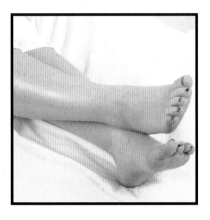

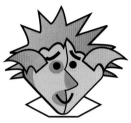

"Did you know that sugar and lemon juice create a sticky substance like wax that is used to remove hair? This technique is called 'sugaring.' which comes from the ancient Egyptians. and is still used today!"

Leg Wax

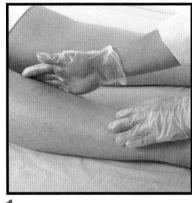

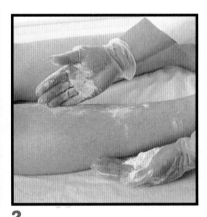

1

2

Leg Wax

1. **Wash and sanitize hands. Drape client. Examine the area to be waxed** for contraindications (problem areas) and continue if no signs are present. **Cleanse area to be waxed** with an antiseptic gel.

2. **Apply powder on area to be waxed** Be sure to apply all over the leg.

3. **Obtain wax** with a clean spatula and **apply at a 45° angle in the direction of the hair growth.** Use sweeping motion when applying the wax. Keep in mind that wax should be applied in rows or sections, since you are covering a much larger area.

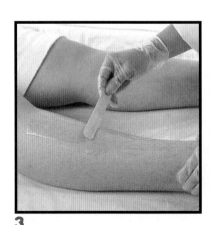

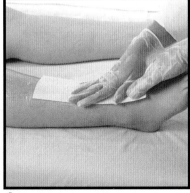

3

4

4. Apply the removal strip. **Press down** in the direction of the hair growth.

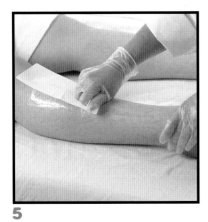

5

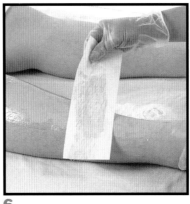

6

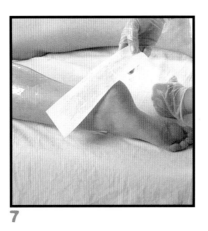

7

5-6. **Pull skin taut** and hold the end of the strip. **Remove the strip quickly in the opposite direction** of the hair growth. **Apply pressure immediately.** Work quickly so that the wax does not get cold and hard while on the leg. **Apply an antiseptic** if slight bleeding or irritation occurs.

7. Remove all the wax from each section before you **repeat procedure** on a new row or section. Once you've completed waxing the top area of both legs, have your client turn over and wax the back of both legs. When you've finished waxing the back of the legs, have your client turn back over. **Apply and remove wax cleanser.** Remove excess product with a towel. **Apply a soothing toner** with cotton. **Tweeze** stray hairs if necessary.

Basic Waxing Completion

Perform after every eyebrow or leg waxing service:

- Offer rebook visit to client
- Recommend retail products for client
- Throw away non-reusable materials used during the waxing service, replace used towels with fresh towels and arrange all products and implements in proper order
- Disinfect your waxing service implements and facial bed
- Wash your hands with liquid antibacterial soap

Permanent Hair Removal

Permanent hair removal, known as electrolysis, uses electric current to damage the cells of the papilla and disrupt hair growth. The goal is to damage enough papilla cells so that either a lighter, finer diameter hair grows back or, ideally, no hair grows from the follicle at all. Several treatments per follicle (exposure to current) are normally required before lasting results are achieved. This is not a one-time service, and many require multiple visits to obtain desired results. In most areas this method is used by a licensed professional called an electrologist. An electrologist has advanced training specifically in the study of electrolysis (or is a medical doctor).

The medical community recognizes three methods of permanent hair removal:

1. Galvanic electrolysis or multiple needle method

2. Thermolysis or high frequency/short-wave method

3. Blend (a combination of galvanic and thermolysis)

Each of these methods has advantages and disadvantages. Remember, advanced training is required to perform electrolysis in most areas.

Galvanic Method

The galvanic electrolysis method destroys the hair by decomposing the papilla. In galvanic electrolysis, multiple wire needles or probes are inserted into the follicle. A low level of current passes into the needle and causes a chemical reaction in the cells of the papilla. The current is typically on from 30 seconds to 2.5 minutes. The instrument has multiple probes that are normally inserted (with minimal discomfort) and activated at one time; for this reason, galvanic electrolysis is sometimes called the "multiple needle" process.

Thermolysis Method

The thermolysis or high frequency/short-wave method involves inserting a single needle (probe) into the follicle. The current travels to the papilla for less than a second, resulting in a coagulation of the cells. The hair is immediately tweezed from the follicle. Because the time and intensity of the current are carefully controlled, preferably by an automatic timer, the client feels only a tiny "flash" of heat. Redness or a slight bump in the skin are normal reactions and disappear in two or three days. The wire used in thermolysis is substantially finer than the electrolysis probe, further reducing client discomfort. This is currently the most popular method of permanent hair removal and is medically recognized as the most effective.

Blend Method

The blend method of hair removal is a combination of galvanic and thermolysis technology. A special instrument designed to combine galvanic current (for best results on resistant follicles) and high frequency current (for faster results) produce the blend. Highly trained electrologists may use this method if the other methods fail. The advantages and disadvantages are similar to those of the individually used methods. The importance of this method is that it offers a "last chance" to clients with excessive or resistant hair growth.

MAKEUP

Now that you've learned what it takes to keep the skin in optimum condition, you are ready to look at how makeup design can enhance your client's overall appearance. Makeup design and trends strongly relate to other fashion mediums, such as clothing and hair. This means that seasonal changes and trends from year to year follow swiftly, one after another. The concepts presented in this chapter are intended to give you the basic skills you'll need to perform makeup services in the salon. The designs you create for your clients in the salon will vary from person to person and will relate to current trends as well as the personal expression of your client. Remember that ideals of beauty vary from culture to culture and in different age groups. As your skill level increases, you may become more interested in other, more specific areas of makeup design. For example, designing makeup for photography, film and theater can be very challenging and rewarding.

Makeup design utilizes an artistic concept called chiaroscuro, an arrangement of light and dark parts, to visually alter the contours of the face. The basic premise of chiaroscuro is that lighter colors stand out and darker colors recede. By applying lighter and darker tones, you can change the apparent contours of the face. Adding light or highlights will accentuate and emphasize areas or features that need to be 'brought out.' Darker tones are applied to shadow or contour areas and features you wish to diminish or minimize. This understanding of the properties of darker and lighter colors allows you to visually alter the shape of the face.

Facial Shapes

The well-proportioned oval face shape has long been considered the ideal or classic facial shape. Standards of beauty have certainly expanded during recent decades, but most corrective makeup and contouring are done to achieve the illusion of an oval face.

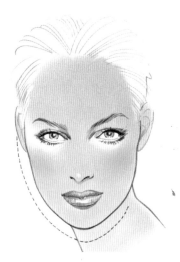

Oval Face

The generally balanced shape and regular features of the oval face will not require much in the way of 'corrective' application. In most instances, **the oval shape represents the ideal, so creating the illusion of an oval face when working on other face shapes can be achieved with corrective makeup.**

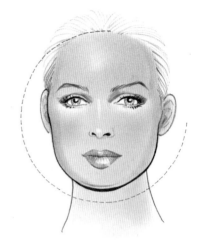

Round Face

Generally a fuller face, the round face, is often characterized by a rounded hairline and chin line as well. Contouring can be used to slenderize the face, adding to the vertical emphasis and making it appear more oval.

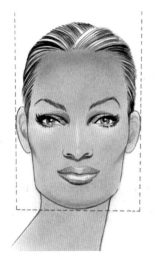

Oblong Face (also known as long)

The oblong facial shape tends to be long and narrow. This face can be visually shortened by applying deeper tones under the chin and horizontally at the hairline. Horizontal lines should be emphasized whenever possible, in brow shape, cheek color and lip shape. Highlighting can be used to add visual width when possible.

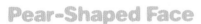

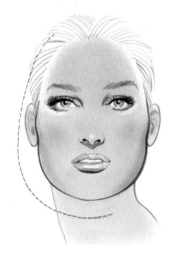

Pear-Shaped Face

A pear-shaped face has a narrow forehead and a wide jaw line. Adding width to the forehead can be achieved with highlighting. Contour to reduce the width at the bottom of the face.

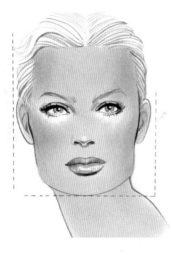

Square Face

The square face is usually characterized by a broad, straight forehead and hairline, with a broad jaw line. The effect can be very angular and almost masculine. Contouring can be done to soften the angularity and reduce the width.

Heart-Shaped Face

The heart-shaped face is characterized by a wider forehead and a narrow jaw or chin line. Width across the forehead can be minimized by contouring while the jaw line can be visually widened with highlighting.

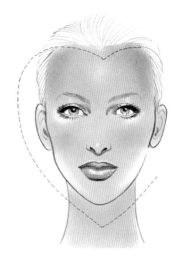

Diamond-Shaped Face

Predominant width through the cheekbones is contrasted by narrow forehead and chin/jaw areas on the diamond-shaped face. Width through the cheekbones can be minimized with contouring and the jaw and forehead can be made to look wider with highlighting.

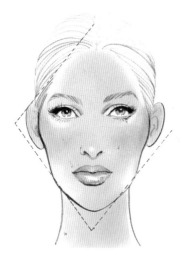

Color Theory

The law of color is equally important in makeup design as it is in hair color design. Remember that all colors are comprised of the three primary colors: red, yellow and blue. Mixing two primaries in equal proportions creates the three secondary colors: green, orange and purple. Mixing primary and secondary colors in equal proportions creates tertiary colors. Colors opposite each other on the color wheel are called complementary colors. For instance, green is the complementary color of red. Complementary colors will neutralize each other when they are mixed together.

Terms You Should Know

HUE is another term for color

TINT is a hue with white added

SHADE is a hue with black added

VALUE is the lightness or darkness of a color

INTENSITY refers to the vibrancy of a color

TONE refers to the warmth or coolness of a color

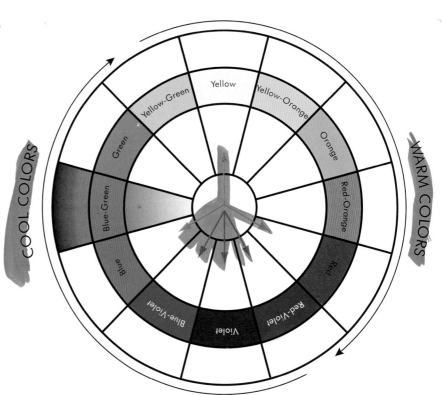

Color Schemes

Monochromatic color schemes use the same color (with variations in value and intensity) throughout the face design.

Analogous color schemes use three colors that are adjacent to each other on the color wheel; often used for daytime face designs. (See pink arrows on color wheel illustration.)

Triadic color schemes use three colors located in a triangular position on the color wheel and are often used for more vibrant face designs. (See blue arrows on color wheel illustration.)

Complementary color schemes use colors that are across from each other on the color wheel in order to achieve the greatest amount of contrast and are often used to enhance eye color.

Warm and **Cool** are terms used to describe the tones found in both skin colors and cosmetic colors. Warm colors have red or yellow tones within them and cool colors have more blue tones within them.

Remember that dark colors seem to recede and diminish the appearance of features or areas, while lighter colors seem to advance, making features or areas appear larger or more prominent.

Makeup Essentials

To perform a professional makeup service, you will need the proper selection of products, implements and equipment. Makeup products are produced by many different manufacturers, are disposable and must be frequently replaced. MSDS guidelines for all products used in the salon must be easily available for your use. Makeup implements are hand-held tools, which must be disinfected or discarded after each use. Makeup equipment includes the furnishings and provisions necessary to provide a professional makeup service.

Makeup Products

PRODUCT	FUNCTION
Cotton	Removes product
Cleanser	Removes dirt, makeup and impurities
Toner	Purifies and restores pH
Moisturizer	Replenishes moisture/oil; protects skin
Concealer	Eliminates discolorations; reduces appearance of blemishes
Foundation	Creates an even skin tone and uniform surface

PRODUCT	FUNCTION
Blush	Adds color or contour
Eye liner	Accentuates and defines shape of eyes
Eye shadow	Accentuates shape and color of eye; contours
Brow pencil/powder	Fills in; corrects shape of eyebrow
Mascara	Defines, lengthens, thickens the eyelashes
Lip liner	Defines natural or corrected shape of the lips
Lipstick	Adds color and texture to the lips
Tissue	Blots the skin; removes excess product
Cotton swabs	Clean up; correct errors

Makeup Implements/Supplies

IMPLEMENT/SUPPLIES	FUNCTION
Head band	Holds client's hair out of the way during application
Towel/makeup drape	Protects client's clothing
Palette	Holds desired amount of product(s)
Spatulas	Remove product(s) from containers
Latex sponges	Apply foundations and concealers; blending; clean up
Tweezers	Shape eyebrows; remove stray hairs
Brushes	Apply makeup; specific to needs
Eyelash curler	Curls and enhances lashes
Mascara wands	Apply mascara
Lash separator	Separates lashes after mascara application

Makeup Equipment

EQUIPMENT	FUNCTION
Mirror	Allows artist to check balance; allows client to follow application
Proper lighting	Allows artist to work accurately and gauge results
Makeup chair	Places client at proper height for makeup application/service

Infection Control and Safety

It is essential that you practice infection control and safety while performing makeup services so that you protect the health and well-being of your clients.

1. Wash and sanitize hands before and after every client.

2. Sanitize brushes after every client.

3. Use disposable applicators whenever possible and discard after use.

4. Avoid using products and makeup directly from containers. Use spatulas to place the desired amount of product on your makeup palette. If more product is needed, remember to use a fresh spatula.

5. Use a fresh drape on every client.

6. Sharpen all pencils before and after each use.

7. Remove product if you see signs of allergic reactions to cosmetic products, such as redness, swelling or inflammation.

8. Avoid excess pressure in and around the eye area.

9. Exercise extra precautions to avoid getting products or implements in the eyes.

10. Keep your fingernails well-groomed to avoid scratching your clients.

Client Consultation

To help you remember the important steps of the consultation process, keep in mind that: Great Artists Always Draw Creatively. Just change your focus to your client's makeup needs.

Greeting

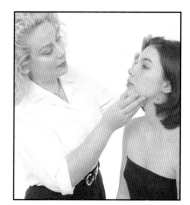

*   Meet the client and greet her with a firm handshake and a pleasant voice.

*   Build rapport and develop a relationship with the client through communication.

*   Assist client in filling out a consultation form.

Ask, Analyze and Assess

*   Ask questions: discover the purpose of the makeup application. Is it a special occasion or has the client come in for a makeup application lesson?

*   Analyze your client's skin tone and skin type.

*   Assess the facts found in the consultation form and in the answers to your questions; thoroughly think through your recommendations.

Agree

- Explain recommended face design and color selections.

- Identify products to be used and price for the service (if different from standard pricing).

- Gain feedback and approval from your client.

- Return to step two (ask, analyze and assess) if your client is hesitant with your recommendations.

Deliver

- Ensure client comfort during service.

- Focus on and deliver the service that was agreed upon.

- If explanations are needed, be clear and precise.

Complete

- Confirm that client is pleased with services rendered (satisfaction/feedback).

- Escort client to retail area and show at least two products used during service.

- Recommend products for future makeup applications.

- Invite client to make a purchase.

- Suggest a time for your client's next visit; schedule appointment if possible.

- Thank your client for visiting the school or salon.

- Record on client record card the products used and recommended.

Makeup Techniques and Products

Although makeup techniques and products can vary according to the occasion, the client's skin type and features, as well as the client's wishes, there are basic guidelines you can follow, which we'll outline in this section. To start, you'll want to keep the following points in mind before and/or during a makeup application:

- Prepare the skin (cleanse, tone and moisturize) before applying any cosmetics. Proper skin care ensures smooth application and better product adherence.

- Facial hair removal and brow shaping are done prior to the application of makeup. Keep in mind that additional shaping and 'filling in' of the brows may occur during the makeup service. Refer to the "Hair Removal" portion of this chapter for more information.

- Whenever appropriate, begin with light, sheer foundations that allow you to add if more coverage is required. A heavy, matte foundation will be more difficult to adjust as you work. Remember that foundation is meant to create an even base on the skin.

- Make use of the proper makeup brushes and applicators when applying cosmetics. Brushes are particularly helpful in that they provide more directional control and can be used effectively to blend colors and soften or smudge harder lines.

- Always apply makeup in appropriate lighting. Keep in mind the lighting in which the makeup will be seen and make adjustments according to the light in which you are working. Fluorescent lighting can be deceiving as it often accentuates any blue or green undertones and cancels out warmer tones. Since evening makeup tends to be more dramatic, you must compensate when working under salon lighting or daylight.

- Makeup design is about creating illusions! By using the principles of light and dark colors, you can highlight attractive features or areas and diminish those that are less attractive. Also, by making the best use of 'shine' and 'matte' products you can enhance or diminish appropriately. Careful blending between lights and darks, as well as shine and matte, will help you to create the most effective illusions.

Brushes

It is important to have a selection of makeup brushes available. Note that brush names may vary among manufacturers.

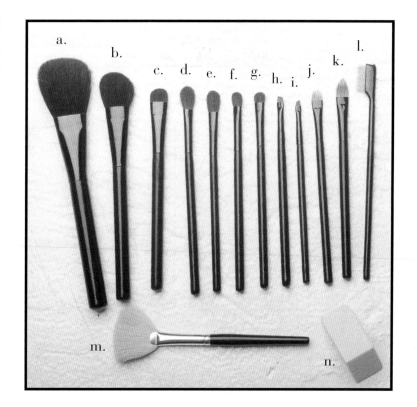

   a.   Large powder brush (dome)

   b.   Contoured brush

   c.   Medium chisel brush

   d.   Large blending brush

   e.   Medium fluff brush

   f.   Small fluff brush

   g.   Small chisel brush

   h.   Angle brush

   i.   Detail angle brush

   j.   Lip brush

   k.   Large camouflage brush

   l.   Eyelash separator

   m.   Fan brush

   n.   Latex sponge

Makeup Corrections/Concealer

Every makeup artist knows the necessity of correcting particular facial imperfections before applying foundation. After preparing the client's skin (cleansing, toning and moisturizing), you'll need to assess the skin for tone and value, as well as for specific problems. Problems such as under-eye circles (often with blue or purple undertones), broken capillaries and blemishes can and should be corrected. If they are not, they may stand out or detract from the completed makeup design.

Concealers are available in cream, pot and stick formulations. They are available in light, medium and dark 'skin tones,' generally with a yellowish base shade. With these tones, you may wish to match the foundation or go one shade lighter. You may also suggest products that offset the skin's natural undertones.

IF UNDERTONE IS:	USE:
Yellow	Violet Base
Red	Green Base
Green	Red Base
Blue/Purple	Yellow/Orange Base

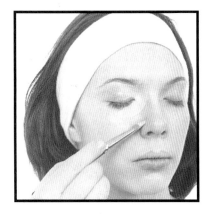 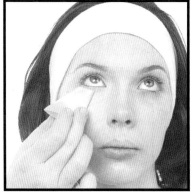 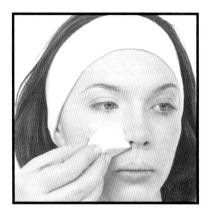

To apply concealer to the eye area, form a half-moon shape that covers the inside edges of the top and bottom of the eye area. Also apply concealer to any darker or shadowed areas of the eye. You may apply with a camouflage brush, but blend with a latex sponge. Apply a minimal amount of pressure to this delicate area to help maintain the elasticity of the skin tissue and prevent wrinkling and creasing. Under the eye, blend toward the bridge of the nose.

To eliminate shadows or discolorations (such as broken capillaries) along the sides of the nose, use a camouflage brush to apply concealer to both sides of the nasal fold, in a triangular shape. Use a latex sponge to blend the concealer into the surrounding skin.

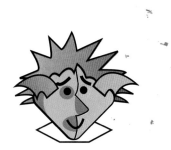

"Remember that makeup applicators must be discarded or disinfected after each use to follow infection control guidelines."

Foundation

When correctly selected and applied, foundations even out skin color and create a smoother, more even skin texture, providing a 'pure canvas' on which to create a makeup design. Foundation is used to correct unwanted skin tones such as sallowness or ruddiness. Unless correction is required, match the foundation to the skin tone. To test a foundation shade to determine if you have chosen the correct color, blend a small amount of foundation on the client's jaw line. The correct color will 'disappear' into the client's skin. Foundation may be considered the most important makeup product, since it creates the canvas on which the other cosmetics appear.

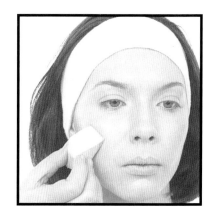

Foundations are available in several forms, the most prevalent of which is liquid form. The liquid form is generally preferred because it offers coverage with a more natural appearance.

Cream foundation has a heavier consistency and is used for additional coverage. Cream foundations require more careful blending than liquid foundations.

Pancake or pan-stick foundations are used for very heavy coverage and are usually applied with water and a sponge. Grease-based foundations also offer very heavy coverage. Both types of 'maximum coverage' foundations are used primarily for photography and theater. They are also used when major corrections are required, such as covering scars or large birthmarks.

In recent years, foundations have become available in a combination of makeup base and powder, which can be found in a compact form. This combination is sometimes called 'one-step' or 'dual finish' makeup because additional powder is not required. Coverage will vary from brand to brand, but is generally on the lighter side, for a more natural effect.

Skin Color Classifications

TYPE	RANGES FROM...
Light Creamy Skin	Light, creamy to slightly peach undertone
Golden Skin	Yellow cast if light to golden tone if tanned
Pink Skin	Pink, light or florid to red undertones
Tan Skin	Light to dark brown; undertone can be red or yellow
Olive Skin	Yellow to yellowish-green color
Brown Skin	Light to dark and may be classified as having brown, red or yellow undertones
Ebony Skin	Dark to quite dark; varies greatly in undertones

Foundation has other applications besides coverage and correction. It is often used to achieve the effects of facial contouring. Lighter shades of foundation are used to highlight a facial feature and darker shades of foundation are used to recess a facial feature. Foundation is also used to complete and correct the lip line.

To apply foundation, place approximately a dime-size amount of product onto your palette. Use your fingertip or a cotton swab to transfer foundation from the palette. Apply to the face, starting in the 'mask' area. The mask area is comprised of the center of the face, especially around the eyes. Measure approximately two-fingers' width around the eyes and near the nose. Then use a latex sponge to blend the product onto the face. Use a pat-and-roll or stippling technique to blend the foundation outward from the mask. Use very gentle pressure as you work. **If too much pressure is applied to the facial skin, broken capillaries can result.** Be sure to blend each section carefully before moving on. Foundation should blend and fade away toward the perimeters of the face, if the mask application is used. This application is used on relatively clear, blemish-free skin that does not require much color correction. **If a more traditional application is used (covering the entire face) or if two shades are used, foundation should blend into the hairline and to the neck, avoiding any lines of demarcation.**

Contouring and Highlighting

Contouring and highlighting can add the illusion of increased dimension to the face and, in some instances, appear to reshape the face. **In makeup application, highlighting the protruding bones can "bring out" these features, while shadowing of the cavities, or recessed areas, can add depth to the face.** Contour means to create an outline, especially of a curving or irregular figure or shape. Heightening the contrasts between lighter and darker tones can create more definition in the planes

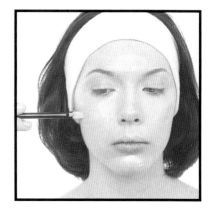

and surfaces of the face. Contour by using a darker shadow to give the appearance of a smaller or receding feature. For example, a wider nose can appear thinner by applying darker tones to the sides of the nose. Highlight by using a lighter tint to create the appearance of a larger or more outstanding feature. Highlighting the receding areas of a weak chin can make the chin seem more prominent and well-proportioned with the rest of the face.

Many cosmetic products can be used to contour the face. The most common products come in powder, liquid and cream forms. Powders create a matte finish, while liquids and creams result in a "glowing" finish. Your client's skin type will help you to determine which type of product will work best for her. Oily skin types usually look best when powders are used. Dryer skin types can benefit from the moisturizing properties often found in liquid or cream formulations. Powders are applied with brushes. A small tapered brush and a shading brush are usually sufficient for all but theatrical contouring. Brushes or sponges may be used to apply liquid and cream contour products.

Remember that contouring needs to be done for subtle effect. Again keep in mind the lighting in which the clients will be seen (i.e. bright lighting may not be very flattering to the 'cosmetic tricks' of highlighting and contouring). Also, products must be blended very well to achieve the most attractive effects.

Eyes

The eyes, often called the windows to the soul, can be the most expressive feature of the face. Many first impressions are based on how well confidence and trust are communicated with the eyes. Since the eyes are such an attention-getting and important feature, you must be sure to use cosmetic artistry very wisely in this area.

The eye area can be divided into thirds. The three areas are the eyelid, the crease area and the brow bone. An eye that is in 'perfect' or ideal proportions would have the following characteristics:

- The area between the base of the lashes and the crease line makes up one-third of the eye.
- The area between the crease line and the eyebrow makes up the remaining two-thirds.
- Well-spaced eyes have the width of one eye between them. 'Close-set' eyes have a space of less (than one eye) between them. 'Wide-set' eyes have a space greater (than one eye).

Eyebrows

Eyebrows 'frame' the eyes and are very important to the balance of any face and makeup design. Refer to the hair removal portion of this chapter for complete procedures on waxing and tweezing.

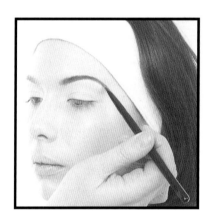

Whether the brows are natural or have been shaped, it may be necessary to shade or fill in to create the most attractive and flattering shape. You can shade or fill in the brows using shadows (powder) or pencils.

Follow these general guidelines for shaping a well-arched eyebrow.

- The brow should begin over the inside corner of the eye.
- The peak, or highest point of the arch, should occur over the outside of the iris of the eye.
- Then imagine a diagonal line from the outside of the nose that extends past the outside of the eye. This point is where the brow should end.

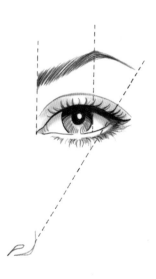

Variations on this basic shape will be appropriate for most face shapes. Keep the natural shape of the brow, as it relates to the client's brow bone, in mind. Extreme changes in brow shape are appropriate for high fashion and theatrical looks.

You can use the shape of the eyebrows to offset imperfections of other facial features. For instance, if the eyes are set too close together, widen the distance between the brows to make the eyes seem more well-spaced. Wide-set eyes can be made to look closer together by extending the brows past the inside corners of the eyes. Straighter, more horizontal brows, with a minimal arch, will help diminish the illusion of length in a long face.

Keep these points in mind when filling in or shading brows:

- Work with sharp pencils and use small, hair-like strokes
- Use two colors to give you a more natural effect and allow you to match hair color more closely
- Make sure you've filled the brow evenly, leaving no sparse areas
- Use a brow brush to soften the edges of the eyebrow
- Strive for symmetry as you work on the other eyebrow

Eyeliner

Eyeliner is used in makeup application to define and emphasize the shape and size of the eyes. Eyeliners come in liquid, pencil and powder formulas. Liquids and powders are usually applied with a brush. Pencil liners are applied to the eye using very short strokes. Eyeliner is usually applied at the lash line. Pencil liners can be applied inside the eyelid as well, but be sure not to cover the tear duct since this may cause injury. Keep in mind that harder lines, such as those achieved with liquid liner, may not be as flattering and are generally reserved for evening or specific fashion makeup designs.

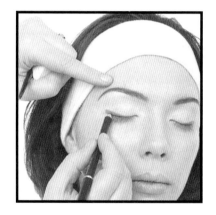

Eye Shadow

Eye shadows come in many forms, including creams, gel, powders and pencils or crayons. Shadows can be used to create a more contoured or exaggerated effect in areas such as the crease. They can also be used to highlight and accentuate areas such as the brow bone. Eye shadow design is often the focal point of a complete makeup design, so you must carefully analyze the client's lifestyle and personality, as well as the occasion for which the makeup is being designed. Blending is especially crucial in this area, since colors are often more intense. Again, it is important to apply very little pressure to the eye area to preserve and protect the delicate skin in this area.

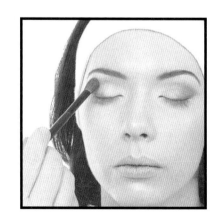

Mascara

Mascara defines, lengthens and thickens the eyelashes. The depth of color used may also serve to enhance and bring out the eye shadow color used. Mascara is available in liquid, cake and cream forms. It is applied with disposable mascara wands and is generally applied to the upper and lower lashes. Note that an eyelash curler may be used prior to the application of mascara to open up the eyes. Use a lash separator after applying mascara to avoid a clumpy look.

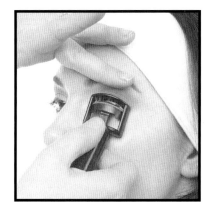 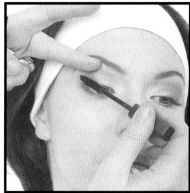 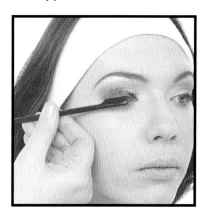

Artificial (false) Lashes

Artificial lashes are not generally worn with day makeup, since they tend to create a more dramatic effect. The exception would be individuals who have lost their lashes or have particularly sparse lashes.

Application of Artificial Strip Lashes

Quality, human hair lashes are the most natural looking. Brown or black will coordinate well enough to be worn with most hair colors. To apply artificial lashes, you will need an appropriate set of lashes, tweezers, scissors and lash adhesive. Follow these general steps to apply:

1. Begin by measuring the upper lash. Start midway between the inside corner of the eye and the curve where the iris begins and measure to the outside corner. If the lash is too long, trim it to fit.

2. Use your fingers to bend the lashes into a horseshoe shape to make them more flexible and easier to fit to the curve of the eyelid.

3. Apply a thin strip (small amount) of eyelash adhesive to the base of the artificial lashes and allow it to set for a few seconds.

4. Apply the lashes. Begin with the shorter, or inside, part of the lashes and position them midway between the inside corner of the eye and the curve where the iris begins. Position the remaining lashes as close to the client's own lashes as possible. You may also work from the outside corner toward the inside corner, so long as the lashes have been accurately measured and trimmed.

5. Apply bottom lashes by using lash adhesive in the same manner as for the upper lashes. Place the lashes under the client's lower lashes, with shorter lashes toward the center of the eye and longer lashes toward the outside.

Application of Semi-Permanent Individual Eyelashes (Eye Tabbing)
Although not done frequently, another method of applying false lashes is known as eye tabbing. Tabbing involves the application of individual, synthetic lashes to the client's own lashes. The application lasts approximately 6-8 weeks, with lashes falling off as the client's own lashes naturally fall out. Lower lashes will not last as long, since the oils in this area will cause the adhesive to break down.

Facial Powder

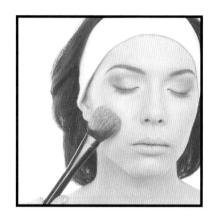

Facial powders are primarily designed to 'set' other makeup products so that they last longer without fading, streaking or rubbing off. They are applied after liquid or creme products, such as foundations or cream blushes. They are applied before powdered blushes or contour colors. The most common forms available are loose and pressed powders. Both forms can be found in translucent and tinted shades. **A colorless (translucent) powder may be worn with any foundation shade since it is designed to allow the skin/foundation shade to show through without imparting any color.** Tinted powders should be used in coordination with matching foundations. They may also be worn successfully by women who do not wear foundation and want only the sheerest coverage. Application with a powder brush (or large dome brush) will yield lighter coverage. For heavier coverage, use a sponge or powder puff. Facial powder is generally applied before mascara.

Blush

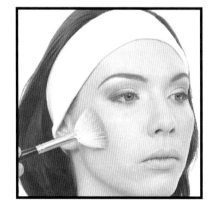

Blush is used to add color to the face, especially to the cheek area. Without blush, the face may appear to be flat or dull, since foundation has evened out skin tone and reduced any natural 'blush.' Blush can also be used to enhance facial contouring.

Blushes are available in liquid, cream, gel and powder forms. Cream and gel products are applied prior to the application of facial powder, usually with a small sponge. Powdered blush is applied after facial powder, usually with a brush. **Liquid cheek color products seem to be suitable for all skin types.** The fairness or darkness of your client's skin will determine the depth of the blush color you recommend. Blush should coordinate with the tones of the rest of the makeup application. Warm eye makeup and lip colors require warmer blush colors, while a cooler makeup design requires a cooler blush color.

The blush color should always be applied for a soft or subtle effect. Apply in a C-shaped motion from the temple to the cheekbone, being careful not to extend beyond the middle of the eye. If blush has been applied too heavily, soften the effect by applying translucent powder over it.

Like many other aspects of makeup design, blush application, particularly placement of color, will follow fashion trends. Be sure the application you choose is the most flattering to your client and not just the fad of the moment.

Lips

Lips, like eyes, deserve special makeup considerations. Generally, a soft, natural look in lip color application is preferred, especially for daytime. **The mouth should not "stand out" above the other facial features.** Fashion trends may call for a stronger mouth at certain times but overall the makeup design should remain proportionally balanced.

Lip Liner

Lip liner is applied to the outer edge of the lips to define the shape of the lips and to prevent lipstick from 'bleeding' onto the skin around the mouth. It may also be used to visually correct imperfections in lip shape. Note that darker colors of lip liner (and lip color) are often chosen for evening to balance with more intense eye makeup design.

Lip Color

The purpose of lipstick is to complete the balance of color. It is usually the last cosmetic to be applied. Be cautious that the lip color you choose does not overpower the amount of color that you have applied to the cheeks and eyes. Lipstick (and lip liner) can correct the shape and size of a mouth to make it more proportionate with the rest of the facial features.

Lip color is available in a variety of forms, the most common of which is lipstick, contained in a cylindrical tube. It is best applied with a lip brush, which allows the contour of the mouth to be carefully followed or reshaped as needed.

Lip glosses tend to have less concentration of color than lipsticks. Glosses impart a shiny appearance and can also be used as highlighters over a lipstick shade. Glosses usually have moisturizing properties and are soothing for dry, chapped lips. They are popular with younger girls who want some color, but not as much as a lipstick.

Some lip products contain sunscreens to block out ultraviolet rays and prevent the lips from becoming chapped. As with all other makeup products, it is a good idea to look at the ingredients of lip color products, as well as the color, before making your selection.

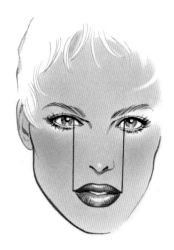

To properly apply makeup to the lips, follow these basic guidelines:

1. Analyze the overall size of the mouth: check the proportions with the other facial features to determine if the mouth is too large or too small.

2. Apply foundation to the lips to block out the natural lip line so that you may create a new one if desired. Blocking out the natural lip color also allows for truer color from lip color products and prevents bleeding of color. Applying powder over the foundation will make lip color last longer.

3. Use a lip liner (pencil) or lip brush to line the lips. For general outlining, use a natural tone, two or three shades darker than the natural lip color or that matches the tone of the lipstick you have chosen.

4. Start lining the upper lip at the outside corners and work from either side toward the center or the 'bow' of the lips. Then line the lower lip from the center toward either side. Note that this is the point at which you may need to 'correct' any imperfections in lip shape. See illustrations that follow.

5. When the lip liner is complete, fill in the shape using the appropriate shade of lip color. Use a sanitized lip brush and work to the edges of the lip shape, but not beyond the lip liner.

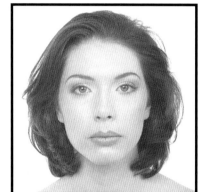

COMPLETED MAKEUP APPLICATION

Lip shapes

An examination of the ideal mouth and lips would reveal:

- A frontal view in which the bottom lip is slightly fuller than the top, with a total shape and size that creates balance and harmony with the rest of the facial features.

- A side view that shows an indentation above the upper lip and below the bottom lip. The top lip, the bottom lip and the chin should extend forward almost equally.

You can use the principles of contouring and highlighting, using darker and lighter colors, to make "corrections" on different lip shapes. Remember to keep corrections as subtle and natural as possible to avoid an overly 'drawn-on' look. Foundation should be applied to the lips prior to corrective lining.

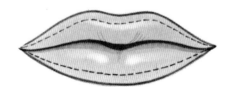

1. **Thin lips.** Use brighter, lighter colors to make them appear fuller. Increase the size of both the upper and lower lips by outlining them with a soft, curving line, just outside the natural lip line.

   a. Thin lower lip—extend the curve of the lower lip to balance the shape of the mouth.

   b. Thin upper lip—build up the curve of the upper lip to balance the shape of the mouth.

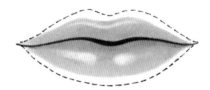

2. **Full lips.** Use a pencil and outline just inside the natural lip line, and minimize fullness by choosing darker, more muted lip colors. Blend carefully within the 'new' lip line.

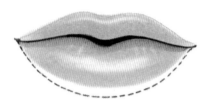

3. **Full bottom lip.** If the bottom lip is a lot fuller than the top or the top lip is too thin or small, mute the lower lip with a deeper color and use a shade or two lighter for the upper lip. Be sure to use colors in the same color family. Line the lower lip to look smaller and leave the upper lip unlined or line it slightly outside the natural lip line.

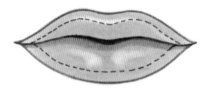

4. **Small mouth.** Build the outside edges of the upper and lower lips by lining slightly outside the natural lip line. Then extend the corners of the mouth outward.

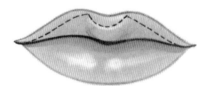

5. **Sharply defined 'cupid's bow.'** As you line the upper lip, round off the sharp peaks and widen the curve of the upper lip.

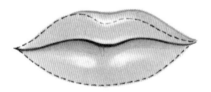

6. **Uneven or crooked lips.** To create a more balanced shape, use lip liner to build up the areas that are not large enough or defined enough.

Corrections for Facial Features

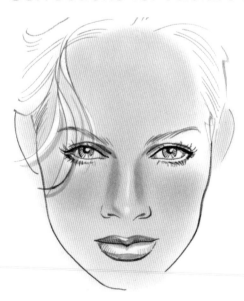

1. **Wide Nose.** To make a wide nose look narrower, apply a darker tone, or shader, along the sides of the nose and a thin line of highlighter down the center of the nose.

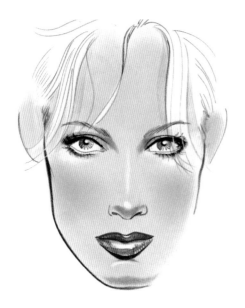

2. **Long Nose.** Visually shorten a long nose by contouring the tip of it.

3. **Prominent Chin.** Make the chin visually recede by contouring the prominent area, blending underneath and onto the throat.

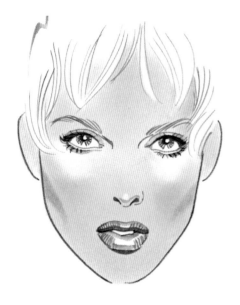

4. **Undefined Cheekbones.** To give the cheekbones more dimension, apply highlighter over the very top of the cheek bone. Then contour the hollow under the cheekbone (where the cheekbones naturally indent). You may also use this technique to create a more dramatic emphasis for already well-defined cheekbones. Avoid creating obvious stripes of contour in an effort to create the illusion.

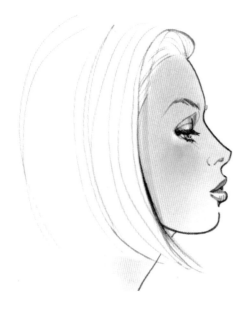

5. **Receding Chin.** To "bring out" a chin that recedes or is weak, apply highlighter on and under the chin.

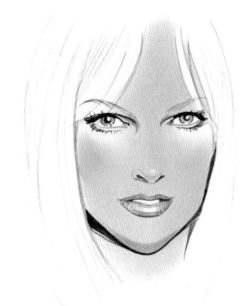

6. **Pointed Chin.** Minimize the point of the chin by softening it with a contouring product or slightly darker foundation.

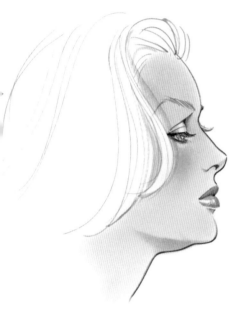

7. **'Double' Chin.** Contour the heavier area to make it recede and appear slimmer.

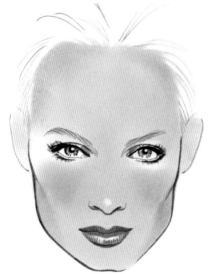

8. **Broad or Square Jaw.** Contour along the jaw and through the sides of the face to minimize width. You may use a deeper foundation than on the rest of the face to help create balance between the upper and lower parts of the face.

9. **High or Broad Forehead.** Contour along the outside edges to narrow the forehead or along the top to visually shorten the appearance of a high forehead.

Brow Design and Placement of Lights and Darks

Brow design and the placement of lights and darks can visually alter the position of the eyes on the face. In this illustration, the eyes are the same distance apart in each of the three sets. Notice how, in the second set, **placing deeper tones toward the inside corners (or toward the nose), and extending the eyebrows beyond the inside corner of the eye makes the eyes seem closer set than they are.** Beginning the eyebrow farther out and using deeper tones toward the outside of the eyes as illustrated in the third set, **creates the illusion of wide-set eyes.** When following fashion trends, be sure that your makeup design is not accentuating less than perfect features.

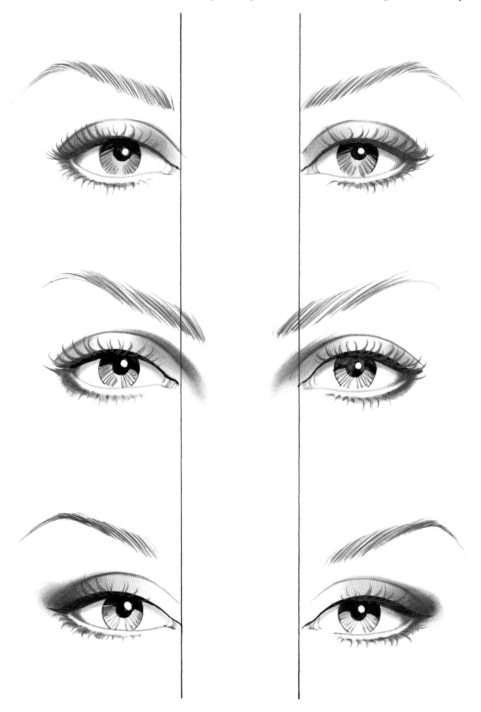

Basic Makeup Application

Although different occasions call for different makeup applications, a daytime makeup application (outlined here) covers the general guidelines. Refer to the images in the preceding portion of this chapter for visual reference.

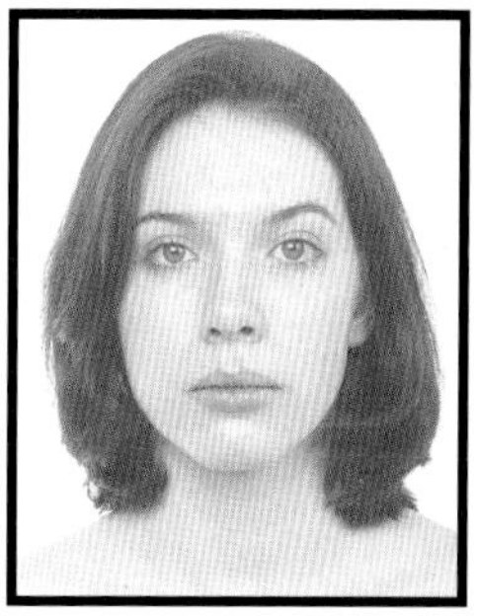

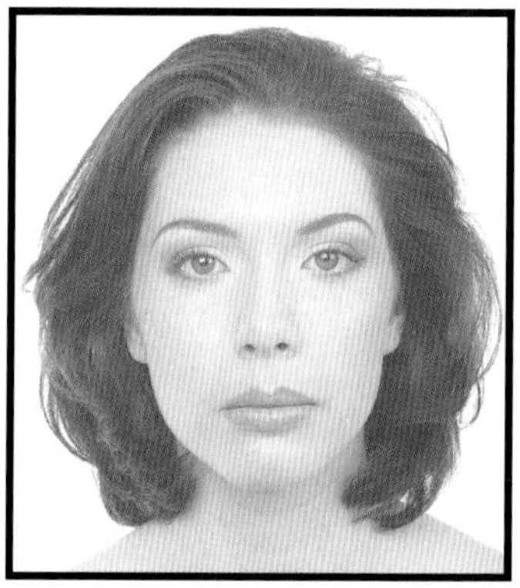

Basic Makeup Application Preparation

Before you start your makeup application, it is important to have your area, products, implements and equipment in proper order prior to your client's arrival. Be sure to take care of the following points:

- Sanitize chair, station and brushes
- Set out brushes, applicators, spatulas and palette, cleaners, toners, moisturizers, cleansing pads, facial tissue, cape, headband, cotton pads, draping sheet or robe, towels, eyelash curler and assorted makeup

Basic Makeup Application Procedure

- Wash and sanitize hands
- Prepare client (drape, including headband, and position chair)
- Consult with client
- Cleanse, tone and moisturize skin
- Analyze skin, face, brows, eyes and lips
- Groom brows if needed (brush and tweeze)
- Select appropriate foundation color
- Apply concealer as needed
- Apply foundation
- Shade brows (brush and fill in as needed)
- Check brows for symmetry
- Apply eyeliner
- Apply eyeshadow(s)
- Apply blush, if cream, liquid or gel
- Apply tinted or translucent powder
- Apply blush, if powder
- Apply mascara
- Apply lip liner
- Apply lip color
- Check coverage, balance accuracy
- Remove draping

Basic Makeup Application Completion

Perform after every makeup service:

- Offer rebook visit to client
- Recommend retail products for client
- Throw away non-reusable materials used during the makeup application service, replace used towels with fresh towels and arrange all products and implements in proper order
- Disinfect your makeup service implements and makeup chair
- Wash your hands with liquid antibacterial soap

Evening Makeup Application

Although many of the actual step-by-step techniques remain the same for an evening makeup application, there are distinct differences. Generally, evening makeup designs are intended to be seen in softer, more indirect lighting than daytime makeup designs. Color is used more intensely and the overall effect is more dramatic. Here are some of the key changes that are made for an evening makeup application.

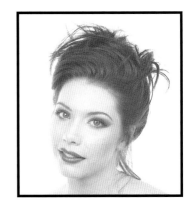

- Darker eyeliner (here, black, grease-based) can be used for more depth of color. The harder edge is then blended slightly with a small detail brush.

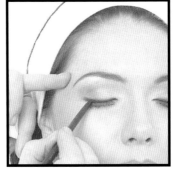
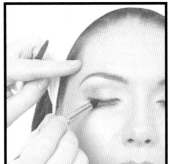

- More intense color is often used on the eyes. Color is sometimes applied to areas that are left more natural in a daytime design. Here, a deep, coppery brown is applied with a 'dabbing' motion, which results in more intense concentration of color.

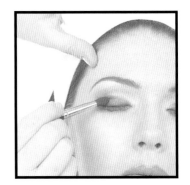

- The color is then worked up and contoured into the crease and slightly beyond for a dramatic effect. Note that there is no harsh line – the shadows should be very well blended.

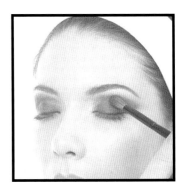

- Color is more often 'wrapped' around the eye for evening, bringing color and emphasis to the area below the eye.

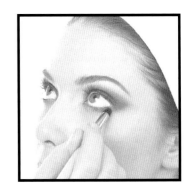

- Another application of eye liner, this time liquid, is used for more definition and drama.

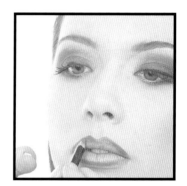

- Note that mascara application is usually heavier for evening.

- Darker colors can be used for a stronger, more defined mouth for evening.

- Stronger eye and lip colors may require stronger cheek color, so carefully check the balance of the face.

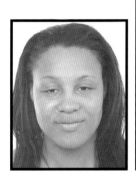
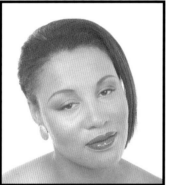

Ethnic (Darker Skin) Makeup Application

Ethnic and darker skin makeup applications require careful consideration. Foundations and concealers must be well chosen, as it is easy to go too light or too cool in your color choice. In general, these skin types can carry off more color than lighter skin colors without looking overly made up. Note that the application shown here is an example of an evening look.

- Extra attention must be paid to color choices on deeper skin tones. Very often, unevenness of tone and depth will need to be corrected.

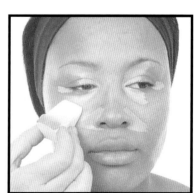

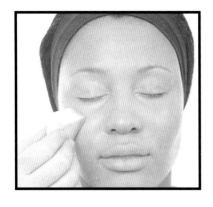

- Yellow-based products are often appropriate for darker skin colors. Concealers and foundations that are too cool will look ashy or gray on these skin colors.

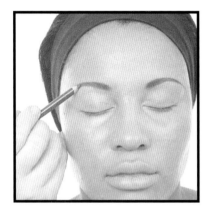

- In this instance, a brow pencil is used to fill in and shape the brows. A pencil will create a stronger, more defined brow than a powder, particularly on this darker skin color.

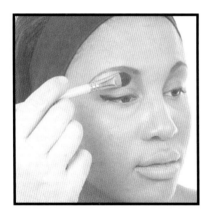

- Regardless of the pattern of application, note that richer, more intense colors can often be used on ethnic skins. Heavily pigmented skin can cause makeup colors to appear faded or washed out if they are too muted or sparingly applied. Keep the overall balance of color in mind as you design your makeup.

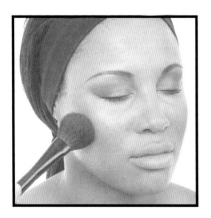

- Cheek color must be in proportion with the rest of the color on the face. Again, remember that more color may need to be applied on darker skin tones in order to be effective. Here blush is applied solely for color and to soften the look, not to contour the area.

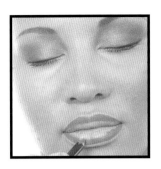
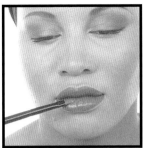

- Follow the basic guidelines for lip shaping. In this case, the lip line is redrawn just inside the natural lip line to subtly minimize the size of the mouth. The deeper tone used to line and fill the lips adds to the effect, while creating harmonious balance through the entire face.

Bridal Makeup Application

It's that once-in-a-lifetime occasion when a woman wants to look more beautiful than she has ever looked. Yet weddings (and brides!) present special challenges to the professional makeup artist. The makeup application needs to last all day and/or evening with minimal upkeep. Many brides wear their hair up for their big day, and that can alter the appearance of the face shape. Brides usually wear white, ivory or other very light colors, which have the effect of draining color from the face, unless the bride is tanned or ethnic.

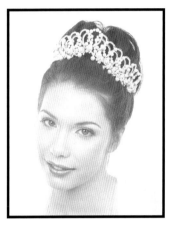
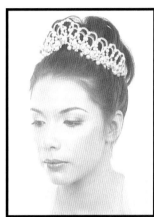

One of the biggest challenges to the professional makeup artist is to create a makeup design that looks naturally beautiful to the naked eye and that can hold up to photography. Most women are photographed more on their wedding day than on any other day in their lives. Here are some specific points to consider when designing makeup for the bridal client:

- Make sure that skin is well prepared – exfoliated earlier if needed. The 'canvas' should be as perfect as possible. Make sure skin is moisturized, but not oily. This precaution is especially important around the eyes. Preparation ensures that the makeup design will look good and helps the makeup to last longer.

- Ideally, the only touch-up products needed should be powder, lip liner and lipstick.

- Foundation (as always) should match and complement the bride's skin tone. Apply the least amount possible for a fresh, natural look. Use concealer on the inside corner of the eyes to hide imperfections.

- Remember that many types of photographic lighting have cool undertones and will bring out cool tones in the makeup design. Stay with a neutral-to-warmer palette.

- On oily skins, avoid face, cheek and eye products with orange or strong yellow undertones. These colors tend to oxidize more on oily skin and turn more yellow.

- Many gowns have lower-cut necklines. Be sure to powder the skin in the exposed areas so that light reflections in the face and the décolletage are similar.

- For longer-lasting cheek color, apply a cream blush (if skin is not oily), followed by an application of powder blush after the face has been powdered.

- Recommend curling the lashes and using waterproof mascara (for obvious reasons!).

- Eyes and brows should be accentuated with definition more than with color.

- Positioning white or very light highlights in the eye area will create a reflection of the dress, which is very effective.

- Brows tend to 'disappear' in photographs, so make sure they are well groomed and defined. For a slightly more dramatic effect that will hold up to photos, suggest more styling on the outside edges.

- There is usually a bit of kissing going on at a wedding, so use good judgment in the design of your lip makeup. Be careful of overly glossy products that may smear and spoil the rest of the makeup.

- Use a long-lasting lip liner (products with silicone are excellent) and apply to the entire lip. Use a color about 2-3 shades darker than the natural lip color and that matches the tone of the lipstick color.

- An extra tip for 'camera-ready' makeup: Be sure not to powder until after the eye makeup is complete. Then clean up under the eye using concealer on a latex sponge or small brush.

She's ready for her big day – and photographs that will bring back special memories.

You likewise are drawing closer to your big day – the time when you begin your work as a professional. You, of course, are building not for just a day but for a lifetime. This chapter has set the foundation for you in the area of skin – skin theory, skin care, hair removal and makeup. The following images show you the multitude of inspirational and exciting possibilities open to you in makeup design.

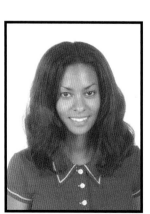

BEFORE

DAY

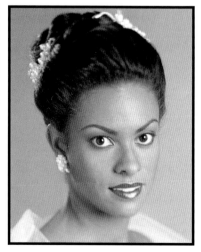

BRIDAL/EVENING

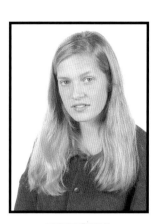

BEFORE

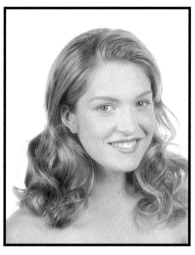

DAY

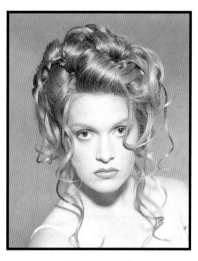

EVENING

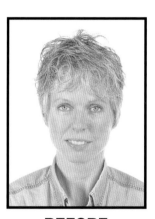

BEFORE

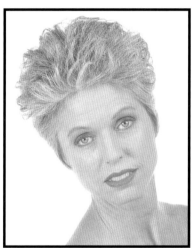

DAY

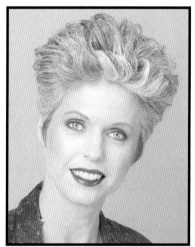

EVENING

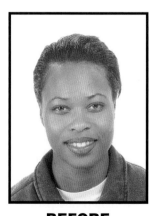

BEFORE

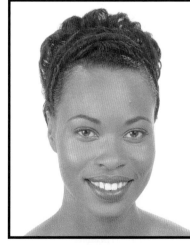

DAY

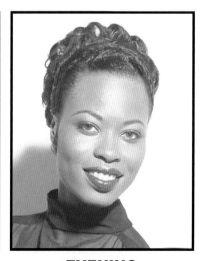

EVENING

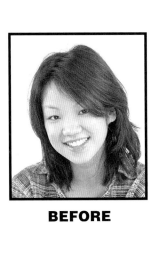
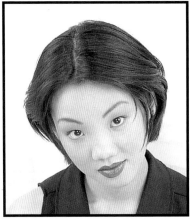
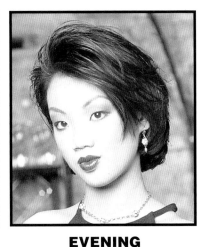

BEFORE   **DAY**   **EVENING**

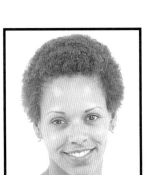
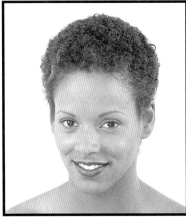
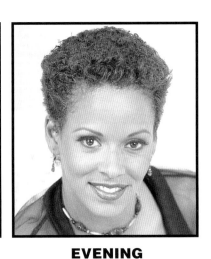

BEFORE   **DAY**   **EVENING**

It's 2 U!

Build Your Critical Thinking Skills

In this chapter you have prepared yourself to meet the following Industry Standards for entry-level cosmetologists:

- Provide basic skin care services
- Perform hair removal services
- Apply appropriate cosmetics to enhance a client's appearance

It's Up to You to know what to do. Using your training to this point, review the following case scenario and think through how you would handle the challenge.

Your last client has just left and you are ready to begin your next client, Ms. Jones. Ms. Jones is busy talking with the receptionist as you approach the desk. It seems that Ms. Jones does not want you to be her stylist today. She is aware that the client you just finished has psoriasis and she is concerned because she knows psoriasis is contagious. What would you do?

INDEX